PROLACTIN
BASIC AND CLINICAL
CORRELATES

Proceedings of the IV
INTERNATIONAL CONGRESS
on PROLACTIN held in
Charlottesville, Virginia on
June 27-29, 1984

Proceedings of the IV
INTERNATIONAL CONGRESS
on PROLACTIN under the
patronage of the International
Society of Neuroendocrinology
in association with the
International Society of
Endocrinology, and held in
Charlottesville, Virginia on
June 27-29, 1984

PROLACTIN
BASIC AND CLINICAL CORRELATES

Edited by

Robert M. MacLeod
Professor of Medicine
University of Virginia
Charlottesville, Virginia

Michael O. Thorner
Professor of Medicine
University of Virginia
Charlottesville, Virginia

Umberto Scapagnini
Professor of Pharmacology
University of Catania
Catania, Italy

Assistant Editor
Susan M. Adams
University of Virginia
Charlottesville, Virginia

FIDIA
RESEARCH
SERIES
Volume 1

LIVIANA PRESS
Padova

SPRINGER VERLAG
Berlin - Heidelberg
New York - Tokyo

FIDIA RESEARCH SERIES

An open-end series of publications on international biomedical research, with special emphasis on the neurosciences, published by LIVIANA Press, Padova, Italy, in cooperation with FIDIA Research Labs, Abano Terme, Italy.

The series will be devoted to advances in basic and clinical research in the neurosciences and other fields.

The aim of the series is the rapid and worldwide dissemination of up-to-date, interdisciplinary data as presented at selected international scientific meetings and study groups.

Each volume is published under the editorial responsibility of scientists chosen by organizing committees of the meetings on the basis of their active involvement in the research of the field concerned.

DISTRIBUTION

Sole distribution rights outside Italy granted to Springer - Verlag.

All orders for the Fidia Research Series should be sent to the following addresses

Italy:
LIVIANA EDITRICE S.p.A. - 1, Via Luigi Dottesio - Padova 35138, Italia.

North America:
SPRINGER - Verlag New York, Inc. - 175 Fifth Avenue - New York, N.Y. 10010, U.S.A.

Japan:
SPRINGER - Verlag, 37-3 Hongo 3-chome, Bunkyo-Ku, Tokyo 113, Japan.

Rest of the World:
SPRINGER - Verlag Berlin, Heidelberger Platz 3, 1000 Berlin 33, FRG

Printed in Italy

ISBN 88-7675-499-7: Liviana Editrice
ISBN 3-540-15594-5: Springer - Verlag Berlin Heidelberg New York Tokyo
ISBN 0-387-15594-5: Springer - Verlag New York Heidelberg Berlin Tokyo

---

LIVIANA Editrice S.p.A. - 1, via Luigi Dottesio, 35138, Padova, Italy.

SCIENTIFIC COMMITTEE

Henry G. Friesen (Canada)
Clark E. Grosvenor (U.S.A.)
Yuzuru Kato (Japan)
Steven W. J. Lamberts (The Netherlands)
Alan S. McNeilly (U.K.)
Eugenio E. Müller (Italy)
Jimmy D. Neill (U.S.A.)
Seymour Reichlin (U.S.A.)
Claude Robyn (Belgium)
Umberto Scapagnini (Italy)
Andree Tixier-Vidal (France)
Richard I. Weiner (U.S.A.)
Wolfgang Wuttke (F.R.G.)

LOCAL ORGANIZING COMMITTEE

Michael J. Cronin
William S. Evans
Ivan S. Login
Alan D. Rogol
Michael O. Thorner
Robert M. MacLeod, Chairman

ACKNOWLEDGMENTS

The participants and organizers of the Fourth International Congress on Prolactin gratefully acknowledge the generous financial support from:

FIDIA S.P.A.	Sandoz Ltd	Schering AG
Abano Terme	Basle	Berlin
Italy	Switzerland	F.R.G.

The Scientific Organizing Committee would like to thank the Rector and the Board of Visitors of the University of Virginia for providing the excellent facilities in which the Congress meetings were held.

PREFACE

The field of endocrinology has experienced unprecedented growth during the last two decades largely due to its unique relationship with many other areas of basic and applied sciences that also are expanding rapidly. The study of the pituitary gland and particularly prolactin is among the most productive sub-specialty areas of endocrinology, because of its association to impinging topics of investigation. In the study of prolactin we observe the fusion of dynamic forces propelling the studies of functional cellular ultrastructure with those of molecular and cellular biology as they more clearly define the mechanisms of hormone secretion. These studies integrate well with those measuring the response of the lactotroph and its function as controlled by neural networks and peripheral regulators. The central and peripheral activities of prolactin are being better understood because the student of metabolism finds common ground with the behavioralist and the comparative endocrinologist due to prolactin's immense spectrum of activities. The reproductive biologist and the neuropharmacologist are exploring ground formerly thought to be the domain of the clinical endocrinologist and the surgeon. This movement toward the interactive study of prolactin is not new and in the recent past a need was perceived for a forum for the purpose of exchanging information on this topic. Such a forum was provided by the organization of the First International Congress on Prolactin held in Brussels, and subsequent Congresses were held in Nice and in 1981, in Athens.

The Fourth International Congress on Prolactin was convened in Charlottesville, Virginia, on June 27, 28, and 29, 1984. The Congress participants were welcomed by President Frank L. Hereford and Professor Edward W. Hook, both of whom provided an historical perspective of the importance that Thomas Jefferson, founder of the University of Virginia, placed on science and medicine. The Congress was a success as measured by the participation of 375 individuals from 27 countries and was organized so that ample time was provided for discussion of the verbal and poster presentations by almost two hundred individuals. A representative number of these presentations have been compiled in this book, which provides an insight into some of the most current concepts about prolactin. The authors of these manuscripts are also members of classically structured scientific disciplines, however as 'prolactinologists' they have experienced the benefits of the information and advances made in other impending areas of biological science. It is expected that the synergistic interaction among these areas will provide for even greater advances in the future.

There is a continuum in the field of prolactin research as demonstrated by the recognition of two individuals who have and will contribute greatly to endocrinology. Dr. Joseph A. Martial, Professor of Biochemistry at the University of Liège, Belgium was recognized for his exciting description of the human prolactin genomic structure, that will be the basis for much applied research in the future. He was awarded the first Sandoz Prize for Research on Prolactin for this outstanding recent achievement.

A pioneer in the field of endocrinology and more particularly in the area of prolactin research was honored for his long and outstanding achievements. Dr. Joseph Meites, Professor of Physiology, Michigan State Universtity, East Lansing, Michigan, has been a leader in this field for forty years and now upon his election to Professor Emeritus he continues to blaze new trails in research. Many of his former students, postdoctoral fellows and colleagues joined together to acknowledge him as a person who has greatly influenced research on prolactin to be one of the most exciting areas of endocrinology today and to give him their best wishes for the future.

The Local Organizing Committee would like to thank all the individuals who helped with many phases of the Congress. We expecially wish to thank Carlos Valdenegro, Suzanne B. O'Dell, Margaret MacQueen, Allan M. Judd, Denis Leong, Pat Williams, Alma Tribble, Linda D. Evans, Jeff Weiss, and John Zysk.

For the Editors
Robert M. MacLeod
University of Virginia

CONTENTS

III. INTRACELLULAR PITUITARY MECHANISMS REGULATING PROLAC-TIN RELEASE

IV. MODIFICATION OF PROLACTIN PRODUCTION BY STEROIDS

IX. EXPERIMENTAL AND CLINICAL EFFECTS OF PROLACTIN ON BEHAVIOR AND BRAIN FUNCTION

X. PATHOGENESIS OF PROLACTINOMAS

XI. CLINICAL AND THERAPEUTIC ASPECTS OF HYPERPROLACTINEMIA

XVI

PROLACTIN
BASIC AND CLINICAL CORRELATES

Proceedings of the IV INTERNATIONAL CONGRESS on PROLACTIN
held in Charlottesville, Virginia on June 27-29, 1984

Prolactin. Basic and clinical correlates
R.M. MacLeod, M.O. Thorner and U. Scapagnini (eds.),
Fidia Research Series, vol. I,
Liviana Press, Padova © 1985

Section I
The functional ultrastructure
of prolactin cells

THE FUNCTIONAL ULTRASTRUCTURE
OF PROLACTIN CELLS: AN OVERVIEW

A. Tixier-Vidal

Groupe de Neuroendocrinologie Cellulaire, College de France
75231 Paris Cedex 05

The biology of prolactin cells was presented as a structural framework for various physiological regulations and intracellular mechanisms and the discussion provided an opportunity for several important advances in this portion of the Congress. A comprehensive view of membrane traffic in prolactin cells and other secretory cells was presented by Marilyn G. Farquhar. The major established routes of membrane traffic were defined and emphasis was given to the key role played by the Golgi complex in sorting secretory, lysosomal, and membrane proteins, and directing them to their correct destinations. Although little is known about the mechanisms involved in these phenomena, recent progress in this area of research, using new immunological probes, was presented. The mannose-6-phosphate groups which serve as a "recognition marker" for the receptor-mediated sorting of lysosomal enzymes have been localized on the cis side of the Golgi complex, that is, opposite from the trans side where granule formation takes place (Farquhar et al.). Several antigens specific for intracellular membranes (rough endoplasmic reticulum, Golgi membranes, lysosomal membranes respectively) have been localized in prolactin cells, thus providing direct evidence for an immunological heterogeneity of intracellular membrane compartments and for their sorting in the Golgi zone (Tougard et al.).

As concerns the subcellular structures involved in the acute release of prolactin, electron microscope immunocytochemical studies performed in lactating rats have suggested that soluble prolactin contained within the rough endoplasmic reticulum and possibly within the Golgi complex may be preferentially released before that in secretory granules (Nikitovitch-Winer et al.). This is consistent with results from previous studies performed with GH_3 cells which showed that small vesicles serve as carriers for the release of prolactin (Tougard et al.). Thus it has come to be accepted that in addition to secretory granules other structures, most probably vesicles, participate in the acute release of prolactin.

New insights into the analysis of prolactin secretion at the single cell level were presented using the "the reverse hemolytic plaque assay" (RHPA). This permits a direct approach to the functional heterogeneity of prolactin cells. The combination of this methodology with autoradiography provided a direct demonstration that the preferential release of newly synthesized [³H]-prolactin is due to lactotrope heterogeneity. These findings can now be correlated with ultrastructure features of individual prolactin cells.

Many other interesting or new aspects of the cell biology of prolactin cells were presented including the preparation of a monoclonal antibody that recognizes a cell surface protein in GH₃ cells (Kapatos and Barker), the autoradiographic identification of prolactin cells by means of specific ligands (Stumpf et al.) and the extractability of bovine and of rat pituitary prolactin (Jacobs' group).

The paracrine interactions elegantly revealed by C. Denef, using culture of anterior pituitary reaggregates, offer a unique opportunity to analyze cell-to-cell interactions which are relevant to tissue organization *in vivo*. The presentation of new developments in these studies of the functional interaction between gonadotropes and lactotropes showed that the response of prolactin cells to angiotensin II is modulated by gonadotropes in an opposite manner depending on the doses and/or the gonadotrope subpopulations. The underlying mechanism of such interactions may be the release of paracrine soluble factors which remain to be characterized.

Prolactin. Basic and clinical correlates
R.M. MacLeod, M.O. Thorner and U. Scapagnini (eds.),
Fidia Research Series, vol. I,
Liviana Press, Padova © 1985

Section I
The functional ultrastructure
of prolactin cells

MEMBRANE TRAFFIC IN PROLACTIN
AND OTHER SECRETORY CELLS

Marilyn Gist Farquhar

Department of Cell Biology, Yale University School of Medicine
New Haven, Connecticut 06510

INTRODUCTION

It has been clear for some time that exocytosis in glandular cells and endocytosis in cultured cells and phagocytes involve membrane fusion-fission events and transport via membrane-carriers. In the last few years we have come to realize that these processes are general properties of all cell types, and that in every cell there is considerable membrane traffic which involves shuttling of membrane between various cell compartments and cell surfaces. For some time our interest has been in studying biosynthetic and recycling membrane traffic in secretory cells. The prolactin cell has proved to be a very useful model for such studies.

In this presentation, I will briefly outline the major established routes of membrane traffic which have been charted so far in prolactin and other cells.

It should be stated at the outset that we have learned a great deal that is applicable to prolactin cells from work on other exocrine and endocrine cell types, but, by the same token, the prolactin cell has taught us some general principles that are applicable to other cells as well.

THE LYSOSOMAL PATHWAY

Let's begin with what is probably the most familiar and the oldest documented route of membrane traffic, i.e, the pathway by which endocytic vesicles formed at the cell surface deliver their contents to lysosomes (route 1 in Fig. 1). Originally it was assumed that both the contents and the membrane of the endocytic vesicle were delivered to lysosomes and degraded. In the meantime this concept has had to be modified in two respects: first, it is now clear that the fate of the membrane and the contents differ — whereas the contents are usually degraded in lysosomes, the membrane recycles (routes

4

2 and 5 in Fig. 1); secondly, we now know that in many cases the incoming vesicles fuse initially with a prelysosomal compartment (route 3 in Fig. 1), usually referred to as an endosome (1) or receptosome (2), which lacks lysosomal enzymes but has a low pH (~ 5.5) (3). This compartment provides an acidic environment in which many ligands such as LDL (4) and many peptide hormones (1,3) dissociate from their receptors, thereby facilitating rapid recycling of receptors to the cell surface (route 5 in Fig. 1) and delivery of the ligand to lysosomes or to other cell compartments (route 4 in Fig. 1).

This lysosomal route is utilized by all known cell types, but lysosomal traffic is heaviest in cultured cells and in phagocytic cells such as macrophages (5). In addition, many, if not most cells, internalize peptide hormones and LDL by receptor-mediated endocytosis and deliver them to lysosomes via this route (2,4).

The existence of the lysosomal pathway has been validated in prolactin cells and other pituitary cell types using nonspecific, electron-dense tracers, such as horseradish peroxidase (HRP)(6) and anionic and cationic ferritins (7). It still remains to be determined whether or not more specific substances such as TRH and dopamine, which bind to receptors on prolactin cells, are internalized by receptor-mediated endocytosis and delivered to lysosomes or other cell compartments. We have obtained autoradiographic evidence (8) that GnRH is internalized into gonadotrophs and delivered to lysosomes after binding to surface receptors.

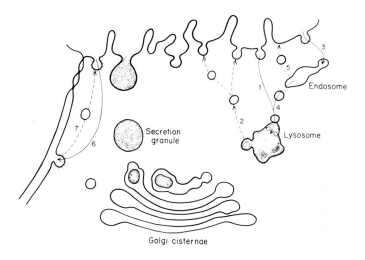

Figure 1. The lysosomal (1-5) and transcellular (6-7) routes of membrane traffic (see text for details). From Farquhar (49).

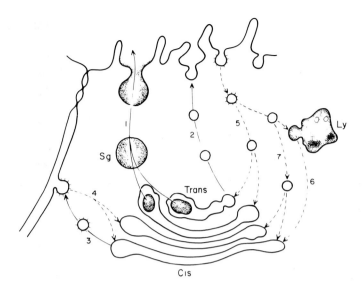

Figure 2. The exocytosis (1-3) and plasmalemma to Golgi (4-7) pathways (see text for details). From Farquhar (49).

THE TRANSCELLULAR ROUTE

For many years it was believed that all endocytic vesicles were destined to fuse with lysosomes. It is now clear that this is not the case and that other options are available. For example, some endocytic vesicles serve to transport ligands across the cell from one cell surface to another (routes 6 and 7 in Fig. 1). Transcellular traffic is the heaviest in endothelial cells of the type present in muscle capillaries where the vesicles serve to shuttle solutes from the lumen to the adventitia and back (9). The transcellular route is also utilized for the transepithelial transport of immunoglobulins, e.g., transport of maternal IgG in the suckling rat intestine (route 6 in Fig. 1) (10) or transport of IgA in the reverse direction in the liver (11), mammary or intestinal epithelium (route 7 in Fig. 1). Such a pathway has not yet been documented in prolactin cells. However, it is of interest that this route has been documented in neurons in which it has been shown that nonspecific tracers such as HRP or lectin-HRP conjugates can be picked up and transported in a retrograde manner through a chain of several neurons (12). In this way neuronal pathways and connections can be traced. The work on neurons demonstrates that transcellular transport provides a mechanism by which ligands (peptide hormones, growth factors, and other regulatory molecules) can be transported over long distances from one cell surface to another and can even be transferred from one cell to another.

THE EXOCYTOTIC PATHWAY

Another familiar route of membrane traffic is the exocytotic pathway (route 1 in Fig. 2) which is now known to be the general mode for release of secretory products from all cell types (13). In fact, exocytosis is the only documented route for release of secretory products. In endocrine and exocrine glandular cells it is one of the major routes of membrane traffic because in such cells secretory granule membranes are continually fusing with the cell surface and discharging their contents. Two types of secretory cells have been distinguished (14): those with a so-called "regulated" pathway, characteristic for exocrine and endocrine glandular cells, which concentrate their products into secretory granules and whose discharge is regulated by specific secretagogues, and those with a so-called "constitutive" or non-regulated pathway, typified by fibroblasts and plasma cells (14). Such cells do not concentrate their secretory products into granules but instead package them in dilute form in small vesicles which are continually discharged by exocytosis (route 2 in Fig. 2) but are not influenced by known secretagogues. The available evidence (reviewed in ref. 15) also suggests that plasmalemmal membrane proteins, especially membrane glycoproteins, are ferried to the appropriate cell surface via small vesicles where they are delivered by exocytosis (routes 2 and 3 in Fig. 2).

Exocytosis was described in prolactin cells over 20 years ago by Sano (16) and Pasteels (17) and has been amply confirmed by others (see ref. 18). It has been established that fusion occurs preferentially with that portion of the prolactin cell surface facing the capillary basement membrane, and that upon discharge the granule contents are rapidly solubilized and disappear from view. Tixier-Vidal and coworkers (19) have provided evidence that exocytosis is also the route used for secretion of prolactin from GH_3 cells, a prolactin secreting cell line which makes very few secretory granules but instead packages the hormone in small vesicles which are continually undergoing discharge by exocytosis. Kelly and coworkers (20,21) have presented data suggesting that two exocytotic pathways, one regulated and the other constitutive, exist simultaneously in AtT-20 cells, an ACTH-secreting mouse cell line. The regulated pathway is slow, cAMP-dependent, and is used for the packaging, storage and discharge of ACTH, proteoglycans and several acidic peptides of unknown function. The constitutive pathway is fast, cAMP- independent, and is used for delivery of a plasma membrane protein (gp70) and several other peptides and sulfated macromolecules. These findings raise the possibility that two distinct exocytotic pathways may also exist in prolactin and other pituitary cells.

In prolactin cells, as in many other cell types, it has been repeatedly observed (see ref. 22) that, after radiolabeling, newly-synthesized hormone is preferentially released over old stored hormone, and this phenomenon has often been postulated to be due to mechanisms of discharge other than exocytosis. We have obtained autoradiographic evidence (22) that heterogeneity within the prolactin cell population may explain this phenomenon, at least in part, that is, a very active subpopulation of prolactin cells synthesizes, concentrates, and secretes prolactin at a very fast rate, and is responsible for this preferential release. A similar conclusion was reached by quite a different approach (reverse hemolytic plaque assay) at this meeting by Neill and coworkers.

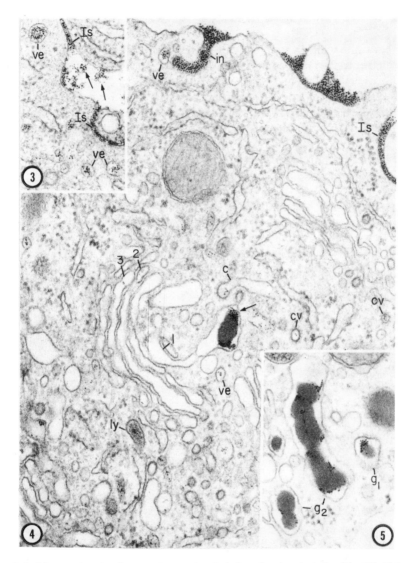

Figures 3-5. Mammotrophs from estrogen-treated females incubated with CF (0.1 mg/ml) demonstrating transport of this tracer via small vesicles to the Golgi complex. Fig. 3 shows that initially (after 15 min of incubation) CF is seen binding to the cell membrane and within numerous transporting vesicles (ve) located in the cytoplasm near the cell membrane. Fig. 4 shows that after 60 min, CF is still seen along the free cell surface (upper right), within membrane invaginations (in), and within smooth (ve) or coated (cv) vesicles, but, in addition, some molecules are now found within the stacked Golgi cisternae, around a forming secretion granule, and in a lysosome (ly). Here, CF molecules are seen in three (1-3) of the stacked Golgi cisternae, and are especially concentrated at the periphery of a granule (arrow) condensing within the transmost cisterna. Several molecules are also present within the coated tip of another smooth cisterna (c). Fig. 4 (60 min) shows CF within immature type I (g_1) and type II (g_2) prolactin granules, sticking to the periphery of the dense content. Figs. 3 and 4 - X 58,000; Fig. 5 - X 53,600. From Farquhar (7).

THE PLASMALEMMA TO GOLGI ROUTE

Another route which was actually discovered in pituitary cells (6,7,23), is the one from cell surface to the Golgi complex (routes 5-7 in Fig. 2) whereby incoming endocytic vesicles fuse directly or indirectly with Golgi cisternae (Figs. 3-6). Our results (7,24,25) indicate that this is a major pathway in both regulated and nonregulated cells which are producing proteins for export, including pituitary prolactin cells (Figs. 3-5) and somatotrophs (Fig. 6), and parotid epithelia (26), plasma cells, and myeloma cells (27). This type of traffic is the heaviest to the trans side of the Golgi stack, i.e., the side on which secretory granules are formed, and indirect evidence indicates that this pathway is connected with the recycling of membrane utilized in the packaging of secretory granules or vesicles.

The significance of this pathway is far-reaching because it provides a mechanism by which surface membrane constituents (e.g., receptors) or bound ligands (e.g., hormones, LDL and other regulatory molecules) can be delivered to a biosynthetic compartment (see Table I) and thereby influence cell metabolism.

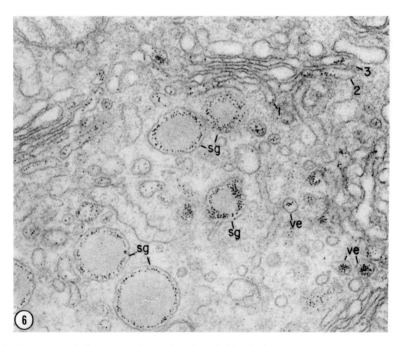

Figure 6. Somatotroph from a male rat incubated 60 min in CF (0.5 mg/ml), demonstrating that endocytic vesicles fuse, directly or indirectly, with Golgi cisternae. Tracer molecules are present within several stacked Golgi cisternae (1-3), within multiple smooth vesicles (ve) in the Golgi region, and within numerous growth hormone secretion granules (sg) of varying size. Note that the CF molecules are located exclusively at the periphery of the dense granule contents. X 67,000. From Farquhar (7).

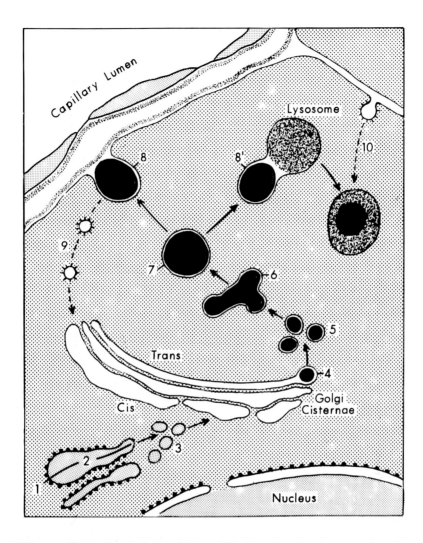

*Figure 7.*Diagram illustrating the intracellular traffic that takes place in connection with the synthesis, packaging and secretion of prolactin, as documented by work from many laboratories. Prolactin is synthesized on ribosomes (1), segregated into rough ER (2), transported by small vesicles (3) to the Golgi complex, passes through the Golgi complex and is concentrated into small immature granules on the trans side of the stack (4). Several of these aggregate (5 and 6) to form the mature secretory granule (7). During active secretion, the latter fuses with the cell membrane by exocytosis (8), its content is discharged into the perivascular spaces and the granule membrane recycles back to the Golgi cisternae (9). When secretory activity is suppressed and the cell must dispose of excess stored hormone, some granules fuse with lysosomes (8') and their content is degraded. Besides these routes, an endocytic pathway from the cell surface to lysosomes has also been demonstrated (10).

Thus, the biosynthetic (ER to Golgi), exocytotic (granules to plasmalemma), crinophagic (granules to lysosomes), and plasmalemma to Golgi routes are heavily utilized in this cell. Modified from Smith and Farquhar (29).

10

To date this pathway has been demonstrated in prolactin cells primarily by use of general tracers such as HRP or cationized ferritin. However, in other cell types we have documented the existence of this pathway using several specific markers, e.g., we have obtained autoradiographic data suggesting that GnRH reaches Golgi elements in gonadotrophs (8). In addition, we have recently obtained immunocytochemical evidence that transferrin (an iron-binding protein that regulates cell growth) and transferrin receptors are internalized at the cell surface and delivered to Golgi cisternae in immunoglobulin-secreting cells (28). Thus, the existence of this route in secretory cells has been documented using both general and specific tracers. Studies on the physiologic consequences of these events are still in their infancy.

THE CRINOPHAGIC PATHWAY: SECRETION GRANULES TO LYSOSOMES

Another pathway which is not as widely known as the others mentioned so far is the crinophagic pathway, that is, the pathway originally discovered in prolactin cells (29) by which secretion granules fuse with lysosomes and their contents are degraded (18,29-31). This pathway (diagrammed in Fig. 7) is utilized primarily when secretion is inhibited. It was originally discovered in prolactin cells from post-lactating rats in which it was demonstrated by morphological and cytochemical techniques that, 24-48

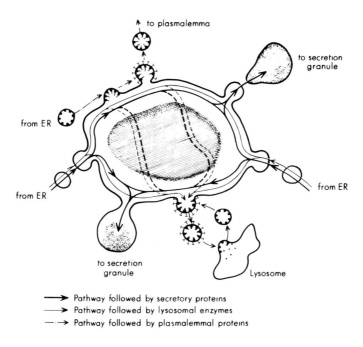

Figure 8. The biosynthetic (solid lines) and recycling membrane (interrupted lines) pathways for transport between the ER and Golgi complex (1 and 2) and the Golgi complex and lysosomes (3-6). From Farquhar (49).

h after suckling pups are removed from their mothers, numerous secretion granules can be seen within lysosomes. Both immature (polymorphous) and mature granules were found within, or in the process of fusing with, *bona fide* lysosomes (i.e., acid phosphatase- and arylsulfatase-positive). It was postulated that this phenomenon, for which corroborative biochemical data has since been obtained (32-34), may serve to regulate the secretory process by incorporating and disposing of undischarged secretion granules. This same phenomenon has since been detected in other pituitary cell types (thyrotropes, gonadotropes, somatotropes, and ACTH cells) (30,31) as well as in other cell types, and it appears to constitute one of several regulatory mechanisms for regulation of hormone secretion.

BIOSYNTHETIC PATHWAYS: ER TO GOLGI AND GOLGI TO LYSOSOMES

It is now clear that the intracellular pathway taken by secretory proteins, originally delineated in the exocrine pancreatic cell, is generally applicable to all cells producing cells for export i.e., all known exocrine and endocrine cell types as well as nonglandular cells such as fibroblasts and plasma cells. In addition, it is now known (reviewed in ref. 15) that lysosomal enzymes and some membrane proteins, primarily glycoproteins, follow the same general pathway initially. All these products are synthesized as preproteins with a "signal peptide" or "leader sequence" which provides a recognition marker that directs attachment of the ribosomes bearing the nascent chain to the rough ER (35). Prolactin is among the numerous proteins shown to contain a signal peptide and has often served as a model for such studies (35). After the ribosomes attach to the membranes of the rough ER, the nascent proteins are segregated within the cavities of the rough ER, and are eventually transported to the Golgi complex (route 1 in Fig. 8). Considerable co-translational and post-translational modification of the proteins takes place in transport through the rough ER.

The discovery of the signal sequence together with the isolation and purification of a "signal recognition protein" (36) which binds to ribosomes and regulates translocation (by allowing translocation in the presence of competent ER membranes and inhibiting protein synthesis in their absence) helped to establish the general applicability of segregation in the ER to secretory products. These developments have served in large part to silence the suggestion, often voiced in the endocrine literature, that secretory products may follow alternative intracytoplasmic routes (i.e., through the cell sol).

After transport of the biosynthetic products (i.e., secretory, membrane and lysosomal proteins) to the Golgi complex they pass through a series of Golgi compartments or subcompartments (route 1 in Fig. 8) where additional post-translational modifications occur. The biosynthetic functions that take place primarily or exclusively in the Golgi complex are listed in Table I. Then, somewhere in the Golgi complex, all these products are sorted and directed to their correct intracellular or extracellular destination, i.e., secretory products are segregated into granules or vesicles to be discharged by exocytosis (route 1 in Fig. 2), lysosomal enzymes are delivered to lysosomes (route 3 or 5 in Fig. 8), and membrane proteins are delivered to the appropriate cell surface (routes 2 and 3 in Fig. 2) or intracellular compartments. We now know (15) that one of the major functions of the Golgi complex is to sort all of this biosynthetic and recy-

Table I - *Functions of the Golgi Complex**

1. *Addition of the Man-6-P recognition marker to lysosomal enzymes*	*Early*
2. *Trimming of N-linked oligosaccharides of glycoproteins (alpha-Mannosidase I)*	*Early*
3. *Addition of terminal sugars (GAL, FUC, SA) of glycoproteins*	*Late*
4. *Sulfation of proteoglycans and glycoproteins*	*Late*
5. *Concentration of secretory proteins*	*Late*
6. *Processing of prohormones*	*Late*

* *Functions are listed in order of their sequence -- i.e., secretory proteins, lysosomal enzymes and membrane glycoproteins pass through the Golgi complex and are progressively modified in transit (see ref. 15).*

cling membrane traffic and direct it to its correct "address".

That the secretory pathway (ER - Golgi - immature granules - mature granules) is taken by prolactin has been amply documented by a variety of techniques, including autoradiography (37,38), immunocytochemistry (19,39), and cell fractionation (18). The detailed kinetics of the process have been determined by autoradiography (37,38). High resolution autoradiographic analysis of the prolactin secretory pathway (38) has further established that the secretory product is concentrated > 200 X by the time it is packaged into granules. The mechanism by which the concentration of prolactin is achieved is not understood, but has been suggested to be initiated by ionic interaction between the hormone and certain negatively-charged sulfated macromolecules (glycoproteins and proteoglycans) known to be present in these (40-43) and other (13,21,43) secretory granules.

TRAFFIC THROUGH THE GOLGI COMPLEX

At present there is considerable interest in the pathways taken by newly synthesized products to and through the Golgi complex. The cytochemical data available (summarized in Table II) plus the biochemical evidence available (44,45) indicate that the membranes of the individual cisternae in the Golgi stack have a different protein composition. At present it is usually assumed that the individual cisternae remain stationary and the products, i.e., the secretory, lysosomal and membrane proteins, enter the Golgi complex on the cis side of the stacked cisternae (the side facing the rough ER) and move sequentially across the stacks, traversing the cisternae one by one, to reach the trans side (the side on which the secretion granules are formed) where sorting is thought to take place. In the case of prolactin, it is clear that concentration and packaging into granules occurs on the trans side, but it is not yet clear whether or not the hormone passes through all the cisternae in the stack (19, 39).

Table II - *Cytochemical Reactions of Golgi Cisternae*

	Cis	Trans
5'-Nucleotidase	+	+ *
Adenylate Cyclase	+	+
Periodic Acid-Silver Methenamine	+	+ *
OsO$_4$ Impregnation	+	−
Acid Phosphatase	−	+
Thiamine Pyrophosphatase	−	+
Galactosyl Transferase**	−	+
Glucose-6-Phosphatase***	−	−

*   A gradient of increasing reactivity from the cis to the trans side was detected.
**   Localized by immunocytochemistry.
*** A marker for the endoplasmic reticulum.

SITES AND MECHANISMS OF SORTING

It is becoming increasingly evident that during these various vesicular transport operations the cell is capable of considerable sorting, i.e., sorting of membrane constituents from fluid contents, sorting of receptors (membrane components) from ligands, as well as sorting of membrane components from one another. The sites identified so far where such sorting can take place include the plasmalemma, the Golgi complex, and endosomes, of which the most familiar is the plasmalemma, where selective binding and internalization of both receptor and ligands is well documented.

Similar events are believed to take place in the Golgi complex but relatively little data are available indicating how this is done and where in the Golgi complex specific events occur (15). It is assumed that, as in the case of other transport operations, transport between the various subcompartments of the Golgi is effected by specific vesicular carriers (see Fig. 9) which have specific receptors for transported species on their inner (cisternal) surfaces and appropriate recognition signals for the receiving compartment on their outer surfaces. In the case of the Golgi, only one type of specific receptor is known, that for the sorting of lysosomal enzymes (46-48). There is evidence that sorting is accomplished through the interaction between a specific carbohydrate recognition marker, mannose-6-phosphate (Man-6-P) present in lysosomal enzymes and Man-6-P receptors present on intracellular membranes. Thus, there is considerable evidence that at least some of the lysosomal enzymes are removed from the secretory pathway, via coated vesicles, a receptor-mediated event comparable to receptor-mediated endocytosis at the cell surface (Fig. 9).

We have recently purified the Man-6-P receptor, raised an antibody to it, and used the antibody to localize the receptor by immunocytochemistry (47). We found that the Man-6-P receptor is concentrated in cis Golgi cisternae of several cell types, i.e., exocrine pancreatic, hepatic and epididymal epithelia (47). Based on these findings we have proposed that the Man-6-P-dependent sorting of lysosomal enzymes occurs on

14

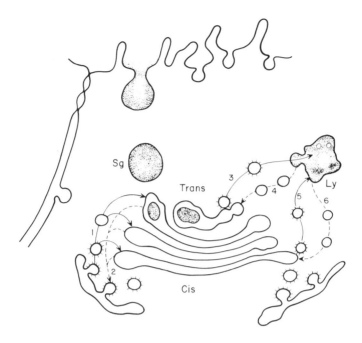

Figure 9. Diagram of a Golgi cisterna viewed *en face* depicting the presumed role of the Golgi complex in sorting and directing biosynthetic traffic of membranes and secretory products. Four types of traffic are depicted: (1) ER - Golgi; (2) Golgi - lysosomes; (3) Golgi - condensing granules or vacuoles; and (4) Golgi - plasmalemma. In all cases, transport is assumed to be effected by vesicular carriers which must possess specific receptors for transported species on their inner (cisternal) surfaces and appropriate recognition signals for the receiving compartment on their outer surfaces. In two cases (types 2 and 3) there is evidence that coated vesicles are involved. In only one case (type 2) is the specific recognition marker (mannose-6-phosphate) known. The large dots attached to the membrane represent the receptor and the small dots the lysosomal enzymes. Lysosomal enzymes bearing Man-6-P receptors are assumed to bind to Man-6-P receptors and to be removed from the secretory pathway by receptor mediated sorting comparable to receptor mediated endocytosis at the cell surface. The enzymes are then transported to lysosomes or endosomes via coated vesicle carriers (47,48) where they dissociate from their receptors (facilitated by low pH) and the receptors recycle back to the Golgi complex. From Farquhar and Palade (15).

the cis side of the Golgi complex (route 5 in Fig. 8) instead of on the trans side (route 3 in Fig. 8) as has been widely assumed up to now. Interestingly, a special subpopulation of coated vesicles appears to serve as the carrier to ferry lysosomal enzymes from cis Golgi cisternae to lysosomes or endosomes (48). Similar studies localizing Man-6-P receptors in prolactin cells are now in progress.

Apart from plasmalemmal and Golgi elements, there appear to be an unknown number of prelysosomal sites (endosomes) involved in the sorting of receptors from ligands (e.g., LDL receptors and LDL or asialoglycoprotein receptors from desialylated glycoproteins) and sorting of different internalized ligands (e.g., IgG from desialylated glycoproteins) takes place (1). The only mechanism known so far that affects the sorting operation is the pH of the receiving compartment (3); however, pH cannot be the only mechanism involved since electrostatic interactions lack the necessary specificity. It seems more likely that specificity is accomplished by appropriate interactions among membrane constituents. For example, binding of ligand to receptors may trigger a conformational change in a membrane protein that triggers membrane fission or exposes a sequence on the cytoplasmic domain of the membrane that recognizes the appropriate receiving compartment and promotes fusion. In such cases, pH may serve to modulate ligand binding or trigger (as in the case of viral entry) (1) the necessary fusion event.

SUMMARY AND CONCLUSIONS

One of the major revelations from research in cell biology during the last few years has been the discovery of the existence of multiple pathways of vesicular membrane traffic, summarized in Figs. 1,2, and 8 (solid lines), plus the demonstration that cells reutilize or recycle the membranes involved in these various transport operations (interrupted lines in Figs. 1,2 and 8).

It has become clear that considerable sorting of membrane constituents and ligands takes place at the plasmalemma (receptor-mediated uptake), in the Golgi complex, and in endosomes. The Golgi complex is the intracellular site where much of the biosynthetic and recycling membrane traffic converges and where products are sorted and directed to their correct destinations.

At present it is evident that the basic pathways of membrane traffic are similar in all cells except that some are emphasized and others deemphasized according to the predominant function of a particular cell type. In phagocytic cells and cells in culture, the lysosomal route (from the plasmalemma to endosomes and lysosomes) is the predominant route, and in some types of endothelial cells transcellular membrane traffic predominates. In exocrine and endocrine secretory cells, including prolactin cells, the biosynthetic, exocytotic, and plasmalemma to Golgi routes (believed to be connected with granule membrane recycling) (24-27) are emphasized. In prolactin cells as well as some other endocrine cells, the crinophagic route appears also to be heavily utilized for regulation of secretion by hormone degradation.

ACKNOWLEDGMENTS

This research was supported by NIH Research Grant AM 17780.

REFERENCES

1. Helenius A, Mellman I, Wall D, Hubbard A. (1983): TIBS 8:245
2. Pastan IH, Willingham MC. (1981): Science 214:504
3. Tycko B, Maxfield FR. (1982): Cell 28:643
4. Goldstein JL, Anderson RGW, Brown MS. (1982): Ciba Fd Symp 92:77

5. Steinman RM, Mellman IS, Muller WA, Cohn ZA. (1983): J Cell Biol 96:1

6. Pelletier G. (1973): J Ultrastruct Res 43:445

7. Farquhar MG. (1978): J Cell Biol 77:R35

8. Duello TM, Nett TM, Farquhar MG. (1983): Endocrinology 112:1

9. Palade GE, Simionescu M, Simionescu N. (1979): Acta Physiol Scand Suppl 463:11

10. Abrahamson DR, Rodewald R. (1981): J Cell Biol 91:270

11. Renston RH, Jones AL, Christiansen WD, Hradek G. (1980): Science 208:1276

12. Brushart TM, Mesulam MM. (1980): Neurosci Lett 17:1

13. Palade GE. (1975): Science 189:347

14. Tartakoff A, Vassali P, Detraz M. (1978): J Cell Biol 79:694

15. Farquhar MG, Palade GE. (1981): J Cell Biol 91:77s

16. Sano M. (1962): J Cell Biol 15:85

17. Pasteels JL. (1963): Arch Biol 74:439

18. Farquhar MG. (1977): In Dellman HD, Johnson JA, Klachko DM (eds) *Comparative Endocrinology of Prolactin*. Plenum Press, New York, pp 37-94

19. Tougard C, Picart R, Tixier-Vidal A. (1982): Biol Cell 43:89

20. Kelly RB, Gumbiner B. (1982): Cell 28:51

21. Kelly RB, Moore HP, Gumbiner B. (1983): J Cell Biol 97:810

22. Walter AM, Farquhar MG. (1980): Endocrinology 107:1095

23. Farquhar MG, Skutelsky E, Hopkins CR. (1975): In Tixier-Vidal A, Farquhar MG (eds) *The Anterior Pituitary Gland*. Academic Press Inc. New York, p 81

24. Farquhar MG. (1981): Methods Cell Biol 23:399

25. Farquhar MG. (1982): Ciba Fd Symp 92:157

26. Herzog V, Farquhar MG. (1977): Proc Natl Acad Sci USA 74:5073

27. Ottosen PD, Courtoy PJ, Farquhar MG. (1980) J Exp Med 152:1

28. Wood J, Farquhar MG. (1984): J Cell Biol, in press

29. Smith RE, Farquhar MG. (1966): J Cell Biol 31:319

30. Farquhar MG. (1969): In Dingle JT, Fell HB (eds) *Lysosomes in Biology and Pathology*. North Holland Publishing Co, Amsterdam, p 462

31. Farquhar MG. (1971): Memoirs Soc Endo 19:79

32. Shenai R, Wallis M. (1979): Biochem J 182:735

33. Dannies PS, Rudnick MS. (1980): J Biol Chem 255 7:2776

34. Nansel DD, Gudelsky GA, Reymond MJ, Neaves WB, Porter JC. (1981) Endocrinology 108:896

35. Blobel G, Walter P, Chong CN, Goldman BM, Erickson AH, Lingappa VR. (1979): Symp Soc Exp Biol 33:9

36. Walter P, Ibrahimi I, Blobel G. (1981): J Cell Biol 91:551

37. Farquhar MG, Reid D, Reid JA. (1978): Endocrinology 102:296

38. Salpeter M, Farquhar MG. (1981): J Cell Biol 91:240

39. Tougard C, Picart R, Tixier-Vidal A. (1980): Am J Anat 158:471

40. Zanini A, Gianattasio G, Nussdorfer G, Margolis RK, Margolis RU, Meldolesi I. (1980): J Cell Biol 86:260

41. Slaby F, Farquhar MG. (1980): Mol Cell Endocrinol 18:33

42. Rosensweig LJ, Farquhar MG. (1980): Endocrinology 107:422

43. Rosa P, Zanini A. (1983): Eur J Cell Biol 31:94

44. Goldberg DE, Kornfeld S. (1983): J Biol Chen 258:3159

45. Dunphy WG, Rothman JE. (1983): J Cell Biol 97: 270

46. Sly WS, Fischer HD. (1982): J Cell Biochem 18:67

47. Brown WJ, Farquhar MG. (1984): Cell 36:295

48. Brown WJ, Constantinescu E, Farquhar MG. (1984): J Cell Biol 98:320

49. Farquhar MG. (1983): Fed Proc 42:2407

Prolactin. Basic and clinical correlates
R.M. MacLeod, M.O. Thorner and U. Scapagnini (eds.),
Fidia Research Series, vol. I,
Liviana Press, Padova © 1985

Section I
The functional ultrastructure
of prolactin cells

SOLUBLE PROLACTIN MAY BE DIRECTLY RELEASED FROM CELLULAR COMPARTMENTS OTHER THAN SECRETORY GRANULES

M.B. Nikitovitch-Winer, S.M. Yu, and R.E. Papka

Department of Anatomy, Medical Center, University of Kentucky,
Lexington, KY 40536-0084

Mammotrophs, the adenohypophysial cells which secrete prolactin, have been extensively studied with light (L/M) and electronmicroscopy (E/M) both *in vivo* and *in vitro*. Their distinctive morphology when examined with E/M has made them an ideal subject for the study of cellular processes involved in synthesis and release of pituitary hormones. With the use of experimental procedures which combine both biochemical and electronmicroscopic methodology, convincing evidence has been presented that the mammotrophs, like other secretory cells, follow the general scheme of protein synthesis and release as proposed by Palade (1). Thus, Farquhar et al. (2) have demonstrated that prolactin is synthesized within the RER and transported to the Golgi complex where it is processed and packaged into secretory granules. It is within these granules that prolactin is stored prior to release by exocytosis in response to appropriate stimuli. The evidence, however, is not convincing that the above described route of synthesis and release of prolactin is the exclusive mode of its secretion. Studies of the release of prolactin in lactating animals led Grosvenor (3) and Nicoll (4) to postulate the existence of temporal phases in this process. After the onset of suckling, they contend that prolactin is first "depleted", then "transformed", and finally released. This postulate implies the possibility that prolactin may be contained in different intracellular compartments ("rapidly" and "slowly releasable pools") which are processed differentially as well as released at different rates depending on a variety of factors.

With the purpose of examining the morphologic substrate which may be the basis for the possible differential storage pools of prolactin, we (5) used E/M to study the immediate morphologic changes that are induced in mammotrophs of lactating rats by resumption of the suckling stimulus applied for varying intervals following prolonged deprivation of this stimulus. We found that when the suckling stimulus was denied for 5-7 h, many mammotrophs contained very dilated cisternae of both the RER and the Golgi apparatus. The most obvious change observed, as a result of re-applying the suckling stimulus for 1 and 3 min, was the collapse of the cisternae which appeared as if they had emptied their content. There was also an apparent fragmentation of the RER-cisternae to form many vesicles of different sizes. These rapid changes in cisternal content, as well as configuration, suggest that the RER cisternae may represent the "easily releasable pool" of prolactin. To investigate further the question of prolactin storage and release, we studied the morphology of pituitaries of lactating animals utilizing immunocytochemical methods as well as conventional E/M. Also, plasma and pituitary prolactin levels were examined and related to the morphologic data.

Lactating Sprague-Dawley rats with litter sizes adjusted to 10 pups/mother at birth were used on days 12-16 of lactation. They were separated from their young for 5-7 h before reuniting them for 1-30 min. Morphologic changes were examined using conventional E/M, the horseradish peroxidase-antiperoxidase (PAP) method of Sternberger (6) both with L/M and E/M (7,8), as well as the colloidal gold immunocytochemistry technique (9) at the E/M level. Following a pilot study examining temporal morphologic changes, the primary times selected were 0-time (indicating the end of the 5-7 h period of removal of pups), 1, 3, 10 and 15 min of suckling. Two days prior to the end of the experiment, intracardiac catheters were inserted and blood samples were obtained through these at designated times prior to sacrifice. At the time of sacrifice, final blood samples were taken and the pituitaries excised. The latter were either used completely for morphologic studies or halved and also used for evaluation of prolactin contents. In additional groups of animals, the pituitary morphology, prolactin content, and prolactin plasma levels were studied at the same designated times after treatment with substances known to inhibit prolactin release such as pergolide mesylate (PM), dopamine, and pentabarbital (PB).

For morphologic studies, the adenohypophyses were processed in the following way: 1) for conventional E/M, the glands were fixed and processed by the method described by Karnovsky (10); 2) for immunocytochemistry, the adenohypophyses were processed, embedded in paraffin, and sectioned at 5-7 um. After deparaffinization, the sections were processed with the PAP method. The following steps were used for L/M: 1) application of NIAMDD rabbit anti-serum to rat prolactin diluted 1:40 for 16 h or 1:1,000 for 48 h, followed by 2) goat anti-rabbit gamma-globulin (Miles Laboratories) diluted 1:10-1:100 for 8 h, and then 3) PAP (Miles Laboratories) diluted 1:50-1:500 for 16 h before processing with 4) 3,3'-diaminobenzidine tetrahydrochloride (Sigma) in 0.002% H_2O_2, pH 7.6, for 20 min. For control staining, normal rabbit serum was used to replace the antiserum in step 1. After appropriate processing, the sections were counterstained in 0.25% azure B, 0.25% methylene blue, and 0.2% sodium borate. The procedure for the immunocytochemistry E/M was identical to steps 1-4 described above for L/M. The following additional steps were performed: sections were washed in 0.1 M cacodylate buffer for 10 min., immersed in 2% osmium tetroxide in cacodylate buffer for 20-30 min., dehydrated, immersed in acetone/Epon 812 mixture, transferred through two 10 min. changes of Epon 812, and examined with L/M. Specific areas of sections were then selected, cut out, immersed in Epon, and placed flat on the tips of precured Epon blocks. Ultrathin sections were viewed by E/M.

The great advantage of the above method is that it permits examination of sections with L/M and selection of specific areas of the section which can then be cut out and processed for E/M. This was of crucial importance since the peripheral part of the adenohypophysis responded most dramatically to the acute stimulus of re-established suckling, and it was thus necessary to select a specific part of the section prior to its study with E/M. The disadvantages of this method are that the secretory granules do not "stain" with this pre-embedding technique and that the morphology is not very distinct. For these reasons, portions of glands were processed in parallel for study with conventional E/M which permits easy visualization of secretory granules and other morphologic detail. The above methods, using the two techniques, supplemented one another. Additionally, some glands were processed using the colloidal gold immunocytochemistry method. Radioimmunoassay procedures were performed according to the method of Niswender et al. (11) using the NIAMDD rat prolactin-RP-2 as standard. Plasma and pituitary samples were processed and prolactin level evaluated. Statistical evaluation of the data was done using analysis of variance. The inter- and intra-assay coefficients of variation were less than 5%.

As Figure 1 illustrates, the prolactin plasma levels were uniformly low at 0-time (5-7 h of separation of dams from pups) and were at basal levels of 16.4 ± 2.0 ng/ml.

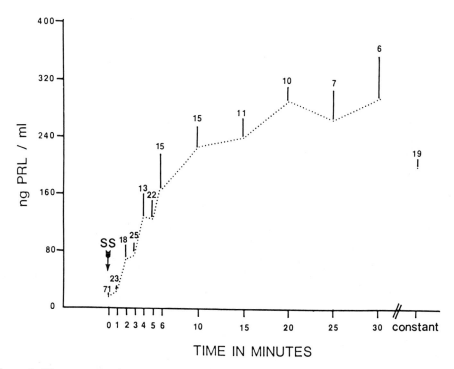

Figure 1. Plasma prolactin concentrations in lactating rats at 0-time and following resumption of the suckling stimulus. Numbers above the vertical lines represent the numbers of lactating rats at each time interval. The vertical lines indicate the standard error of the mean. Constant = continuously lactating rats.

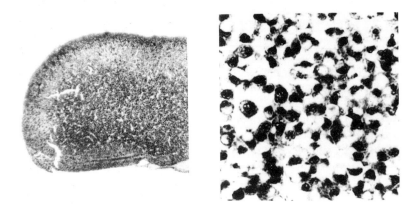

Figure 2. Low power overview of part of the adenohypophysis of a lactating rat (PAP-L/M, X25). Note the distribution of mammotrophs (dark dots of IM) into a large central area and a narrow peripheral rim. IM = immunoreactive material.

Figure 3. Higher magnification of a pituitary at 0-time, (PAP-L/M. X400). The IM is distributed either as a clump or diffusely throughout the cytoplasm. The nuclei and all other cells besides the mammotrophs appear clear.

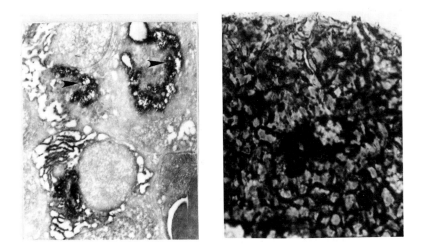

Figure 4. Three mammotrophs are represented, two of which have the IM clumped within the Golgi area (arrowheads) whereas the third one has IM also diffusely dispersed within the cytoplasm surrounding the RER (PAP-E/M, X3500).

Figure 5. The meshwork of spaces filled with IM is evident in this view of the periphery of the gland taken from an animal at 3 min of resumed suckling (PAP-L/M, X400).

Following the re-establishment of suckling, prolactin plasma levels increase to 74.2 ± 18.6 ng/ml at 3 min of suckling, and within 10 min of suckling reach the concentration of 223.2 ± 32.8 ng/ml. In animals which continued to suckle without interruption (constant suckling rats), the prolactin plasma levels were 190.0 ± 13.4 ng/ml. Prolactin plasma levels remained at basal levels at all times studied in animals treated with PM, dopamine, and PB (not shown). The pituitary prolactin content, during constant suckling, was 2.21 ± 0.05 ug/mg wet weight. It was increased at 0-time to 6.67 ± 0.65 ug/mg wet weight and remained at that level at 3 and 10 min of re-suckling. Despite the fact that statistically significant increases in plasma levels of prolactin are observed within 3 and 10 min of resumption of suckling, no change of pituitary content was observed at those times, indicating that prolactin synthesis is keeping pace with its release.

Figure 2 shows a low power field of a section processed with PAP and examined with L/M (PAP-L/M). It can be observed that mammotrophs are distributed throughout a large central area and a peripheral rim, separated by an area sparse in mammotrophs. Figure 3, using higher magnification, shows more clearly the immunoreactive material (IM) within the specific prolactin cells. In some cells the IM is diffusely distributed throughout the cytoplasm; in others it is primarily clumped in the vicinity of the "pale appearing" nucleus. Specimens processed with PAP and viewed with E/M (PAP-E/M) reveal that some mammotrophs contain the IM distributed throughout the cytoplasm in the vicinity of the RER cisternae whereas in others the IM is primarily located within the Golgi area as seen in Figure 4. Immediately following the reinstitution of the suckling stimulus after 5-7 h of its deprivation, one observes, with PAP-L/M, that the periphery of the adenohypophysis fills with IM forming a network between adjacent cells. This change begins at 1 min, reaches its maximum at 3 min (Fig. 5) and is markedly reduced by 10 min of renewed suckling. This pattern of IM distribution was seen without exception in every gland examined at 3 min of suckling taken from animals in which prolactin release had occurred. By contrast no IM was ever present surrounding mammotrophs in the same area of the gland at 0-time, nor when animals were pre-treated with dopamine, PM, or PB prior to the return of the pups (Fig. 6). The PAP-E/M shows (Fig. 7) that the IM seen with L/M at 3 min of re-suckling is located within the extracellular spaces (ECS). The intensity of the diffuse intracellular IM was observed with L/M to decrease at 3-5 min suckling (not shown). The change of configuration of the RER cisternae following onset of suckling is seen in Figure 8. Many vesicles with circular and very irregular profiles are seen and some appear to have undergone exocytosis. The extrusion of secretory granules begins around 5 min and becomes more massive at 10 and 15 min of resumed suckling. This process of exocytosis is shown in Figure 9, where prolactin has been labeled with grains of colloidal gold. Two labeled vesicles of different density are seen undergoing exocytosis. The colloidal gold immunocytochemistry has been very useful in identifying at least 2 different types of mammotrophs, as judged by the sizes and shapes of their secretory granules (Fig. 10). In this post-embedding procedure, the heaviest labelling is seen in secretory granules. In some cells significant numbers of grains are found outlining the Golgi cisternae. RER cisternae and ECS also contain grains of colloidal gold but they are fewer in numbers. However, even though the background labelling is very low (see Fig. 9), it is not possible to ascertain at this time whether this labelling within RER and ECS is specific.

The present work has given suggestive morphologic evidence that the re-application

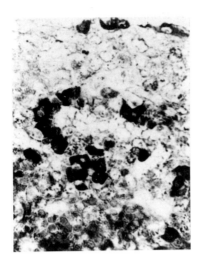 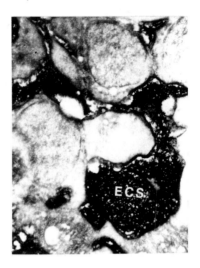

Figure 6. No meshwork of spaces filled with IM is seen in this section of the gland taken from an animal treated with PM prior to the 3 min of resumed suckling (PAP-L/M, X420).

Figure 7. This E/M of the periphery of the gland at 3 min of resumed suckling reveals the dilated ECS filled with IM (PAP-E/M, X3400). ECS / extracellular spaces.

of the suckling stimulus after a 7-hour interruption immediately triggers the release of prolactin-IM into the ECS of the periphery of the adenohypophysis. From here it is slowly cleared within the first 10 min of suckling. This preferential localization of prolactin-IM into the ECS of the periphery of the gland is puzzling at the moment. The difference in dopaminergic tone in the portal vessels supplying the periphery of the adenohypohysis compared to that of vessels supplying the center of the gland, as reported by Porter's group (12), may be responsible for this differential regional response. The demonstration of this apparent accumulation of prolactin-IM within ECS suggests an increase in concentration of prolactin in the external milieu immediately surrounding mammotrophs. These changes in extracellular prolactin concentrations *in vivo* tend to support the concept of mammotroph autoregulation suggested by Kadowaki et al. (13) on the basis of their *in vitro* work.

Concomitant with and following the appearance of IM within the ECS, intracellular IM appears to decrease in intensity and the previously swollen RER cisternae seem to lose their content in some cells. In others, the endoplasmic reticulum cisternae assume a different topography and the newly formed vesicular cisternae give, at times, the appearance of undergoing exocytosis. In addition, the plasma prolactin levels increase several fold in concentration by 3 min of renewed suckling. All these acute changes are seen before any appreciable release of prolactin secretory granules is observed. Taken together, these observations give circumstantial evidence that, as a result of an acute stimulus, prolactin may first be released from intracellular compartments other than secretory granules. Only after this first surge of release has occurred, do secretory granules seem to be recruited to supply further secretion in order to maintain minute-

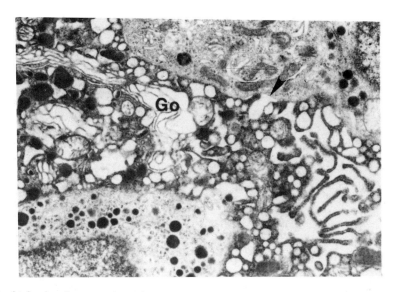

Figure 8. At 3 min of resumption of suckling many mammotrophs contain very active looking Golgi areas and the RER which assumes a multivesicular configuration. Note at the arrowhead the appearance of confluence of one of these vesicles with the ECS (Conventional E/M, X9800).

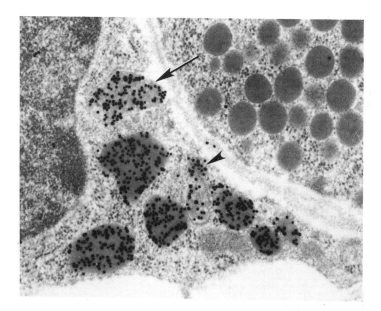

Figure 9. Exocytosis is clearly seen (arrow) in this section processed with colloidal gold immunocytochemistry. Note the vesicle of lower density (arrowhead) which is also extruding its content. The cell above is a growth hormone producing cell. Note the low background over that cell (E/M, X30400).

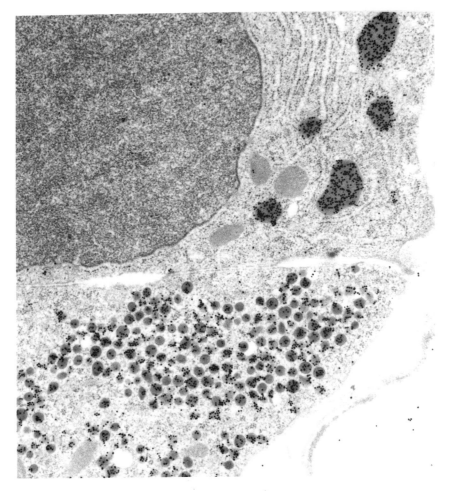

Figure 10. Note the drastic difference in the size of secretory granules of these adjacent cells which both reacted with the second antibody complexed with the colloidal gold (E/M, X29.500).

to-minute plasma prolactin levels at a constant, optimal concentration throughout the duration of suckling. It is possible that the above described events which take place prior to granule release provide the morphologic background for the "depletion-transformation" phase of prolactin postulated by Grosvenor and by Nicoll. The indication that cellular compartments other than secretory granules may participate directly in the release process is not unique to mammotrophs. Rothman (14), in a series of publications, has provided a great deal of evidence suggesting that even in the exocrine pancreas enzyme release may occur via additional routes different from the secretory granules. Walker and Farquhar (15) have demonstrated that newly synthesized prolactin is preferentially released over the older synthesized hormone but deduce that this still occurs through secretory granule release. They suggest that the differential rate of release is due to the heterogeneity of the mammotrophs. Indeed, Tixier-Vidal's group (16), and our present work, also demonstrate clearly the existence of at least two types of these cells. The functional meaning of the heterogeneity is still unclear. It is hoped that the colloidal gold technique will help clarify this point as well as provide a marker to determine with certainty whether prolactin, in some circumstances, may be released through pathways that bypass the secretory granules. Since IM was only seen within the ECS and in areas of the mammotroph other than secretion granules when the PAP pre-embedding technique was used, we are in the process of developing a similar procedure using colloidal gold, which provides a more refined localization of the IM. It is of interest to note that Tixier-Vidal's group (16) has also demonstrated positive staining over the "ground cytoplasm" when pre-embedding immunocytochemical methods are used but not with post-embedding methods.

ACKNOWLEDGMENTS

We thank Dr. A.F. Parlow and the Rat Pituitary Hormone Program of the NIADDK for the generous gifts of rat antigens and antisera and Mrs. Merle Wekstein for excellent technical assistance.

REFERENCES

1. Palade G. (1975): Science 189:347
2. Farquhar MG, Reid JJ, Daniell LW. (1978): Endocrinology 102:296
3. Grosvenor CE, Mena F, Whitworth NS. (1979): Endocrinology 105:884
4. Nicoll CS. (1972): Gen Comp Endocrinology (Suppl) 3:86
5. Chang NG, Nikitovitch-Winer MB. (1976): Cell Tiss Res 166:399
6. Sternberger LA. (1970) *Immunocytochemistry*, ed 2. John Wiley and Sons, Inc., New York, p 104
7. Yu SM, Nikitovitch-Winer MB. (1980): Anat Rec 199(3):286a (Abstract)
8. Yu SM, Nikitovitch-Winer MB. Program of the 64th Annual Meeting of the Endocrine Society, 1981, p 303 (Abstract)
9. Roth J, Bendayan M, Orci L. (1978): J Histochem Cytochem 26:1074
10. Karnovsky MJ. (1965): J Cell Biol 27:137a
11. Niswender GD, Chen CL, Midgley AR, Meites J, Ellis S. (1969): Fed Proc 33:237
12. Reymond MJ, Speciale SG, Porter JC. (1983): Endocrinology 112:1958
13. Kadowaki J, Ku N, Oetting WS, Walker AM. (1984): Endocrinology 114:2060
14. Rothman SS. (1975): Science 190:747
15. Walker AM, Farquhar MG. (1980): Endocrinology 107:1095
16. Tougard C, Picart R, Tixier-Vidal A. (1980): Am J Anat 158:471

Prolactin. Basic and clinical correlates
R.M. MacLeod, M.O. Thorner and U. Scapagnini (eds.),
Fidia Research Series, vol. I,
Liviana Press, Padova © 1985

Section I
The functional ultrastructure
of prolactin cells

AUTORADIOGRAPHIC STUDIES WITH [3H]-LISURIDE, [3H]-DOPAMINE, AND [3H]-DOMPERIDONE IN PITUITARY AND BRAIN

W. E. Stumpf, W. M. Detmer, M. Sar, R. Horowski* and R. Dorow*

Department of Anatomy, University of North Carolina, Chapel Hill, NC 27514
*Research Laboratories of Schering AG, Berlin (West), Germany

INTRODUCTION

Biochemical receptor binding studies with dopamine and dopaminergic agonists and antagonists provided evidence not only for various subtypes of dopamine receptors, but also for possible differential interaction with receptors to serotonin and catecholamines. Lisuride, an ergot derivative, has been shown to interact with D-1 and D-2 dopamine receptors as well as with alpha- and beta-adrenergic receptors (1). This is based on specific binding of lisuride to diverse structures known to contain D-1 dopamine receptors, such as a cell-free homogenate of the neostriatum, or D-2 dopamine receptors in the intermediate lobe of the rat pituitary. The lisuride mediated inhibition of alpha-MSH release is not due to enhanced adenylate cyclase activity (1). Similarly, in the anterior lobe of the pituitary, lisuride mediated inhibition of prolactin release appears to be related to the activation of D-2 dopamine receptors. In contrast, binding in the neostriatum is thought to occur on D-1 dopamine receptors. Because of the multiple and varied sites of action of dopamine agonists and antagonists, the use of non-disruptive histochemical procedures can be expected to contribute to the clarification of compound specific sites and mechanisms of action.

In the present experiments autoradiography has been used for identification of sites of [3H]-lisuride uptake and retention in brain and pituitary with some comparison to [3H]-dopamine and [3H]-domperidone.

[3H]-lisuride, spec. act. 26.4 Ci/mM (Schering AG Berlin), dissolved in ethanol was injected i.v. under ether anesthesia. Two male Sprague Dawley rats each received 1.7 ug, 3.0 ug or 3.5 ug/100 g bw of [3H]-lisuride and were sacrificed 30 min or 1 hr afterwards.

[3H]-dopamine, spec. act. 47 Ci/mM (Amersham), was dissolved in 0.02 M acetic acid-ethanol (1:1) and injected subcutaneously at 3.3 ug/100 g bw into three female Sprague Dawley rats, which were sacrificed 15 or 30 min afterwards.

[3H]-domperidone, spec. act. 43.4 Ci/mM (Amersham) was dissolved in ethanol.

Six male Sprague Dawley rats were injected i.v. with 1.76 ug/100 g bw of [³H]-domperidone and were killed 15, 30 or 60 min afterwards.

In addition, two groups of 3 CF-1 albino mice at day 20 of lactation were injected with [³H]-dopamine or [³H]-lisuride and sacrificed 30 min afterwards.

Competition studies included unlabeled lisuride or dopamine, 2 rats each and 1 mouse each, at 1000 times higher dose, injected prior to the radioactively labeled lisuride or dopamine.

Pituitaries from all animals and brains from 3 rats with [³H]-lisuride and from 2 rats each with [³H]-dopamine or [³H]-domperidone were removed, frozen, sectioned, and thaw-mounted on dried emulsion coated slides. After exposure of 4-6 months, autoradiograms were photographically processed and stained with methylgreen-pyronin after Stumpf and Sar (2).

Quantitative evaluation of brain autoradiograms was done with [³H]-lisuride treated rats, using a computer program for automated counting of silver grains in selected brain areas using a Zeiss inverted microscope with a television camera in line with an Artek counter, Model 982, and an Apple IIe computer. Background counts were subtracted and measurements expressed as number of silver grains per 1000 u² over a given brain region divided by the number of silver grains over the corpus callosum.

PITUITARY

After injection of [³H]-lisuride to rats and mice, at 30 min as well as at 1 hour, radioactivity is observed in the anterior, intermediate and neural lobe. The general level of radioactivity is highest in the intermediate lobe, moderate in the anterior lobe, and lowest in the neural lobe. In certain areas of the anterior lobe, including a region close to the intermediate lobe, strong accumulations of radioactivity can be seen in one or several cells frequently found bordering sinusoids (Fig. 1). It appears that some of the high level radioactivity is associated with cells and their immediate vicinity, and it is difficult to decide where the center of highest radioactivity lies. Other cells in the anterior lobe contain varying degrees of radioactivity. In the intermediate lobe as well as in the neural lobe, the radioactivity is diffuse and no specific cellular or subcellular accumulation can be recognized.

After competition with unlabeled lisuride there is some reduction of radioactivity, but there is no apparent reduction in the clusters in the anterior lobe. When autoradiograms were stained with antibodies to ovine beta-LH, bovine beta-TSH, or ovine prolactin, the cells associated with the center of clustered radioactivity remained unstained (Figs. 4-6). It appears, however, that the cytoplasm of some prolactin positive cells contains more radioactivity than the cytoplasm of cells stained with LH or TSH antibodies.

After injection of [³H]-dopamine, the highest concentration of radioactivity is seen in the neural lobe. It appears that this radioactivity is not concentrated in glial cells but arranged in patches, which are heterogeneously distributed and more frequently close to the border of the intermediate lobe, from where strands of radioactivity appear to continue into the intermediate lobe, apparently following blood vessels and connective tissue septa. In the intermediate lobe, the cells bordering the neural lobe con-

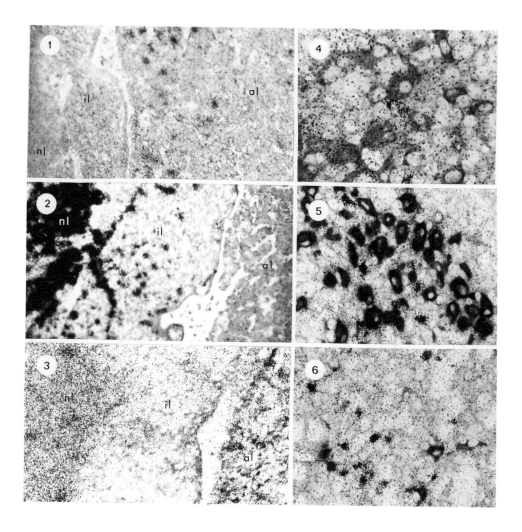

Figures 1-6. Autoradiograms of rat pituitary after [³H]-lisuride (Figs. 1, 4-6), [³H]-dopamine (Fig. 2) and [³H]-domperidone (Fig. 3), showing different patterns of concentration of radioactivity. The clusters of radioactivity in the anterior lobe with [³H]-lisuride do not correspond to cells immunostained with antibodies to ovine prolactin (Fig. 4), ovine beta LH (Fig. 5) and bovine beta TSH (Fig. 6). NL neural lobe, IL intermediate lobe, AL anterior lobe. Magnifications: x 95 (Figs. 1-3), x 350 (Fig. 4), x 200 (Figs. 5 and 6).

tain more radioactivity than those bordering the anterior lobe. The latter cells and the cells between the septa contain relatively low levels of radioactivity. In the anterior lobe a diffuse level of radioactivity exists, which is higher than the level of radioactivity in the intermediate lobe, with the exception of the patchy or strand-like regions usually associated with septa.

After [^{3}H]-domperidone injection, the distribution of radioactivity appears similar to the distribution observed after [^{3}H]-dopamine injection. Levels of radioactivity are very high in the neural lobe with special, point-like accumulations within the neuropil. In the intermediate lobe, radioactivity is high only along connective tissue septa, while between such strands radioactivity levels are low. The strands of radioactivity appear to arise from the neural lobe, from where they taper off toward the border with the anterior lobe. In the anterior lobe diffuse radioactivity exists with occasional circumscribed areas with high levels of radioactivity similar to those observed with [^{3}H]-lisuride.

BRAIN

After injection of [^{3}H]-lisuride using different doses and time intervals, a similar pattern of concentration and retention of radioactivity is obtained in certain areas in the brain. Results were quantitatively evaluated and are depicted in the table; examples of autoradiograms are depicted in Figures 7-12. The highest concentration of radioactivity is seen in the choroid epithelium (not listed); lower concentrations were seen in the median eminence and caudate-putamen. High levels of concentration exist also in certain nuclei of the dorsal thalamus, lamina IV of the cortex, globus pallidus, certain layers of the hippocampus, substantia nigra (not listed) and stratum griseum superficiale of the superior colliculus (not listed). Regions of the hippocampus show generally low levels of concentration when compared with cortex, hypothalamus, and amygdala.

After injection of [^{3}H]-dopamine, accumulation of radioactivity is seen only in the median eminence and choroid plexus. However, throughout the brain a low level of radioactivity above background exists.

A similar distribution is seen after [^{3}H]-domperidone injection, with relatively low uptake in brain tissues, except for the median eminence and choroid plexus.

DISCUSSION

The results of the present studies demonstrate a distinct pattern of distribution of radioactivity in brain and pituitary, which is characteristic for the individual "dopamine agonist" and "dopamine antagonist". As expected, after [^{3}H]-dopamine or [^{3}H]-domperidone injection, little radioactivity enters the brain, except for regions outside of the blood brain barrier, such as, the choroid plexus, the median eminence, the pineal and the subfornical organ. After [^{3}H]-lisuride injection, by contrast, a high uptake of radioactivity is visible at 30 min and 60 min in all regions of the brain studied, with highest uptake - in addition to the median eminence and choroid plexus - in the caudate-putamen, certain regions of the dorsal thalamus, lamina IV of the cortex, stratum griseum superficialis of the superior colliculus, the central gray of the midbrain and

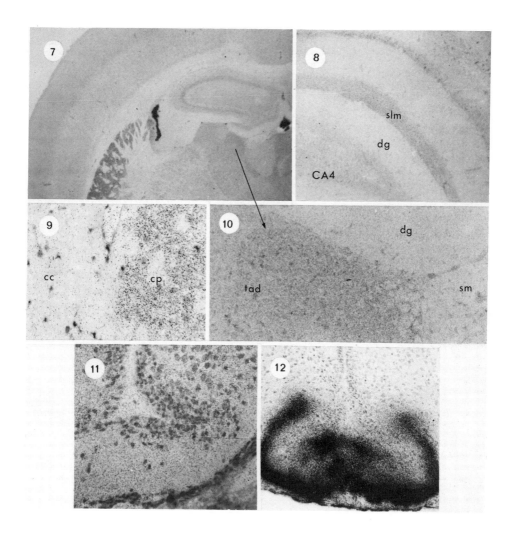

Figures 7-12. Autoradiograms of rat brain after injection of [³H]-lisuride (Figs. 7-11) or [³H]-dopamine (Fig. 12), showing accumulation of radioactivity in cortex (Fig. 7), caudate-putamen cp (Figs. 7 and 9, cc corpus callosum), hippocampus (Figs. 7 and 8) with stratum lacunosum-moleculare slm (Fig. 8), thalamus (Figs. 7 and 10) with higher magnification of nucleus anterodorsalis tad (Fig. 10, dentate gyrus dg, stria medullare sm) and median eminence (Figs. 11 and 12). Note the difference in accumulation of radioactivity in the median eminence with [³H]-lisuride (Fig. 11) and [³H]-dopamine (Fig. 12). Magnifications: x 12 (Fig. 7), x 100 (Fig. 8), x 250 (Figs. 9-11), x 150 (Fig. 12).

Table I. - *Concentration of Radioactivity in Brain Regions after Injection of [³H]-Lisuride (quantitative assessment of autoradiograms)*

Structure	1.7 ug/100 g bw-30 min *SG/1000 u^2	**Ratio	3.0 ug/100 g bw-30 min SG/1000 u^2	Ratio
Corpus Callosum	14.59 ± 1.70	1.00	17.93 ± 0.83	1.00
Cortex parietalis				
lamina 1	34.34 ± 2.95	2.35	40.07 ± 5.60	2.23
lamina 2	30.97 ± 4.83	2.12	35.79 ± 4.37	2.00
lamina 3	36.78 ± 2.69	2.52	41.37 ± 3.66	2.31
lamina 4	43.75 ± 4.04	3.00	46.24 ± 0.86	2.58
lamina 5	35.89 ± 4.34	2.46	37.27 ± 3.93	2.08
lamina 6	36.77 ± 4.67	2.52	38.65 ± 2.45	2.16
Hippocampus				
CA1 str oriens	29.51 ± 4.91	2.02	28.72 ± 1.00	1.60
CA1 str radiale	29.09 ± 1.67	1.99	30.16 ± 3.38	1.68
CA1 str lac-mol	34.37 ± 1.70	2.36	47.51 ± 6.06	2.65
GD str mol	28.51 ± 1.35	1.35	24.50 ± 1.23	1.37
CA4	35.77 ± 3.60	2.45	45.24 ± 3.59	2.52
Caud-Putamen	70.16 ± 10.98	4.81	80.68 ± 7.54	4.03
Glob Pallidus			43.98 ± 2.69	2.20
Thalamus				
Org Subfornicale				
n periventricul	44.56 ± 7.29	3.05	53.43 ± 2.27	2.67
n thal ant-dors			63.31 ± 8.02	3.17
n thal lateral				
Hypothalamus				
n paraventricul				
n suprachiasm			32.78 ± 1.74	1.64
ant hypoth area			48.85 ± 4.48	2.44
n arcuatus	31.04 ± 2.69	2.13	42.57 ± 3.65	2.37
n ventromedialis	34.36 ± 3.77	2.36		
n dorsomedialis	35.45 ± 4.22	2.43		
EM outer	51.09 ± 3.34	3.50	91.59 ± 3.63	5.11
EM inner			72.08 ± 2.16	4.02
Amygdala				
n medialis	41.99 ± 4.57	2.82		

* SG = silver grains (mean ± standard deviation)
** Ratio is expressed as silver grain density over structure divided by silver grain density over corpus callosum

Concentration of Radioactivity in Brain Regions after Injection of [³H]-Lisuride
(continued)

Structure	3.5 ug/100g bw-60 min	
	SG/1000 u²	Ratio
Corpus Callosum	27.75 ± 4.16	1.00
Cortex parietalis		
lamina 1		
lamina 2	79.61 ± 9.85	2.87
lamina 3	77.89 ± 3.84	2.81
lamina 4	87.94 ± 12.30	3.17
lamina 5	70.15 ± 4.73	2.53
lamina 6	70.75 ± 12.34	2.55
Hippocampus		
CA1 str oriens		
CA1 str radiale		
CA1 str lac-mol		
GD str mol		
CA4 str mol		
Caud-Putamen	127.27 ± 4.57	4.59
Glob Pallidus	74.06 ± 14.20	2.67
Thalamus		
Org Subfornicale	84.75 ± 10.94	3.05
n pervientricul	85.52 ± 9.78	3.08
n thal ant-dors		
n thal lateral		
Hypothalamus		
n paraventricul	66.49 ± 4.09	2.40
n suprachiasm		
ant hypoth area		
n arcuatus		
n ventromedialis		
n dorsomedialis		
EM outer		
EM inner		
Amygdala		
n medialis		

the substantia nigra. Although our study of brain regions is incomplete, some of the results correspond to expectations compatible with classification of lisuride as a "dopamine agonist", especially regarding the strong localization in the caudate-putamen and substantia nigra. The high concentration of radioactivity in the periventricular thalamus, the anterodorsal nucleus of the thalamus in conjunction with lamina IV of the cortex is noteworthy, as is the concentration in the stratum lacunosum-moleculare in CAI of the hippocampus, the latter contrasting with the low uptake in the dentate gyrus. Since the stratum lacunosum-moleculare has been reported to carry noradrenergic fibers and since the hippocampus is believed to be devoid of dopaminergic innervation (3), lisuride may bind to noradrenergic elements in this region. Of interest also is the intense labeling of the thalamic nucleus anterodorsalis, the nucleus interanterodorsalis and the nuclei periventriculares, all structures considered to belong to thalamic regions related to the limbic allocortex (4).

In the pituitary, after injection of [³H]-dopamine and its antagonist [³H]-domperidone, the highest concentration of radioactivity is seen in the neural lobe in small individual or confluent patches or strands which can be followed into the intermediate lobe. This appears to correspond to the course of dopaminergic fibers which have been shown to exist in both lobes (5) and may reflect presynaptic uptake, which does not seem to exist for [³H]-lisuride. By contrast, the high cellular distribution of radioactivity in the intermediate lobe after [³H]-lisuride - different after [³H]-dopamine and [³H]-domperidone - may reflect target cell receptor uptake. Indications of such uptake exist also in the anterior lobe in prolactin cells and possible other cells. The occurrence of clusters of strong radioactivity at certain sinusoids and bordering cells is puzzling, since they remain visible in competition studies. The specific nature of this clustered radioactivity remains to be elucidated, because of difficulties in the evaluation of the autoradiograms, such as the irregular distribution of such clusters, their absence in large portions of the anterior lobe, and their lack of conspicuous association with lactotropes. The existence of neurosecretory nerve fibers in the anterior lobe is still controversial, although contact of fibers with anterior pituitary cells in defined regions of the pars distalis has been described (6-8). Since the clusters of radioactivity are seen at and in cells near sinusoids, where nerve fibers have been reported to exist, it is likely that these clusters represent uptake by such fibers. Our data on the distribution of [³H]-dopamine and [³H]-lisuride in the pituitary suggest that lisuride is likely to bind to receptors which correspond only in part to those of dopamine.

In conclusion, autoradiographic studies with the dopamine agonist [³H]-lisuride, [3H]-dopamine, and the dopamine antagonist [³H]-domperidone show different patterns of distribution in the brain and pituitary. In the pituitary, after [³H]-dopamine and [³H]-domperidone, the highest concentration exists in the neural lobe and in specific regions of the intermediate lobe. In the anterior lobe, radioactivity is not confined to lactotropes. Occasional clusters of radioactivity were seen near sinusoids not associated with lactotropes, gonadotropes or thyrotropes. In the brain, after [³H]-lisuride injection, the highest uptake is seen in the caudate-putamen, a region known to be rich in dopamine receptors. High uptake also exists in areas where dopamine receptors are believed to be absent, such as the hippocampus. After [³H]-dopamine and [³H]-domperidone injection, radioactivity is accumulated only in areas outside of the blood brain barrier.

ACKNOWLEDGMENTS

This work was supported by U.S. PHS grant NS 09914 and a grant from Schering AG, Berlin.

REFERENCES

1. Cote TE, Eskay RL, Frey EA, Grewe CW, Munemura M, Tsuruta K, Brown EM, Kebabian JW. (1983) In: Calne DB, Horowski R, McDonald RJ, Wuttke, W (eds): *Lisuride and Other Dopamine Agonists*. Raven Press, New York, p 45
2. Stumpf WE, Sar M. (1975) In: Methods in Enzymology, Academic Press, New York, vol 36:135
3. Creese I, Hamblin MW, Leff SE, Sibley DR. (1983) In: Iversen LL, Iversen SD, Snyder SH (eds) *Biochemical Studies of CNS Receptors*. Plenum Press, New York, p 81
4. Hajdu F, Hassler R. (1973): Exp Brain Res 17:216
5. Baumgarten HG, Bjorklund H, Holstein AF, Nolin A. (1972) Z Zellforsch 126:483
6. Theret C, Tamboise E. (1963): Ann Endocrinol Paris 24:421
7. Kurosumi K, Kobayashi Y. (1980): Archivum Histologicum Japonicum 43:141
8. Westlund KN, Childs GV. (1982): Endocrinology 111:1761

Prolactin. Basic and clinical correlates
R.M. MacLeod, M.O. Thorner and U. Scapagnini (eds.),
Fidia Research Series, vol. I,
Liviana Press, Padova © 1985

Section I
The functional ultrastructure
of prolactin cells

IMMUNOCYTOCHEMICAL IDENTIFICATION OF MEMBRANE COMPARTMENTS INVOLVED IN SECRETORY PROCESS AND ENDOCYTOSIS IN PROLACTIN CELLS

C. Tougard, D. Louvard*, R. Picart, and A. Tixier-Vidal

Groupe de Neuroendocrinologie Cellulaire, College de France,
75231 Paris Cedex 05 *Unite de Biologie des Membranes,
Institut Pasteur, 75724 Paris Cedex 15, France.

The importance of intracellular membrane traffic in many cell processes such as protein secretion, biogenesis of membrane domains, and endocytosis has been recognized increasingly during the past few years. Studies performed with various cell types and with different approaches have led to the concept that all these processes are mediated by vesicular traffic and that the cells reutilize or recycle vesicular containers rather than resynthesizing them (1). Several intracellular pathways have been revealed, most of which converge in the Golgi zone where secretory products and membrane components are sorted and directed to their final sites of insertion. However, the mechanisms for sorting and directing such traffic are still unknown. Among the various approaches which may contribute to the resolution of these problems, the immunocytochemical localization of membrane constituents in specific cell structures represents an important step. This was recently made possible with the development of immunological probes: antibodies specific to several membrane components of the dog pancreas rough endoplasmic reticulum (A-RER) (2), antibodies specific to a 135 Kd protein of rat liver Golgi apparatus (A-Golgi) (2) and antibodies specific to a 100 Kd protein of rat liver lysosomal membranes (A-Ly-M) (3,4).

We have applied these antibodies to prolactin cells in culture where morphology can be easily correlated with prolactin secretion. Normal prolactin cells were used as a reference system for identification of immunostained intracellular membrane compartments. The correlation with functional studies were performed on clonal, tumor derived GH_3/B_6 cells which have the advantage of offering homogeneous populations of prolactin cells. Previous studies in both cell types have permitted localization of prolactin in all of the membrane compartments classically involved in the biosynthetic pathway of secretory products: rough endoplasmic reticulum (RER), saccules and vesicles of the Golgi complex, and secretory granules. In that respect, GH_3 cells behave exactly as normal prolactin cells, except that they have very few and small secretory granules. However they possess small vesicles loaded with prolactin which may serve as carriers for the release of prolactin (5,6).

MEMBRANE COMPARTMENTS INVOLVED IN THE BIOSYNTHETIC PATHWAY

Immunoperoxidase staining was performed according to Tougard et al. (7). When applied to normal prolactin cells, the A-RER labeled the membrane of all of the RER cisternae, including the perinuclear cisternae. The same localization was observed in GH₃ cells (Fig. 1) (7). No modification in the distribution of the A-RER stained membranes was found after stimulation of prolactin release by thyroliberin (TRH) or after inhibition of prolactin secretion by monensin (7).

In normal prolactin cells, the A-Golgi labeled the membrane of some Golgi saccules, mostly the medial saccules and, with a decreasing intensity, the inner saccules of the trans face (Fig. 2). In addition they labeled the membrane of small vesicles, mainly located in the Golgi zone, as well as that of lysosome-like structures. In contrast, the secretory granule membrane was unstained, except at the level of very few segregating

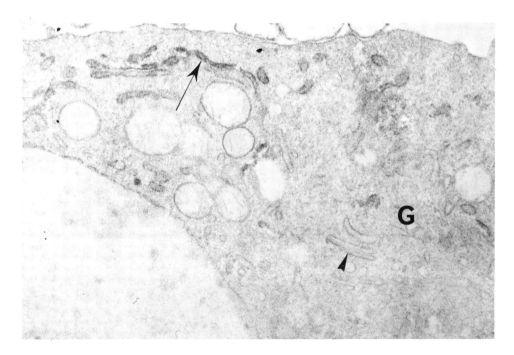

Fig. 1. A GH₃ cell was immunostained with A-RER antibodies. The reaction product labeled short and discontinuous cisternae (arrows). In the Golgi zone (G) the membranes of saccules and vesicles were not stained. However a slight deposit was observed on one face of elongated cisternae which might represent transitional elements (arrowhead) (X 24.000).

secretory material (Fig. 2). In some cells, the A-Golgi labeled discrete areas of the plasma membrane and a few vesicles beneath the plasma membrane. In GH$_3$ cells, the same structures were stained with the A-Golgi (7).

The stimulation of prolactin release by TRH was correlated with interesting modifications in the organization of the A-Golgi stained membranes in GH$_3$ cells (7). These modifications consisted mainly of an extension of the Golgi zone and an increase in the number of small immunoreactive vesicles dispersed in the cytoplasm and beneath the plasma membrane. Some of these vesicles were observed fusing with the plasma membrane. These modifications induced by TRH treatment are in favor of an increas-

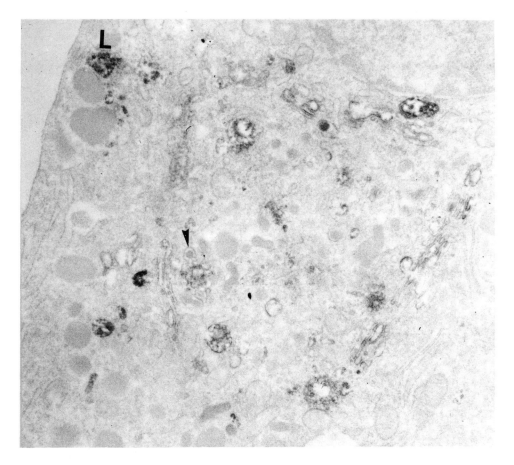

Fig. 2. A normal prolactin cell was immunostained with A-Golgi antibodies. The reaction product was observed on Golgi saccules mostly located in a medial position. The membrane of secretory granules was unstained. However, inside the Golgi zone a slight deposit was seen on the membrane of segregating secretory material (arrowhead). Small vesicles located inside the Golgi zone as well as in the cytoplasm were also labeled. In addition lysosome-like structures (L) were strongly stained (X 21.000).

ed membrane flow, concomitantly to the acute stimulation of prolactin release. This interpretation is consistent with the results obtained in previous studies using other approaches (8,9).

The inhibition of basal prolactin release induced in GH_3 cells by monensin treatment was correlated previously with a storage of prolactin in large dilated vacuoles which accumulated in the disorganized Golgi zone of those cells (10). The membranes of most of these large vacuoles were stained with the A-Golgi, indicating that they derived from a Golgi subcompartment. Moreover, the A-Golgi also labeled the small vesicles which were induced by TRH even in the presence of monensin (7). This is an important observation since monensin did not prevent the TRH-induced stimulation of prolactin release (10). Thus the A-Golgi labeled both a monensin-sensitive and a monensin less sensitive smooth membrane compartment, suggesting the existence of several intracellular routes for the release of prolactin.

MEMBRANE COMPARTMENTS INVOLVED IN THE ENDOCYTIC PATHWAY

The endocytic pathway was followed in GH_3 cells using as a tracer cationized ferritin (CF). Following binding at 4 C, CF particles were found associated into clusters exclusively located at the cell surface. After transfer of the cells at 37 C, CF particles were progressively internalized. At 15 min, CF was seen on small pits and small vesicles beneath the plasma membrane. From 15 min onwards, CF was also found in large, electron lucent structures which often, but not always, resembled multivesicular bodies. From 30 min onwards they were also found in large structures which were acid phosphatase positive and thus represent secondary lysosomes. In the Golgi zone, CF was found exclusively in small vesicles.

To identify membrane compartments involved in this pathway we used two immunological probes: anti-lysosomal membrane antibodies (A-Ly-M) described above (3,4) and anti-clathrin antibodies (11).

When applied to normal prolactin cells (Fig. 3) the A-Ly-M labeled the membranes of large structures which looked like secondary lysosomes and those of some multivesicular bodies. It also labeled some saccules in the Golgi stacks as well as some vesicles. In contrast, neither the secretory granule membrane nor the plasma membrane were stained. The same localizations were found in GH_3 cells using the same technical procedure (Fig. 4) (12).

The membrane of the small pits and vesicles involved in the first steps of CF endocytosis exhibited an immunoreactive clathrin coat, but was unstained with the A-Ly-M. In contrast the membrane of the large electron lucent structures involved in the second step of CF endocytosis was lightly but significantly stained with A-Ly-M (Fig. 4). In parallel experiments these structures were found devoid of acid phosphatase activity. As could be expected the lysosome-like structures which were loaded with CF at a later stage of endocytosis were strongly stained with the A-Ly-M (12).

These observations revealed the existence in the endocytic pathway of GH_3 cells of a prelysosomal compartment which possesses on its membrane a 100 Kd antigen immunologically related to a gastric purified H^+, K^+-ATPase (3,4). Thus it might represent an acidified prelysosomal compartment, the existence of which has been recently

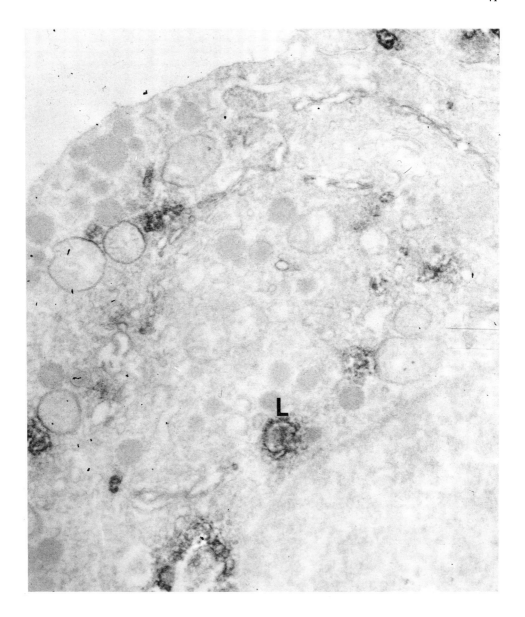

Fig. 3. A normal prolactin cell was immunostained with A-Ly-M antibodies. The membrane of lysosomes (L) was strongly labeled. The reaction product was also found on the membrane of 1 or 2 Golgi saccules, mostly located in a medial position. The membrane of small vesicles was also labeled. In contrast neither the secretory granule membrane nor the plasma membrane were stained (X 30.000).

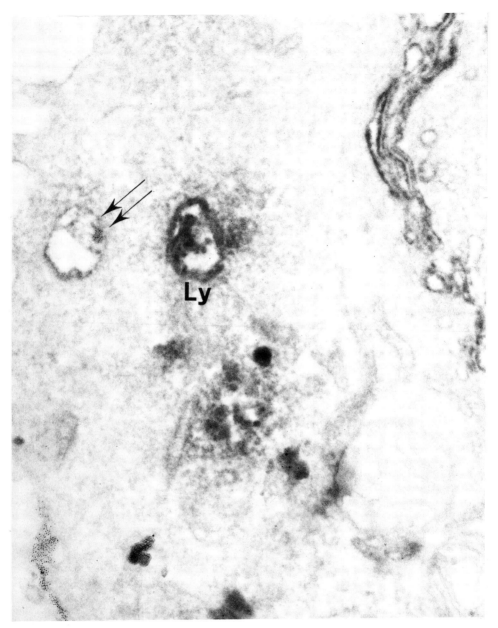

Fig. 4. A GH₃ cell has been incubated for 15 min at 37 C after binding of CF at 4 C and was then stained with A-Ly-M antibodies. CF particles are seen in some patches at the cell surface which is not stained with the A-Ly-M. Inside the cells CF clusters are seen associated with the membrane of a large electron lucent structure (endosome? or nascent multivesicular body?) which is stained with the A-Ly-M (double arrows). In addition the A-Ly-M also stained other structures which do not contain CF: lysosomes (Ly) and in the Golgi zone several saccules in a medial position as well as some vesicles (X 60.000).

shown in several cell types using various approaches (13,14). The absence of the 100 Kd antigen on the membrane of the small pits and vesicles involved in the first step of CF internalization is a matter of speculation. Further studies using other experimental conditions are needed to clarify that point. This is however a minor point as compared to the strong evidence for the existence of an acidified prelysosomal compartment in GH$_3$ cells. This may have important functional implications in view of the numerous ligands which interact with its plasma membrane to regulate prolactin secretion.

CONCLUSION

Using various immunological probes which were previously shown to have a narrow specificity for defined membrane components we have shown an immunological specificity of membrane compartments involved in the two most important routes of intracellular membrane traffic in prolactin cells: the biosynthetic pathway and the endocytic pathway. In both cases a very subtle subcompartmentalization of membranes has been revealed.

As concerns the biosynthetic pathway, the most interesting and original findings were obtained with the A-Golgi which recognized one membrane polypeptide (135 Kd) of rat liver Golgi apparatus and which stained most Golgi membranes in normal rabbit kidney (NRK) cells (2). In prolactin cells these antibodies recognized only a subcompartment of the Golgi saccules as well as small vesicles. In contrast, they did not recognize the secretory granule membrane, a very interesting negative finding which suggests a change in membrane composition or conformation, at an early step of the packaging of secretory material. Another important aspect of the usefulness of the ''Golgi probe'' concerns its application to the analysis of membrane flow in relation with an alteration of the secretory activity, either a stimulation by TRH, or a blockade by monensin (7).

As concerns the endocytic pathway, the A-Ly-M which is specific to a 100 Kd polypeptide of the lysosomal membrane allowed us to show the existence in prolactin cells of a prelysosomal compartment which may be similar to the acidified prelysosomal compartment recently identified in other cell types. Further studies are needed to explore the functional meaning of this compartment by using other ligands, more physiological than CF, to follow the endocytic pathway. Of great interest also is the presence of the 100 Kd lysosome polypeptide in structures which possess the 135 Kd Golgi polypeptide, such as the lysosome membrane and most probably some Golgi saccules, whereas this polypeptide is absent on secretory granule membranes. This illustrates directly the role of the Golgi zone in the sorting out of membrane components.

For the future the use of immunological probes to analyze membrane traffic opens the possibility of analyzing the molecular mechanisms involved in the sorting and the direction of membrane components and secretory products in prolactin cells.

ACKNOWLEDGMENTS

We acknowledge the excellent technical assistance of Mrs. E. Rosenbaum, Miss A. Bayon, and Mr. C. Pennarun. This work was supported by grants from the Centre

National de la Recherche Scientifique (E.R. 89 and ATP "Pharmacologie des Recepteurs des Neuromediateurs").

REFERENCES

1. Farquhar MG. (1963) In: *Methods in Enzymology: Biomembranes*, Part L, *Membrane Biogenesis: Processing and Recycling*, vol 98:1
2. Louvard D, Reggio H, Warren G. (1982): J Cell Biol 92:92
3. Reggio H, Harms E, Bainton D, Coudrier E, Louvard D. (1982): J Cell Biol 95:413a
4. Reggio H, Bainton D, Harms E, Coudrier E, Louvard D. J Cell Biol, in press
5. Tougard C, Picart R, Tixier-Vidal A. (1980): Am J Anat 158:471
6. Tougard C, Picart R, Tixier-Vidal A. (1982): Biol Cell 43:89
7. Tougard C, Louvard D, Picart R, Tixier-Vidal A. (1983): J Cell Biol 96:1197
8. Gourdji D, Kerdelhue B, Tixier-Vidal A. (1972): C R Acad Sci 274(D):437
9. Tixier-Vidal A, Brunet N, Gourdji D. (1979) In: *Hormones and Cell Culture*. Cold Spring Harbor Conf. Cell Proliferation 6:807
10. Tougard C, Picart R, Morin A, Tixier-Vidal A. (1983): J Histochem Cytochem 31:745
11. Louvard D, Morris C, Warren G, Stanley K, Winkler F, Reggio H. (1983): EMBO J 2:1655
12. Tougard C, Louvard D, Picart R, Tixier-Vidal A. submitted
13. Tycko B, Maxfield FR. (1982): Cell 28:643
14. Galloway CJ, Dean GE, Marsh M, Rudnick G, Mellman I. (1983): Proc Natl Acad Sci USA 80:3334

Prolactin. Basic and clinical correlates
R.M. MacLeod, M.O. Thorner and U. Scapagnini (eds.),
Fidia Research Series, vol. I,
Liviana Press, Padova © 1985

Section I
The functional ultrastructure
of prolactin cells

A MONOCLONAL ANTIBODY THAT RECOGNIZES A CELL-SURFACE PROTEIN ON GH₃ CELLS

G. Kapatos, J. Massetta and J. L. Barker

Laboratory of Neurophysiology, National Institute of Neurological
and Communicative Disorders and Stroke
National Institutes of Health
Bethesda, Maryland 20205

Clonal mammalian cell lines, by virtue of their homogeneity, have promoted progress towards elucidating the biochemical bases of many biological processes. Our understanding of the molecular mechanisms involved in the regulation of peptide synthesis-secretion coupling within prolactin-containing cells of the anterior pituitary has, for example, expanded dramatically since the introduction of the GH_3 cell line (1). These prolactin and growth hormone-secreting cells derived from the rat pituitary are known to express a wide variety of membrane receptors for an assortment of hormones and neurotransmitter substances (2). GH_3 cells are also electrically excitable, exhibiting several classes of ion channel mechanisms (3). The physiological actions of these membrane macromolecules appear linked both to each other and to the metabolism of prolactin (4). The surface of GH_3 cells can thus be thought of as a homogeneous source of specialized membrane proteins that are essential for intercellular communication, and therefore common to other communicative cell types such as neurons. The same properties have led us to utilize these cells as a complex immunogen with the ultimate goal of generating a panel of monoclonal antibodies (mAb) that would bind with, identify, and possibly alter the function of specific receptor and ion channel determinants on live cells. Immunoreagents such as these would then permit investigation of the molecular biology of the target proteins within the confines of a model peptidergic cell system. To perform these initial immunological studies we have exploited the analytical power of flow cytometry, a technique that not only permits quantitative multiparametric determinations of the properties of individual living cells, but also the isolation of cell subpopulations for culture and further study.

We have utilized an *in vitro* immunization protocol to generate mAbs to the cell surface of GH_3 cells (5). The GH_3/B_6 cell line, passage number 12, was obtained from Dr. B. Dufy, Bordeaux, France. Cells were cultured under an atmosphere of 7.5%

CO_2-92.5% air in 75 cm² poly-lysine coated tissue culture flasks with bicarbonate-buffered Hams F10 medium supplemented by the addition of 15% heat inactivated horse serum, 2.5% fetal calf serum, and 50 ug/ml gentamycin. Medium was changed twice weekly. Prior to immunization a culture of these cells, grown in a 75 cm² flask to approximately 75% confluence, was fixed by the following protocol. After aspiration of culture medium, cultures were washed extensively with sterile Hanks buffered saline solution (HBSS), immersed in 4% buffered paraformaldehyde, pH 7.5, for 1 hour at room temperature, and then again washed extensively with HBSS. Dulbeccos modified Eagles medium (DMEM) was then added to the flask, which was incubated overnight at 37 C in order to scavange unreacted formaldehyde and insure freedom from contamination. To this fixed and washed culture was added a suspension of spleen cells derived from Balb/c mice. Cultures were incubated in DMEM containing 5% fetal calf serum, 2 mM L-glutamine, 1mM sodium pyruvate, 4.5 g/L D-glucose, 25 mM HEPES, 10% non-essential amino acids, 50 uM mercaptoethanol and 50% by volume allogeneic thymocyte conditioned medium generated by a 48 hour culture of Balb/c and C57bl thymocytes. Following 4-7 days in culture, spleen cells were harvested, fused at a ratio of 1:1 with SP2/0-Ag14 myeloma cells, and hybridomas selected by established techniques (6). Hybridoma supernatants were screened by an enzyme linked immunosorbent assay (ELISA) performed on GH_3 cells grown and fixed in 96 well microtest plates. From this immunization and screening protocol 23 hybridomas secreting mAbs directed against GH_3 cells were isolated. It has, however, been observed that mAbs generated against fixed antigens may not recognize the same antigen in its native configuration. We then determined by fluorescence activated cell sorting (FACS) techniques whether this panel of mAbs were also reactive with live GH_3 cells. This screening procedure entailed the following: Cultures of GH_3 cells were harvested with Versene (1:5000), and 50,000 cells in HBSS-1% bovine serum albumin (HBSS-BSA) were added to each well of a 96 well microtest plate. The plate was centrifuged and the cell pellets resuspended in undiluted hybridoma culture supernatant. Control wells received culture supernatant conditioned by the parental myeloma cell line. After incubating for 1 hour at 4 C, microplates were again centrifuged, supernatants discarded, the cell pellet washed by resuspension in HBSS-BSA followed by centrifugation and resuspension of the pellet in HBSS-BSA containing fluorescein (FITC)-labelled goat anti-mouse immunoglobulin (Ig). After 1 hour and the wash procedures described above, cells were resuspended in 0.5 ml of HBSS-BSA and analyzed on a Becton Dickinson FACS 440 equipped with a 5 watt argon-ion laser tuned to excite at 488 nm at a power output of 400 milliwatts. Details of the flow cytometric analysis will be presented later. Of the 23 hybridomas originally found to be positive by ELISA, 9 were also observed to produce fluorescence signals above background. These 9 mAbs presumably recognize cell-surface antigens present on live GH_3 cells, and meet our first requirement for investigating mAb effects on GH_3 cell function. One of these 9 hybridomas, labelled Gl, was chosen for further analysis and cloned by the method of limiting dilution. Gl was produced in ascites fluid of pristane treated Balb/c mice. The mAb was purified from ascites fluid by a combination of salt fractionation, molecular sieve chromatography, and ultrafiltration techniques. High performance liquid chromatographic analysis of this preparation indicated a Ig purity of approximately 80% at a protein concentration of 5 mg/ml. Ig chain sub-typing showed Gl mAb to be of the IgMk class.

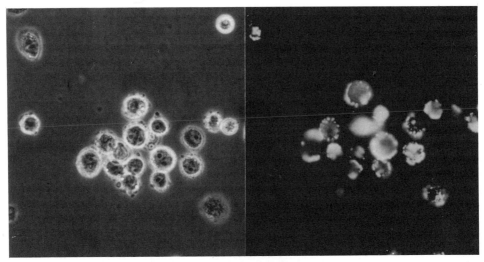

Figure 1. Phase contrast (left) and fluorescence (right) photomicrographs of the same field of live GH₃ cells reacted at 4 C with Gl and FITC-labelled secondary antibody. Cells were photographed before equilibrating to room temperature. Note the cell-surface labelling pattern, and the unlabelled cells in the upper right and left center of the field.

Immunocytochemical visualization of Gl-antigen is presented in Figure 1. The technique of indirect immunofluorescence was performed on live cultures of GH₃ cells maintained at 4 C and the identical field of cells was photographed under both phase-contrast and fluorescence optics. Note the diffuse fluorescent cell-surface labelling pattern. Comparison of the phase-contrast and fluorescence photomicrographs also indicated that not all cells were reactive for Gl. Substitution of Gl with a control mAb of the same Ig class as Gl, MOPC104E, did not produce any labelling. When cultures reacted at 4 C with Gl and secondary antibody were permitted to equilibrate to room temperature, a sequence of patching, capping, and shedding of antigen-antibody complexes could be observed. This expulsion of antigen is reminiscent of the type of ligand-receptor modulation known to occur with numerous hormone and growth-factor receptors (7).

The antigen recognized by Gl was determined by the immunoblotting technique (8). A crude membrane fraction from GH₃ cells prepared in the presence of protease inhibitors was electrophoresed under denaturing and reducing conditions (9). Proteins separated according to their apparent molecular weight (mw) were then electrically transferred to nitrocellulose, and this replica was incubated overnight with Gl. Bound Gl mAb was visualized by reaction with a peroxidase-coupled secondary antibody and peroxidase substrates. Figure 2 illustrates that Gl reacted primarily with a protein exhibiting an apparent mw of 41,000 daltons. Incubation of an identical replica with the control mAb, MOPCl04E, demonstrated that this was a specific interaction.

These flow cytometric, microscopic and biochemical observations show that Gl antigen is a cell-surface macromolecule. We decided to utilize flow cytometric techni-

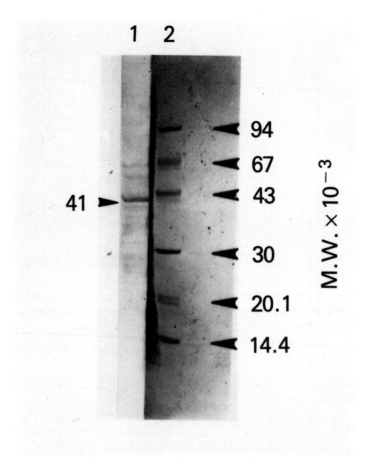

Figure 2. Gl antigen was identified by the technique of immunoblotting. Proteins were electrophoresed in SDS-polyacrylamide with the discontinuous buffer system of Laemmli (9) and then transferred to the nitrocellulose membrane shown here (8). Lane 1 contained a crude membrane fraction prepared from GH_3 cells and was reacted with Gl, peroxidase-labelled secondary antibody and peroxidase substrates. Lane 2 received protein standards and was stained with Amido Black. Note that Gl reacted primarily with a protein exhibiting an apparent molecular weight of 41,000.

ques in an attempt to characterize the biological properties of the cell-bound antigen in the hope of ultimately elucidating its function. Before these analyses were undertaken, however, we first established optimum Gl mAb and FITC-labelled secondary antibody dilutions necessary for specifically labelling live GH_3 cells in suspension for FACS analysis.

Sterile conditions were maintained in preparing GH_3 cells for flow cytometry and sorting. Confluent cultures were treated with Versene, and the cells suspended by agitation. Cell viability, determined with a hemocytometer and trypan blue exclusion, averag-

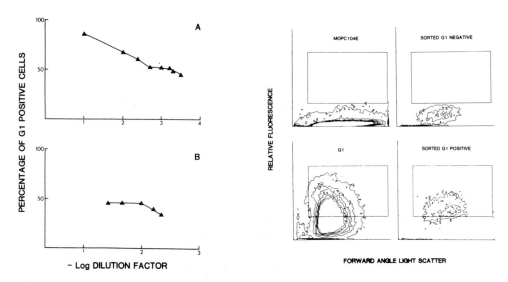

Figure 3. Gl mAb and secondary antibody titration curves were determined by flow cytométry. Data from 50,000 cells were analyzed to determine the percentage of cells positive for Gl at each respective antibody dilution. Dilutions are presented in negative logarithmic form. In 3A, suspensions of cells were reacted with dilutions of Gl ranging from 1/10 to 1/3000. All cells were then incubated with a 1/50 dilution of FITC-labelled secondary antibody. In 3B, cells previously reacted with a 1/500 dilution of Gl were incubated with dilutions of FITC-labelled secondary antibody ranging from 1/25 to 1/250.

Figure 4. Flow cytometric analyses and sorting of GH$_3$ cells. Cells reacted with Gl and FITC-labelled secondary antibody were analyzed for forward angle light scatter and fluorescent intensity. Data from 50,000 cells are presented as dual parameter contour maps. On the left, note the increased fluorescence relative to MOPC104E of cells incubated with Gl. The rectangle in each figure represents the Gl positive sorting gate window. Reanalysis of sorted Gl positive and negative cells is displayed on the right. Note that only Gl positive sorted cells fall within the sort window, and show that there is essentially no overlap between sorted populations.

ed 80%. Cells were harvested by centrifugation, resuspended in HBSS-BSA at concentration of 1 million cells/ml and incubated at 4 C with dilutions of Gl ranging from 1/10 to 1/3000. Cells were then pelleted, washed extensively, and reacted with a 1/50 dilution of an FITC-labelled f(ab')2 fragment of goat anti-mouse Ig which was IgM specific. After pelleting and washing, cells were filtered and the number positive for Gl at each mAb dilution determined by flow cytometry. Fifty thousand cells were analyzed at each mAb dilution. Figure 3A displays the percentage of cells positive for Gl as a function of the mAb dilution factor. The number of immunoreactive cells was found to reach a plateau at mAb dilutions between 1/1500 and 1/500. We interpret this as indicating that all binding sites have been occupied. In contrast, dilutions of 1/2000 or greater did not appear to complex all G1 antigen. The percentage of G1-positive cells began to increase linearly at dilutions less than 1/250. We interpret the binding on this portion of the dilution curve to be nonspecific. The dilution of FITC-labelled secondary antibody required to saturate maximal Gl mAb binding is displayed in Figure 3B. Cells incubated with a saturating concentration of Gl (1/1000) were reacted with dilutions of secondary antibody ranging from 1/25 to 1/250, and then analyzed by flow cytometry. Optimum quantitation of bound mAb was found to require a dilution of secondary antibody of no greater than 1/100. All further flow cytometric analyses were therefore performed at a cell density of 1 million/ml, a 1/1000 dilution of Gl, and a 1/50 dilution of FITC-labelled secondary antibody.

Actual flow cytometric data of GH_3 cells reacted with Gl or control mAb are presented in Figure 4. Data are displayed as dual parameter contour maps. Forward angle light scatter (FALS) an indication of cell size, is plotted on the abscissa. Fluorescence intensity (FI), a value proportional to the number of antibody molecules bound and therefore proportional to the amount of antigen found on the cell surface, is plotted on the ordinate. Contour levels indicate cell frequencies, and are equally spaced. Cell suspensions incubated with MOPC104E and FITC-labelled secondary antibody, or secondary antibody alone, exhibited a single broad peak of FALS indicating that GH_3 cells in suspension vary appreciably in size and/or shape. Nevertheless, cellular FI was relatively constant across the distribution of FALS. A dramatic increase in the number of cells displaying FI above control levels became apparent, however, when the suspension was incubated with Gl. In this experiment approximately 70% of the cells were reactive for Gl, and labelling was relatively constant across the FALS parameter. Under these conditions Gl positive and negative cells could be routinely separated by FACS as long as precautions were taken to maintain the starting cell suspension at 4 C during the entire staining and cell sorting procedure. A typical Gl positive gate window for sorting is shown as a rectangle in figure 4. A Gl negative gate window encompassed all cells exhibiting a FI identical to the MOPCl04E condition. Reanalysis of these two sorted populations by flow cytometry is also shown in Figure 4. Here it can be observed that the sorted populations do not overlap in the FI dimension but display identical FALS, and that the positive population falls primarily within the designated gate window. Cell purities greater than 95% were typical. This level of purity was independently confirmed by fluorescence microscopy and cell counting.

Our ability to isolate Gl positive and Gl negative cells for growth in culture permitted us to address the question of whether these two cell populations are phenotypically distinct with respect to Gl antigen expression, or whether, for example, they differ only with regard to cell life cycle. If the former were correct, the question of what function, if any, the Gl antigen might play in cellular homeostasis might be more easily addressed. The following experiment was performed. Gl positive and negative cells were isolated by FACS and grown in culture. Upon reaching confluency these cultures were again put in suspension and reacted with Gl followed by analysis and sorting. The results from this experiment indicated that the ratio of Gl positive to Gl negative cells was essentially identical in both sorted populations, and equivalent to the starting material. When these previously sorted Gl positive and Gl negative cells were again sorted, grown in culture to confluency, and analyzed for Gl expression, the same data were obtained. This experiment indicated that Gl antigen was not, therefore, expressed by a phenotypically distinct population of GH_3 cells, but was related to some other aspect of cellular development.

Further characterization of the Gl antigen involved manipulations known to modify cell-surface macromolecular structure. Two conditions were chosen for these experiments: 1) Protease or glycosidase treatments were carried out to remove cell-surface proteins and sialic acid residues, respectively. To perform the former, cells were incubated with 0.1% trypsin at 37 C for 30 mintues prior to termination of the reaction by the addition of a two-fold molar excess of soybean trypsin inhibitor. 2) Alternatively, cells were incubated with 50 IU of neuraminidase from Vibrio cholerae in the presence of soybean trypsin inhibitor. Following either of these manipulations cells were reacted with MOPC104E or Gl and then FITC-labelled secondary antibody. Neither of these treatments altered the pattern of FALS or FI typically associated with MOPC104E. Figure 5 illustrates the effect of these treatments on indirect immunofluorescent detection of Gl antigen. Again, flow cytometric data are presented as dual parameter contour maps. Mild proteolysis of the cell-surface produced a level of cellular FI identical with MOPC104E, completely eliminating Gl labelling. This indicates that Gl antigen is a protein, a conclusion supported by the biochemical evidence exhibited in Figure 2. In contrast, the treatment of cells with neuraminidase prior to Gl staining increased the number of cells positive for Gl. This effect occurred without increasing the overall cellular level of FI. The number of binding sites on cells already positive for the an-

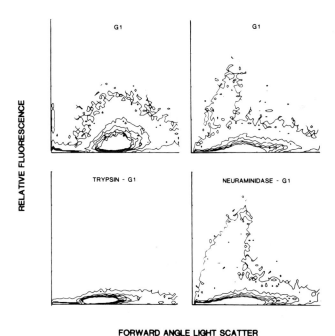

Figure 5. Flow cytometric analyses of the effects of protease and glycosidase treatment on Gl labelling. Data from 50,000 cells are presented as dual parameter contour maps. Two separate experiments are shown. On the left, mild trypsinization completely eliminated Gl staining. On the right, neuraminidase treatment significantly increased the number of cells positive for Gl.

tigen was therefore not increased. This indicates that the removal of sialic acid residues by neuraminidase treatment may serve to unmask Gl antigenic sites, but only on cells that were negative for antigen prior to enzyme treatment.

In summary, our results show that we have successfully produced a panel of mAbs, by an *in vitro* immunization protocol, which react with antigens on the surface of live GH_3 cells. One of these mAbs, labelled Gl, recognizes a glycoprotein of 41,000 mw which upon crosslinking by antibody is shed from the cell. This antigen is not present on the surface of all GH_3 cells. The percentage of positive cells in cultures grown to different states of confluency or from different passage numbers ranged anywhere from 40 to 70%. Gl antigen was not expressed as a cellular phenotype but appeared related to some other aspect of cell function. Further characterization of the antigen indicated that at any one time there may actually be three populations of cells present in confluent cultures: a predominant cell type which expresses Gl antigen in a state normally accessible to the mAb, a second on which the antigen is masked by cleavable sialic acid residues, and a third where antigen is either present but cannot be unmasked by removal of carbohydrate or where no antigen is expressed at all. Work in progress will hopefully determine whether the presence of Gl antigen on the cell-surface is indeed related to differences in membrane composition during the cell cycle. Future research will also concentrate on elucidating the function, if any, that the Gl antigen may play in GH_3 cell physiology, with particular emphasis being placed on peptide content and secretion. Our task will certainly be made easier by the ability to isolate by flow cytometry preparative amounts of pure populations Gl positive and Gl negative cells for immediate characterization.

REFERENCES

1. Tashjian AH Jr, Yasumura Y, Levine L, Sato GH, Parker ML. (1968): Endocrinology 82:342
2. Dannies PS, Tashjian AH. (1973): J Biol Chem 248:6174
3. Dufy B, Barker JL. (1982): Life Sci 30:1933
4. Kaczoroski GJ, Vandlen RL, Katz GM, Reuben JP. (1983) J Membr Biol 71:109
5. Click RE, Benck L, Alter BJ. (1972): Cell Immun 3:264
6. Kohler G, Milstein C. (1975): Nature, Lond 256:495
7. Pastan JH, Willingham MC. (1981): Science 214:504
8. Towbin H, Staehelin T, Gordon J. (1979): Proc Natl Acad Sci USA 76:4350
9. Laemmli UK. (1970): Nature 227:680

Prolactin. Basic and clinical correlates
R.M. MacLeod, M.O. Thorner and U. Scapagnini (eds.),
Fidia Research Series, vol. I,
Liviana Press, Padova © 1985

Section I
The functional ultrastructure
of prolactin cells

PARACRINE INTERACTION IN ANTERIOR PITUITARY

Carl Denef

Laboratory of Cell Pharmacology, Department of Pharmacology,
University of Leuven, School of Medicine, Campus Gasthuisberg,
B-3000 Leuven, Belgium

Intercellular communication is regarded as a fundamental mechanism of integrated responses in endocrine tissues (1-4). Although experimental data are still fragmentary, there is growing evidence that one cell type may influence neighboring cells by the release of paracrine factors. Recently we have presented evidence that such factors might also exist in rat anterior pituitary (5-7). A functional interaction was demonstrated between gonadotrophs and lactotrophs and gonadotrophs were found capable of secreting a factor with prolactin releasing activity. These data support the concept that the different pituitary cell types do not behave as individually functioning units responding to hypothalamic and peripheral hormonal inputs but that they are organized in a highly integrated circuit of humoral factors in the microenvironment. It is likely that paracrine factors act as rapid and ultra-short loop feedback signals thereby providing a refined control of local homeostasis in the tissue.

The present paper further illustrates these viewpoints in the light of new findings. As before, the biotechnology used was superfused reaggregate cell culture (7,8).

GONADOTROPHS STIMULATED BY LHRH CAN TRANSMIT A SIGNAL TO THE LACTOTROPHS ELICITING PROLACTIN RELEASE

In superfused pituitary cell aggregates consisting of an enriched population of lactotrophs and gonadotrophs obtained by gradient sedimentation at unit gravity, the decapeptide LHRH stimulates not only LH and FSH release but also basal as well as dopamine-inhibited prolactin release. The peptide shows activity from a concentration as low as .01 nM. The extent of stimulation increases with the proportional number of gonadotrophs in the co-culture (1-35%) whereas no stimulation of prolactin release occurs in a lactotroph-enriched population in which only small gonadotrophs in a proportion of less than 1% are demonstrable by immunocytochemical methods.

The gonadotroph-mediated prolactin response to LHRH is a phenomenon only occuring under certain conditions. It has been seen in all experiments run so far with aggregates from 14-day-old female rat pituitary after 4 days in culture. In contrast, in pituitary cell aggregates from adult female or male rats, no such response is detectable after 4 days in culture. A prolactin response to LHRH does, however, occur at 12 days in culture or at 4 days when a lactotroph-rich population from the adult is co-cultured with gonadotrophs from the 14-day-old female. Since no differences in the aggregation process and ultrastructural quality can be detected between the different aggregate preparations, these data suggest that gonadotrophs from 14-day-old rats are in a different functional state than those of the adult and that the latter may acquire such a state after a more prolonged time in culture.

The prolactin response to LHRH is seen when aggregates are cultured in serum-supplemented as well as in chemically defined (8) serum-free medium (unpublished observations). The addition of testosterone (0.1-100 nM), estradiol (0.01-1 nM) or 5 alpha-dihydrotestosterone (1-100 nM) to the culture medium for 10 days strongly inhibits the prolactin response to LHRH, the order of potency being testosterone > estradiol > 5 alpha-dihydrotestosterone. The response is slightly inhibited when T_3 (0.5-5 nM) or dexamethasone is added to the culture medium (unpublished data). Thus, it appears that a more physiological environment (presence of steroid and thyroid hormones) decreases and may eventually suppress the LHRH-stimulated gonadotroph-lactotroph interaction.

GONADOTROPHS CAN RELEASE A SUBSTANCE WITH PROLACTIN RELEASING ACTIVITY

Medium conditioned by aggregrates prepared from a highly enriched population of large gonadotrophs (70-75% pure) also stimulates prolactin release, suggesting that gonadotrophs are capable of secreting a humoral substance with prolactin releasing activity. Although there is no direct proof yet that the prolactin secretion elicited by LHRH in gonadotroph-lactotroph co-cultures is mediated through the same factor releasable from gonadotrophs incubated as a relatively pure population, the experimental data at least provide evidence that paracrine interaction in the anterior pituitary is plausible.

The nature of the humoral factor(s) involved remains unknown. LH, FSH, prolactin, or LHRH itself can be excluded, however, as candidates. Preliminary evidence obtained from ultrafiltration experiments indicates the molecular weight is below 10,000 (unpublished observations).

CULTURED GONADOTROPH-RICH AGGREGATES CONTAIN ANGIOTENSIN I-LIKE IMMUNOREACTIVITY (AI-LI)

Gonadotrophs in situ have been shown to contain substance P (9), ACTH (10), enkephalins (11,12), TRH (12), and angiotensin-II (14). Some of these peptides may originate from internalization (15) but angiotensin may be synthesized by the gonadotroph as renin-LI also has been found in this cell type (16). Using a specific anti-AI antiserum (17) we have found substantial amounts of AI-LI in 1 M acetic acid extracts of gonadotroph-rich aggregates cultured either in serum-supplemented or in serum-free chemically-defined medium for up to 30 days (Schramme, Lijnen, and Denef, unpublished). The amount ranges from 8 to 39 pg/100 ug protein. AI-LI is also present in lactotroph-enriched/gonadotroph-poor aggregates but ranges only between 2 and 12 pg/100 ug protein. Using a specific antiserum against AII (18), AII-LI is also detectable but in much smaller amounts (2 - 7 pg and 0.5 - 3 pg/100 ug protein in gonadotroph-rich and lactotroph-rich aggregates respectively).

AI IS A POTENT STIMULATOR OF PROLACTIN RELEASE FOLLOWING CONVERSION TO AII

AII has been shown to stimulate prolactin release in monolayer cultures (19) as well as in superfused anterior pituitary cell aggregates (20,21). The response is concentration-dependent between 0.1 - 10 nM and stimulation can be blocked by saralasin, an AII receptor antagonist. In more recent experiments we have found that concentrations as low as .01 nM AII are also slightly stimulatory. Subnanomolar concentrations of AII are also effective in stimulating prolactin release in the presence of a strongly inhibitory concentration of dopamine (10 nM).

Prolactin release is also stimulated by AI, the activity of the peptide being comparable to that of AII. However, 1 uM of two competitive angiotensin converting enzyme (ACE) inhibitors, captopril and teprotide, inhibit the effect of 0.1 nM AI completely and inhibit by 60 percent that of 1 nM AI, indicating that the activity of AI arises from prior conversion to AII. This conversion appears to occur at a very fast rate since AI stimulates prolactin release with potency, intrinsic activity, and rate of response comparable to that of AII. Thus, ACE activity seems to be very high in our reaggregate culture. This is not surprising since it has been demonstrated that the anterior pituitary has considerable ACE activity *in vivo* (22).

EVIDENCE FOR MODULATION OF AII ACTION BY "HELPER" AND "SUPPRESSOR" GONADOTROPHS

Aguilera et al. (19) showed that specific binding sites for AII are most probably located on lactotrophs since the highest density of these binding sites was found in lactotroph-rich populations separated by centrifugal elutriation (19). Thus, there is evidence that the prolactin response to AII is brought about by a direct action of AII on lactotrophs. However, we have found that the efficacy of AII in different pituitary cell populations separated by gradient sedimentation at unit gravity (23), and established in culture as reaggregates, differs widely and is not highest in the lactotroph-enriched populations (7). Using preparations from adult male rats, the magnitude of the prolactin response to AII increases with the proportion of gonadotrophs in the different populations whereas no correlation is found with the distribution of lactotrophs, thyrotrophs, corticotrophs, or somatotrophs (7). Thus, either the prolactin cells are functionally heterogeneous or the gonadotrophs may be considered "helper" cells, potentiating the prolactin response to AII. Evidence that gonadotrophs are directly involved in enhancing the AII effect has been obtained from co-culture experiments. When cells from the gonadotroph-richest population (70% gonadotrophs) are mixed with those of a lactotroph-enriched population virtually devoid of gonadotrophs and co-cultured as reaggregates, the prolactin response increases significantly (7). Thus, the stimulatory effect of AII in a gonadotroph-free population can be enhanced by adding gonadotrophs.

We have also studied the effect of AII in similarly separated cell populations from 14-day-old female rats. In this animal model the proportion of gonadotrophs in the pituitary is considerably higher than in the adult (5). This proportional number increases steadily from top to bottom of the sedimentation gradient but reaches much higher values than in the corresponding gradient fractions from adult rats. In such a unit gravity sedimentation gradient the prolactin response to 0.1 nM AII increases with the proportion of gonadotrophs. Most surprisingly, however, the response to 10 nM AII becomes weaker in the most enriched fraction containing all the largest gonadotrophs. We interpret these findings by advancing the hypothesis that gonadotrophs can potentiate the response of lactotrophs to AII but that they may also engage in inhibitory interactions. Up to a certain proportion of these cells, stimulation would prevail but when they are present in higher numbers stimulation would gradually be overruled by inhibition. If this hypothesis is correct, a higher concentration of AII would be expected also to favor the inhibitory interaction and this is indeed found. In order to confirm the latter hypothesis co-culture experiments have been performed. The population with the lowest responsiveness to AII becomes more responsive when it is mixed with a small number of large gonadotrophs taken from the gonadotroph-richest population. A final proportional number as low as 1 - 5% of these large gonadotrophs is effective (7). This potentiating effect, however, fades when the proportion of gonadotrophs in the co-culture is raised to 15% (7). Thus, the latter findings support the hypothesis that gonadotrophs - especially the large gonadotrophs - are capable of functioning as ''helper'' as well as ''suppressor'' cells of the lactotrophs' responsiveness to AII.

To further test the hypothesis, cells from the gonadotroph-richest population were mixed and co-cultured with the gonadotroph-deprived population and exposed to low and high concentrations of AII. When exposed to 0.1 nM AII the prolactin response is somewhat more pronounced in the co-culture condition, but when exposed to 10 nM AII the prolactin response is considerably lower in the co-culture situation (unpublished results).

PROPOSED ROLE FOR ANGIOTENSIN

Angiotensin-like immunoreactivity has been shown in the gonadotrophs and lactotrophs (14), and we have consistently found pg amounts of AI immunoreactivity in acid extracts of reaggregate cell cultures from a highly enriched population of gonadotrophs using a highly selective AI antiserum. If this material is released by appropriate stimuli in the close vicinity of lactotrophs there may be an effective response even with minute amounts of the peptide. Thus, the present findings are consistent with the hypothesis that angiotensin may have a local regulatory role in the pituitary.

Moreover, AII does not seem to behave as a classical releasing factor as it is capable of amplifying as well as blunting its own action presumably through a gonadotroph-lactotroph cell-to-cell communication mechanism. In preliminary experiments we have found evidence that the "helper" and "suppressor" activity of these cells is mediated by the release of humoral factor(s). When AII is superfused in medium previously conditioned for 1 h with the gonadotroph-rich aggregates, the prolactin response enhances severalfold. These data indicate that AII may not only be involved in paracrine actions on its own but also in controlling the release of other presumptive autocrine or paracrine agents.

ACKNOWLEDGMENTS

The excellent technical assistance of R. Dewals, A. De Wolf and M.J. Vanderheyden and secretarial work of M. Bareau are gratefully acknowledged. The authors are grateful to the U.S. National Hormone and Pituitary Program and the National Institute of Arthritis, Diabetes and Digestive and Kidney Diseases and Dr. A.F. Parlow for providing rat prolactin RIA kits.

This work was supported by grants from "Geconcerteerde Onderzoeksakties," F.G.W.O. and Queen Elisabeth Medical Foundation.

REFERENCES

1. Fletcher WH, Anderson NC Jr, Everett JW. (1975): J Cell Biol 67:469
2. Guillemin R. (1981) In: *Intragonadal Regulation of Reproduction*. Academic Press, New York, p 1
3. Hsueh AJW, Jones PB. (1983) Ann Rev Physiol 45:83
4. Kirsch TM, Vogel RL, Flickinger GL. (1983) Endocrinology 113:1910
5. Denef C, Andries M. (1983): Endocrinology 112:813
6. Denef C. In: Proceedings of the 3rd European Workshop on Pituitary Adenomas. Blackwell Scientific, London, in press
7. Denef C. (1984): Hormone Res, in press
8. Denef C, Baes M, Schramme C. (1984): Endocrinology 114:1371
9. Morel G, Chayvialle JA, Kerdelhue B, Dubois PM. (1982): Neuroendocrinology 35:86
10. Childs GV (Moriarty), Ellison DG, Ramaley JA. (1982): Endocrinology 110:1676
11. Braas KM, Wilber JF, Childs GV. (1980): J Cell Biol 87:173a
12. Childs GV (Moriarty), Ellison DG, Foster L, Ramaley JA. (1981): Endocrinology 109:1683
13. Childs GV (Moriarty), Cole DE, Kubek M, Tobin RB, Wilber JF. (1978): J Histochem Cytochem 26:901
14. Steele MK, Brownfield MS, Ganong WF. (1982): Neuroendocrinology 35:155
15. De Palatis LR, Khorram O, Ho RH, Negro-Vilar A, McCann SM. (1984): Life Sci 34:225
16. Naruse K, Takii Y, Inagami T. (1981): Proc Natl Acad Sci USA 78:7579
17. Lijnen PJ, Amery AK, Fagard RH. (1978): J Lab Clin Med 92:35
18. Steele MK, Negro-Vilar A, McCann SM. (1981): Endocrinology 109:893
19. Aguilera G, Hyde CL, Catt KJ. (1982): Endocrinology 111:1045
20. Schramme C, Denef C. (1983): Neuroendocrinology 36:483
21. Schramme C, Denef C. (1984): Life Sci 34:1651
22. Saavadra JM, Fernandez-Pardal J, Chevillard C. (1982): Brain Res 245:317
23. Denef C, Swennen L, Andries M. (1982): Int Rev Cytol 76:225

Prolactin. Basic and clinical correlates
R.M. MacLeod, M.O. Thorner and U. Scapagnini (eds.),
Fidia Research Series, vol. I,
Liviana Press, Padova © 1985

Section II
Influence of brain factors
on prolactin secretion

INFLUENCE OF BRAIN FACTORS ON PROLACTIN SECRETION: AN OVERVIEW

Yuzuru Kato

Second Medical Clinic, Department of Medicine, Kyoto University
Faculty of Medicine, Sakyo-ku, Kyoto 606, Japan

The hypothalamic regulation of prolactin secretion has been one of the most interesting areas of prolactin research. The secretion of prolactin from the anterior pituitary is tonically inhibited by a hypothalamic inhibitory factor (PIF). Numerous studies have substantiated the role of dopamine as PIF. Prolactin release from the pituitary is also stimulated by a hypothalamic prolactin releasing factor (PRF). Some candidates for PRF have been proposed, including thyrotropin releasing hormone (TRH), vasoactive intestinal peptide (VIP), and peptide histidine isoleucine (PHI). Various neurotransmitters in the brain are also involved in the final common pathway for regulating PIF and PRF release from the hypothalamus.

As discussed in detail in this section, our understanding of the hypothalamic mechanisms involved in the neuroendocrine control of prolactin secretion during various physiological states has been further advanced. Kordon et al. classified the mode of actions of hypothalamic signals involved in the neural control of prolactin secretion into three groups. The first group of neurohormones acts at a specific site on the pituitary cells to stimulate or inhibit the secretion of hormones. The second group acts by selectively uncoupling receptors of PRF or PIF from secretory processes. The third group acts at the hypothalamic level by presynaptic modulation of the release of neurohormones into the hypophysial portal system. Multiple anatomical and pharmacological interactions within the hypothalamic neuronal network may indicate that the regulation of prolactin release can be viewed as a coded pleiotropic communication system.

VIP is supposed to play a physiological role as a PRF. Shimatsu et al. clearly showed that prolactin secretion induced by serotonergic stimulation in the brain is mediated, at least in part, by hypothalamic VIP release into the hypophysial portal blood in the rat.

Shin et al. found that intravenous injection of neurophysin II increased plasma prolactin concentration in estradiol primed male rats and proposed neurophysin II as a PRF. However, the direct action of neurophysin on the pituitary gland was not obtained in the rat with pituitary grafts in the kidney. PHI can stimulate prolactin release from the pituitary cells *in vivo* and *in vitro* in the normal male rats, suggesting a more probable role as a PRF (Ohta et al.).

Certain neuropeptides in the hypothalamus may inhibit prolactin secretion. Khorram et al. reported that endogenous alpha-MSH of central origin had an inhibitory role in the release of prolactin in the rat. Kabayama et al. have shown that gastrin releasing peptide (GRP), a new member of the gut-brain peptides, inhibits prolactin secretion possibly by stimulating the release of dopamine from the hypothalamus into the hypophysial portal blood in the rat. Orstead et al. have reported that stalk-median eminence extracts from female hamsters contain specific prolactin synthesis-inhibiting factor (PSIF), which is regulated by the pineal gland.

Prolactin. Basic and clinical correlates
R.M. MacLeod, M.O. Thorner and U. Scapagnini (eds.),
Fidia Research Series, vol. I,
Liviana Press, Padova © 1985

Section II
Influence of brain factors
on prolactin secretion

NEURAL CONTROL OF PROLACTIN SECRETION

Claude Kordon, Dolores Wandscheer, Christine Shu, Daniel Rotten, Sophia V. Drouva, Alain Enjalbert, Jacques Epelbaum, Joel Bockaert, and Hubert Clauser.

Unité 159 de Neuroendocrinologie de l'INSERM, 75014 Paris, France.

The recent discovery of several hitherto unsuspected factors able to affect prolactin secretion, *in vivo* as well as *in vitro*, calls for a reappraisal of our view on prolactin regulation; the original concept of a simple balance between releasing and inhibiting factors is no longer adequate. This raises two major issues which will be dealt with in the present minireview: How are so many signals integrated at the membrane level? What can be said about their physiological relevance?

HYPOTHALAMIC CONTROL OF PROLACTIN: A PLEIOTROPIC NEURONAL NETWORK

Hypothalamic structures concerned with neuroendocrine control were originally assumed to exhibit a relatively simple wiring pattern: a final common neural pathway, made of neurosecretory axons projecting to the median eminence, is driven by a cascade of afferent neurons wired in series. Neurotransmitters were thus assumed to be sequentially involved in the processing of neuroendocrine information. For instance, in certain experimental designs, opiate effects on prolactin were presented as the consequence of initial changes in 5-HT turnover rates, which, in turn, could monitor dopamine release (1).

In fact, as in most other CNS structures, neuronal connections within the hypothalamus are more complex. Tuberoinfundibular neurons send numerous collaterals to at least 5 different structures (median eminence and neurohypophysis, septum, preoptic area, amygdala, striatum), as documented by lesion experiments or electrophysiological mapping methods (2). Extrahypothalamic (nigrostriatal, mesencephalic) neurons can also send collaterals both to neurosecretory cell bodies and to the median eminence (3). The system is thus organized as a network rather than as converging afferent circuits. This allows a very large number of reciprocal interactions to occur both at the perikaryal and the presynaptic levels of the neuronal elements of the network.

Several such interactions have been characterized *in vitro*. To mention only those which concern prolactin control, opiates have been shown to block stimulus secretion coupling of somatostatin (4) and TRH (5); VIP affects somatostatin release (6) and 5-HT, VIP release (7). These actions are likely to involve axo-axonal contacts, a concept now widely accepted although no conventional post-synaptic morphological differentiation has been found so far on hypothalamic axons. Other presynaptic interactions are strongly suggested by turnover studies (opiate influences on dopamine turnover, for instance) (8).

Changes in neurohormonal control levels, whether induced by sensory or somesthetic reflexes or by feed-back regulation, are thus unlikely to involve only one of the many neural signals recognized by the prolactin cell. At any given time, rather, pituitary responses are controlled by multiple simultaneous changes in the neurohumoral (and humoral) environment of the cell. Most factors participating in this environment are not selective of the prolactin cells, but are also affecting other pituitary cell types (examples: thyrotrophs, lactotrophs, and somatotrophs are targets for TRH and somatostatin; thyrotrophs and lactotrophs are targets for dopamine). In that sense, they are pleiotropic, which means that they signal several functions at the same time. Only combined elements of full messages are target selective: selectivity does not rely simply on concentration changes of a given neurohormone, but on multiple fluctuations of all factors involved. The pattern of factor combinations can thus be looked at as a coding system.

INTEGRATIVE AND COUPLING MECHANISMS ON THE PITUITARY CELL

The complexity of hypothalamic neuronal networks is thus matched by a diversity of neural signals able to affect pituitary cells. The prolactin cell is a particularly good example of this, since at least twelve different substances have been shown to affect it directly *in vitro*. For most of them, corresponding specific, saturable binding sites have been identified (Table I). Although binding is usually performed on heterogeneous adenohypophyseal membrane fractions, studies using cells purified by unit gravity sedimentation methods (Fig. 1A) show that some ligands can be selectively recognized by certain cell types. For instance, binding of [³H]-spiperone, a dopaminergic ligand, appears coincident with the sedimentation profile of prolactin cells (and possibly, at the bottom of the gradient, with that of thyrotrophs), whereas binding of LHRH is correlated with heavier fractions (Fig. 1B).

How are signals decoded and integrated by the cell into a consistent message? So far, two major coupling systems have been identified, either of which can be triggered by binding of neurohormones to separate receptors.

Adenylate cyclase coupling

A few receptors have been clearly shown to enhance production of cyclic nucleotides. Available evidence relies on direct measurement of enzyme activation or of cAMP accumulation, on the fact that series of agonist or antagonist analogs of a neurohormone exhibit superimposable potency ratios on binding, cyclase, and secre-

Table I - *Type, level and mode of action of transmitters and neurohormones on PRL secretion*

TRANSMITTER OR HORMONE	IN VIVO EFFECT on PRL	IN VIVO EFFECT on ME release	on pituitary cells	BINDING SITES on homogenates	on PRL cells	MAJOR RECEPTOR COUPLING	REFERENCES
Benzodiazepines	↘		↘¹	+			39
Bombesin	↗		↗		+		40,41
Dopamine	↘		↘	+	+	AC	9,10
GABA	↘ & ↗	↘ DA	↘	+		Cl?	42-47
Neurotensin	↗		↗				48,49
Opiates	↗	↘ DA ↘ SRIF ↘ TRH	↗²			Ga?	4,5 8,50
Serotonin	↗	↗ VIP	O				7,34
Somatostatin	↘		↘³	+		AC	13,14,51,52
TRH	↗		↗	+	+	PL	21,53-55
VIP	↗	↘ SRIF	↗		+	AC	6,12,56,57

¹ Through potentiation of GABA;
² through blunting of DA inhibition;
³ through blunting of TRH of VIP stimulation. AC, adenylate cyclase; Cl, chlorine channels (inferred from other tissues); GABA, GTPase (inferred from other tissues); ME, median eminence; PL, phospholipases; VIP, vasoactive intestinal peptide.

tion (9, 10) (Fig. 2), and on the dependency of binding towards GTP or analogs of the guanyl nucleotide (Fig. 3), a recognized property of cyclase coupled receptors (11).

Using those methods, binding of VIP to its receptor was shown to stimulate pituitary adenylate cyclase (12), whereas D_2-dopamine (9, 10) and somatostatin receptors (13, 14) were recently proven to be negatively coupled with the enzyme. It is of interest to note that high basal levels of cyclase activity coincide, after gradient sedimentation of dispersed pituitary cells, with fractions containing prolactin (and possibly GH) cells (Fig. 1C); that is, those cell types submitted to a predominant, cyclase-dependent inhibitory influence of the brain.

Receptor coupling to phospholipase activity

Phospholipids can act as substrates to several enzymes, each of which can cleave these molecules in several ways and give rise to signals of known biological potency. For instance, phosphatidylethanolamine can be methylated into monomethyl- and dimethyl- forms, and finally, into the trimethylated phosphatidylcholine, a process which locally alters membrane microviscosity (15). Phospholipase C can generate diacylglycerol (DAG), an activator substrate for protein kinase C (16); recombination of DAG with phosphate yields phosphatidic acid (PA), a molecule believed to behave as a Ca^{2+} ionophore (17). However, more recently, the function of Ca^{2+} mobilizers has been

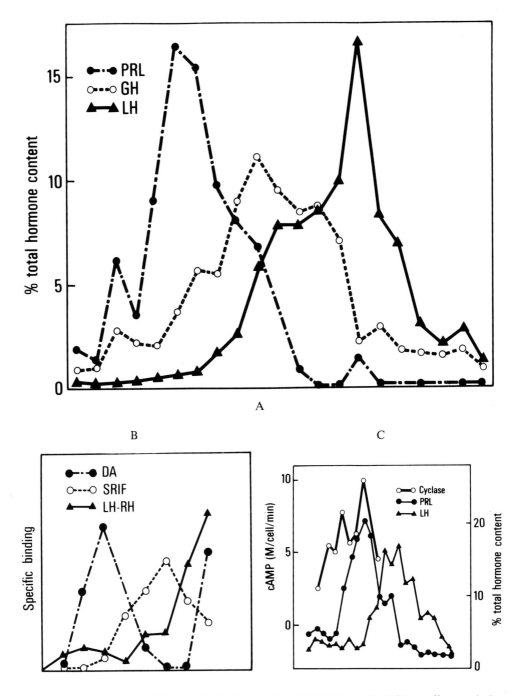

Figure 1. Fractionation of dispersed pituitary cells on LACS (1 to 4% BSA gradient at 1 g).
A: Hormonal profiles. B: Profiles of [³H] spiperone, [¹²⁵I]-Tyr-SRIF and [¹²⁵I]-LHRH binding.
C: Profiles of basal adenylate cyclase activity.

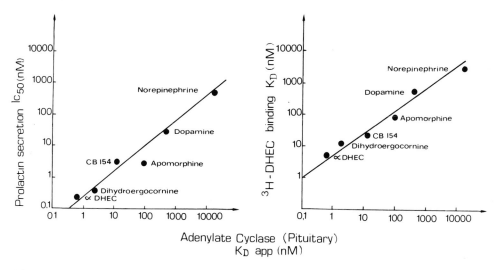

Figure 2. Potency ratios of dopamine agonists on inhibition of pituitary adenylate cyclase on one hand, and of in vitro prolactin release (left diagram) or of [³H]-dihydroergocryptin binding to pituitary membranes on the other hand (right diagram). Note the good correspondence of both curves.

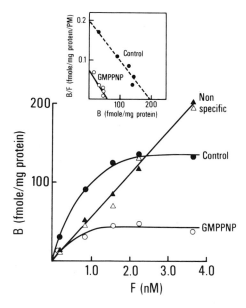

Figure 3. Effect of GMPPNP on non-specific and specific binding of [³H]-spiperone to pituitary membranes.

preferentially attributed to the inositol polyphosphates, which are alternate cleavage products of polyphosphoinositides by specific phospholipases of the C type (18). Consequently to the action of phospholipase C and the influx of Ca^{2+}, A_2 phospholipases are stimulated; these enzymes hydrolyze phosphatidylinositol or phosphatidic acid and release arachidonic acid, a precursor to leukotrienes and prostaglandins.

The hypothesis that secretory signals can be coupled with phospholipases was mostly studied in blood platelets (19), although increased cleavage of phosphatidylinositol under the influence of acetylcholine was also observed long ago in the CNS (20). The approach is delicate and has not been applied often to the pituitary for reaction products are labile and very readily recycled. Changes in the prolactin response to neurohormone can also be evaluated after pharmacological inhibition of phospholipase A_2 or of prostaglandins or leukotriene biosynthesis. But agents used to block these enzymes are not fully reliable; blockade of phospholipase A_2, usually induced by p-bromo-p-phenacylbromide (PB), was mostly documented so far on free enzymes prepared from snake venoms or the pancreas (22,23) and only checked indirectly on organized membranes (24). Besides, the drug also elicits non-specific effects, including a possible inhibition of phospholipase C (25).

Combining data obtained with several methods strongly suggests that TRH stimulation of prolactin is accompanied by a transient increment in PA and DAG (21,26), reaction products of phospholipase C. Phospholipase A_2 could also be involved, possibly as a consequence of an initial phospholipase C activation, since inhibition of the former enzyme by PB has been reported to suppress TRH induced prolactin secretion (27).

Whatever its actual mechanism of action, PB seems to have more general effects on lactotrophs than on somatotrophs. After a 15 minute incubation period with the drug, basal secretion rates of prolactin are decreased (Fig. 4). The effect of TRH is also decreased (Figs. 4 and 5); this fits with the hypothesis that TRH action is mediated by phospholipids rather than by adenylate cyclase. But the prolactin releasing activity of VIP, which is correlated with cyclase stimulation (12), is also attenuated by PB (Fig. 5). Even the inhibitory effect of dopamine on prolactin is diminished after PB treatment (Fig. 6).

Recent observations by Cronin suggest that pituitary adenylate cyclase can be manipulated with immediate consequence on prolactin release (28). This situation contrasts with that observed for somatotrophs, in which cyclase activation by GRF appears more directly related to secretion (29): in parallel, interference with phospholipid metabolism is totally ineffective on basal (Fig. 7) or on GRF stimulated (Fig. 5) release of GH. On that basis, Cronin postulated that receptor coupling to the enzyme and to exocytosis of prolactin could be related in a looser way than previously assumed.

But an apparently less rigid correlation between cAMP production and secretion can also be accounted for by a different hypothesis. Each neuropeptide recognized by the prolactin cell might end up in activating more than one reciprocally interactive coupling mechanism. Their mode of action at that level thus seems also pleiotropic. Although the process is not yet well understood in the pituitary, it could be comparable to that described in other tissues: guanylate and adenylate cyclic nucleotides can exhibit an inhibitory feed-back on phospholipase C in blood platelets (30); on the other hand, prostaglandins, one of the major end products of phospholipase A_2, can stimulate adenylate cyclase in many tissues including the pituitary (31). This could also explain

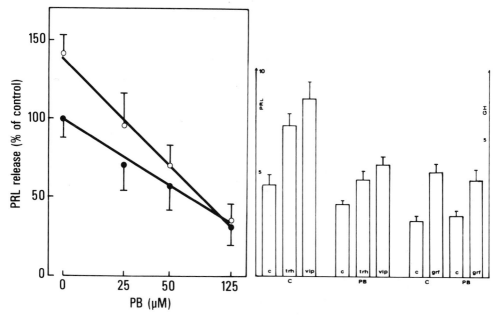

Figure 4. Effect of increasing concentrations of p-bromo-phenacylbromide (PB) on basal and TRH (10 uM) stimulated release of prolactin in vitro. PB was applied for 15 min, and the pituitaries were consequently washed for 1 hour before testing the peptide during a 1 hour incubation.

Figure 5. Differential effects of PB (50 uM) on TRH on VIP stimulation of prolactin and on GRF stimulation of GH. Same experimental conditions as in Fig. 4.

why TRH has been reported to stimulate production of the cyclic nucleotide (12), but not in a synchronous and well correlated manner.

In addition, steroids can also affect enzymatic activities correlated with phospholipid metabolism. After treatment with estradiol, pituitary cell membranes incorporate more [3H]-methionine into methylated forms of phosphatidyl-ethanolamine than in untreated controls (32). (Table II).

Table II - *Effect of estradiol implantation (5 days) on [3H]-methyl incorporation into phospolipids of pituitary membranes (pmol/mg prot/h)*

Phospholipid	Ovex Controls	Ovex Estradiol
Phosphatidyl-N-monomethyl-ethanolamine	.51 ± .05	2.05 ± .24
Phosphatidyl-N-N-dimethyl-ethanolamine	.76 ± .09	4.78 ± .55
Phosphatidylcholine	.80 ± .06	5.42 ± .56

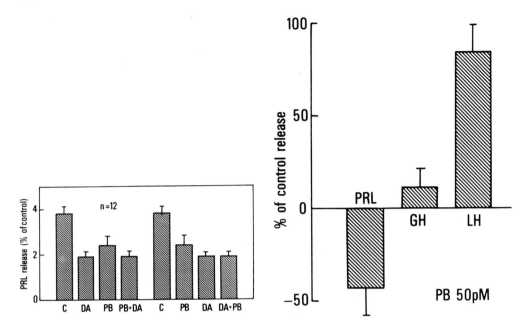

Figure 6. Effect of PB (50 uM) on dopamine inhibition of prolactin. Same conditions as in Fig. 4.

Figure 7. Differential effects of PB (50 uM) on basal release of prolactin, GH and LH. Same conditions as in Fig. 4.

PHYSIOLOGICAL RELEVANCE OF NEUROHORMONES INVOLVED IN PROLACTIN CONTROL

Dopamine is the most conspicuous prolactin regulating factor. Its tonic inhibition of the hormone explains why blockade of its release or of its receptors has marked effects on prolactin secretion under almost any circumstance. Dopamine can thus be assumed to be important for the homeostatic control of prolactin; this role is achieved by an original reciprocal feed-back interaction between the pituitary hormone and the tuberoinfundibular transmitter: a decrease in dopamine turnover increases prolactin release; this, in turn, stimulates dopamine release (33) and thus antagonizes the initial change in prolactin release rate (that is, it tends to reset initial levels of the hormone). Both the prolactin cell and the tuberoinfundibular neuron are regulated in that way; dopamine neurons terminating in the median eminence appear devoid of presynaptic autoreceptors, responsible for feedback regulation of other central dopaminergic neurons; they depend upon prolactin levels to regulate their activity.

In spite of its major involvement, dopamine has not been shown to trigger prolactin responses to known neurogenic stimuli. For example, release induced by stress or suckling increases dopamine turnover, as shown by indirect turnover studies (34). If the transmitter were to account for the elevated plasma levels measured under these physiological situations, a decreased rather than an increased turnover should be expected. The role of other substances should thus be examined. Unfortunately, few data are available as yet, because antagonists to most peptides involved in prolactin regulation are still to be discovered.

A mediation of endogenous opiates in the prolactin response to stress has clearly been established by previous studies. Stress releases at the same time pituitary ACTH and beta-endorphin (35); blockade of opiate effects by naloxone does not impair the ACTH and the beta-endorphin response to the stressful stimulus, but abolishes the prolactin response. In that case, hypothalamic morphinomimetic peptides, or, more likely, pituitary beta-endorphin can be viewed as "paracrine entrainers" of the prolactin component of the hormonal stress response.

It was tempting to investigate whether the circadian release of prolactin, which can be amplified by chronic oestrogenization of the animal and whose initial rising phase under these conditions is synchronous with that of ACTH and beta-endorphin (36), was not entrained by a similar mechanism. This however does not seem to be the case; chronic implants of naloxone, which block the morphine alleviation of nociceptive responses (tail flick test) over a long period of time, elevate basal prolactin levels and induce a slight delay in the circadian fluctuation, but do not affect its rhythmic pattern (Table III) (Rotten D, unpublished data).

Table III - *Effect of naloxone (NAL) implants on circadian fluctuations of prolactin (ng/ml plasma) in estradiol-treated female rats*

Time	0900	1100	1300	1500	1700
Control	90 ± 10	225 ± 45	602 ± 80	625 ± 45	380 ± 25
NAL	180 ± 65	260 ± 80	370 ± 85	525 ± 80	510 ± 90

In contrast, manipulation of GABA synaptic transmission by blockade of GABA transaminase totally suppresses the circadian pattern of prolactin release. Dexamethasone is also able to modulate prolactin fluctuation, mainly by uncoupling its VIP-induced release (37).

CONCLUSION

The relative importance of each endogenous neurohormone participating in the "coding system" of prolactin control is still poorly understood. The lack of structural antagonists for most neuropeptides involved, as well as a multiplicity of sites of action exhibited by some factors (examples: SRIF, opiates, or GABA acting both presynaptically within the median eminence and on the pituitary cell itself), explain why assessment of their role still relies on indirect, often inconclusive methods. Notwithstanding this, dopamine seems clearly involved in feed-back regulation; opiates and possibly GABA are probably most important in resetting prolactin levels under stressful conditions. The observation that opiates seem to uncouple presynaptic depolarization from its exocytotic consequence on several hypophysiotrophic factors (dopamine, TRH, SRIF, LHRH ...) suggests that morphinomimetic peptides act by inducing a pharmacological hypothalamo-hypophyseal deconnection during stress.

REFERENCES

1. Spampinato S, Locatelli V, Cocchi D, Vissentini L, Bajusz S, Ferri S, Muller EE. (1979): Endocrinology 105:163
2. Renaud L. (1981): Neuroendocrinology 33:186
3. Palkovits M. (1981): Neuroendocrinology 33:123
4. Drouva S, Epelbaum J, Tapia-Arancibia L, Laplante E, Kordon C. (1981): Neuroendocrinology 32:163
5. Tapia-Arancibia L, Astier H. (1983)
6. Epelbaum J, Tapia-Arancibia L, Besson J, Rotsztejn WH, Kordon C. (1979): Eur J Pharmacol 58:493
7. Shimatsu A, Kato Y, Matsushita N, Katakami H, Yanaihara N, Imura H. (1982): Endocrinology 111:338
8. Ferland L, Fuxe K, Eneroth P, Gustafsson JA, Skett P. (1977): Eur J Pharmacol 43:89
9. Enjalbert A, Bockaert J. (1983): Mol Pharmacol 23:576
10. Giannattanasio G, De Ferrari ME, Spada A. 1981 Life Sci 28:1605
11. Rodbell M. (1980): Nature 284:17
12. Gourdji D, Bataille D, Vauclin N, Grouselle D, Rosselin G, Tixier-Vidal A. (1979): FEBS Letters 104:165
13. Borgeat P, Labrie F, Drouin J, Belanger A, Immer K, Seetany K, Nelson V, Gotz M, Schally AV, Coy DH, Coy ES. (1974): Biochem Biophys Res Comm 56:1052
14. Enjalbert A, Rasolonjanahary R, Moyse E, Kordon C, Epelbaum J. (1983): Endocrinology 113:822
15. Strittmatter WJ, Hirata F, Axelrod J. (1981) In: Dumont J, Greengard P, Robiron GA (eds) *Advances in Cyclic Nucleotide Research.* Raven Press, New York, vol 14:83
16. Castagna M, Takai Y, Kaibuchi K, Sano K, Kikkawa U, Nishizuka Y. (1982): J Biol Chem 257:7847
17. Putney JW Jr, Weiss SJ, Van de Walle CM, Haddas RA. (1980): Nature 284:345
18. Streb H, Irvine RF, Berridge MJ, Schultz I. (1983): Nature 306:67
19. Laychock SG, Putney JW Jr. (1982): In: *Cellular Regulation of Secretion and Release,* Academic Press, New York, p 53
20. Schacht J, Agranoff BW. (1974): In: Schacht J, de Robertis F (eds) *Neurochemistry of Cholinergic Receptors.* Raven Press, New York, p 121
21. Rebecchi MJ, Kolesnick RN, Gershengorn MC. (1983): J Biol Chem 258:227
22. Vallee E, Gougat J, Navarro J, Delahayes JF. (1979): J Pharm Pharmacol 31:588
23. Verheij HM, Volwerk JJ, Jansen EHJM, Puyk WC, Dijkstra BW, Drenth J, de Hass GH. (1980): Biochemistry. 19:743
24. Vargaftig BB, Fouque F, Chignard M. (1980): Thrombosis Res 17:91
25. Hofmann SL, Prescott SM, Mayerus PW. (1982): Arch Biochem Biophys 215:237
26. Martin TF. (1983): J Biol Chem 258:14816
27. Canonico PL, Schettini G, Valdenegro CA, MacLeod RM. (1983): Neuroendocrinology 37:212
28. Cronin MJ, Moyers GA, MacLeod RM, Hewlett EL. (1983): J Cycl Nucl and Prot Phosphoryl Res 9:245

29. Cronin MJ, Hewlett EL, Evans WS, Thorner MO, Rogol AD. (1984): Endocrinology 114:904
30. Takai Y, Kaibuchi K, Sano K, Nishizuka Y. (1982): J Biochem (Japan) 91:403
31. MacLeod RM Lehmeyer JE. (1970): Proc Natl Acad Sci 67:1172
32. Drouva SV, Laplante E, Phan T, Camalin JC, Le Fur G, Kordon C. (1983): Neurosci Lett, suppl. 14:98
33. Lofstrom A, Jousson G, Wiesel FA, Fuxe K. (1976): J Histochem Cytochem 24:130
34. Mena F, Enjalbert A, Carbonell L, Priam M, Kordon C. (1976): Endocrinology 99:445
35. Rossier J, French E, Rivier C, Shibasaki C, Guillemin R, Bloom FE. (1980): Proc Natl Acad Sci 77:666
36. Szafarczyk A, Hery M, Laplante E, Ixart G, Assenmacher I, Kordon C. (1980): Neuroendocrinology 30:369
37. Rotsztejn WH, Dussaillant M, Noubou F, Rosselin G. (1981): Proc Natl Acad Sci 78:7584
38. Enjalbert A, Hugues JN, Moyse E, Peillon F, Shu C, Epelbaum J. (1984): 4th International Congress on Prolactin, Charlottesville, Virginia (abstract)
39. Schettini G, Cronin MJ, O'Dell SB, MacLeod RM. (1984): Brain Res 291:343
40. Westendorf JM, Schonbrunn A. (1982): Endocrinology 110:352
41. Westendorf JM, Schonbrunn A. (1983): J Biol Chem 258:7527
42. Enjalbert A, Ruberg M, Arancibia S, Fiore L, Priam M, Kordon C. (1979): Endocrinology 105:823
43. Lamberts SWJ, MacLeod RM. (1978): Proc Soc Exp Biol Med 158:103
44. Grandison L, Guidotti A. (1979): Endocrinology 105:754
45. Schally AV, Redding TW, Arimura A, Dupont A, Linthicum GL. (1977): Endocrinology 100:681
46. Vijayan E, McCann SM. (1978): Brain Res 155:35
47. Racagni G, Apud JA, Locatelli V, Cocchi D, Nistico G, Di Giorgio RM, Muller EE. (1979): Nature 281:575
48. Vijayan E, McCann SM. (1979): Endocrinology. 105:64
49. Enjalbert A, Arancibia S, Priam M, Bluet-Pajot MT, Kordon C. (1982): Neuroendocrinology 34:95
50. Enjalbert A, Ruberg M, Arancibia S, Priam M, Kordon C. (1979): Nature 280:595
51. Enjalbert A, Epelbaum J, Arancibia S, Tapia-Arancibia L, Bluet-Pajot MT, Kordon C. (1982): Endocrinology
52. Enjalbert A, Tapia-Arancibia L, Rieutort M, Brazeau P, Kordon C. (1982): Endocrinology 110:1634
53. Gourdji D, Kerdelhue B, Tixier-Vidal A. (1982): C R Acad Sci (Paris) 274:437
54. Grant G, Vale W, Guillemin R. (1972): Biochem Biophys Res Commun 46:28
55. Tashjian AH, Barowsky NJ, Jensen DK. 1971 Biochem Biophys Res Commun 43:516
56. Bataille D, Peillon F, Besson, Rosselin G. (1979): C R Acad Sci (Paris) 288:1315
57. Ruberg M, Rotsztejn WH, Arancibia S, Besson J, Enjalbert A. (1978): Eur J Pharmacol 51:319

Prolactin. Basic and clinical correlates
R.M. MacLeod, M.O. Thorner and U. Scapagnini (eds.),
Fidia Research Series, vol. I,
Liviana Press, Padova © 1985

Section II
Influence of brain factors
on prolactin secretion

INVOLVEMENT OF VASOACTIVE INTESTINAL POLYPEPTIDE IN SEROTONERGIC STIMULATION OF PROLACTIN SECRETION IN RATS

Akira Shimatsu, Yuzuru Kato, Hikaru Ohta, Katsuyoshi Tojo, Yasuhiro Kabayama, Tatsuhide Inoue, and Hiroo Imura.

Second Medical Clinic, Department of Medicine,
Kyoto University Faculty of Medicine, Sakyo-ku, Kyoto 606, Japan.

Vasoactive intestinal polypeptide (VIP) is currently viewed as a putative prolactin releasing factor (PRF) (1,2) since it is present in the hypothalamus (3), secreted into hypophysial portal blood (4,5), and stimulates prolactin secretion, at least in part, by acting directly at the pituitary level (6-9). However, the physiological role of endogenous VIP in regulating prolactin secretion remains to be determined. We have previously reported that brain serotonergic mechanisms play a stimulating role in regulating VIP release from the hypothalamus (10,11) and prolactin secretion from the pituitary (12,13). In the present study, we report the possible involvement of VIP in prolactin secretion induced by serotonergic stimulation using an immunoneutralization method.

Wistar strain male rats weighing 230-250 g were anesthetized with urethane (150 mg/100 g BW, ip) after overnight fasting. Test substances were injected into a jugular vein or into a lateral ventricle and blood samples of 0.6 ml were withdrawn from the jugular vein immediately before and 10, 20, and 40 min after the injection as described previously (6). Anti-VIP rabbit serum (AVS) or normal rabbit serum (NRS) was injected into a jugular vein in a volume of 0.5 ml/rat 30 min before the administration of the test substances. Plasma samples were separated promptly and kept at -20 C until assayed. Prolactin concentrations in the plasma were measured by specific radioimmunoassay using a kit supplied from the NIADDK (6,13). NIADDK-rat prolactin RP-1 was used for the standard. The VIP binding capacity of AVS-treated rat plasma was determined *in vitro* by calculating the bound percent of [^{125}I]-VIP (approximately 40 pg) added to 0.1 ml of rat plasma diluted to 1:20 according to the radioimmunoassay for VIP (5). Student's t test was used for the statistical evaluation.

AVS (KRV-1) was generated in a rabbit against the synthetic VIP-bovine thyroglobulin conjugate with glutalaldehyde. The anti-serum was specific for VIP, showing no cross-reactivity with porcine intestinal peptide histidine isoleucine (PHI), secretin, glucagon, thyrotropin releasing hormone and rat growth hormone releasing factor (GRF). Its avidity and binding capacity were 4.2 x 10⁹ l/mol and 7.2 nmol/ml, respectively.

As shown in Figure 1, intravenous injection of VIP (10 ug/rat) caused a significant increase in plasma prolactin levels in control animals pretreated with NRS. Plasma levels raised by VIP were significantly suppressed in animals pretreated with AVS (mean ± SE integrated prolactin release: NRS 101.2 ± 33.7 ng/ml *vs* AVS 34.4 ± 6.4 ng/ml, p < 0.05). On the other hand, prolactin release induced by domperidone (1 ug/100 g BW, iv), a peripheral dopamine receptor blocker, was not affected by AVS treatment (integrated prolactin release: NRS 152.5 ± 23.8 ng/ml *vs* AVS 168.6 ± 34.0 ng/ml). These findings indicate the AVS which we used was capable of antagonizing specifically the stimulating effect of VIP on prolactin release *in vivo*.

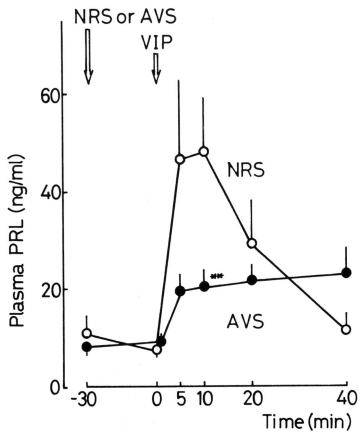

Fig. 1. Effects of intravenous injection of VIP (10 ug/rat) on plasma prolactin levels in urethane-anesthetized rats pretreated with anti-VIP rabbit serum (AVS) or normal rabbit serum (NRS). NRS and AVS were given intravenously (0.5 ml/rat) 30 min before the injection of VIP. Mean (± SE) values of 4 and 7 rats are shown. Statistical difference is shown by asterisk (** p < 0.02 *vs* NRS).

The intraventricular administration of serotonin (5HT, 1 ug/rat) resulted in a significant increase in plasma prolactin levels in rats pretreated with NRS. 5HT-induced prolactin release was markedly blunted in animals pretreated with AVS (integrated prolactin release: NRS 547.0 ± 121.1 ng/ml *vs* 30.7 ± 8.0 ng/ml, p < 0.01) as shown in Figure 2. Prolactin release induced by intravenous injection of 1-5-hydroxytryptophan (1-5HTP, 5 mg/100 g BW), a precursor of 5HT, was also blunted in animals pretreated with AVS compared with NRS (integrated prolactin release: NRS 493.2 ± 81.8 ng/ml *vs* AVS 304.0 ± 36.5 ng/nl, p < 0.05) (Fig. 3). Basal levels of plasma prolactin were not affected by AVS or NRS in each experiment. Diluted rat plasma obtained 70 min after the injection of AVS was capable of binding 79.4 ± 0.6% of [^{125}I]-VIP added *in vitro*.

It is well known that the administration of 5HT or its precursor, 5HTP, stimulates the secretion of prolactin (12-16). The mechanism by which 5HT influences the release

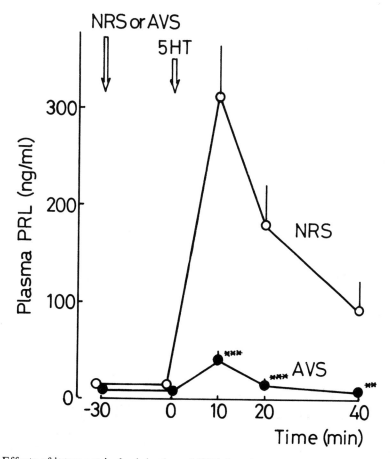

Fig. 2. Effects of intraventricular injection of 5HT (1 ug/rat) on plasma prolactin levels in rats pretreated with AVS or NRS. Mean (± SE) values of 6 rats are shown. Statistical differences are shown by asterisks (** p < 0.02, *** p < 0.01 *vs* NRS).

of prolactin remains to be elucidated. 5HT does not stimulate prolactin release from the anterior pituitary *in vitro* (16) and prolactin release induced by 5HTP is blunted in rats with extensive hypothalamic ablation (12), suggesting that the site of action of 5HT is not the pituitary gland. It has been postulated that 5HT may stimulate prolactin release by inhibiting the release of prolactin inhibiting factor (PIF) and/or by stimulating the release of PRF from the hypothalamus. Recently Pilotte and Porter (17) demonstrated that dopamine levels in rat pituitary stalk plasma were reduced by 5HT administration, whereas dopamine infusion did not prevent the 5HT-induced prolactin release. We have reported that 5HTP caused a further increase in plasma prolactin levels in rats pretreated with either alpha-methyl-p-tyrosine or reserpine (13). These findings support the hypothesis that 5HT causes the release of a hypothalamic PRF which stimulates prolactin secretion from the pituitary (18).

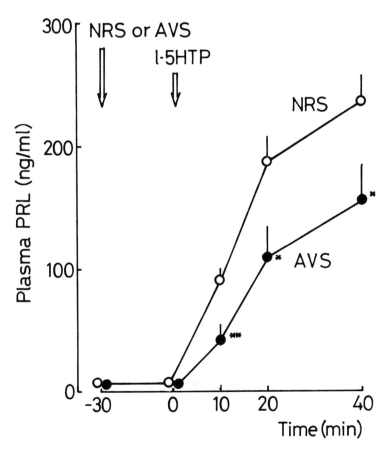

Fig. 3. Effects of intravenous injection of 1-5HTP (5 mg/100 g BW) on plasma prolactin levels in rats pretreated with AVS or NRS. Mean (± SE) values of 5 rats are shown. Statistical differences are shown by asterisks (* p < 0.05, ** p < 0.02 *vs* NRS).

We have previously reported that the concentration of VIP in rat hypophysial portal plasma was significantly increased by the intraventricular injection of 5HT or by the intravenous injection of 5HTP (10). We have also reported that VIP release from the hypothalamus is stimulated by 5HT *in vitro* (11). VIP stimulates prolactin release from the pituitary *in vitro* and antagonizes the inhibitory effects of dopamine and gamma-aminobutyric acid on prolactin secretion (6-9). It is postulated, therefore, that hypothalamic VIP may be involved in 5HT-induced prolactin secretion.

In the present study, we showed that plasma prolactin response to serotonergic stimulation was significantly suppressed by AVS which was injected intravenously to neutralize circulating VIP activity. We also found that prolactin release induced by 5HT was blunted by AVS which was injected into a lateral ventricle or infused into a single hypophysial portal vessel (19, 20). These findings strongly suggest that hypothalamic VIP is involved, at least in part, in mediating serotonergic stimulation of prolactin secretion in the rat.

ACKNOWLEDGMENTS

Supported in part by grants from the Ministry of Education and the Ministry of Health and Welfare, Japan.

REFERENCES

1. Neill JD. (1980): In: Martini L, Ganong WF (eds) *Frontiers in Neuroendocrinology*. Raven Press, New York, vol 6:129
2. Kato Y, Matsushita N, Shimatsu A, Imura H. (1982) In: Shizume K, Imura K, Shimizu N (eds) Proc 7th Asia and Oceania Congress of Endocrinology. Excerpta Medica, Amsterdam, p 136
3. Samson WK. (1982) In: Said SI (ed) *Vasoactive Intestinal Peptide, Advances in Peptide Hormone Research Series*. Raven Press, New York, vol 1:91
4. Said SI, Porter JC. (1979): Life Sci 24:227
5. Shimatsu A, Kato Y, Matsushita N, Katakami H, Yanaihara N, Imura H. (1981): Endocrinology 108:395
6. Kato Y, Iwasaki Y, Iwasaki J, Abe H, Yanaihara N, Imura H. (1978): Endocrinology 103:554
7. Ruberg M, Rostejn WH, Arancibia S, Besson J, Enjalbert A. (1978): Eur J Pharmacol 51:319
8. Shaar CJ, Clemens JA, Dininger NB. (1979): Life Sci 25:2071
9. Matsushita N, Kato Y, Shimatsu A, Katakami H, Yanaihara N, Imura H. (1983): Life Sci 32:1263
10. Shimatsu A, Kato Y, Matsushita N, Katakami H, Yanaihara N, Imura H. (1982): Endocrinology 111:338
11. Shimatsu A, Kato Y, Matsushita N, Katakami H, Ohta H, Yanaihara N, Imura H. (1983): Brain Res 264:148
12. Ohgo S, Kato Y, Chihara K, Imura H, Maeda K. (1976): Endocrinol Jpn 23:485
13. Matsushita N, Kato Y, Katakami H, Shimatsu A, Imura H. (1981): Proc Soc Exp Biol Med 168:282
14. Kamberi IA, Mical RS, Porter JC. (1971): Endocrinology 88:128
15. Lu KH, Meites J. (1973): Endocrinology 93:152

16. Lamberts SWJ, MacLeod RM. (1978): Endocrinology 103:287
17. Pilotte NS, Porter JC. (1981): Endocrinology 108:2137
18. Clemens JA, Roush ME, Fuller RW. (1978): Life Sci 22:2209
19. Kato Y, Katakami H, Matsushita N, Shimatsu A, Ohta H, Kabayama Y, Imura H. (1983): Biomed Res 4 (Suppl):233
20. Shimatsu A, Kato Y, Ohta H, Tojo K, Kabayama Y, Inoue T, Yanaihara N, Imura H. (1984): Proc Soc Exp Biol Med 175:414

Prolactin. Basic and clinical correlates
R.M. MacLeod, M.O. Thorner and U. Scapagnini (eds.),
Fidia Research Series, vol. I,
Liviana Press, Padova © 1985

Section II
Influence of brain factors
on prolactin secretion

VASOACTIVE INTESTINAL PEPTIDE CAUSES A CALCIUM-DEPENDENT STIMULATION OF PROLACTIN SECRETION WITHOUT ALTERING ELECTROPHYSIOLOGICAL MEMBRANE PROPERTIES IN GH$_4$C$_1$ CELLS.

E. Haug[1], T. Bjoro[1], O. Sand[2], J. Gordeladze[3] and K.M. Gautvik[3,4]

[1]Hormone Laboratory, Aker Hospital, [2]Department of Biology, University of Oslo
[3]Institute for Surgical Research, Rikshospitalet,
[4]Institute of Medical Biochemistry, University of Oslo, Oslo, Norway.

The hypothalamus exerts its influence on the anterior pituitary gland by secretion of stimulatory and inhibitory substances reaching their target cells through the pituitary portal circulation. Unlike the other pituitary hormones the release of prolactin is tonically inhibited by the hypothalamus (1), and various observations have suggested that dopamine is involved (2,3). However, changes in dopamine secretion probably play an integral part in a complex mechanism, probably including other hypothalamic hormones (4). Vasoactive intestinal peptide (VIP), originally isolated from hog intestine (5), is supposed to play a physiological role as a hypothalamic hormone which stimulates prolactin secretion (6-10). The present contribution describes recent studies of the effects of VIP on the GH$_4$C$_1$ clonal cell line, and gives a comparison of the effects of VIP and TRH on the GH$_4$C$_1$ cells.

THE GH CELL SYSTEM

In 1968 Tashjian et al. (11) reported the establishment of three strains of epithelial cells from a transplantable rat pituitary tumor. The cell strains, which are referred to collectively as GH cells, produce both prolactin and growth hormone (GH). Both hormones are immunologically indistinguishable from authentic rat hormones and have retained their biological activity (11,12). Although the cells are of tumor origin they have the ability to respond to several hypothalamic and steroid hormones, as well as to a range of other secretagogues, in a manner analogous to normal anterior pituitary cells (13,14). The GH$_4$C$_1$ cell strain used in this study produces predominantly prolactin and only small amounts of GH.

EFFECTS OF VIP ON PROLACTIN RELEASE

The acute release of prolactin from the GH_4C_1 cells was measured using a perifusion system based on the method of Lowry and McMartin (15). A suspension of GH_4C_1 cells was obtained from monolayer cultures. The cells were stacked in a Bio-Gel P-2 column confined within a 5 ml syringe (10), continuously perfused at a rate of 0.25 ml/min, and the fractions were collected at 2 min intervals. The experiments were conducted at 37 C. The cells were exposed to the peptides during 4 min periods, and Figure 1 shows that VIP and TRH caused an instantaneous increase in prolactin release. VIP was always less effective than TRH on a molar basis. The maximum effect of TRH, obtained at 10 nM, was always higher (1.2 - 3.0 fold, n = 12) than for VIP. Figures 1 and 5 show that increasing concentrations of VIP caused a dose-related increase in prolactin release with half-maximal and maximal effects at 80 nM and 10 uM, respectively.

The concentrations of VIP necessary to stimulate prolactin release from the GH_4C_1 cells are in agreement with the dose-response relationship demonstrated using rat hemipituitaries (7, 16). Gourdji et al. (9) using GH_3/B_6 cells, and Dorflinger and Schonbrunn (17) using GH_4C_1 cells, however, found that 10 nM VIP stimulated prolactin release maximally. This discrepancy may at least partly reflect a dilution of VIP during the passage through the perifusion system used in this study (10).

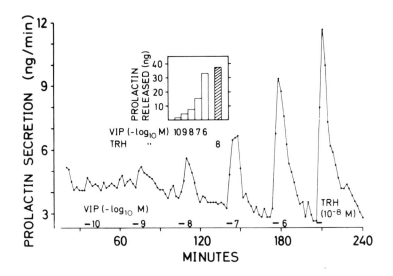

Figure 1. Prolactin release from perifused Bio-Gel P-2 columns containing about 70 x 10⁶ GH_4C_1 cells. Thick lines indicate 4 min infusion pulses of VIP and TRH (adjusted for the time-lag due to the dead volume of the system). Prolactin was measured in the eluate, and secretion expressed as the amount of hormone released during 1 min. The inset represents the total prolactin released (ng) in excess of basal secretion. (From ref. 10).

Somatostatin (SRIH) is another hypothalamic factor released to the portal circulation of the pituitary, and this peptide has been shown to almost completely inhibit TRH-stimulated prolactin release (14). Figure 2 shows that SRIH gradually decreased basal prolactin secretion rate to about 60% of pretreatment levels, and in the presence of SRIH the prolactin responses elicited by VIP were drastically reduced. These observations are in agreement with the report of Westendorf and Schonbrunn (18), and suggest that SRIH may inhibit both basal and stimulated prolactin secretion by direct action on the lactotropes.

ON THE ROLE OF CALCIUM IN THE REGULATION OF PROLACTIN RELEASE

Measurements of hormone release have shown that the exocytosis of secretory granules from most peptide-producing endocrine cells is triggered by influx of extracellular Ca^{2+}. Electrophysiological experiments have demonstrated that anterior pituitary cells are able to generate Ca^{2+}-dependent action potentials (19-21). It has been suggested therefore that the entry of extracellular Ca^{2+} is associated with the Ca^{2+}-dependent action potentials.

In the case of the enhancement of prolactin release from GH cells induced by TRH there is experimental evidence in favor of this idea. TRH-stimulated prolactin release is dependent on extracellular Ca^{2+} (10,14), and it is inhibited by blockers of voltage-

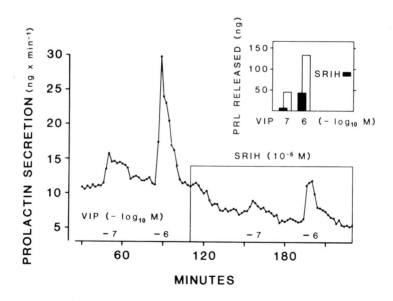

Figure 2. Prolactin release from perifused GH_4C_1 cells exposed to 4 min infusion pulses of VIP in the absence or presence of SRIH. The inset represents the total prolactin released in excess of basal secretion.

sensitive calcium channels (10,22). Figure 3 shows the effects of VIP, TRH, and KCl on prolactin release alone and in combination with $CoCl_2$ and verapamil or during calcium-free conditions. In calcium-free medium the effects of VIP and high K^+ were completely abolished. Normal responses were regained when Ca^{2+} was added to the perfusion medium. Co^{2+} and verapamil, two commonly used blockers of voltage-sensitive calcium channels, completely inhibited prolactin release induced by VIP, TRH, and high K^+. Verapamil also caused a gradual decrease in basal prolactin secretion to about 30%, while Co^{2+} was less effective. The inhibitory effects of these calcium channel blockers on stimulated as well as basal prolactin secretion were reversible.

LACK OF ELECTROPHYSIOLOGICAL EFFECTS OF VIP

The electrophysiological effects of TRH on GH cells previously have been described in detail (19,21,23,24). Application of TRH causes a biphasic membrane response: an initial hyperpolarization followed by a late depolarization leading to increased firing rate in spontaneously active cells or induction of action potentials in previously silent cells. TRH thus leads to an increased influx of Ca^{2+} through voltage-sensitive calcium channels in the GH cells. Figure 4 gives an example of the response to TRH.

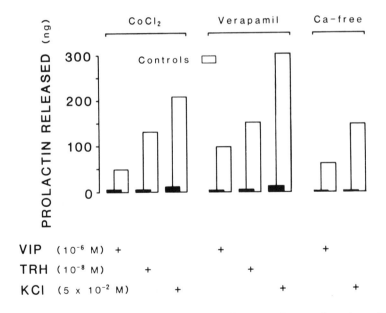

Figure 3. Prolactin release from perifused GH_4C_1 cells exposed to 4 min pulses of VIP, TRH or KCl. The experiments were performed in the absence or presence of either 1M $CoCl_2$ or 0.1M verapamil or in culture medium with (1.3 mM Ca^{2+}) or without Ca^{2+}. Values are given as the total prolactin released in excess of basal secretion. Controls represent prolactin released in response to VIP, TRH, or KCl in the absence of blockers and in Ca-containing medium.

The data presented so far show a striking similarity both in the time-course of the prolactin release induced by VIP and TRH, and the Ca^{2+} dependency of this release. It was thus reasonable to suggest a similar mode of action for these two peptides. Cells in monolayer culture were penetrated by microelectrodes, and the peptides were applied to the cell surface by pressure ejection through micropipettes (14, 24). Figure 4 shows that VIP had no visible effect on the electrical membrane properties of GH_4C_1 cells. The spontaneously active cell was continuously exposed to VIP from the time indicated by the arrow. After 1.5 min exposure to VIP, TRH was ejected through a second delivery pipette, and the cell showed the normal, biphasic membrane response leading to increased firing frequency. This lack of membrane response to VIP is in agreement with a recent report by Dufy et al. (25), who showed that VIP has no effect on the action potentials of GH_3/B_6 cells.

EFFECTS OF VIP ON ADENYLYL CYCLASE ACTIVITY

It is accepted that two of the key factors regulating the intracellular secretory machinery in most cells are Ca^{2+} and the adenylyl cyclase-cyclic AMP system. A TRH-responsive adenylyl cyclase has recently been described in GH cells (26), and a good correlation exists between cyclic AMP formation in intact GH_4C_1 cells and prolactin release in response to TRH (27). However, since full expression of the effect of TRH is also dependent on extracellular Ca^{2+}, the cyclic AMP and the calcium-signalling systems appear to act in concert to promote prolactin secretion after TRH treatment (14).

Figure 5 shows the dose-response effect of VIP on adenylyl cyclase activity in the presence of 40 uM guanosine triphosphate (GTP). Adenylyl cyclase activity was measured in cell homogenates as described elsewhere (26). VIP caused a dose-dependent increase in the enzyme activity with half-maximal and maximal effects at about 50 nM and 1 uM, respectively. A close correlation was found between adenylyl cyclase activation and VIP enhanced prolactin release.

Figure 6 shows that maximal stimulation of adenylyl cyclase activity by VIP was 5-fold higher than that for TRH and equal to fluoride stimulation. A preincubation period of 20 min nearly abolished the responsiveness to a second treatment with TRH. VIP, however, significantly increased adenylyl cyclase activity also following a proceding incubation with the peptide, although the second response was reduced to 40% of the first response. Preincubation with TRH had no effect on the response to the second treatment with VIP and vice versa.

DISCUSSION

Our results demonstrate that the hypothalamic peptides TRH and VIP have similar but not identical modes of actions on the prolactin-secreting GH_4C_1 cells.

The enhanced Ca^{2+} influx through the voltage-sensitive calcium channels, linked to the increased action potential activity, is probably essential for the prolactin release induced by TRH (14, 19, 21, 22, 24). [For contrasting views see Gershengorn et al., this volume and Martin et al., this volume. --Eds.] VIP, on the other hand, has no

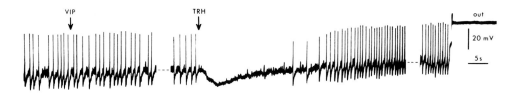

Figure 4. Lack of membrane response to continuous VIP application by ejection from a micropipette filled with 100 uM VIP and positioned 40 um from the penetrated cell. Start of the VIP stimulation is indicated by arrow. The second arrow indicates start of TRH application by ejection from a second micropipette filled with 1 uM TRH and positioned at the same distance from the cell. The electrode was withdrawn from the cell in the last part of the recording. Broken lines indicate 1 min interceptions of the recording. (From ref. 10).

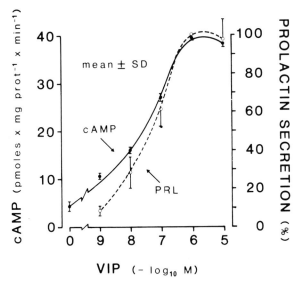

Figure 5. VIP dose-response curves for the adenylyl cyclase activity and for prolactin secretion. Enzyme activity was measured in GH_4C_1 cell homogenates treated with VIP (20 min, 35 C) at the concentrations indicated. Prolactin release was calculated from perifusion experiments (n = 5), and the responses are expressed as total PRl released above basal secretion by 4 min pulses of VIP at the concentrations indicated. The responses are given as percentage of the response to 1 uM VIP, which was included in all experiments.

effect on the Ca-dependent action potentials. It is possible that VIP enhances Ca^{2+} influx in GH_4C_1 cells through agonist-gated channels independently of the action potentials, as demonstrated for exocrine cells (28). The blockers of voltage-sensitive calcium channels, like Ca^{2+} and verapamil, have poor specificity and may also inhibit

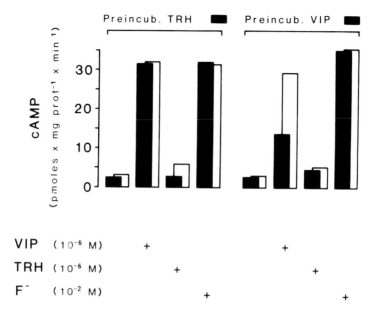

Figure 6. Adenylyl cyclase activity in GH_4C_1 particulate fractions treated for a 20 min period (30 C) with VIP, TRH, and fluoride (F^-) at the concentrations indicated (open columns). Filled columns give the adenylyl cyclase activity in fractions preincubated (20 min, 30 C) with either 1 uM TRH or VIP 1 uM. After preincubation, the particulate fraction was washed twice, resuspended in buffer and treated for a second period (20 min, 30 C) with VIP, TRH and fluoride (F^-) at the concentrations indicated. Controls received vehicle only during the preincubation period.

agonist-gated channels (29). However, the existence of such channels has never been shown in endocrine cells.

Alternatively, VIP may inhibit the uptake of Ca^{2+} into the intracellular stores. In the normal state of cellular equilibrium, the continuous influx of Ca^{2+} through the voltage-sensitive calcium channels is compensated by an effective uptake of Ca^{2+} into mitochondria and endoplasmic reticulum, keeping the cytosolic Ca^{2+} concentrations at about 10 uM. Increased cytosolic Ca^{2+} concentrations, leading to exocytosis, may be achieved either by increased influx or reduced uptake into the intracellular stores. In both cases the enhancement of cytosolic Ca^{2+} will be abolished by blocking the influx through the calcium channels.

VIP is far more potent than TRH in increasing the cellular cyclic AMP concentration. We are now focusing our attention on the possible relation between the VIP-induced adenylyl cyclase activation and increased cytosolic Ca^{2+} concentration. It is tempting to speculate that one possible action of cyclic AMP may turn out to be at the level of Ca^{2+} uptake into intracellular stores. Such a mechanism has been suggested previously for the facilitatory action of cyclic AMP on the release of insulin from beta cells (30, 31).

ACKNOWLEDGMENTS

Financial support has been received from the Norwegian Society for Fighting Cancer. We thank Miss Nina Gjerlaugsen, Mrs. Berit Ingebrigtsen, and Mrs. Aasa Stokland for skilled technical assistance and Mrs. Kjersti Gunneng for typing the manuscript.

REFERENCES

1. Everett JW. (1954): Endocrinology 54:685
2. MacLeod RM. (1976): In: Martini L, Ganong WF (eds) *Frontiers in Neuroendocrinology.* Raven Press, New York, vol 4:169
3. Ben-Jonathan N, Oliver C, Weiner HJ, Mical RS, Porter JC (1977) Endocrinology 100:452
4. de Greef WJ, Plotsky PM, Neill JD. (1981): Neuroendocrinology 32:229
5. Said SI, Mutt V. (1970): Science 169:1217
6. Ruberg M, Rotsztejn WH, Arancibia S, Besson J, Enjalbert A. (1978): Eur J Pharmacol 51:319
7. Enjalbert A, Arancibia S, Ruberg M, Priam M, Bluet-Pajot MT, Rotsztejn WH, Kordon C. (1980): Neuroendocrinology 31:200
8. Rotsztejn W, Benoist L, Besson J, Beraud G, Bluet-Pajot MT, Kordon C, Rosselin B, Duval J. (1980): Neuroendocrinology 31:282
9. Gourdji D, Bataille D, Vauclin N, Grouselle D, Rosselin G, Tixier-Vidal A. (1979): FEBS Lett 104:165
10. Bjoro T, Haug E, Sand O, Gautvik KM. (1984): Mol Cell Endocrinol, in press
11. Tashjian AH Jr, Yasumura Y, Levine L, Sato GH, Parker ML. 1968: Endocrinology 82:342
12. Haug E, Gautvik KM. (1976): Acta Endocrinol (Copenh) 82:282
13. Tashjian AH Jr. (1979): Methods Enzymol 58:527
14. Haug E, Gautvik KM, Sand O, Iversen JG, Kriz M. (1982): In: McKerns KW, Pantic V (eds) *Hormonally Active Brain Peptides.* Plenum Publ Corp, New York, p 537
15. Lowry PJ, McMartin C. (1974): Biochem J 142:287
16. Shaar CJ, Clemens JA, Dininger NB. (1979): Life Sci 25:2071
17. Dorflinger LJ, Schonbrunn A. (1983): Endocrinology 113:1551
18. Westendorf JM, Schonbrunn A. (1982): Endocrinology 110:352
19. Kidokoro Y. (1975): Nature 258:741
20. Taraskevich PS, Douglas WW. (1977): Proc Natl Acad Sci USA 74:4064
21. Ozawa S, Sand O. (1978): Acta Physiol Scand 102:330
22 Tan K-N, Tashjian AH Jr. (1984): J Biol Chem 259:427
23. Dufy B, Vincent J-D, Fleury H, du Pasquier P, Gourdji D, Tixier-Vidal A. (1979): Science 204:509
24. Sand O, Haug E, Gautvik KM. (1980): Acta Physiol Scand 108:247
25. Dufy B, Israel JM, Zyzck E. (1982): Neuroendocrinol Lett 4:245
26. Gautvik KM, Gordeladze JO, Jahnsen T, Haug E, Hansson V, Lystad E. (1983): J Biol Chem 258:10304
27. Gautvik KM, Kriz M, Jahnsen T, Haug E, Hansson V. (1982): Mol Cell Endocrinol 26:295
28. O'Doherty J, Stark RJ. (1982): Am J Physiol 242:G513
29. Botelho SY, Dartt DA. (1980): J Physiol 304:397
30. Sehlin J. (1976): Biochem J 156:63
31. Matthews EK. (1979): Symp Soc Exp Biol 33:225

Prolactin. Basic and clinical correlates
R.M. MacLeod, M.O. Thorner and U. Scapagnini (eds.),
Fidia Research Series, vol. I,
Liviana Press, Padova © 1985

Section II
Influence of brain factors
on prolactin secretion

THE ROLE OF ALPHA-MELANOCYTE STIMULATING HORMONE (alpha-MSH) AS AN INHIBITORY MODULATOR OF PROLACTIN SECRETION IN THE RAT.

Omid Khorram, Joa C. Bedran de Castro, and Samuel M. McCann.

Department of Physiology, University of Texas Health Science Center, Dallas, Texas 75235

Alpha-melanocyte stimulating hormone (alpha-MSH) is a tridecapeptide with a clear physiological role in adaptive color changes in lower vertebrates. The function of this peptide in mammalian species has yet to be elucidated. This review is a summary of our efforts directed at determining whether this neuropeptide, which is localized extensively throughout the nervous system (1), in particular, in the hypophysiotropic area and in the hypophysial portal blood (2), has a role in regulating the secretion of prolactin from the anterior pituitary gland.

In an initial study (3), we demonstrated that injection of alpha-MSH into the third ventricle of ovariectomized (OVX), freely moving rats induced a dose-dependent depression of basal levels of plasma prolactin. The peptide was more effective in lowering the stress-induced prolactin release and was also effective in inhibiting prolactin secretion in OVX rats primed earlier with estrogen. Furthermore, we found no effect of the peptide at the pituitary level on the basis of incubation of the peptide with hemipituitaries or dispersed pituitary cells. Thus, the inhibition of prolactin release by alpha-MSH appears to be exerted on structures near its site of injection in the third ventricle. Since administration of dopamine receptor blockers prior to the injection of alpha-MSH blocked the inhibitory effect of the peptide on PRl secretion, we proposed that alpha-MSH activates the tuberoinfundibular dopaminergic neurons, which in turn would inhibit prolactin release from the pituitary gland. We obtained similar effects of alpha-MSH on pulsatile release of luteinizing hormone (4).

While our experiments were in progress, a number of groups demonstrated that the brain contains multiple forms of alpha-MSH, the predominant species being des-acetyl alpha-MSH (5,6). Thus it became important to determine if des-acetyl alpha-MSH was also active in lowering plasma prolactin. The result of this experiment is shown in Figure 1. In this experiment, des-acetyl alpha-MSH was infused into the third ventri-

cle of OVX, freely moving rats. The peptide lowered plasma prolactin relative to prein-
jection levels within five min. The amount of inhibition obtained with des-acetyl alpha-
MSH was similar to that obtained with alpha-MSH. These results thus supported our
hypothesis that alpha-MSH of central origin (probably hypothalamic) is an inhibitor
of prolactin release.

Our attempts were then focused on establishing the physiological importance of
alpha-MSH-induced inhibition of prolactin release by passive immunization studies.
Specific antisera were raised against alpha-MSH and fully characterized by radioimmunoassay for their crossreactivity with ACTH and related peptides, and by gel filtration chromatography (7). The antiserum used in these passive immunization studies
(KDM-1) cross-reacted 36% with des-acetyl alpha-MSH and did not cross-react with
ACTH (1-39), ACTH (1-24), beta-MSH, alpha-MSH, and beta-endorphin. In the experiments involving intraventricular injections of the antisera, sera from rabbits im-
munized against alpha-MSH or normal rabbit serum (NRS) were purified by ammonium
sulfate precipitation and the globulin fraction was used. In the intravenous (iv) injections of the antiserum, the whole serum was used.

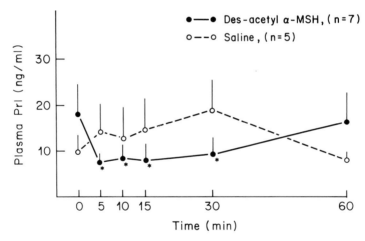

Figure 1. The effect of 3rd ventricular (IVT) injection of Des-acetyl alpha-MSH on plasma prolactin levels of OVX, freely moving rats. *: $p < 0.05$ relative to time 0.

The results of the passive immunization studies are depicted in Figures 2 and 3.
In this experiment, OVX rats were injected 24 h prior to the experiment with 5 ul of
the globulin fraction of KDM-1 or NRS. On the day of the experiment one blood sample was withdrawn. As seen in Figure 2, a single injection of KDM-1 significantly elevated
plasma prolactin levels 24 h later. After the initial blood sample was taken the animals
received a second IVT injection of KDM-1 or NRS (5 ul). Beginning 25 min after this
injection, blood samples were withdrawn every 10 min for 3 h (Fig. 3). Anti-MSH induced a clear increase in the amplitude of prolactin pulses ($p < 0.01$), mean plasma
prolactin ($p < 0.01$), and the area under the secretion curve of prolactin ($p < 0.01$).

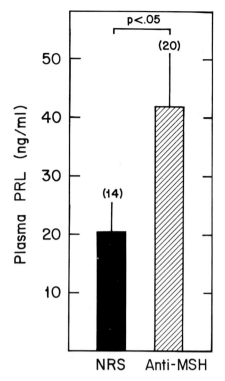

Figure 2. Effect of IVT injection of 5 ul of globulins prepared from NRS and anti-serum (KDM-1) on plasma levels of prolactin 24 h after the injection.

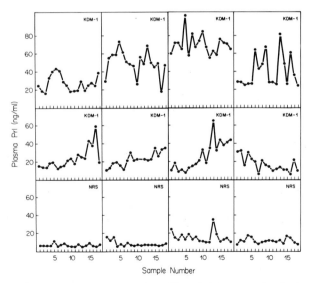

Figure 3. Representative three-hour hormonal profiles of the same animals shown in Fig. 2 after a second IVT injection of NRS or anti-serum (KDM-1).

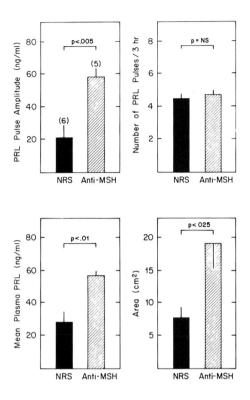

Figure 4. Summary of various parameters of pulsatile release of prolactin represented in Fig. 3.

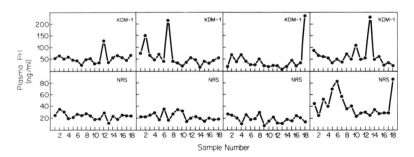

Figure 5. Representative three-hour profiles of prolactin after two IV injections of KDM-1 or NRS (0.2 ml) administered 24 h apart. Note the difference in scale between the two treatment groups.

The number of prolactin pulses was unaffected (Fig. 4). These results indicate that endogenous brain alpha-MSH exerts a tonic inhibitory effect on prolactin secretion.

The effect of iv injections of anti-MSH (0.2 ml) was also determined, employing the same experimental protocol as in the IVT injections. The results of these experiments are shown in Figures 5 and 6. The area under the secretion curve of prolactin and the amplitude of prolactin pulses were significantly increased following the iv injections of anti-MSH; however, the number of pulses of prolactin was unaffected. The fact that both routes of administration of the antiserum were effective in stimulating the secretion of prolactin suggests that the alpha-MSH neurons involved in inhibiting the release of prolactin lie in an area outside the blood-brain barrier. The median eminence could be one potential site of interaction between the alpha-MSH and dopaminergic terminals.

In further experiments, we investigated the potential role of alpha-MSH in the stress-induced release of prolactin (8). Ovariectomized rats were injected in the third ventricle with 5 ul of either anti-MSH (KDM-1) or NRS (globulin fraction of each) 24 h before the experiment and on the day of the experiment. Twenty-five minutes after the second injection of KDM-1 or NRS, the animals were subjected to 1.5 min of ether exposure and blood samples were withdrawn at various times thereafter. As depicted in Figure 7, ether exposure significantly ($p < 0.025$) elevated plasma prolactin levels within 5 min in the NRS-injected rats, but had no effect in the antiserum-injected rats. Plasma

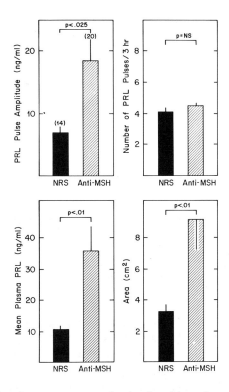

Figure 6. Summary of various parameters of pulsatile release of prolactin represented in Fig. 5.

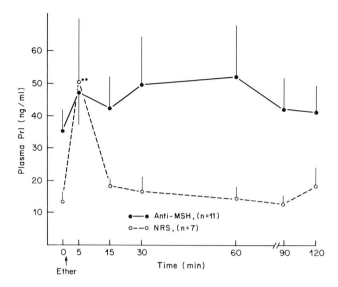

Figure 7. Effect of IVT injection of KDM-1 or NRS on the stress-induced release of prolactin. *: p < 0.025 relative to time 0.

prolactin levels in the antiserum-treated rats were significantly higher than the corresponding levels in the NRS-injected rats at 15, 30, 60 (p < 0.05), 90 (p < 0.025), and 120 min (p < 0.05). These results, along with our demonstration of the greater effectiveness of MSH in inhibiting prolactin release in the stressed rat (3), support the hypothesis that MSH released under stressful conditions may have a role in restoring the high levels of prolactin to baseline levels.

In summary, our studies indicate that brain alpha-MSH serves as an inhibitory modulator of prolactin secretion in a mammalian species, the rat. This inhibition is mediated by dopamine and operates under basal and stressful conditions, when prolactin levels are elevated. Beta-endorphin, a peptide related to alpha-MSH and derived from a common precursor, has a physiologically important stimulatory effect on prolactin secretion (9). In contrast to alpha-MSH, beta-endorphin affects prolactin release via inhibition of the activity of the tuberoinfundibular dopaminergic neurons (10). Thus the intriguing question raised is how two neuropeptides found in the same neurons and presumably released at the same time produce opposite effects on the secretion of prolactin. Recently a second alpha-MSH containing neuronal system with cell bodies in the dorso-lateral hypothalamus has been described (11). Unlike the arcuate alpha-MSH cell bodies which contain both alpha-MSH and beta-endorphin, this newly described group of cell bodies does not contain beta-endorphin or beta-lipotropin (11). Thus, selective release of alpha-MSH can be obtained if this group of neurons is involved in modulating the secretion of prolactin. Alternatively, a differential sensitivity of the dopaminergic neurons to alpha-MSH and beta-endorphin may lead to an initial deactivation followed by activation of these neurons by beta-endorphin and alpha-MSH respectively. Thus alpha-MSH, by opposing the action of beta-endorphin, could prevent a hyperprolactinemic state which would be the case if the effect of beta-endorphin went unopposed. So our future experiments will be directed at determining the interaction between alpha-MSH and beta-endorphin in regulating the release of prolactin.

REFERENCES

1. O'Donohue TL, Miller RL, Jacobowitz DM. (1979): Brain Res 176:101
2. Oliver C, Mical RS, Porter JC. (1977): Endocrinology 101:598
3. Khorram O, Mizunuma H, McCann SM. (1982): Neuroendocrinology 34:433
4. Khorram O, DePalatis LP, McCann SM. (1984): Endocrinology 114:227
5. Evans CJ, Lorenz R, Weber E, Barchas JD. (1982): Biochem Biophys Res Comm 106:910
6. Jegou S, Tonon MC, Vaudry H, Pelletier G. (1983): Brain Res 260:91
7. Khorram O, McCann SM. (1984): Biol of Neonate (in press)
8. Khorram O, Bedran De Castro JC, McCann SM. (1984): Proc Natl Acad Sci (in press)
9. Ragavan VV, Frantz AG. (1981): Endocrinology 109:1769
10. Moore KE, Johnston CA. (1982): In: MacLeod RM, Muller EE (eds) Neuroendocrine Perspectives vol 1:23
11. Watson SJ, Akil H. (1980): Brain Res 182:217

Prolactin. Basic and clinical correlates
R.M. MacLeod, M.O. Thorner and U. Scapagnini (eds.),
Fidia Research Series, vol. I,
Liviana Press, Padova © 1985

Section II
Influence of brain factors
on prolactin secretion

THE MAJOR PROLACTIN RELEASING ACTIVITY FROM BOVINE POSTERIOR PITUITARY IS IDENTIFIED AS NEUROPHYSIN-II.

S.H. Shin, M.C. Obonsawin, and S. Vincent.

Department of Physiology, Queen's University, Kingston, Canada K7L 3N6

For the last several years, we have been trying to define the physiological role of the prolactin releasing factor (PRF) using mostly physiological and pharmacological techniques (1-3). Evidence suggests that the PRF plays an important role in prolactin release, particularly in the case of acute stress (1,2). In order to chemically isolate and characterize the PRF, the prolactin releasing activity of an acetic acid extract of freshly frozen bovine hypothalamic tissue was compared to that of an acetic acid extract of bovine posterior pituitary tissue. Both extracts were tested in estradiol primed rats. Posterior pituitary tissue was used because vasopressin stimulates prolactin release by a direct action on the lactotroph (4). The posterior pituitary extract stimulated prolactin release in estradiol primed male rats while the equivalent amount of hypothalamic extract did not show any noticeable stimulatory effect on prolactin release. We have therefore attempted to isolate the active component of the posterior pituitary extract using classical fractionation techniques.

ISOLATION OF THE PROLACTIN RELEASING ACTIVITY FROM THE POSTERIOR PITUITARY

Male Sprague-Dawley rats (Charles River, CD, Canadian Breeding Farm and Laboratories) were acclimatized in a controlled environment with illumination for 14 h daily (06:00 - 20:00 h) and a temperature of 25 ± 1 C. Purina Lab Chow and tap water were supplied ad libitum.

In vitro experiments were performed as described previously (5). Adenohypophyses were dispersed with trypsin (6). Cell recovery was 2-3 million cells per adenohypophysis. The cells were suspended in an appropriate volume of Dulbecco's modified Eagle's medium (Gibco) to make a cell suspension of 0.3 - 0.4 million cells per milliliter. 0.5 ml of the cell suspension was distributed to each well of a MultiWell Tissue Culture plate (24 well) (Falcon). After the cells had been maintained in culture for 2 days under

5% CO2 - 95% air at 35 C, the prolactin releasing activity of the extracts was tested.

To test the activity of the extracts *in vivo*, normal male rats and hypophysectomized male rats (Canadian Breeding Farm and Laboratories) with an adenohypophysis grafted under the kidney capsule (7), were implanted with a silastic capsule containing estradiol (60 mg) 3 or more weeks before the experiment (8). An indwelling cannula was inserted into the right atrium as previously described (9).

The fractions derived from the posterior pituitaries were dissolved in 0.9% sterile saline and were administered as a bolus injection through the atrial cannula.

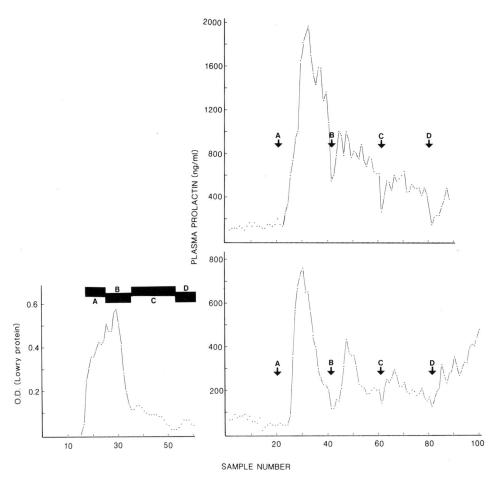

Figure 1. The optical density (O.D.) profile of bovine posterior pituitary extract filtered on a Sephadex G-25 column (left panel) and the effects of the fractions (equivalent of 2 posterior pituitaries) on prolactin release in extradiol primed male rats (right panel). The effects of bolus injections (arrow) of fraction groups A, B, C, and D on prolactin release in the rats were monitored by taking blood samples every 2 min (sample number x 2 = min). Each panel shows the result from an individual rat. Each datum point represents the mean value of a triplicate assay.

Approximately 70 ul of blood were withdrawn through the indwelling cannula every 2 min. The plasma samples were harvested as previously described (10) and triplicate samples of 10 ul plasma were assayed using an RIA kit for rat prolactin, supplied by the NIADDK (National Hormone and Pituitary Program). The coefficient of variation for interassay and intraassay variability were 14.6 and 7.2% respectively. Maximum sensitivity was 0.03 ng per tube. The quantity of prolactin was expressed in terms of NIADDK-rPRL-3.

Fractionation of the posterior pituitary tissue extract

Bovine posterior pituitaries, custom ordered from Bockneck Ltd, Toronto, were collected immediately after animal slaughtering and frozen individually on dry ice. They were then thawed in our laboratory at 0-3 C and cleared of other attached tissue such as small pieces of anterior pituitary. One batch of posterior pituitaries had a wet weight of 100 g. The mean weight of a single posterior pituitary was approximately 0.4 g. The posterior pituitaries were homogenized in a blender in 500 ml of chilled 1 M acetic acid and extracted for 24 h at 4 C. The extract was centrifuged at 10,000 x g for 30 min and eluted with 1 M acetic acid on a Sephadex G-25 fine column (3 x 90 cm).

A Lowry protein assay (11) showed that proteins were localized in fractions 17-34 (Fig. 1). The fractions after gel filtration on Sephadex G-25 were arbitrarily divided into 4 groups (A:17-24, B:25-34, C:35-52, D:53-60) and the prolactin releasing activity of each group (equivalent to 2 neurohypophyses) was tested in estradiol primed normal male rats. Prolactin releasing activity was found in the protein groups (Group A:17-24 and Group B:25-34) (Fig. 1).

Vasopressin can stimulate prolactin release (4). According to Schally et al. (12) vasopressin (molecular weight of 1000 dalton) is located in group C. However, the prolactin releasing activity of group C is only marginal when compared to that of groups A or B (Fig. 1).

ISOLATION OF PROLACTIN RELEASING ACTIVITY FROM OTHER PROTEINS

In order to purify and characterize the active component, the protein fractions (17-34) were subfractionated by gel filtration on Sephadex G-75. The fractions were pooled, the lyophilized powder was redissolved in 10 ml of 1 M acetic acid, applied on a Sephadex G-75 superfine column (3 x 40 cm), and eluted with 1 M acetic acid. Two major peaks were separated. The second peak is commonly known as the neurophysin fraction. The Sephadex G-75 fractions were subdivided into 4 groups (A:13-17, B18-23, C:24-28, D:29-35) and each group of fractions (equivalent to 2 neurohypophyses) was tested for its prolactin releasing activity. The major activity was found in the neurophysin fractions, fraction groups C and D (Fig. 2).

When the fractions from groups C and D were pooled and injected into estradiol primed normal male rats, they showed a dose-response relationship (Fig. 3). However, they did not stimulate prolactin release when administered to hypophysectomized rats with a grafted pituitary under the kidney capsule (Fig. 4).

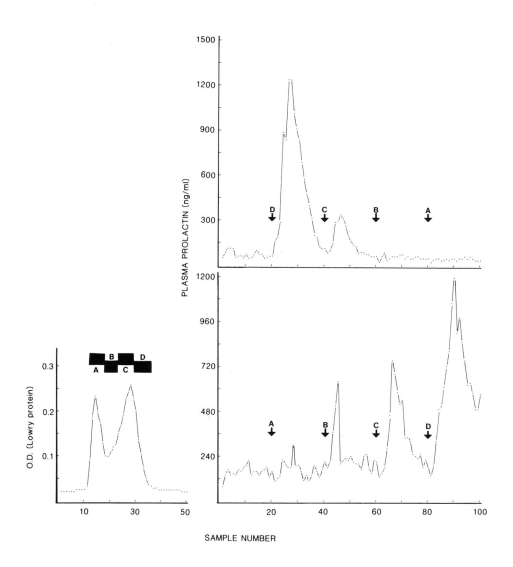

Figure 2. The optical density (O.D.) profile of the posterior pituitary protein fractions after filtration on Sephadex G-75 (left panel) and the effects of the G-75 fractions (equivalent of 2 posterior pituitaries) on prolactin release on estradiol primed male rats (right panels). The effects of bolus injections (arrow) of fractions groups A, B, C, and D in estradiol primed male rats were monitored by taking blood samples every 2 min (sample number x 2 = min). Each panel shows the results from an individual rat. Each datum point represents the mean value of a triplicate assay.

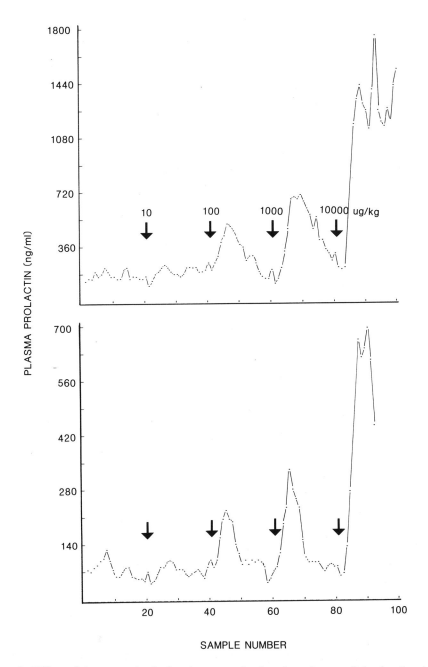

Figure 3. Effect of the neurophysin fraction on prolactin release in estradiol primed male rats. 10, 100, 1000, and 10000 ug/kg neurophysin (arrow) was injected as a bolus and plasma prolactin concentration was monitored by taking blood samples every 2 min (sample number x 2 = min). Each panel shows the results from an individual rat. Each datum point represents the mean value of a triplicate assay.

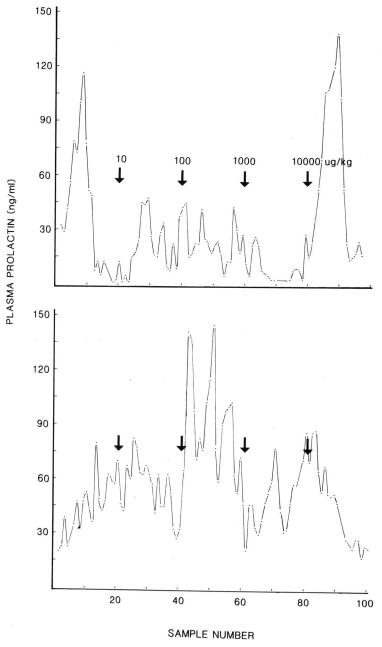

Figure 4. Effect of the neurophysin fraction on prolactin release in estradiol primed, hypophysectomized rats with an anterior pituitary grafted under the kidney capsule. 10, 100, 1000, and 10000 ug/kg neurophysin (arrow) was injected and plasma prolactin concentration was monitored by taking blood samples every 2 min (sample number x 2 = min). Each panel shows the results from an individual rat. Each datum point represents the mean value of a triplicate assay.

ISOLATION OF THE PROLACTIN RELEASING ACTIVITY
FROM THE NEUROPHYSIN FRACTION

After the gel filtration on Sephadex G-75, the biologically active (neurophysin) fraction was subfractionated by DEAE ion exchange chromatography. DEAE Sephadex A-25 (1.6 x 27 cm) was equilibrated with pyridine (0.823 M) acetate (pH 6.0). The second peak (the neurophysin fraction) fractionated on the Sephadex G-75 column was lyophilized, redissolved in 4 ml pyridine acetate buffer (pH 6.0), adjusted to pH 6.0 by adding 1 M NaOH, and discontinuously eluted with the pyridine (0.823 M) acetate buffer pH 6.0, pH 5.5 and 1 M acetic acid (13). The protein concentration was monitored by the Lowry protein assay.

We obtained neurophysin-I and neurophysin-II (Fig. 5) by a well established method developed by Breslow et al. (13). Polyacrylamide gel electrophoresis (PAGE) (14,15) separated the neurophysin fraction into 2 bands. The NP-I fraction showed 2 bands, a major band (NP-I) and second minor band, while the NP-II fraction presented only one band. PAGE was performed on a 7% gel (6 x 80 mm) at pH 9.5, with 5 mA/tube. The protein was stained with 0.25% Coomassie blue and the excess dye was removed by diffusion in an acetic acid:methanol:water (15:10:175) solution.

NP-I and NP-II were injected into estradiol primed male rats as a bolus. NP-I at doses of 10, 100, and 1000 ug/kg did not show any consistent dose-response relationship. However, NP-II elevated plasma prolactin to a much higher concentration than did NP-I, and, unlike NP-I, showed a dose-response relationship (Fig. 5). The lowest dose of NP-II needed to increase plasma prolactin concentration was 10 ug/kg. However, neither NP-I nor NP-II had any effect on prolactin release from dispersed adenohypophysial cells in a primary monolayer culture (Fig. 6). The results from the ectopic pituitary experiments and the *in vitro* experiments indicate that neurophysin does not stimulate prolactin release by acting directly on the lactotroph, but does so through an intermediary step.

PLASMA CONCENTRATION OF NEUROPHYSIN

The minimum effective dose of NP-II needed to elevate plasma prolactin concentration is 10 ug/kg in the estradiol-primed rat. A high concentration of vasopressin (approximately 14 ng/ml) is detected in the monkey portal blood (16). Since the molecular weight of NP is 10 times that of vasopressin, the concentration of NP expressed as weight/volume will also be 10 times higher (140 ng/ml) than that of vasopressin, if the two were released in an equimolar ratio. However, the mean concentration of NP in portal blood is 60 ng/ml in the monkey (16). Assuming that there is 50 ml of plasma per kg body weight, then the theoretical maximum plasma concentration of NP after an injection of 10 ug/kg is 200 ng/ml plasma. Therefore the dose is reasonably within the physiological concentration, since the stimulation of prolactin release would require a plasma concentration of neurophysin several times higher than that of basal concentration.

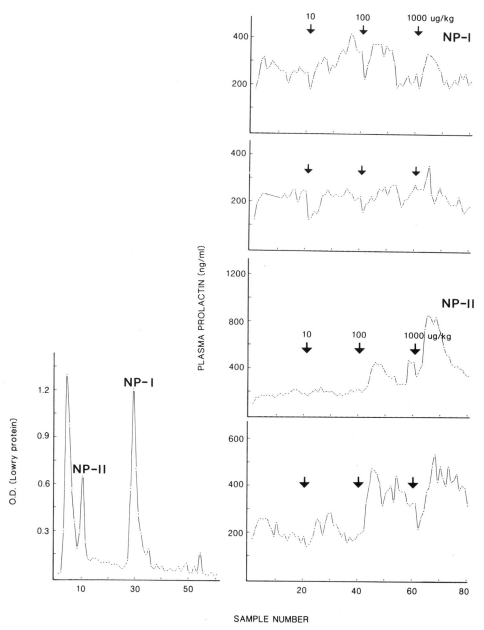

Figure 5. The optical density (O.D.) profile of neurophysins separated by ion exchange chromatography on DEAE Sephadex A-25 column (left panel). Neurophysin-I and neurophysin-II were prepared by discontinuous gradient elution. 10, 100 and 1,000 ug/kg of neurophysin-I (2 upper right panels) and neurophysin-II (2 lower right panels) were injected by a bolus (arrow) and plasma prolactin concentration was monitored by taking blood samples every 2 min (sample number x 2 = min). Each panel shows the results from an individual rat. Each datum point represents the mean value of a triplicate assay.

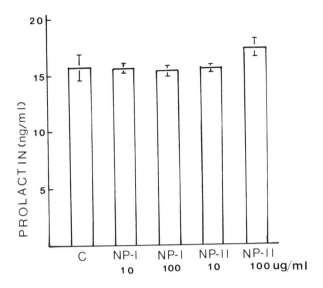

Figure 6. Effect of neurophysins-I and -II fractions on prolactin release from dispersed adenohypophysial cells in a primary cell culture. Samples (50 ul) of medium were obtained after a 1 h incubation. There were 6 wells for each condition, and the samples from each well were assayed in triplicate. Vertical bars represent mean ± SEM.

SUMMARY

There are several candidates for the PRF. One of the components of hypothalamic extracts known to have a stimulatory effect on prolactin release is thyrotropin releasing hormone (TRH) (17). However, TRH is not likely the sole nor major physiological PRF (1,8). Another strong candidate for the PRF is vasoactive intestinal polypeptide (VIP) (18) but further study is required before VIP can be accepted as the PRF.

During the course of our effort to identify and characterize the PRF, we have noticed that the neurohypophysis, an anatomical extension of the hypothalamus, has a strong stimulatory effect on prolactin release and that the major stimulatory activity was in the NP-II fraction.

Neurophysin is the carrier protein for neurohypophysial hormones. There are two major neurophysins, NP-I and NP-II. NP-I is the specific carrier protein for oxytocin and NP-II for vasopressin. Vasopressin and NP-II are synthesized in the hypothalamus as a single prohormone (19), transported down to the neurohypophysis (20, 21), and released together (22). It has been the general view that the physiological role of NP-II is that of carrier protein for vasopressin, and that the NPs do not have any major physiological effect.

These experiments have shown that neurophysin can stimulate prolactin release in the estrogen primed normal male rat. However, neurophysin does not have any effect on a monolayer culture of dispersed adenohypophysial cells nor on the ectopic pituitary under the kidney capsule, and thus we conclude that neurophysin acts indirectly to stimulate prolactin release. Therefore, neurophysin is not a PRF but does have a powerful effect on prolactin release.

ACKNOWLEDGMENTS

This work was supported by the Medical Research Council of Canada. Appreciation is expressed to Drs. A.F. Parlow and S. Raiti for supplying the prolactin radioimmunoassay kits through the NIAMDD Rat Pituitary Hormone Distribution Program, and to Miss Angela Street for excellent secretarial assistance.

REFERENCES

1. Shin SH. (1978): Life Sci 23:1813
2. Shin SH. (1979): Life Sci 25:1829
3. Shin SH. (1980): Neuroendocrinology 31:375
4. Shin SH. (1982): Neuroendocrinology 34:55
5. Shin SH. (1978): Life Sci 22:67
6. Hymer WC, Kraicer J, Bencosme SA, Haskill JS. (1972): Proc Soc Exp Biol Med 141:966
7. Shin SH, Reifel CW. (1981): Neuroendocrinology 32:139
8. Piercy M, Shin SH. (1980): Neuroendocrinology 31:270
9. Shin SH, Chi HJ. (1979): Neuroendocrinology 28:73
10. Chi HJ, Shin SH. (1978): Neuroendocrinology 26:193
11. Lowry OH, Rosebrough NJ, Farr AL, Randall RJ. (1951): J Biol Chem 193:265
12. Schally AV, Nair RMG, Redding TW, Arimura A. (1971): J Biol Chem 246:7230
13. Breslow E, Aanning HL, Abrash L, Schmir M. (1971): J Biol Chem 246:5172
14. Davis BJ. (1964): Ann NY Acad Sci 121:404
15. Ornstein L. (1964): Ann NY Acad Sci 121:321
16. Zimmerman EA, Carmel PW, Husain MK, Ferin M, Tannenbaum M, Frantz AG, Robinson AG. (1973): Science 182:925
17. Tashjian AH, Barowsky NJ, Jensen DK. (1971): Biochem Biophys Res Commun 109:382
18. Kato Y, Matsuhita N, Shimatsu A, Imura. (1983): In: Shizume K, Imura H, Shimazu N (eds) Endocrinology, International Congress Series 598 Excerpta Medica, Amsterdam p 136
19. Gainer H, Sarne Y, Brownstein MJ. (1977): J Cell Biol 73:366
20. Scharrer E, Scharra B. (1954): Rec Prog Hormone Res 10:183
21. Sachs H. Fawcett P, Takabatake Y, Portanova R. (1969): Rec Prog Hormone Res 25:447
22. Johnston GI, Hutchinson IS, Morris BJ, Day EM. (1975): Ann NY Acad Sci 248:272

Prolactin. Basic and clinical correlates
R.M. MacLeod, M.O. Thorner and U. Scapagnini (eds.),
Fidia Research Series, vol. I,
Liviana Press, Padova © 1985

Section II
Influence of brain factors
on prolactin secretion

STIMULATION BY GASTRIN RELEASING PEPTIDE AND NEUROTENSIN OF DOPAMINE RELEASE FROM RAT HYPOTHALAMUS: POSSIBLE INHIBITORY CONTROL OF PROLACTIN SECRETION

Yasuhiro Kabayama, Yuzuru Kato, Akira Shimatsu, Norio Matsushita, Hikaru Ohta, Katsuyoshi Tojo, and Hiroo Imura

Second Medical Clinic, Department of Medicine,
Kyoto University Faculty of Medicine
Sakyo-ku, Kyoto 606, Japan

The secretion of prolactin is tonically inhibited by the hypothalamus. Numerous studies have substantiated the role of hypothalamic dopamine as prolactin-inhibiting factor (PIF) (1). However, the regulation of dopamine release from the hypothalamus remains to be fully elucidated.

Gastrin releasing peptide (GRP), a 27 amino acid, was initially isolated from porcine gastrointestinal tract (2) and subsequently GRP-like immuno-reactivity was found in the rat hypothalamus (3). We have previously reported that rat prolactin release induced by a Met[5]-enkephalin analog, FK33-824, was inhibited by intraventricular injection of synthetic GRP (4). GRP did not affect either plasma prolactin levels produced by a high *in vivo* dose of domperidone, a dopamine antagonist, or prolactin release from the pituitary *in vitro*. FK33-824 stimulates prolactin secretion in the rat by inhibiting dopamine release from the median eminence (5). These findings suggest an involvement of dopamine in the inhibitory action of GRP on prolactin secretion.

Neurotensin (NT), a tridecapeptide originally isolated from bovine hypothalami (6), has a variety of actions on pituitary function. Prolactin secretion is stimulated by intravenous injection of NT in rats (7-9), whereas intraventricular injection of NT suppresses basal prolactin secretion (9) and prolactin release induced by stress (10) and 5-hydroxytryptophan, a precursor of serotonin (11). We also found that intraventricular injection of NT suppressed prolactin release induced by FK33-824 in conscious male rats (Fig. 1). Interruption of dopamine neurotransmission by either alpha-methyl-p-tyrosine or spiroperidol attenuated the inhibitory effect of NT on prolactin release (11), suggesting that the central dopaminergic system mediates the prolactin-inhibitory effect of NT.

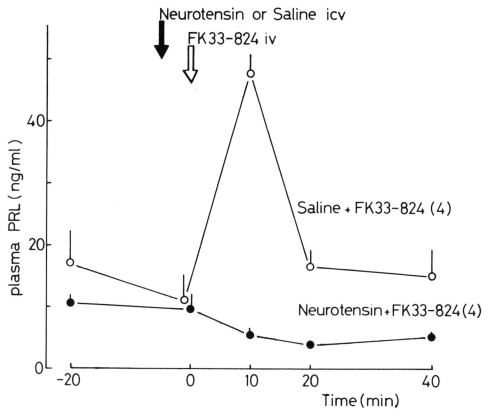

Figure 1. Effect of intraventricular injection of neurotensin on prolactin release induced by intravenous injection of FK33-824, a Met[5]-enkephalin analog, in conscious male rats. Neurotensin (3 nmol/rat) was injected into the lateral ventricle 3 min before the iv injection of FK33-824 (10 ug/100 g BW) in the rat with chronically implanted intraventricular and intraatrial catheters. In control animals, saline (10 ul/rat) was injected icv before FK33-824 injection.

We further examined the effects of GRP and NT on dopamine release from the rat hypothalamus *in vitro*. Wistar strain male rats weighing 250-300 g were sacrificed by decapitation, and hypothalamic fragments, defined by the anterior margin of the optic chiasm, the anterior margin of the mammillary bodies, the lateral hypothalamic nuclei, and a depth of 1.5 mm from the attachment of the stalk, were dissected. The fragments were bisected midsagittally and 16 hypothalamic halves (8 hypothalami equivalents) were placed on a Sephadex G-25 column, which was perifused with Krebs-Ringer bicarbonate buffer containing 10 mM glucose and 0.1% bovine serum albumin (KRBG, pH 7.4), saturated with a 95% O_2-5% CO_2 mixture, as described previously (12). The flow rate was 330 ul/min and fractions eluting from the perifusion column were collected every 5 min. Synthetic porcine GRP (Peninsula Lab, Belmont, Calif.) and NT (Peptide Res. Foundation, Mino, Japan) were dissolved in KRBG. KRBG solutions with high potassium (K^+) concentrations (20 mM and 56 mM) were obtained by substituting the equivalent amount of Na$^+$ with K$^+$. Calcium-free medium was prepared by replacement of CaCl$_2$ in KRBG with MgCl$_2$. The hypothalamic fragments were stimulated with a 5-min pulse of high K$^+$ with or without GRP (1 - 10 uM) and a 10-min pulse of GRP (1 uM) or NT (10 uM).

The dopamine concentration in the effluent was measured by high performance liquid chromatography and electro-chemical detection method after extraction with alumina according to a modification of the method described by Kissinger et al. (13) as shown in Figure 2. The minimum detectable dopamine concentration in this assay was 20 pg. The intra- and inter-assay coefficients of variation averaged 2.9% and 3.3%, respectively.

Statistical significance was evaluated by Student's t test, and one-way analysis of variance in combination with Duncan's new multiple range test.

ASSAY PROCEDURE

Sample 1.65
```
            5% EDTA , Na2S2O5                       100 µg
    |       3,4-dihydroxy benzylamine                 2 ng
            0.1 M Tris HCl PH 8.6                      4 ml
Shaking for 20 min.
    |
Aqueous layer was removed
    |
Alumina was washed with distilled water 3 times
    |
Alumina with 3 ml distilled water was applied on 0.2 um Microfilter
MF-1 ( BAS )
    |
Centrifugation 3000 rpm for 5 min.
    |       0.2 N HCl 100 µl
Vortex
    |       incubation 10 min. at room temperature
Centrifugation 3000 rpm for 5 min.
    |       0.2 N HCl 100 µl
Vortex
    |       incubation 10 min. at room temperature
Centrifugation 3000 rpm for 5 min.
    |
HPLC-ECD          SAMPLE      : 100 µl / 200 µl
                  COLUMN      : Yanapak ODS-T
                  CARRIER     : 0.1 M Citrate buffer
                                10% Methanole
                                0.08% 1-Octane sulfonic acid
                  Temperature : 25 - 28°C
                  FLOW RATE   : 1 ml / min.
                  DETECTOR    : electrochemical detector with
                                two glassy carbon electrodes
                                ( YANAKO VMD 501 )
                                0.525 - 0.700 V vs Ag / AgCl
```

Figure 2. Assay procedure for dopamine measurement in the effluent of the rat hypothalamic fragment perifused.

The spontaneous release of dopamine from rat hypothalamic fragments was rather stable after 60 min of preperifusion and then gradually decreased during the perifusion period of 100 min. When the hypothalamus was perifused with KRBG containing 20 mM K$^+$, dopamine release was rapidly increased (peak dopamine values: 20 mM K$^+$, 64.0 ± 5.2 vs 15.3 ± 1.56 pg/hypothalamus/5 min, p< 0.01) (Fig. 3). Dopamine release was increased more in hypothalamic fragments that were stimulated by a high dose of K$^+$ (56 mM) (1326 ± 284 pg/hypothalamus/5 min vs 20 mM K$^+$, p < 0.01). When calcium ions were removed from the perifusion medium, basal dopamine release and high K$^+$ (20 mM)-induced dopamine release were blunted.

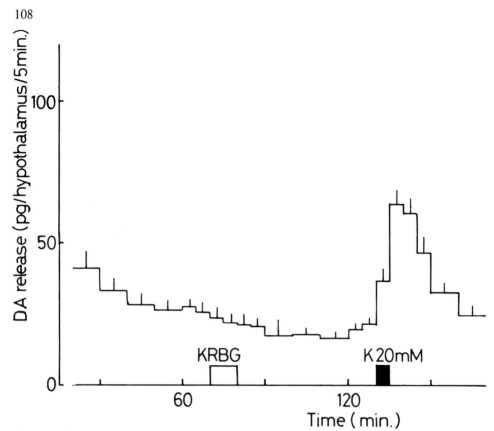

Figure 3. Spontaneous dopamine release from perifused rat hypothalamus and the effect of a high concentration (20 mM) of potassium (K^+). Values are the mean ± SE of dopamine released (pg/hypothalamus/5 min).

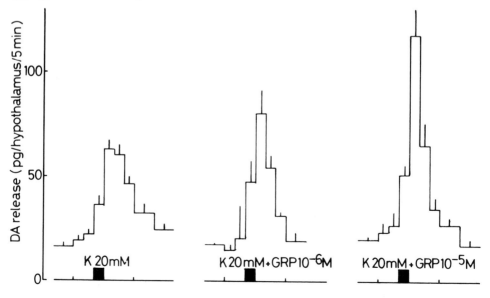

Figure 4. Effects of concomitant addition of high K^+ (20 mM) and GRP (1 uM and 10 uM) on dopamine release from perifused rat hypothalamus.

Dopamine release induced by high K$^+$ (20 mM) was significantly enhanced by concomitant addition of GRP (1 uM and 10 uM) in a dose-related manner (GRP 1 uM + 20 mM K$^+$, 80.2 + 4.0 and GRP 10 uM + 20 mM K$^+$, 115.9 $\pm$ 13.7 pg/hypothalamus/5 min) (Fig. 4).

GRP (10 uM) alone significantly stimulated basal dopamine release from the hypothalamic fragment perifused (GRP, 39.5 $\pm$ 2.8 vs KRBG, 25.3 $\pm$ 5.0 pg/hypothalamus/5 min, p < 0.05) (Fig. 5, 6).

Dopamine release from the hypothalamic fragments was also stimulated by NT (10 uM) infused for 10 min (NT 37.3 $\pm$ 5.9 vs KRBG 21.9 $\pm$ 3.1, p < 0.05) (Fig. 6).

In summary, using a perifusion system, we demonstrated the release of dopamine from rat hypothalamus by depolarizing concentrations of K$^+$ in a dose-related and Ca^{2+}-dependent manner. Dopamine release induced by high K$^+$ was enhanced by GRP in a dose-related manner. Basal dopamine release was also stimulated by GRP and NT.

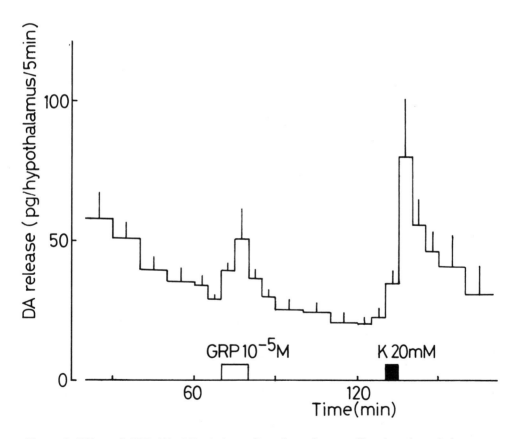

Figure 5. Effect of GRP (10 uM) on dopamine release from perifused rat hypothalamus.

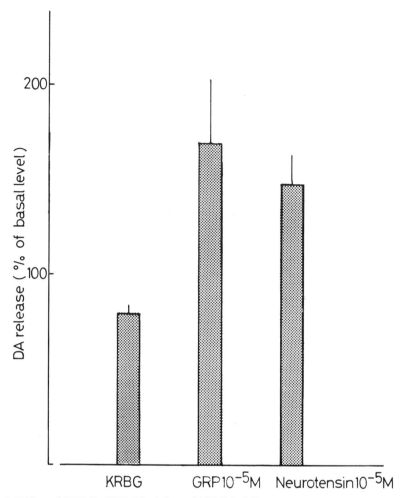

Figure 6. Effect of KRBG, GRP (10 uM), and NT (10 uM) on dopamine release from perifused rat hypothalamus. Values are the mean ± SE of % of basal levels.

The physiological significance of these findings remains to be further investigated. However, intraventricular injection of GRP (4) and NT (9-11) inhibits prolactin secretion in the rat and dopamine antagonists suppress prolactin secretion (4,11). Taking these studies together it is suggested that GRP and NT inhibit prolactin secretion by stimulating dopamine release from the hypothalamus into the hypophysial portal blood in the rat.

ACKNOWLEDGMENTS

This study was supported in part by grants from the Ministry of Education and the Ministry of Health and Welfare, Japan.

REFERENCES

1. Weiner RI, Ganong WF. (1978): Physiol Res 58:905
2. McDonald TJ, Journvall H, Nilsson G, Vabne M, Ghater MA, Bloom SR, Mutt V. (1979): Biochem Biophys Res Commun 90:227
3. Roth KA, Weber E, Barchas JD. 1982 Brain Res 251:277
4. Matsushita N, Kato Y, Katakami H, Shimatsu A, Yanaihara N, Imura H. (1983): Proc Soc Exp Biol Med 172:118
5. Matsushita N, Kato Y, Katakami H, Shimatsu A, Imura H. (1982): Endocrinol Jpn 29:277
6. Carraway R, Leeman SE. (1973): J Biol Chem 250:1907
7. Rivier C, Brown M, Vale W. (1977): Endocrinology 100:751
8. Kato Y, Abe H, Iwasaki Y, Iwasaki J, Imura H. (1978): Proc 6th Asia & Oceania Congr Endocrinol 1:341
9. Maeda K, Frohman L. (1978): Endocrinology 103:1903
10. Tache Y, Brown M, Collu R. (1979): Endocrinology 105:220
11. Koening JI, Mayfield MA, MacCann SM, Krulich L. (1982): Neuroendocrinology 35:277
12. Shimatsu A, Kato Y, Matsushita N, Katakami H, Yanaihara N, Imura H. (1983): Endocrinology 110:2113
13. Kissinger PT, Refshauge R, Dreiling R, Adams RN. (1973): Anal Lett 6:465

Prolactin. Basic and clinical correlates
R.M. MacLeod, M.O. Thorner and U. Scapagnini (eds.),
Fidia Research Series, vol. I,
Liviana Press, Padova © 1985

Section II
Influence of brain factors
on prolactin secretion

PRESENCE OF PROLACTIN SYNTHESIS-INHIBITORY FACTOR ACTIVITY IN THE HAMSTER STALK-MEDIAN EMINENCE: EFFECTS OF BLINDING AND PINEALECTOMY

K. Michael Orstead and David E. Blask

Department of Anatomy, College of Medicine
The University of Arizona
Tucson, Arizona

The photoperiodic environment plays an important role in the secretion of prolactin in a number of mammalian species, particularly those that are seasonally breeding animals (1,2). The Syrian hamster (*Mesocricetus auratus*) represents one species in which the long-term control of prolactin is intimately linked with the effects of photoperiod on seasonal reproductive physiology (3,4).

In both male and female hamsters that are either blinded or exposed to short photoperiod, pituitary levels of immunoreactive prolactin are consistently reduced by as much as 80% compared with normal animals, while blood levels have been reported to be either decreased or unaltered (5,6). In general, the effects of short photoperiod or light-deprivation on prolactin are either partially or completely prevented by removal of the pineal gland (3,5).

Little is known about the neuroendocrine control of prolactin synthesis, storage, or secretion in either normal or light-deprived hamsters. Therefore, the purpose of the present investigation was to determine whether stalk-median eminence extracts from normal female hamsters contain prolactin-release inhibitory factor (PIF) activity and whether PIF activity is altered by light-deprivation, either alone or in combination with pinealectomy.

A large group of adult female hamsters were divided into the following three subgroups: Intact, blind plus sham-pinealectomized (Blind-Sham) and blind plus pinealectomized (Blind-Pinx). Blinding was performed by bilateral orbital enucleation. Pinealectomy was accomplished by techniques described previously (7). The sham procedure was identical to that for pinealectomy, except the pineal was not removed. All operations were performed under ether anesthesia. After surgery, the animals were housed in a light:dark cycle of 14:10 for 12 weeks.

Upon sacrifice, truncal blood was collected and the serum stored frozen until assayed

114

for prolactin. Neutralized, acidic stalk-median eminence (SME) extracts were prepared from each of the three groups of hamsters using a modification of a protocol previously described (8). Briefly, following decapitation and removal of the brain, the SME region of the mediobasal hypothalamus was excised; the vertical depth of the cut was approximately 0.5 mm. Each SME region, which weighed approximately 2.0 mg, was placed into a glass homogenization tube containing ice-cold 0.1 N HCl; the SME regions from 54 animals in each group were pooled in 3.0 ml HCl for a concentration of 18 SME/ml. The pooled SME regions were homogenized and then centrifuged. The extracts were neutralized to pH 7.6 with NaOH. Appropriate dilutions of the stock SME extracts were made with Kreb's Ringer bicarbonate buffer containing 100 mg% glucose (KRB) to obtain final concentrations of 0.5, 1.0, 2.0, and 4.0 eq of SME/ml.

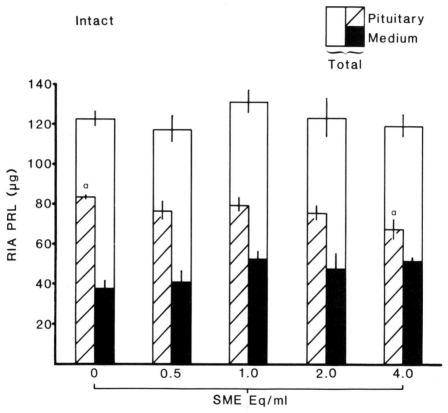

Figure 1. The mean total (open bars), pituitary (cross-hatched bars), and media (solid bars) amounts of immunoreactive prolactin (RIA-PRL) contained in vials following the incubation of anterior pituitaries from adult female hamsters with increasing concentrations of equivalents (Eq) of stalk median eminence (SME) extracts from Intact female hamsters. There were 6 vials per group and 3 hemipituitaries per vial. Total amounts (medium + pituitaries) of prolactin are expressed as ug/vial, pituitary prolactin as ug/gland and media prolactin as ug/ml. Vertical lines from top of bars represent SEM. Prolactin levels with the same superscript represent values that are significantly different from one another. Pituitary: a, p < 0.05.

Anterior pituitary glands from adult female hamsters were hemisected and the hemipituitaries distributed among incubation vials containing 1 ml of KRB such that there were 3 hemipituitaries per vial. Following a 1 h preincubation period the media were replaced with 1 ml of KRB containing 10 uCi of [³H]-leucine and various concentrations of SME as listed above; control vials did not contain SME. The hemipituitaries were incubated in either the presence or absence of SME for an additional 2 h. At the end of the incubation the pituitaries were homogenized in 0.1 M PBS and stored frozen with the media for subsequent determination of newly synthesized as well as immunoreactive prolactin.

Labeled prolactin was assayed by polyacrylamide disc gel electrophoresis followed by liquid scintillation spectrophotometry of the prolactin band (9,10). Prolactin synthesis was defined as the total amounts (medium + pituitaries) of [³H]-leucine incorporated into prolactin *in vitro*.

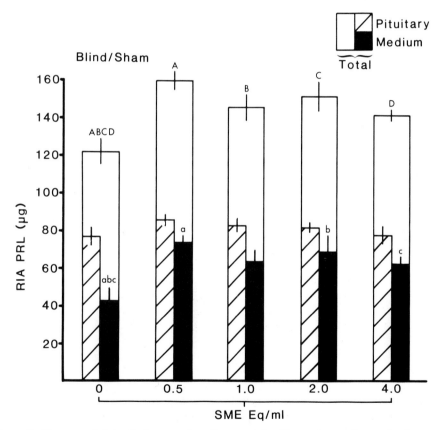

Figure 2. The mean total, pituitary, and media amounts of immunoreactive prolactin contained in vials following the incubation of anterior pituitaries from adult female hamsters with increasing concentrations of equivalents (Eq) of stalk median eminence (SME) extracts from Blind-Sham female hamsters. For further details refer to the legend of Figure 1. Total: A, p < 0.005; B-D, p < 0.05. Medium: a-c, p < 0.05.

Immunoreactive prolactin levels in sera, media, and pituitaries were measured with the use of a recently-developed homologous radioimmunoassay for hamster prolactin (11).

Surprisingly, at no concentration tested did the addition of SME extracts obtained from intact female hamsters either inhibit or stimulate the release of immunoreactive prolactin *in vitro* (Fig. 1). However, SME from Blind-Sham hamsters, compared with controls, stimulated the release of prolactin at each dose tested. Additionally, the total amount (media + pituitaries) of immunoreactive prolactin was significantly greater in the vials containing the SME from Blind-Sham animals than in the control vials (Fig. 2). Figure 3 reveals that SME extracts from Blind-Pinx hamsters, like extracts of the Intact group, neither stimulated nor inhibited the release of prolactin.

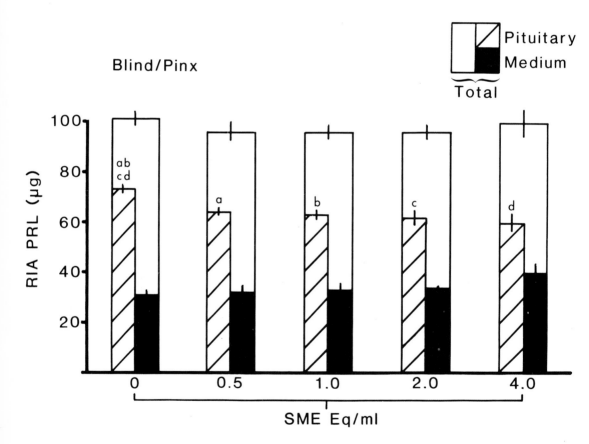

Figure 3. The mean total, pituitary and media amounts of immunoreactive prolactin contained in vials following the incubation of anterior pituitaries from adult female hamsters with increasing concentrations of equivalents (Eq) of stalk median eminence (SME) extracts from Blind-Pinx female hamsters. For further details refer to the legend of Figure 1. Pituitary: a-d, $p < 0.005$.

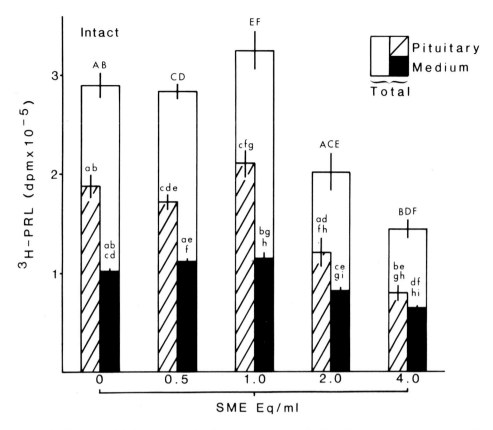

Figure 4. The mean total (open bars), pituitary (cross-hatched bars) and media amounts (solid bars) of newly-synthesized [³H]-prolactin contained in vials following the incubation of anterior pituitaries from adult female hamsters with increasing concentrations of equivalents (Eq) of stalk median eminence (SME) extracts from Intact female hamsters. Total amounts (medium + pituitaries) of [³H]-prolactin are expressed as dpm/vial, pituitary as dpm/gland and medium as dpm/ml. There were 6 vials per group and 3 hemipituitaries per vial. Vertical lines from top of bars represent SEM. [³H]-prolactin levels with the same superscript represent values that are significantly different from one another. Total: A-F, p < 0.001. Pituitary: a,b,e-g, p < 0.001; c,h, p < 0.05; d, p < 0.005. Medium: a,b, p < 0.05; c-h, p <0.001; i, p < 0.005.

In Figure 4 it can be seen that exposure of pituitaries to SME extract from Intact hamsters (2.0 or 4.0 eq/ml) resulted in a significant reduction, relative to controls, in the incorporation of [³H]-leucine into newly synthesized prolactin. Interestingly, prolactin synthesis actually appeared to be stimulated in pituitaries exposed to 1.0 SME eq/ml. In contrast, SME extracts from Blind-Sham hamsters only inhibited the incorporation of [³H]-leucine into prolactin by about 21% at the highest concentration of extract (Fig. 5). Unlike the extracts from Intact animals (Fig. 4), 1.0 SME eq/ml from Blind-Sham hamsters did not stimulate incorporation of tritiated-leucine into prolactin

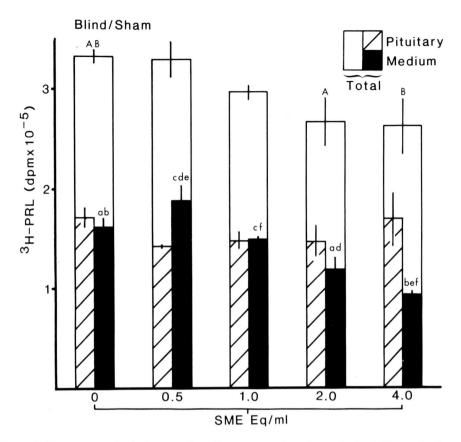

Figure 5. The mean total, pituitary, and media amounts of newly-synthesized [³H]-prolactin contained in vials following the incubation of anterior pituitaries from adult female hamsters with increasing concentrations of equivalents (Eq) of stalk median eminence (SME) extracts from Blind-Sham female hamsters. For further details refer to the legend of Figure 4. Total: A,B, p < 0.05. Medium: a,c, p < 0.05; b,d,e, p < 0.001; f, p < 0.005.

(Fig. 5). Figure 6 reveals that SME tissue extracts from Blind-Pinx hamsters markedly inhibited prolactin synthesis at the two highest concentrations similar to the inhibition produced by the extracts from Intact animals.

Serum levels of immunoreactive prolactin from Blind-Sham SME donor animals were significantly decreased by about 66% as compared with both Intact and Blind-Pinx hamsters (data not shown). Additionally, the amount of stored immunoreactive prolactin, as well as newly synthesized prolactin, was decreased by about 88% in the pituitaries of the Blind-Sham SME donors as compared with pituitaries of Intact controls. While pinealectomy prevented the blinding-induced decrease in stored immunoreactive prolactin it did not, however, alter the blinding-induced suppression of [³H]-leucine incorporation into newly synthesized prolactin (unpublished data).

The results of the present investigation indicate that the Syrian hamster differs from the albino rat with respect to the neuroendocrine control of prolactin. For example, whereas either hypothalamic or SME extracts from rats inhibit the release of immunoreactive prolactin from the anterior pituitary gland *in vitro* (12), this does not seem to be the case in hamsters. This is indeed puzzling inasmuch as the transplantation of hamster anterior pituitary glands beneath the kidney capsule results in a hypersecretion of prolactin (13) as occurs in the rat. Ostensibly, these findings indicate that, like the rat, the hypothalamus of the hamster exerts a tonic inhibitory control over the secretion of immunoreactive prolactin. Indeed, an earlier study employing

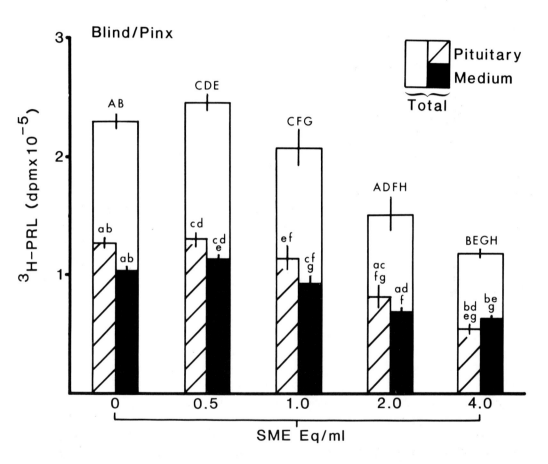

Figure 6. The mean total, pituitary, and media amounts of newly-synthesized prolactin contained in vials following the incubation of anterior pituitaries from adult female hamsters with increasing concentrations of equivalents (Eq) of stalk median eminence (SME) extracts from Blind-Pinx female hamsters. For further details refer to the legend of Figure 4. Total: A,B,D-G, p < 0.001; C,H, P < 0.05. Pituitary: a-e, p < 0.001; f, p < 0.01; g, p < 0.05. Medium: a,b,d-g, p < 0.001; c, p < 0.005.

neutralized acid extracts of whole hypothalamus from female hamsters demonstrated that release of immunoreactive prolactin was inhibited *in vitro* (14). Discrepancies between this study and our own may reflect methodological differences, such as the amount of hypothalamic tissue used as well as the incubation time which was shorter in the Donofrio et al. study (14).

Unexpectedly, extracts of SME from Intact hamsters inhibited the incorporation of [^{3}H]-leucine into newly synthesized prolactin in a dose-dependent manner. We are unaware of any report of similar effects of rat SME extracts on prolactin synthesis. These results suggest that the hamster SME contains a factor(s) which preferentially inhibits the synthesis of prolactin rather than the release of its storage form(s). This prolactin-synthesis inhibitory factor (PSIF) activity could be due to one or more substances present in the extracts (dopamine? GABA?). It could also be argued that these extracts may be stimulating the degradation of prolactin in addition to inhibiting its synthesis (15). However, the use of a relatively short incubation time makes this possibility less likely since it takes dopamine, a stimulator of prolactin degradation, several hours to increase prolactin degradation (15,16). Still another possibility is that the extracts could have altered the uptake of tritiated-leucine by pituitary glands (17).

Interestingly, blinding resulted in a decrease in PSIF activity in SME extracts, since the inhibition of incorporation of [^{3}H]-leucine into newly synthesized prolactin was not as great as in pituitaries exposed to intact SME extracts. Additionally, SME extracts from the Blind-Sham group exhibited prolactin-releasing factor (PRF) activity since the release and total amount of immunoreactive prolactin was increased in pituitaries exposed to these extracts. Since the mediobasal hypothalamic content of immunoreactive TRH is increased in blind female hamsters versus normal hamsters (18), it is possible that PRF activity detected in extracts from blind animals is due to increased TRH. The suppressed prolactin synthesis, storage, and secretion observed in blind animals (unpublished results) might be explained on the basis of an increased release of a PSIF coupled with an inhibition of release of a PRF (TRH?). This could account for the decrease in PSIF activity as well as the increase in PRF activity in SME extracts from Blind-Sham hamsters.

The PSIF activity in SME extracts from Blind-Pinx hamsters was virtually identical to activity observed in extracts from Intact animals. Moreover, like the extracts from the intact group, SME extracts from the Blind-Pinx group did not exhibit the PRF activity seen in the Blind-Sham animals. These data indicate that the blind-induced alterations in SME PSIF and PRF activities are mediated by the pineal gland.

In conclusion, this is the first study to demonstrate the presence of PSIF activity in SME extracts from normal hamsters. Our data suggest that there may be fundamental differences between the hamster and the rat with regard to neuroendocrine regulation of prolactin. Additionally, we have provided the first evidence that light-deprivation and pinealectomy influence the level of bioassayable hypothalamic prolactin-regulating activities. Finally, this study suggests that the marked inhibition of prolactin synthesis, storage, and secretion in light-deprived female hamsters may involve a pineal-induced alteration in the synthesis and/or release of hypothalamic substances that regulate the activity of the prolactin cell in this seasonally-breeding, photoperiodically-sensitive species.

ACKNOWLEDGMENTS

Supported in part by a University of Arizona Graduate Student Research Development Grant. The authors wish to thank Dr. Frank Talamantes of the University of California, Santa Cruz, for the generous supply of hamster prolactin antiserum and purified hamster prolactin used in the RIA.

REFERENCES

1. Reiter RJ. (1980): Endocr Revs 1:109
2. Kennaway DJ, Obst JM, Dunstan EA, Friesen HG. (1981): Endocrinology 108:639
3. Reiter RJ. (1975): J Exp Zool 191:111
4. Reiter RJ, Johnson LY. (1974): Neuroendocrinology 14:310
5. Reiter RJ, Johnson LY. (1974): Horm Res 5:311
6. Borer KT, Kelch RP, Corley K. (1982): Neuroendocrinology 35:13
7. Hoffman RA, Reiter RJ. (1965): Anat Rec 153:19
8. Ratner A, Meites J. (1964): Endocrinology 75:377
9. Reisfield RA, Lewis UJ, Williams DE. (1962): Nature (Lond.) 195:281.
10. MacLeod RM, Lehmeyer JE. (1974): Endocrinology 94:1077
11. Soares MJ, Colosi P, Talamantes F. (1983): Proc Soc Exp Biol Med 172:379
12. Talwalker PK, Ratner A, Meites J. (1963): Am J. Physiol 205:213
13. Bartke A, Goldman BD, Bex FJ, Kelch RP, Smith MS, Dalterio S, Doherty PC. (1980): Endocrinology 106:167
14. Donofrio RJ, Reiter RJ, Sorrentino S, Blask DE, Talbot JA. (1973/74): Neuroendocrinology 13:79
15. Maurer RA. (1980): Biochemistry 19:3573
16. Dannies PS, Rudnick MS. (1980): J Biol Chem 255:2776
17. Dannies PS. (1982): Biochem Pharmacol 31:2845
18. Vriend J, Wilber JF. (1983): Horm Res 17:108

Prolactin. Basic and clinical correlates
R.M. MacLeod, M.O. Thorner and U. Scapagnini (eds.),
Fidia Research Series, vol. I,
Liviana Press, Padova © 1985

Section II
Influence of brain factors
on prolactin secretion

EPISODIC AND PULSATILE SECRETION OF PROLACTIN IN THE LACTATING RAT

Gyorgy Nagy, Balint Kacsoh and Bela Halasz

2nd Department of Anatomy, Semmelweis University Medical School
Tuzolto u. 58 Budapest, Hungary H-1450

It is well established that the separation of the maternal rat from her pups causes a rapid and marked decrease of plasma prolactin levels (1,2) and that after some hours of separation, suckling stimulus results in a very rapid increase in plasma prolactin concentration (3-6). If the non-suckling period is longer than 12 h or less than 4 h the hypophyseal depletion mechanism becomes refractory to the stimulus (7). Under normal conditions, pups are attached to the nipples for more than 12 hours/day. The frequency of suckling is about 50-80 times a day (8). The young suckle continuously for several hours independently whether or not they obtain milk. It is generally assumed that during lactation the levels of plasma prolactin are constantly high.

Recent data indicate that there are circadian rhythms in plasma prolactin (9) and corticosterone concentrations (9,10) of lactating rats.

It is well known that prolactin is secreted in a pulsatile manner in freely behaving female and male rats (11-15). Less is known about the secretion pattern of prolactin during free lactation. Therefore the aim of this study was to determine the pattern of prolactin in freely behaving lactating rats and to investigate the role of the serotonergic and norepinephrinergic system in this pattern.

Primiparous lactating Wistar strain rats were used on days 8-10 of lactation (the day of parturition was considered as day 1). They were housed in individual cages in an air conditioned room with alternating 14 h light: 10 h darkness. The animals received food and water ad libitum. Litter size was reduced to 8 on the second day postpartum. Serial blood samples were taken from freely behaving mothers between 08.30 and 10.20 and between 14.30 and 16.30 at 10 min intervals or between 08.30 and 09.40 and between 14.30 and 15.30 at 5 min intervals. At each time 100-150 ul of blood was withdrawn via chronic cannula implanted into the right jugular vein two or three days prior to testing. The cannulation technique and blood sampling procedure are described elsewhere (16). To study the role of the serotonergic system neurotoxin lesion of the dorsal raphe nucleus (DR) and hypothalamic suprachiasmatic region (SCR) were performed on day 2 of lactation by microinjecting 5.5 ug 5,7-dihydroxytryptamine (5,7-DHT, Sigma Chemical Co.,) in 2 ul 0.5% ascorbic acid in saline within 10 min using a Hamilton microsyringe. Twenty minutes prior to the injection of 5,7-DHT the animals received 25 mg/kg, ip. desmethylimipramine (DMI) in saline to prevent norepinephrine depletion. FLA-63, a specific dopamine-beta-hydroxilase (DBH) inhibitor was injected (25 mg/kg, ip.) 2 or 26 h prior to the blood sampling to investigate the role of the norepinephrinergic system.

In freely behaving lactating rats the individual curves exhibited marked fluctuations both in the morning (Fig. 1) and afternoon (Fig. 2) sampling periods. During the morning period the mean prolactin level gradually decreased. In the afternoon two episodic bursts could be separated, one around 15.00 and another one around 16.00 h. The time period between the peak values was 54 ± 6.8 min. The ANOVA test showed the mean afternoon curve to be non-significant ($p > 0.05$), presumably because the individual secretion patterns were not synchronous. The mean prolactin level in the morning (175.5 ± 15.8 ug/L) was significantly lower ($p < 0.01$) than in the afternoon (505.1 ± 32.0 ug/L).

There are pulsatile fluctuations in plasma prolactin levels both in the morning period and during the afternoon episode.

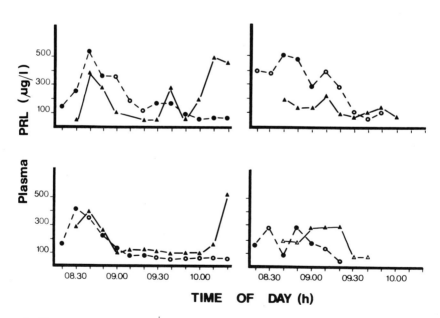

Figure 1. Changes in plasma prolactin levels within a two hour period (from 08.30 to 10.30) in the morning, sampling every 10 min; 8 individual prolactin curves. (solid symbols, mother is in contact with her pups; empty symbols, absence of contact).

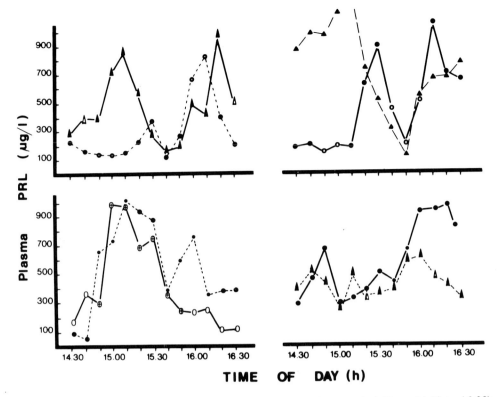

Figure 2. Changes in plasma prolactin levels within a two hour period (from 14.30 to 16.30) in the afternoon, sampling every 10 min; 8 individual prolactin curves. (solid symbols, mother is in contact with her pups; empty symbols, absence of contact).

Figure 3 shows two representative cases, sampling at 5 min intervals between 08.30 and 09.40 h and between 14.30 and 15.30 h. When the amplitude and period time were calculated we found that the period time was nearly equal in the morning (18.5 ± 0.8 min) and the afternoon (13.5 ± 0.9 min), and the amplitude in the morning was smaller than that calculated in the afternoon. The fluctuations (episodic and pulsatile) were not under a strict control of the suckling stimulus; there were low hormone levels when the pups were suckling the nipples and also elevated values when the mother was away from her pups (Figs. 1, 2, 3).

In the next experiment we investigated the effect of the injection of 5,7-DHT into the dorsal raphe nucleus (DR) and into the hypothalamic suprachiasmatic region (SCR) on the afternoon prolactin pattern. Figure 4 demonstrates that the episodic secretion pattern was not modified by sham operation (Fig. 4a). Also, 6-7 days after DR lesion the individual curves show marked fluctuations but the episodic bursts are concentrated around 15.00 h. (Fig. 4b). 5,7-DHT injection into the SCR did not cause any change in the episodic pattern of the afternoon prolactin levels (Fig. 4c).

In rats pretreated with FLA-63 2 h prior to blood sampling, the afternoon prolactin episode was completely suppressed. Injection of the enzyme inhibitor 26 h prior to testing did not cause any change (Fig. 5b,c).

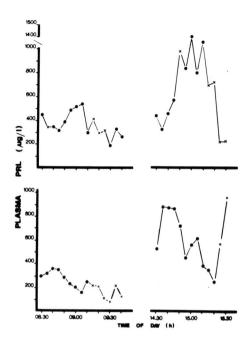

Figure 3. Two individual prolactin curves comparing the morning secretion pattern and the afternoon pattern (5 min intervals).

The present findings are in agreement with the previously described (9) lactationary circadian plasma prolactin rhythm in the rat.

Further, prolactin seems to be secreted in episodes. We found one episode in the morning, that was followed by gradual decay to low levels reaching the daily trough. In the afternoon, two episodes of high amplitude were observed; the interepisode level being much higher than the daily minimum.

We could not detect correlation between suckling activity and prolactin values. If the mother is separated from her litter, there is a complete block in prolactin release lasting about 3-7 minutes and it is followed by a partial block of prolactin secretion (2). This phenomenon could be called "separation-induced prolactin decrease". After separation, the suckling stimulus results in a rapid elevation in plasma prolactin levels (3-6).

The contradiction between this experiment and the above mentioned literary data can be resolved by supposing different regulatory mechanisms of prolactin in freely behaving lactating rats and in separation-suckling stimulus experimental conditions. The suckling-induced prolactin response can be prevented by inhibiting the serotonergic (17-21) but not the norepinephrinergic (22) system. Further, in female rats intracerebroventricular administration of 5,7-DHT had no effect on the ability to release prolactin at proestrus or during lactation although brain serotonin (5-HT) levels were 35% of control levels (23). Intracerebroventricularly administered 5-HT elevates prolactin in-

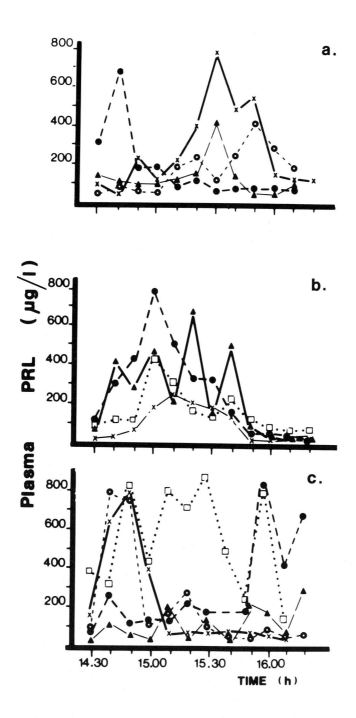

Figure 4. Individual plasma prolactin levels between 14.30 and 16.30 in controls (a), and in rats injected with 5,7-DHT (5-5 ug/rat) into the DR (b), or into the SCR (c), 6-7 day earlier.

128

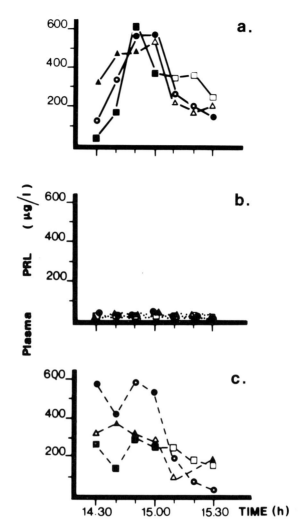

Figure 5. Individual plasma prolactin levels between 14.30 and 15.30 in controls (a), and in rats pretreated with FLA-63 (25 mg/kg bw. ip.) 2 h (b), and 26 h (c), prior to sampling.

dependently of the dopamine concentration in the portal circulation (24), probably through some prolactin-releasing factor(s). There are evidences that DR is involved in the serotonergic mediation of prolactin release (25-27). Also, the serotonergic afferents to the SCR are a major target of 5-HT fibers concerned with rhythmic regulation (28-31). These afferents are necessary to generate the afternoon prolactin surge, at least in ovariectomized, estrogen-treated non-lactating rats (32). On the other hand our present findings show that pharmacological lesion of the serotonergic elements of the DR or SCR does not affect the high afternoon prolactin levels during lactation (Fig. 4).

Since a number of pharmacological studies indicate that norepinephrinergic neurons may play a stimulatory role in the phasic release of the adenohypophyseal hormones (13,33-34), it is not surprising that FLA-63, a specific dopamine-beta hydroxylase inhibitor causing a 50-60% decrease of hypothalamic norepinephrine content (35), prevented the afternoon prolactin episodes (Fig. 5).

In summary, free lactation is characterized by episodic and pulsatile prolactin secretion. Prolactin changes appear to be independent from the actual suckling activity. These findings confirm our previous suggestion (9,16) that the control of prolactin secretion during free lactation is different from that occurring when separation- and suckling-induced changes are examined.

ACKNOWLEDGMENTS

We would like to thank Dr. Albert Parlow and NIAMDD for providing us with the rat prolactin kit. The excellent technical assistance of Mrs. I. Balazs and Mrs. I. Dukony are gratefully acknowledged.

REFERENCES

1. Chiocchio SR, Cannata MA, Cordero Funes JR, Tramezzani JH. (1979): Endocrinology 105:544
2. Nagy G, Halasz B. (1983): Neuroendocrinology 37:459
3. Kwa HG, Verhofstadt F. (1968) In: Gaul C (ed) Progress in Endocrinology. Excerpta Medica, Amsterdam, p 979
4. Amenomori Y, Nellor IE. (1969): Fed Proc 28:505
5. Krulich L, Kuhn E, Illner P, McCann SM. (1970): Fed Proc 29:579
6. Terkel J, Blake CA, Sawyer CH. (1972): Endocrinology 91:49
7. Grosvenor CE, Mena F. (1982) In: Muller EE, MacLeod RM (eds) *Neuroendocrine Perspectives*. Elsevier Biomedical Press, New York, vol 1:69
8. Tindal IS. (1978) In: Larson BL (ed) *Lactation*. London Academic Press, New York, vol 4:67
9. Kacsoh B, Nagy G. (1983): Endocrinologia Exp 17:301
10. Tachi N, Tomogane H, Yokoyama A. (1981): Physiol Behav 27:481
11. Willoughby IO, Brazean P, Martin B. (1977): Endocrinology 101:1298
12. Shin SH, Chi HJ. (1979): Neuroendocrinology 28:73
13. Negro-Vilar A, Ojeda SR, Advis JP, McCann SM. (1979): Endocrinology 105:86
14. Wiersma I. (1981): Neuroendocrinology 33:288
15. Sarkar DK, Miki N, Meites J. (1983): Endocrinology 113:1452
16. Nagy G, Kacsoh B, Halasz B. (1984): Neuroendocrinology (in press)
17. Kordon C, Blake CA, Terkel J. Sawyer CA. (1973/74): Neuroendocrinology 13:213
18. Gallo RV, Rabii J, Moberg GP. (1975): Endocrinology 97:1096
19. Rowland D, Steel M, Moltz H. (1978): Neuroendocrinology 26:8
20. Mena F, Enjalbert A, Carbonell L, Priam M, Kordon C. (1976): Endocrinology 99:445
21. Barofsky A-L, Taylor I, Massari VJ. (1983): Endocrinology 113:1894
22. Carr LA, Conway PM, Voogt JL. (1977): Brain Research 133:305
23. Clemens IA, Smalstig EB, Fuller RW. (1977): Fed Proc 36:277
24. Pilotte NS, Porter JC. (1981): Endocrinology 108:2137
25. Advis JP, Simpkins JW, Bennett I, Meites J. (1978): Life Sci 24:359

26. Van de Kar LD, Bethea CL. (1982): Neuroendocrinology 35:225
27. Fesler RG, Deyo SN, Meltzer HY, Miller RJ. (1984): Brain Research 299:231
28. Meyer DC, Quay WB. (1976): Endocrinology 98:1160
29. Szafarczyk A, Ixart G, Malaval F, Nouguier-Soule J, Assenmacher I. (1979): J Endocrinol 83:1
30. Dunn JD, Johnson DC, Castro AJ, Swenson R. (1980): Neuroendocrinology 31:85
31. Hery M, Dusticier G, Faudon M, Barrit MC, Hery F. (1981): J Physiol (Paris) 77:497
32. Kawakami M, Arita J, Yoshioka E. (1980): Endocrinology 106:1087
33. Weiner R, Ganong WF. (1978): Physiological Reviews 58:905
34. Gallo RV. (1980): Neuroendocrinology 30:122
35. Simonyi A, Kanyicska B, Szentendrei T, Fekete MIK. (1984): European Journal of Pharmacology 98:285

Prolactin. Basic and clinical correlates
R.M. MacLeod, M.O. Thorner and U. Scapagnini (eds.),
Fidia Research Series, vol. I,
Liviana Press, Padova © 1985

Section II
Influence of brain factors
on prolactin secretion

STIMULATION OF PROLACTIN SECRETION
BY PEPTIDE HISTIDINE ISOLEUCINE (PHI) IN THE RAT
IN VIVO AND *IN VITRO*

Hikaru Ohta, Yuzuru Kato, Katsuyoshi Tojo, Akira Shimatsu, Tatsuhide inoue, Yasuhiro Kabayama, and Hiroo Imura

Second Medical Clinic, Department of Medicine, Kyoto University
Faculty of Medicine, Sakyo-ku, Kyoto 606, Japan

Peptide histidine isoleucine (PHI), one of the newly identified brain-gut peptides, consists of 27 amino acids and has a remarkable sequence homology with vasoactive intestinal polypeptide (VIP) (1). Both PHI and VIP may be derived from a common precursor molecule (2,3). We have previously reported the coexistence of PHI and VIP in rat hypophysial portal blood and their concentrations were about 7 times higher than in the peripheral blood (4).

It is well known that VIP stimulates prolactin secretion by acting, at least in part, directly at the pituitary in the rat (5-7) and other species (8-10). The stimulating effect of PHI on prolactin release was recently reported in incubated rat anterior pituitary cells (11,12). However, the role of PHI in regulating the secretion of prolactin remains to be fully elucidated.

In the present study, we examined the effect of PHI on prolactin secretion in the rat *in vivo* and *in vitro*. Male Wistar rats weighing 250-300 g were used throughout the experiments. In *in vivo* experiments, drugs were administered into the lateral ventricle in a volume of 10 ul/rat or intravenously in a volume of 0.1 ml/100 g BW in urethane-anesthetized rats (5) or in conscious animals with chronically implanted intraatrial and intraventricular catheters (13). Blood samples of 0.5 ml were collected from the jugular vein immediately before and at intervals of 5 to 20 min after the injection of test substances. In *in vitro* experiments, prolactin release from dispersed rat anterior pituitary cells was studied using the superfusion method described previously (7). Rats were sacrificed by decapitation and anterior pituitary cells were dispersed with 0.5% trypsin. After incubation for 48 h at 37 C, the cells (5×10^6) were placed on a small Sephadex G-25 column and superfused with Krebs-Ringer bicarbonate buffer containing 10 mM glucose and 0.1% bovine serum albumin at a constant flow rate of 330 ul/min. The perfusate was collected every 5 min. The cell column was stimulated by drugs as a 5 min pulse without changing the flow pressure. Prolactin concentrations in the plasma and the perfusate were measured by specific radioimmunoassay using a kit supplied from the NIAMDD (7). The NIAMDD rat prolactin-RP-1 was used as the standard. Statistical differences were evaluated by Student's t test and Duncan's new multiple range test.

Intraventricular injection of porcine PHI-27 (200 ng, 1 ug, and 5 ug/rat) resulted in a dose-related increase in plasma prolactin levels in urethane- anesthetized male rats and the mean (± SE) peak values of plasma prolactin were 17.4 ± 1.1, 77.9 ± 13.9 and 229.3 ± 3.7 ng/ml, respectively (Fig. 1A). Intraventricular administration of PHI-27 also raised plasma prolactin levels in conscious rats (Fig. 1B). Saline solution injected intraventricularly as a control did not affect plasma prolactin levels in these animals.

Intravenous injection of PHI-27 (10 ug/100 g BW) significantly raised plasma prolactin levels in both anesthetized and conscious rats compared with saline injection (Fig. 2A,B).

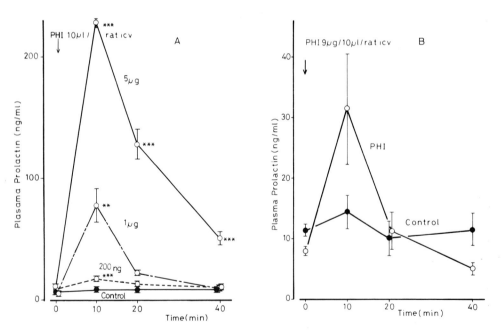

Figure 1. Effects of intraventricular injection of PHI on plasma prolactin levels in male urethane-anesthetized (A) and in conscious rats (B). PHI-27 was injected in doses of 200 ng, 1 ug and 5 ug per rat in anesthetized rats and in a dose of 9 ug per rat in conscious rats. All values represent mean ± SE of 5-8 animals in each group. Arrow shows the time of injection. * P < 0.05 vs saline control, ** P < 0.01 vs control, *** P < 0.001 vs control.

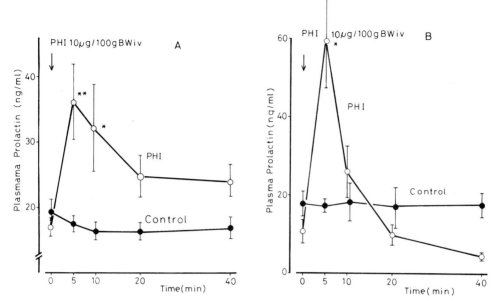

Figure 2. Effects of intravenous injection of PHI (10 ug/100 g BW iv) on plasma prolactin levels in male urethane-anesthetized (A) and conscious rats (B). * P < 0.05 vs saline control, ** P < 0.01 vs control.

In *in vitro* studies, prolactin release from superinfused rat anterior pituitary cells was stimulated by addition of PHI (1-100 nM) in a dose-related manner as shown in Figure 3. The mean (± SE) maximum changes of prolactin release expressed as percent of respective basal prolactin release were 146 ± 12, 16 ± 13 and 182 ± 19%, respectively (Fig. 4). In this system, VIP (10 nM) also raised prolactin release (196 ± 16%) and the potency to stimulate prolactin secretion was as great as that of PHI.

We have previously reported that VIP stimulated prolactin secretion in the rat when VIP was injected intraventricularly or intravenously *in vivo* (5) and when VIP was added to the superfused anterior pituitary cells in *vitro* (7,10), suggesting a direct action of VIP to stimulate the secretion of prolactin from the pituitary. These findings are on the same line of other reports (6,8,9,14,15).

PHI is found in the median eminence (16). We have reported that PHI as well as VIP is highly concentrated in the hypophysial portal blood (4). It is interesting to examine the effect of PHI on the secretion of prolactin from the pituitary. We have first demonstrated in the present study that either intraventricular or intravenous injection of PHI stimulates prolactin release in both anesthetized and conscious male rats *in vivo*. We have also found that prolactin release from superfused rat anterior pituitary cells is stimulated by PHI *in vitro*.

Recently, the stimulating action of PHI-27 on prolactin secretion from the incubated rat anterior pituitary cells was reported from two other laboratories (11,12). Werner

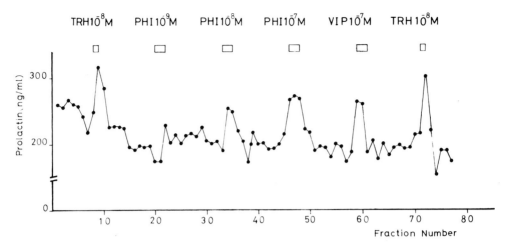

Figure 3. Effects of TRH (10 nM), PHI (1-100 nM) and VIP (100 nM) on prolactin release from superfused rat anterior pituitary cells. A representative experiment is shown.

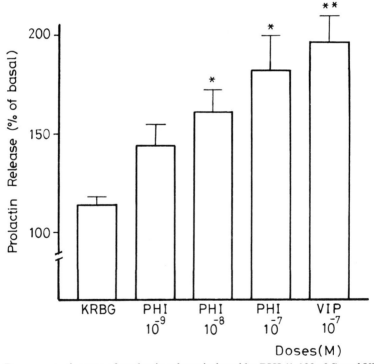

Figure 4. Dose-responsiveness of prolactin release induced by PHI (1-100 nM) and VIP (100 nM) from superfused rat anterior pituitary cells. Values represent mean ± SE maximum changes of prolactin release expressed by % of respective basal prolactin release. * P < 0.05 vs KRBG control, ** P < 0.01 vs control.

et al. (11) reported that the effect of PHI to stimulate prolactin release from rat pituitary cells was much greater than that of VIP. In contrast, Samson et al. (12) reported that PHI stimulated rat prolactin release to the same extent as that of VIP. In the present study, we also showed the stimulation by PHI of rat prolactin secretion is as great as that of VIP. The discrepancy between the reports may be explained by the purity of the peptide.

It is concluded that PHI has a stimulating action on rat prolactin secretion and at least a part of the effect may be a direct effect on the pituitary. However, further studies are required to elucidate the physiological role of PHI as a prolactin releasing factor in rats and other species.

ACKNOWLEDGMENTS

Supported in part by grants from the Ministry of Education and the Ministry of Health and Welfare, Japan.

REFERENCES

1. Tatemoto K, Mutt V. (1981): Proc Natl Acad Sci 78:6603
2. Bloom SR, Christofides ND, Delamarter J, Buell G, Kawashima E, Polak JM. (1983): Lancet ii:1163
3. Itoh N, Obata K, Yanaihara N, Okamoto N. (1983): Nature 304:547
4. Shimatsu A, Kato Y, Ohta H, Kabayama Y, Inoue T, Tojo K, Imura H. (1983): Neurosci Lett 43:259
5. Kato Y, Iwasaki Y, Iwasaki J, Abe H, Yanaihara N, Imura H. (1978): Endocrinology 108:395
6. Ruberg M, Rotsztejn WH, Arancibia S, Besson J, Enjalbert A. (1978): Eur J Pharmacol 51:319
7. Matsushita N, Kato Y, Shimatsu A, Katakami H, Yanaihara N, Imura H. (1983): Life Sci 32:1263
8. Frawley LS, Neill JD. (1981): Neuroendocrinology 33:79
9. Ottesen B, Nyboe AA, Gerstenberg T, Ulrichsen H, Manthorpe T, Fahrenkrug J. (1981): Lancet ii:696
10. Kato Y, Matsushita N, Shimatsu A, Imura H. (1982) In: Shizume K, Imura H, Shimizu N (eds) Endocrinology. Excerpta Medica, Amsterdam, p 136
11. Werner S, Hulting A-L, Hokfelt T, Eneroth P, Tatemoto K, Mutt V, Maroder L, Wunsch E. (1983): Neuroendocrinology 37:476
12. Samson WK, Lumpkin MD, McDonald JK, McCann SM. (1983): Peptides 4:817
13. Kato Y, Hiroto S, Katakami H, Matsushita N, Shimatsu A, Imura H. (1982): Proc Soc Exp Biol Med 169:95
14. Vijayan E, Samson WK, Said SI, McCann SM. (1979): Endocrinology 104:53
15. Shaar CJ, Clemens JA, Dininger NB. (1979): Life Sci 25:2071
16. Hokfelt T, Fahrenkrug J, Tatemoto K, Mutt V, Werner S. (1982): Acta Physiol Scand 116:469

Prolactin. Basic and clinical correlates
R.M. MacLeod, M.O. Thorner and U. Scapagnini (eds.),
Fidia Research Series, vol. I,
Liviana Press, Padova © 1985

Section II
Influence of brain factors
on prolactin secretion

PARTICIPATION OF BRAIN HISTAMINE IN THE PROLACTIN RESPONSE TO STRESS

A. M. Seltzer and A. O. Donoso

Laboratorio de Investigaciones Cerebrales, Facultad de C. Medicas, UNC.
Mendoza, Argentina

In mammals, prolactin secretion is inhibited tonically by the tuberoinfundibular dopamine-containing system. The amine, released into the pituitary portal vessels, acts directly on prolactin cells (1). Noradrenaline and other brain monoamines would not be essential for the tonic control of prolactin secretion (2).

Stress can overcome the tonic inhibition; consequently it enhances the prolactin discharge toward the systemic circulation. The stress-induced prolactin release has been associated with the activation of monoaminergic fibers projecting from caudal encephalic areas. This effect can be depressed by deafferentation or chemical lesioning of the neural pathways entering the mediobasal hypothalamus (3,4). These pathways are known to contain noradrenergic, serotonergic, and histaminergic fibers (5,6).

The notion that stress may affect brain histamine turnover (7) stimulated studies to ascertain the significance of histamine in the induced secretion of prolactin. In this contribution, we present results obtained from rats treated with a histamine-depleting drug and selective antihistamines. Acute restraint was used as stressor. A possible interrelationship of noradrenaline and histamine was also examined.

Adult male rats were immobilized in small wire cages for 15 min. At the completion of experiments, animals were killed by decapitation and blood collected from the trunk, in a time of less than 10 sec. Prolactin in plasma was determined by radioimmunoassay. One-way analysis of variance and Duncan's new multiple range test were used for statistical evaluation of data.

HISTAMINE AND RESTRAINT STRESS

Figure 1 shows the results of an experiment combining restraint with ip injections of oc-fluoromethyl-histidine (FH). This drug inhibits brain histamine synthesis (79% histamine depletion in hypothalamus, 4 h after injection). FH treatment blunted the increase of plasma prolactin levels. Prolactin levels in these rats were significantly lower ($p < 0.01$) than in controls injected ip with physiological saline. Results thus indicate that histamine depletion impairs the prolactin response to restraining stress.

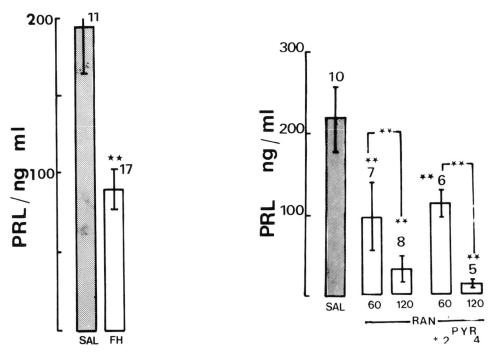

Figure 1. Effect of oc-fluoromethyl-histidine (FH) on plasma prolactin levels of stressed rats. Drug was injected ip in doses of 20 mg/kg, 4 h before restraining. SAL = saline; ** $p < 0.01$ vs SAL. Number of animals at top of columns.

Figure 2. Antihistamine effect on plasma prolactin levels of rats submitted to stress. RAN = ranitidine; PYR = pyrilamine ip; SAL = saline. ** $p < 0.01$ vs SAL. Significance between columns pointed out by arrows ** $p < 0.01$.

Further evidence was obtained in the experiment shown in Figure 2. Ranitidine, an H_2 selective histamine antagonist (8), was injected intraventricularly (IVT) in doses of 120 ug/rat, 10 min before restraining. This treatment fully prevented the increase of plasma prolactin levels. Smaller doses of ranitidine (60 ug/rat) produced partial effects. Ranitidine probably acted at central sites, because the drug does not cross the blood-brain barrier. Indeed, the antagonistic action was absent when ranitidine was injected ip, even at large doses (90 mg/kg). It is of some interest that ranitidine was able to prevent completely the increase of plasma prolactin, while FH led only to a decrease of the prolactin release induced by restraint. Such a difference might be due to the fact that ranitidine induces an extensive blockade of postsynaptic histamine receptors, while a resistant pool of histamine (i.e., the mast cells pool) which may be released by stress, remains after FH injection (9). Figure 3 shows that the H_1-histamine an-

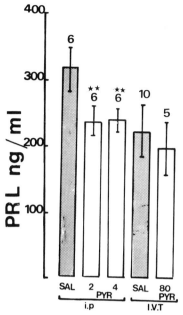

Figure 3. Plasma prolactin increase in rats treated with pyrilamine (PYR) prior to restraint. Drug was injected ip or IVT at doses indicated at bottom of the figure. SAL = saline. ** p < 0.01 vs SAL. Number of animals at top of columns.

tagonist pyrilamine exhibited a minor but significant (p < 0.01) inhibitory effect on plasma prolactin increase if injected ip prior to stress. However, this drug had no action if given IVT. As demonstrated elsewhere pyrilamine, at the doses used, is effective in blocking other effects of histamine (10). Pyrilamine ip was found to be ineffective even to affect the ranitidine action (see Fig. 2).

HISTAMINE-NORADRENALINE INTERRELATIONSHIP

The findings shown above indicate that depletion and antagonism of brain histamine impair the prolactin response to stress. As is known, IVT injection of either histamine or noradrenaline enhances prolactin release in rats (11,12). Therefore, it was considered of interest to examine the effect of noradrenaline depletion on the prolactin release induced by restraint. As shown in Table 1, the treatment with DDC (diethyldithiocarbamate), a noradrenaline-synthesis inhibitor, suppressed the post-restraint increase of plasma prolactin levels. This agrees with previous reports (13) concerning other drugs (FLA-64) in rats subjected to stress.

Outlined results led to the proposal that stress acts through a linkage of noradrenaline and histamine. Such a hypothesis gives rise to several questions. 1) Are both amines essential for a consistent response of prolactin to stress? It appears to be so since the selective depletion of one of these amines can block this response to stress.

Table 1. *Noradrenaline depletion and plasma prolactin increase in rats subjected to restraint. DDC was injected ip in doses of 350 mg/kg, 3h before stress*

Group	Plasma Prolactin ng/ml RP-1
Saline (7)	287.0 ± 42.6[1]
DDC (5)	12.5 ± 0.8**

[1] Mean ± SEM.
** p < 0.01 vs SAL. In parentheses: number of animals.

2) Does the occurrence of side-effects of antihistamines on the noradenaline system or vice versa favor such a hypothesis? This is unlikely because ranitidine was reported to have no effect on adrenergic receptors (8) and FH does not alter catecholamine synthesis (9). On the other hand, DDC is a well known dopamine-beta- hydroxylase inhibitor that blocks the conversion of dopamine to noradrenaline (14). 3) Is there a cascading transmitter function in which histamine or noradrenaline are the first steps affected by stress? To answer this, further experiments are in progress. Recent data

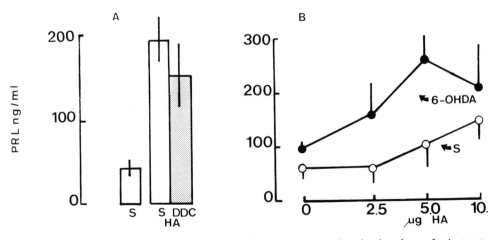

Figure 4. Effects of noradrenaline depletion on histamine-induced prolactin release. In A, treatment with DDC (350 mg/kg, ip) 3 h before histamine injection (5 ug/rat IVT, 15 min before killing). S = saline. Open columns indicate controls (n = 10, before and after histamine). The filled column, histamine injection in DDC-treated rats (n = 5). In B, rats treated with 6-OHDA (8 ug bilaterally into the mediobasal hypothalamus, 1 week before) or saline. Histamine was injected IVT, 15 min before blood sampling. Each point corresponds to 6 rats.

from our laboratory in slightly stressed (handled) rats suggest that the action of histamine on prolactin does not require noradrenaline mediation. This is shown in Figure 4. Male rats treated with DDC or lesion of catecholamine nerve endings in the mediobasal hypothalamus by means of 6-hydroxydopamine (6-OHDA), showed a consistent plasma prolactin release to increasing log doses of histamine IVT. Even though the threshold-effective dose of histamine in these rats was lower than for controls, its overall action was quantitatively similar (2-way ANOVA; F: non sign. difference). The apparently high plasma prolactin levels in 6-OHDA-lesioned rats might be due to an increased reaction to handling.

CONCLUSIONS

The reported findings indicate that brain histamine may integrate a chain of neurotransmitters for activation of prolactin discharge elicited by stress. The effect of histamine seems to occur mainly through H_2 receptor sites.

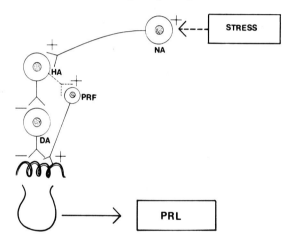

figure 5

Since depletion and antagonism of both histamine and noradrenaline did cancel the stress-induced prolactin surge, a link between these transmitters may occur. Whether the histamine path is directly stimulated by stress, or the noradrenergic cells are involved first, remains to be worked out. Preliminary data support the second view and suggest that histaminergic pathways are closer to the final neural step. Histamine or noradrenaline might be integrated with the tuberoinfundibular dopaminergic system or a prolactin-releasing factor in order to induce the prolactin surge upon stress. This is shown diagrammatically in Figure 5.

REFERENCES

1. MacLeod RM. (1976) In: Martini L, Ganong, WF (eds) Frontiers in Neuroendocrinology 4:169
2. Weiner RI, Ganong, WF. (1978): Physiol Revs 58:905
3. Krulich L, Hefco E, Aschenbrenner, JE. (1975): Endocrinology 96:107
4. Fenske M, Wuttke W. (1976): Brain Res 104:63
5. Moore RY, Bloom FE. (1979): Ann Rev Neurosc 2:113
6. Schwartz JC. (1977): Ann Rev Pharmacol Toxicol 17:325
7. Verdiere M, Rose C, Schwartz JC. (1977): 129:107
8. Brittain RT, Jack D, Price BJ. (1981): Trends Pharmacol Sci 2:310
9. Garbarg M, Barbin G, Rodergas E, Schwartz JC. (1980): J. Neurochem 35:1045
10. Seltzer AM, Donoso AO. (1982): Neuroendocrinol Lett 4:299
11. Donoso AO. (1980): J Endocrinol 76:193
12. Vijayan E, McCann SM. (1978): Neuroendocrinology 25:150
13. Krulich L, Marachlewska-Koj A. (1976): Fed Proc 35:555 (Abstract)
14. Goldstein M. (1966): Pharmacol Rev 18:77

Prolactin. Basic and clinical correlates
R.M. MacLeod, M.O. Thorner and U. Scapagnini (eds.),
Fidia Research Series, vol. I,
Liviana Press, Padova © 1985

Section II
Influence of brain factors
on prolactin secretion

A SURVEY OF PINEAL INDOLES AND ANALOGUES WHICH AFFECT PROLACTIN SECRETION IN THE ADULT MALE SYRIAN HAMSTER

M.K. Vaughan, A.P. Holtorf, J.C. Little*, T.H. Champney and R.J. Reiter

Department of Cellular and Structural Biology, Division of Neuroendocrinology
University of Texas Health Science Center
San Antonio, Texas 78284

The Syrian hamster (*Mesocricetus auratus*) is a photosensitive, seasonally-breeding rodent whose reproductive organs undergo a profound involution when the animal is exposed to artificial or natural photoperiods of less than 12.5 hrs light/day (1). This impressive response is known to be pineal-mediated and, interestingly, can be induced or prevented by the appropriate timing, dose, and duration of exposure to various pineal indoleamines. Prolactin is a key hormone in this dramatic response; depressed levels of pituitary and plasma prolactin are correlated with complete gonadal degeneration in males of this species. Concomitantly, testicular regression induced by short photoperiods is accompanied by a precipitous decline in gonadal LH/hCG and prolactin receptors (2,3). The present minireview concentrates on the identification of pineal indoles and their analogues which affect prolactin and summarizes the current theories on their mechanisms of action.

A. DAILY AFTERNOON INJECTIONS OF INDOLES

In 1976, Tamarkin and coworkers (4) reported that afternoon injections (at the end of the light phase) of the pineal indoleamine, melatonin, duplicated the effects of short non-stimulatory photoperiods in the hamster; morning injections were ineffective. This fortuitous discovery of an afternoon melatonin-sensitive "critical period" was a major breakthrough in pineal physiology. Accumulated evidence now indicates

---

* Present address: Department of Biology, Abilene Christian University, Abilene, Texas

144

that prolactin plays a pivotal role in this response. The transplantation of prolactin-secreting homologous pituitaries under the renal capsule partially or completely prevents gonadal degeneration due to afternoon melatonin injections or short photoperiod (5-7).

Melatonin belongs to a unique family of pineal indoles; the biochemical mechanisms relating to the multitude of factors controlling their synthesis, secretion, and metabolism are considered at length elsewhere (8). Initially, it was unknown whether the prolactin-suppressing effects of melatonin were unique or were shared by other structurally related indoles. To evaluate this question, Sackman and coworkers (9) treated hamsters in long stimulatory photoperiods (14:10 LD) with afternoon injections of 25 ug of melatonin, 5-methoxytryptophol, N-acetylserotonin, or 6-hydroxymelatonin for 50 days. Pituitary prolactin contents and plasma concentrations were significantly depressed by injections of either melatonin or its immediate precursor, N-acetylserotonin. Since pinealectomy completely prevented the action of these two indoles, the authors concluded that an intact pineal was necessary for the observed effects.

A more recent study by Richardson and collaborators (10) expanded the list of indoles that were ineffective in eliciting either the suppression of prolactin or the gonadal inhibitory response. In this study, groups of hamsters were maintained in a 14:10 light:dark cycle (lights on 0600 h) and received daily afternoon injections (1700 h) of fresh indolic solutions prepared in ethanolic saline. Groups of hamsters received either vehicle or 25 ug/day of melatonin, N-acetylserotonin, 6-hydroxymelatonin, 5-hydroxy-tryptophol, or 5-methoxytryptophol for 10 weeks. As in the experiment mentioned above (9), these authors confirmed that melatonin suppressed plasma prolactin levels, whereas injections of 6-hydroxymelatonin and 5-methoxytryptophol were ineffective. A newly-tested indole, 5-hydroxytryptophol, also failed to modify prolactin release (Fig. 1). In

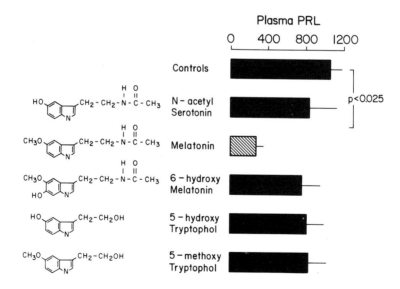

Figure 1. Effect of various pineal indoles on plasma prolactin levels in adult male Syrian hamsters. Indoles were administered sc daily at 1700 h. Results are expressed in terms of standard hamster anterior pituitary. Means ± S.E.M. are indicated. (Data from ref. 9)

contrast to the experiment of Sackman and coworkers (9), Richardson and his group (10) found N-acetylserotonin to be ineffective in depressing plasma prolactin levels.

In a second experiment, Richardson and coworkers (10) studied the effects of various synthetic analogues of pineal indoles on pituitary and plasma prolactin levels after 7 weeks of treatment. As in their first experiment, the indoles were injected sc daily into adult male hamsters maintained in a 14:10 LD photoperiod. The animals received diluent or 25 ug/day of hexanoyl methoxytryptamine, acetyl methoxytryptophol, propionyl methoxytryptophol, or 6-chloromelatonin; the effects of these compounds were measured against those produced by the injections of melatonin, the natural pineal indole, in another group of animals. The results from this experiment clearly indicated that 6-chloromelatonin was as effective as melatonin in reducing the pituitary content and concentration of prolactin; correspondingly, the gonads of these animals were depressed in weight. Interestingly, two of the synthetic analogues, hexanoyl methoxytryptamine and acetyl methoxytryptophol, increased the prolactin concentration in the pituitary (Fig. 2).

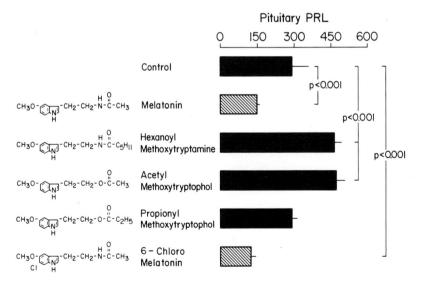

Figure 2. Effect of various synthetic analogues of pineal indoles on pituitary prolactin levels in adult male Syrian hamsters. Indoles were administered sc daily at 1700 h. Means ± S.E.M. are indicated. (Data from ref. 9)

5-Methoxytryptamine (5MT), a methylated indole formed directly from its precursor, serotonin, by hydroxyindole-0-methyltransferase, is present in the pineal gland of several mammalian species (11). This compound has received considerable attention lately since, in some instances, it causes testicular atrophy (12, 13); however, its effects on prolactin have not been examined heretofore. In the present experiment, male hamsters were divided into groups of 9-10 animals each and maintained in 14:10 LD (lights on 0600 h). Groups of hamsters received daily sc injections (1700 h) of 5, 15, 25, 50, 100, or 200 ug of 5MT for 12 weeks; the control group received only alcoholic-saline vehicle. The results, expressed in terms of a pool of standard hamster anterior pituitaries (SHAP), are presented in Table 1.

These results indicate that 5MT can, indeed, suppress plasma prolactin levels when administered daily over an extended period of time. Interestingly, the gonads from these hamsters were significantly reduced in weight only by the 200 ug injections of 5MT (13). This suggests that other factors (possibly hormonal) besides prolactin may need to be altered before degeneration can occur.

Table 1. *Effect of various doses of 5-methoxytryptamine on plasma prolactin in adult male Syrian hamsters. Means ± S.E.M. are indicated*

Treatment	Dose ug	Plasma Prolactin ug SHAP/ml
Controls	Vehicle	4.420 ± 0.690
5-methoxytryptamine	5	0.984 ± 0.087*
	15	0.807 ± 0.156*
	25	0.447 ± 0.141*
	50	0.648 ± 0.138*
	100	0.528 ± 0.084*
	200	0.777 ± 0.105*

* $P < 0.001$ vs controls

In summary, many but not all of the indoles present in the pineal have now been tested for their ability to depress pituitary and plasma prolactin levels when administered as daily afternoon injections in the hamster. It would appear that melatonin and 5-methoxytryptamine are among the most potent of the natural indoles tested to date.

B. COUNTER-ANTIGONADOTROPHIC EFFECTS OF PINEAL INDOLES

In 1974, Reiter and coworkers (14) described what is now called the counter-antigonadotrophic effect of melatonin. This effect is produced by the implantation of a melatonin-beeswax pellet into hamsters that are exposed to natural or short photoperiodic conditions or are receiving afternoon injections of melatonin. The pellet releases the indole at a constant but slow rate, completely preventing the fall in pituitary and plasma prolactin and the ensuing gonadal degeneration. One theory concerning this unusual effect invokes the downregulation of receptors by the continuous availability of melatonin; this theory will be explored more fully in the next section.

Since a melatonin pellet prevents the effects of afternoon injections of melatonin, we wondered if a melatonin pellet could also overcome the action of other indoles (e.g. 5MT, 6-chloromelatonin) injected each evening; a positive answer to this question might imply that the various indoles were acting at a common site. To test this intriguing question, we injected groups of male hamsters with 25 ug/day of 5MT or the synthetic analogue of melatonin, 6-chloromelatonin, at 1700 h. Subgroups of these indole-injected animals received biweekly implantation of a melatonin-beeswax pellet (1:24 mg). The results shown in Figure 3 clearly indicate that melatonin pellets completely prevent the fall in pituitary prolactin that accompanies afternoon injections of 5MT or 6-chloromelatonin alone.

Several other indoles (5-methoxytryptophol, 6-hydroxymelatonin, N-acetyl serotonin, 5-hydroxytryptophol) have been evaluated for their ability to produce this counterantigonadotrophic response when presented in pellet form to light-deprived hamsters (15, 16). Two of these indoles (5-methoxytryptophol and 6-hydroxymelatonin) were significantly effective in preventing the pituitary fall in prolactin.

Recently, Pevet and Haldar Misra (17) reported that 5MT, like melatonin, prevented involution of the gonads in dark-exposed animals. Subsequent experiments in our

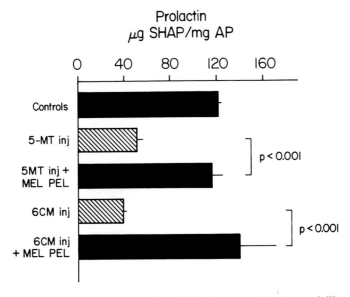

Figure 3. Adult male Syrian hamsters received daily afternoon injections of diluent, 25 ug/day 5-methoxytryptamine (5MT), or 6-chloromelatonin (6CM). Additionally, groups of 5MT and 6CM-injected hamsters received biweekly subcutaneous implants containing 1 mg melatonin (MEL). Results are expressed in terms of standard hamster anterior pituitary. Means ± S.E.M. are indicated.

laboratory confirmed their original observation, that pellets containing 1 mg 5MT were effective in preventing short-day induced testicular regression; however, a dose-response curve comparing the minimal effective dose of 5MT and melatonin indicated that melatonin was the more potent of the two indoles. One question which had remained unanswered was whether any of these indoles, besides melatonin itself, could prevent the effects of afternoon-injected melatonin on the neuroendocrine-reproductive axis. To test this question, 4 groups of hamsters were administered 25 ug of melatonin each afternoon (1700 h); a control group received diluent only. Of the 4 groups receiving melatonin injections, 3 groups additionally received a biweekly implant of a beeswax pellet that contained 1 mg of melatonin, 5MT, or 6-chloromelatonin. As can be seen in Figure 4, 5MT in this experiment did not prevent the fall in pituitary prolactin.

This observation was somewhat surprising to us since 5MT at this dose had been effective previously in light-deprived hamsters. One important implication of such a finding is that afternoon melatonin treatment and exposure of hamsters to less than 12.5 hrs light/day are not equivalent treatments physiologically as we had thought previously. Alternatively, the hamster may exhibit a differential sensitivity to 5MT (perhaps due to season, temperature, or nutrition) and the dosage released from the pellet may not have been sufficient to overcome the effects of the melatonin injections.

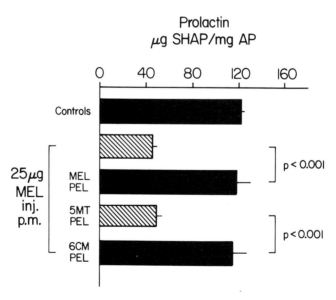

Figure 4. Adult male Syrian hamsters received daily afternoon injections of 25 ug melatonin (MEL). Three groups of MEL-injected animals also received biweekly subcutaneous implants of a pellet containing either 1 mg MEL, 5-methoxytryptamine (5MT) or 6-chloromelatonin (6CM). Results are expressed in terms of standard hamster anterior pituitary. Means ± S.E.M. are indicated.

C. THEORIES REGARDING THE MECHANISM OF ACTION

The observation that chronic implants of indoles (melatonin, 6-chloromelatonin, 5-methoxytryptophol) counteract the effects of short photoperiod or daily injections of melatonin has spawned several theories regarding the mechanism of action of such compounds. One proposal (14) suggested that the chronic availability of melatonin changed the time at which the neuroendocrine-reproductive axis was sensitive to inhibition by daily acute melatonin injections. A corollary premise would be that melatonin injections in the late afternoon mimicked the effects of short photoperiods by bringing into phase two previously unsynchronized neural elements which could be dissociated subsequently by chronic availability of certain indoleamines.

Another theory currently in vogue concerns the saturability and sensitivity of the presumed melatonin receptors. Endogenous melatonin is a hormonal product of the pineal gland; the indole has a nyctohemeral rhythm in blood, CSF, urine, and the pineal itself. Considering the rhythmic release of the indole, teleological reasoning suggests that its receptors might be most sensitive to its presence early in the scotophase; conversely, the receptors would be least sensitive at the beginning of the photophase, since they would have just experienced a prolonged period of stimulation in darkness. A pulse of melatonin late in the afternoon presumably would stimulate the receptors during their most sensitive period and would be equivalent to advancing the dark phase by several hours. Thus, the repeated afternoon injections of indoles would convince the animal hormonally that he was "seeing" less than 12.5 hrs light/day. However, a pellet providing a constant release of even very low amounts of indole would saturate and desensitize the receptors at all times, a condition generally known as downregulation. Thus, the receptors would be persistently refractory to the afternoon pulse of melatonin injections or to the short photoperiod itself. It is clear from the discussion presented in earlier sections that indoles other than melatonin affect the reproductive endpoints measured. If the downregulation theory is to be retained as a viable working hypothesis of the action of indoles, then one must propose that it be expanded to include the premise that indoles other than melatonin which effectively produce or mask the effect of afternoon injections of melatonin may 1) bind to the melatonin receptor or, alternately, 2) have their own unique receptors. The locus of these presumed receptors is thought to be in the hypothalamus; however, attempts at their localization have met with varied success (1). Certainly, at this point it is still too early to speculate on the cellular location of the indoleamine receptors or their possible interrelationship with the pathways mediating prolactin release and/or inhibition.

One further hypothesis which pertains directly to the involvement of indoleamines in the secretion of prolactin is that proposed by Vriend (18). Several years ago, Vriend and Reiter (19) noticed that hamsters with regressed testes had significantly lower levels of prolactin and thyroxine. In fact, treatments (injections, pellets, short photoperiods) which modified the reproductive system had similar effects on the neuroendocrine-thyroid axis. Since TRH releases prolactin as well as TSH, Vriend (18) reasoned that the indoles or short photoperiods were acting through a common site (perhaps the TRH neuron). Results from our laboratory have confirmed his original observations; additionally, we have examined the effects of the same indoles presented in the preceding sections on T_4 release in the hamster (20,21) and have shown that TRH can act directly to release prolactin in this species (22). Basically, we find that those indoles which are effective in modifying the reproductive axis work on the thyroid axis as well.

Testing the TRH hypothesis in the hamster may present unique problems, due to the timing of injections. Theoretically, administration of TRH on a daily basis should release prolactin which in turn should totally or partially prevent gonadal degeneration. Preliminary attempts in our laboratory to test this hypothesis by administration of TRH late in the afternoon have not been successful; however, a recent abstract by Chen and coworkers (23) suggests that TRH injections at the beginning of the photophase are effective. It should be noted that the three theories presented herein are not mutually exclusive; however, they will form the basis for future studies into the mechanism of action of indoles in this species.

ACKNOWLEDGMENTS

This work was supported by NSF Grant PCM 8304706.

REFERENCES

1. Vaughan MK. (1981): Int Rev Physiol 24:41
2. Bex FJ, Bartke A. (1977): Endocrinology 100:1223
3. Klemcke HG, Bartke A, Borer KT. (1983): Biol Reprod 29:605
4. Tamarkin L, Westrom WK, Hamill AI, Goldman BD. (1976): Endocrinology 99:1534
5. Richardson BA, Petterborg LJ, Vaughan MK, King TS, Reiter RJ. (1982) In: Reiter RJ (ed) The Pineal and Its Hormones. Alan R. Liss, New York, 129
6. Matthews MJ, Benson B, Richardson DL. (1978): Life Sci 23:1131
7. Bartke A, Goldman BD, Bex FJ, Kelch RP, Smith MS, Dalterio S, Doherty PC. (1980): Endocrinology 106:167
8. Klein DC, Auerbach DA, Namboodiri MAA, Wheler GHT. (1981) In: Reiter RJ (ed) The Pineal Gland. CRC Press, Boca Raton, vol 1:199
9. Sackman JW, Little JC, Rudeen PK, Waring PJ, Reiter RJ. (1977): Horm Res 8:94
10. Richardson BA, Vaughan MK, Petterborg LJ, Johnson LY, King TS, Smith I, Reiter RJ. (1983): J Neural Transm 56:187
11. Beck O, Jonsson G, Lundman A. (1981): Arch Pharmacol 318:49
12. Pevet P, Haldar-Misra C, Ocal T. (1981): J Neural Transm 51:303
13. Reiter RJ, Holtorf A, Champney TH, Vaughan MK. (1984): J. Pineal Res 1:91
14. Reiter RJ, Vaughan MK, Blask DE, Johnson LY. (1974)'; Science 185:1169
15. Reiter RJ, Vaughan MK. (1975): Endocr Res Commun 2:299
16. Reiter RJ, Vaughan MK, Blask DE, Johnson LY. (1975): Endocrinology 96:206
17. Pevet P, Haldar-Misra C. (1982): J Neural Transm 55:69
18. Vriend J. (1983): Pineal Res Rev 1:183
19. Vriend J, Reiter RJ. (1977): Horm Metab Res 9:231
20. Vaughan MK, Richardson BA, Johnson LY, Petterborg LJ, Powanda MC, Reiter RJ, Smith I. (1983): J Neural Transm 56:279
21. Vaughan MK, Richardson BA, Petterborg LJ, Holtorf AP, Vaughan GM, Champney TH, Reiter RJ. (1984): Neuroendocrinology (in press)
22. Vaughan MK, Johnson LY, Richardson BA, Brieno EG, Reiter RJ. (1984): Neuroendocr Lett 6:49
23. Chen HJ, Targovnik J, McMillan L, Randall S. (1983): 13th Ann Mtg Neurosci Abst 212.12, p 731

Prolactin. Basic and clinical correlates
R.M. MacLeod, M.O. Thorner and U. Scapagnini (eds.),
Fidia Research Series, vol. I,
Liviana Press, Padova © 1985

Section III
Intracellular pituitary mechanisms
regulating prolactin release

INTRACELLULAR PITUITARY MECHANISMS
REGULATING PROLACTIN RELEASE: AN OVERVIEW

M. Cronin and C. Grosvenor

University of Virginia School of Medicine, Charlottesville, VA 22908
University of Tennessee College of Medicine, Memphis, Tenn 38163

The search for intracellular signals in mammotrophs elicited by hypothalamic and gonadal hormones has intensified dramatically since the last International Congress on Prolactin. This section exemplifies these efforts in that phospholipid metabolites, cyclic AMP and gonadal steroids alter the rate of prolactin release from both normal and tumor-derived pituitary cells in culture. The limitations intrinsic to measuring common intracellular signal molecules or surface receptors in a multiple cell type preparation are relevant to the studies employing hemipituitaries, monolayer cultures or membrane preparations of the normal anterior pituitary gland. Accordingly, the cell type responsible for the measured changes in phospholipid or cyclic AMP can only be inferred. The use of enriched or clonal prolactin cells derived from pituitary tumors avoids this dilemma and offers a unique opportunity to dissect intracellular mechanisms. However, this model suffers from the transformed and abnormal nature often found in tumor cells. Thus, the burden of proof rests with the investigator of tumor cells if extrapolation to the normal mammotroph is a goal. Circumspection in this regard appears warranted. Finally, in the one electrophysiological study in this section, the argument was tendered that membrane conductance (resistance) changes may be crucial for the expression of dopaminergic inhibition of prolactin release.

Drs. Gershengorn, Martin, Canonico and colleagues experimentally approached the relationship between surface receptor activity, phospholipid and calcium metabolism and prolactin release. They measured intrinsic changes after cell surface receptor activation. Drs. Camoratto and Grandison utilized pharmacological agents to inhibit or stimulate enzymes involved in phospholipid and cyclic AMP (respectively) generation in GH_3 clonal tumor cells; the effects of these agents on prolactin release were monitored.

In the GH_3 clonal model, thyrotrophin releasing hormone (TRH) stimulated prolactin release in at least two distinct phases. So-called Phase I occurred in the first minute and was correlated with an increase in a nonmitochondrial source of intracellular free calcium as measured by Quin 2. Synchronized with this event was the phosphorylation of a 97,000 dalton protein by a calcium-dependent protein kinase. This first phase was not blocked by drugs that inhibit calcium uptake from extracellular sources. Importantly, polyphosphoinositides and diacylglycerol concentrations were increased seconds after addition of TRH and inositoltrisphosphate itself stimulated calcium release from the endoplasmic reticulum in permeabilized GH₃ cells.

Phase II of TRH stimulated prolactin release occurred from 5-60 min and was less dependent than Phase I on intracellular sources of calcium. On the other hand, chelating extracellular calcium or blocking plasmalemma calcium channels partially annulled this later release process. One can mimic this phase (without going through Phase I) with phorbal esters and diacylglycerol that activate a C kinase, or by the addition of phospholipase C which converts phosphatidylinositol to polyphosphoinositides and diacylglycerol. These results led to the supposition that C kinase activation is necessary for the full expression of this secretory event. Probably related to this is the observation that TRH stimulated the phosphorylation of several C kinase-dependent proteins whose functions are enigmatic.

In a related study Koike et al showed that synthetic diacylglycerol increased the release of prolactin from cultured anterior pituitary cells; a result mimicked by phospholipase C and a phorbol ester. The presence of dopamine reduced the stimulatory effect of these agents suggesting that catecholamines may function to inhibit prolactin release at a step distal to these stimulatory processes.

Neurotensin also stimulates prolactin release from rat hemipituitary glands, as discussed by Dr. Canonico, offering an interesting contrast to the TRH data of Drs. Gershengorn and Martin. It was demonstrated that this peptide uniquely stimulated phosphatidylinositol breakdown in a concentration and a time associated manner. The secretory effect was not protein synthesis dependent (acute cycloheximide) and apparently limited to prolactin release, as there was no change in luteinizing hormone, follicle stimulating hormone or growth hormone release. It was suggested that the neurotensin receptor may activate mechanisms similar to those described for the TRH receptor.

In the studies of Drs. Camoratto and Grandison, the association between cyclic AMP and phospholipid metabolism was addressed in GH₃ cells. The vasoactive intestinal peptide (VIP) receptor has been well described as associating with adenylate cyclase in a stimulatory mode. VIP and forskolin, which enhances adenylate cyclase activity, both increase the rate of prolactin release from GH₃ cells. By blocking phospholipase A2 or arachidonic acid metabolism, basal as well as VIP- and forskolin-stimulated prolactin release was inhibited. These data can be interpreted in several ways including: 1) that increased cyclic AMP levels can normally alter the phospholipid metabolism required for normal prolactin release; 2) that an optimal phospholipid configuration of the membranes is important for secretion, irrespective of the activity of the cell surface receptors. In a fascinating counterpoint to this latter interpretation, Judd and co-workers speculate that a proper calcium tonus is required to establish dopaminergic inhibition of prolactin release in transplantable MtTW15 rat pituitary tumors. From earlier work, it was known that these tumors harbored dopamine receptors which, when activated, could inhibit phosphatidylinositol turnover and adenylate cyclase activity. In spite of these apparently normal proximal effects, there was no change in prolactin release; it was noted then that the basal rate of prolactin release from the tumors was roughly an order of magnitude less than measured in normal mammotrophs. By artificially increasing the intracellular calcium concentration with ionophore A23187 and the calcium channel activator maitotoxin, the rate of prolactin release was increased in these tumor cells. More importantly, the addition of dopamine or the potent dopaminergic agonist bromocriptine now inhibited this enhanced rate of prolactin release. Thus, altered intracellular calcium status may be the primary lesion in these tumor cells. This tumor does not appear to be relevant to most human microprolactinomas, as the vast majority of these respond to dopamine agonists by reducing prolactin release. However, a subset of microadenomas or the resistant macroadenomas may espress such an anomaly in calcium metabolism.

Because alterations in cyclic AMP levels are also correlated with changes in prolactin release as noted above, it is important to probe this potential mechanism in parallel with the other putative mechanisms now undergoing scrutiny. Cronin and colleagues discovered that the addition of a bacterial adenylate cyclase to pituitary cell cultures markedly enhanced both cyclic AMP levels and prolactin release in normal and clonal pituitary cells (Eukaryotic adenylate cyclase is too fragile to use in such protocols at present). Thus, this enzyme is sufficient to initiate mechanisms involved in prolactin release.

The fact that an electrical current is generated when calcium and other ions pass through a membrane channel has been treated as an epiphenomenon by many prolactin cell physiologists and biochemists over the decade. It is now well documented that TRH induces membrane hyperpolarization from a calcium-activated potassium conductance increase in GH clonal cells. Because these clones do not express the dopamine receptor phenotype, the association of dopamine receptor activity with electrophysiological parameters has had to await enriched or purified populations of normal mammotrophs. An alternative approach was taken by Drs. Israel, Jaquet, and Vincent, recognizing that many human prolactinomas contain a high density of mammotrophs that are responsive to dopamine agonists. They are among the first to measure increased prolactinoma cell membrane conductance with the addition of low concentrations of dopamine. The reversal potential of -100 mV strongly suggests the participation of potassium as has been extensively documented in GH clonal cells. It remains to be demonstrated that normal mammotrophs behave in the same way.

Prolactin. Basic and clinical correlates
R.M. MacLeod, M.O. Thorner and U. Scapagnini (eds.),
Fidia Research Series, vol. I,
Liviana Press, Padova © 1985

Section III
Intracellular pituitary mechanisms
regulating prolactin release

INTRACELLULAR MECHANISMS OF CALCIUM-MEDIATED STIMULATION OF PROLACTIN SECRETION BY THYROTROPIN-RELEASING HORMONE

Marvin C. Gershengorn

Division of Endocrinology and Metabolism, Department of Medicine,
Cornell University Medical College and The New York Hospital,
New York, New York, USA.

Thyrotropin-releasing hormone (thyroliberin, TRH) stimulation of prolactin secretion from GH cells, cloned rat pituitary tumor cells, is dependent on calcium ion (Ca^{2+}) and it has been suggested that an elevation of the concentration of free Ca^{2+} in the cytoplasm ($[Ca^{2+}]_i$) serves to couple stimulation to secretion (1; for review, see 2) in a manner similar to that originally proposed by Douglas for secretion from chromaffin cells (3). Recently, this hypothesis was supported by the direct demonstration that TRH stimulates a rapid elevation of $[Ca^{2+}]_i$ in GH cells (4-5-6). In order to understand the intracellular, molecular mechanisms that mediate the elevation of $[Ca^{2+}]_i$, it was important to determine a) the pool(s) from which calcium was mobilized and b) the mediator(s) of this effect. In this manuscript, I present evidence from our own studies that TRH causes elevation of $[Ca^{2+}]_i$, at least in part, by mobilizing calcium from a nonmitochondrial, intracellular pool(s) and that this action is mediated by inositoltrisphosphate ($InsP_3$), one of the products of hydrolysis of phosphatidylinositol(4,5)bisphosphate [$PtdIns(4,5)P_2$] by a phospholipase C (or phosphodiesterase).

In order to begin to define the pool(s) of calcium involved in TRH action, we first determined whether TRH mobilized calcium from an intracellular store(s). One approach to demonstrate whether intracellular or extracellular Ca^{2+} is involved in the action of TRH is to lower the concentration of Ca^{2+} in the incubation medium during TRH stimulation. Using this experimental design, previous workers found that TRH stimulation of prolactin secretion was abolished from pituitary cells incubated for prolonged periods in medium to which no Ca^{2+} was added or in medium containing Ca^{2+} chelators. However, this did not prove that extracellular Ca^{2+} is required for the TRH effect because these conditions deplete cellular Ca^{2+}. Important insights could be obtained, however, from studies in which TRH-induced prolactin release was measured from cells which were incubated in medium with low Ca²⁺ concentrations for short periods of time prior to TRH addition. Clearly, if TRH were to stimulate prolactin secretion from cells incubated in medium with very low Ca²⁺ concentrations, that is, under conditions of a Ca²⁺ gradient favoring outward flow of Ca²⁺, it would strongly suggest that influx of extracellular Ca²⁺ was not required for stimulated release to occur. Since this experimental design would permit valuable conclusions to be drawn, we (7) studied the effect of varying the extracellular Ca²⁺ concentration of K⁺ (50 mM). Stimulation of pituitary hormone release by K⁺ depolarization is due to influx of extracellular Ca²⁺. In a critical experiment, we examined the effects of lowering the extracellular Ca²⁺ concentration to below that present free in the cell cytoplasm on ⁴⁵Ca²⁺ efflux and prolactin release elicited by TRH. The effects of a 1 min pulse of 1 uM TRH and 50 mM K⁺ were compared in perifusion medium containing 1,500 uM (control) and 2.8 uM Ca²⁺ and in medium in which the concentration of unbound or free Ca²⁺ was lowered to 0.02 uM by adding 33 uM EGTA to medium without added Ca²⁺ (Fig. 1). We found that the increment in prolactin release elicited by 50 mM K⁺ in medium with 2.8 uM Ca²⁺ was less than 3% of that in medium with 1,500 uM Ca²⁺ and there was no detectable increment in prolactin release in medium with 0.02 uM free Ca²⁺. In contrast, TRH enhanced prolactin release under all conditions; prolactin release stimulated by TRH was 50% and 35% of control in medium with 2.8 uM Ca²⁺ and 0.02 uM free Ca²⁺, respectively. These suboptimal responses, however, may

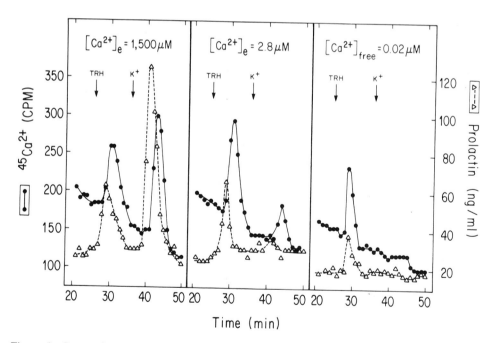

Figure 1. Comparison of the effects of TRH and 50 mM K⁺ on ⁴⁵Ca²⁺ efflux and prolactin secretion from GH₃ cells perifused with medium containing 1,500 and 2.8 uM Ca²⁺ and 0.02 uM free Ca²⁺. (Reproduced from Gershengorn et al. (6).)

have been due to loss of Ca^{2+} from a critical cellular pool(s) induced by the low Ca^{2+} medium. More recently, we (8) studied prolactin release from cells incubated in medium containing 120 mM K^+ and 2 mM EGTA which abolished both the electrical and Ca^{2+} concentration gradients that usually promote Ca^{2+} influx. TRH stimulated prolactin release and $^{45}Ca^{2+}$ efflux from cells incubated under these conditions. In static incubations, TRH stimulated prolactin secretion from (mean ± SE) 11.4 ± 1.2 to 19 ± 1.8 ng/ml in control incubations and from 3.2 ± 0.6 to 6.2 ± 0.8 ng/ml from cells incubated in medium with 120 mM K^+ and 2 mM EGTA. Hence, extracellular Ca^{2+} was necessary for K^+-stimulated release but it was not required for TRH-stimulated $^{45}Ca^{2+}$ efflux or prolactin secretion. Similar conclusions were drawn from experiments in which Ca^{2+} influx was inhibited with the organic channel blocking agent verapamil (11).

In order to implicate cytoplasmic Ca^{2+} as the coupling factor between TRH stimulation and prolactin secretion in cells incubated under conditions that abolished influx of extracellular Ca^{2+} (as described above), it was necessary to measure $[Ca^{2+}]_i$

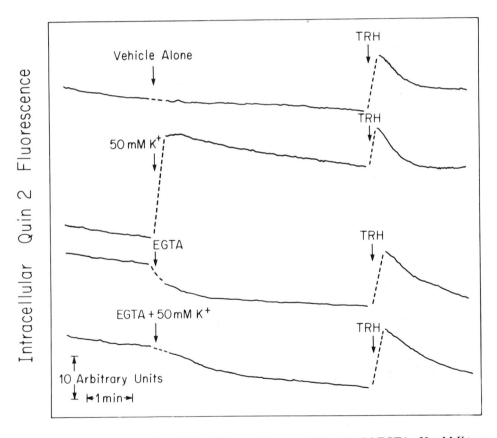

Figure 2. Effects of incubating GH$_3$ cells in medium containing 3 mM EGTA, 50 mM K^+, or both to dissipate the electrochemical driving force for Ca^{2+} influx on the TRH-induced elevation of $[Ca^{2+}]_i$ measured with Quin 2. (Reproduced from Gershengorn and Thaw (4).)

directly. We (4) measured $[Ca^{2+}]_i$ in GH_3 cells with the intracellularly trapped fluorescent indicator, Quin 2 (9,10). In unstimulated cells incubated in medium containing 1.5 mM Ca^{2+}, $[Ca^{2+}]_i$ was 118 ± 18 nM. TRH (1 uM) caused a rapid, transient elevation of $[Ca^{2+}]_i$ to a level estimated to be at least 500 nM which appeared to return towards the unstimulated level by 1.5 to 2 min (Fig. 2). High extracellular K^+ caused an elevation of $[Ca^{2+}]_i$ which was greater and longer in duration than that caused by TRH. When cells were incubated in medium containing 3 mM EGTA, the K^+ depolarization-induced increase in $[Ca^{2+}]_i$ was abolished. By contrast, TRH still caused an increase in $[Ca^{2+}]_i$ in cells preincubated in medium with 3 mM EGTA or 50 mM K^+, or both; as stated above, incubation of cells in medium with EGTA and high K^+ abolishes the electrochemical driving force for Ca^{2+} influx. These data demonstrated that Ca^{2+} influx is not required for the acute elevation of $[Ca^{2+}]_i$ or stimulated prolactin secretion induced by TRH in GH_3 cells. Hence these data were consistent with the notion that in GH_3 cells TRH causes mobilization of Ca^{2+} from an intracellular pool(s) to elevate $[Ca^{2+}]_i$ and stimulate prolactin secretion.

To demonstrate an effect of TRH on cellular Ca^{2+} more directly and then begin to characterize this pool(s), we utilized chlortetracycline, a fluorescent probe of Ca^{2+} in lipid domains (12, 13). We showed that cellular fluorescence of chlortetracycline was caused by both Ca^{2+}- and Mg^{2+}-chlortetracycline complexes. TRH, but not other peptides, caused a rapid decrease in chlortetracycline fluorescence (Fig. 3) which was not due to enhanced loss of chlortetracycline from the cells; half-maximal effect occurred with 10-30 nM TRH. The decrease in fluorescence elicited by TRH appeared to be specific for Ca^{2+}-chlortetracycline complexes. Although other factors could have affected the fluorescence, the very close parallels between the effects of TRH on $^{45}Ca^{2+}$ efflux (see above) and chlortetracycline fluorescence suggest that the decrease in the fluorescence caused by TRH is best explained by displacement of cellular membrane-bound Ca^{2+}.

It is known that agents with local anesthetic activity intercalate into biological membranes and compete with and displace Ca^{2+} from negatively charged sites (14). In particular, procaine-like anesthetics, such as tetracaine, and other drugs such as trifluoperazine and propranolol at high doses have been shown to displace Ca^{2+} complexed with the acidic headgroups of phospholipids within membranes. We (15) utilized these agents to probe membrane-bound Ca^{2+} in intact GH_3 cells. We showed that these agents caused a decrease in cellular ^{45}Ca content and cell-associated chlortetracycline fluorescence intensity and markedly inhibited TRH-stimulated loss of chlortetracycline fluorescence (Fig. 3) and prolactin secretion. We suggested that the loss of cellular Ca^{2+} was due to displacement of Ca^{2+} from membrane binding sites and that inhibition of TRH action by these agents may have been secondary to the loss of membrane-associated Ca^{2+}. These observations that TRH may be affecting Ca^{2+} bound to acidic phospholipids, such as the inositol lipids, were consistent with the hypothesis of Michell (16, 17) that stimulants, like TRH, that act by affecting cellular calcium metabolism to elevate $[Ca^{2+}]_i$ also stimulate the turnover of inositol phospholipids ("PI response"). Hence, we explored the possibility that stimulation of phosphoinositide metabolism by TRH may be an early event in the sequence that leads to stimulation of prolactin secretion.

Hokin and Hokin (18) first demonstrated that acetylcholine stimulated phospholipid metabolism in the exocrine pancreas. Since these initial observations, a vast literature

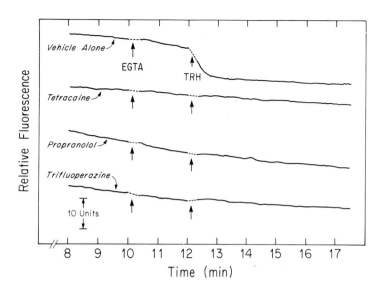

Figure 3. Effects of tetracaine, propranolol and trifluoperazine on TRH-induced decrease in membrane-bound Ca^{2+} monitored with chlortetracycline in GH_3 cells. (Reproduced from Thaw et al. (14).)

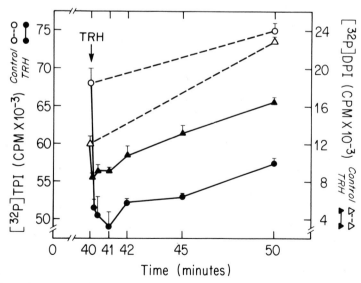

Figure 4. Effect of TRH on [^{32}P]PtdIns(4,5)P_2 ([^{32}P]TPI) and [^{32}P]PtdIns4P ([^{32}P]DPI) in GH_3 cells. (Reproduced from Rebecchi and Gershengorn (24).)

has accumulated which demonstrates that a wide variety of ligand-receptor interactions which are associated with mobilization of cellular Ca^{2+} or stimulation of influx of extracellular Ca^{2+}, or both, perhaps leading to elevation of $[Ca^{2+}]_i$ in many cell types, results in loss of phosphatidylinositol (PtdIns) and formation of phosphatidic acid (PtdA) (16). Although these findings are consistent with a cycle of PtdIns to diacylglycerol to PtdA conversion, as originally suggested (18), it has recently been suggested that these ligands may initiate their action by stimulating hydrolysis of PtdIns $(4,5)P_2$, not PtdIns, by a phospholipase C (phosphodiesterase) (17, 19). The decrease in the level of PtdIns commonly observed after stimulation by this class of ligand is proposed to be due to conversion of PtdIns into phosphatidylinositol(4)monophosphate (PtdIns4P) and then into PtdIns$(4,5)P_2$ by inositol lipid kinases.

In early studies, we (20) and others (21-23) demonstrated that TRH stimulates [^{32}P]-labeling of PtdA and PtdIns in GH$_3$ cells. We (24) subsequently provided evidence that TRH affected inositol lipid metabolism by stimulating a phospholipase C that resulted in a fall in the level of PtdA. On the basis of an increase in inositolmonophosphate (InsP), we suggested that the intital event in TRH-stimulated inositol lipid metabolism may be the hydrolysis of PtdIns by a specific phospholipase C; however, we considered the possibility that TRH stimulation may have been initiated by enhanced hydrolysis of PtdIns$(4,5)P_2$ and/or PtdIns4P.

More recently, we (25), Martin (26) and MacPhee, Drummond and colleagues have investigated whether TRH affects PtdIns$(4,5)P_2$ and PtdIns4P metabolism in GH$_3$ cells and whether this may have resulted from stimulation of a phospholipase C that hydrolyzes PtdIns$(4,5)P_2$. In our studies, we labeled GH$_3$ cells with [^{32}P]orthophosphate or with [^{3}H]inositol. Figure 4 illustrates the time course of the effect of TRH on [^{32}P]PtdIns$(4,5)P_2$ and [^{32}P]PtdIns4P in GH$_3$ labeled with [^{32}P]orthophosphate for 40 min; under these conditions, phospholipids are not labelled to isotopic steady-state. TRH caused a rapid decrease by 15 s in the levels of [^{32}P]PtdIns$(4,5)P_2$ and [^{32}P]PtdIns4P to 76% and 71% of control, respectively. After 1 min, [^{32}P]PtdIns$(4,5)P_2$ and [^{32}P]PtdIns4P increased again at a rate similar to that in control cells. In agreement with our previous observations and not shown here, the levels of [^{32}P]PtdA increased markedly by 15 s after TRH addition and that of [^{32}P]PtdIns did not increase until after 2 min. In cells labelled to isotopic steady-state with [^{32}P]orthophosphate, TRH caused a decrease in PtdIns$(4,5)P_2$ from 33 ± 2.3 pmol/106 cells to 22 ± 1.1 pmol at 30 s.

We also measured the effects of TRH on the levels of PtdIns$(4,5)P_2$ and PtdIns4P in cells labeled with [^{3}H]inositol for 48 h, a time that we (24) had shown previously is sufficient to label PtdIns to isotopic steady-state. The relative content (means $\pm$ SD) of inositol lipids in control GH$_3$ cells prelabelled with [^{3}H]inositol was: PtdIns$(4,5)P_2$, $2.5 \pm 1\%$; PtdIns4P, $2.8 \pm 1\%$; lysophosphatidylinositol, $6.2 \pm 1\%$; PtdIns, $88 \pm 1\%$. TRH stimulated rapid loss by 15 s of [^{3}H]PtdIns$(4,5)P_2$ and [^{3}H]PtdIns4P to 60% and 65% of control, respectively: the nadirs in the levels of [^{3}H]PtdIns$(4,5)P_2$ and [^{3}H]PtdIns4P were at 45 s and 60 s, respectively (Fig. 5). After 1 min in the continued presence of TRH, the levels of [^{3}H]PtdIns$(4,5)P_2$ and [^{3}H]PtdIns4P increased but remained below control for at least 5 min. Concomitant with the fall in [^{3}H]PtdIns$(4,5)P_2$ and [^{3}H]PtdIns4P and in agreement with our previous observations (24), TRH caused a decrease in [^{3}H]PtdIns to 86% of control by 2 min; there was no measurable change

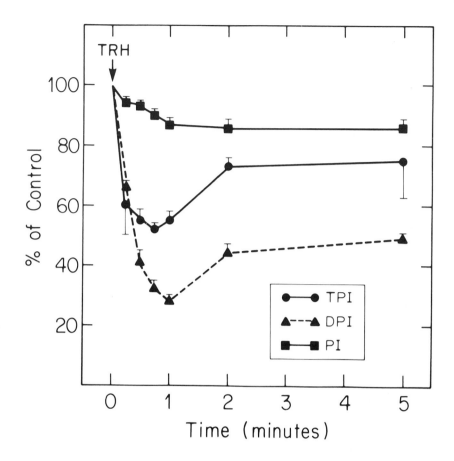

Figure 5. Effect of TRH on the levels of PtdIns(4,5)P$_2$ (TPI), PtdIns4P (DPI), and PtdIns (PI), in GH$_3$ cells. (Reproduced from Rebecchi and Gershengorn (24).)

in the level of [^{3}H]lysophosphatidyl- inositol (results not shown). The effect of TRH to decrease [^{3}H]PtdIns(4,5)P$_2$ was concentration-dependent; half-maximal effect occurred with approximately 5 nM TRH (results not shown), a concentration similar to that needed for half-maximal loss of [^{3}H]PtdIns (24).

We had previously observed that TRH caused increases in the levels of inositolmonophosphate (InsP), diacylglycerol, and PtdA in GH$_3$ cells and suggested that TRH may stimulate inositol lipid hydrolysis specifically by stimulating the activity of a phospholipase C which hydrolyzed PtdIns (24). We also presented evidence that strongly suggested that the diacylglycerol and PtdA formed during TRH stimulation were derived from inositol lipids. However, we considered the possibility that TRH could have stimulated a phospholipase C specific for either PtdIns(4,5)P$_2$ or PtdIns4P) because diacylglycerol can be formed by hydrolysis of PtdIns(4,5)P$_2$, PtdIns4P, or PtdIns and InsP can be formed directly from the hydrolysis of PtdIns or by dephosphorylation from inositolbisphosphate (InsP$_2$), a product of phospholipase C hydrolysis of PtdIns(4,5)P$_2$. Hence, to identify the initial reaction stimulated by TRH, it was important to monitor the levels of all the inositol sugars in GH$_3$ cells during TRH stimulation. In particular, InsP$_3$ was measured because it is the only sugar that is a specific reaction product in the metabolism of the inositol lipids; that is, InsP$_3$ appears only to be formed by hydrolysis of PtdIns(4,5)P$_2$ by a phospholipase C in mammalian cells.

The inositol sugars were measured in cells prelabelled to isotopic steady-state with [^{3}H]inositol. In unstimulated cells the relative content (means $\pm$ SD) of the inositol sugars was: [^{3}H]InsP$_3$, 1.3 $\pm$ 0.1%; [^{3}H]InsP$_2$, 3.9 $\pm$ 0.1%; [^{3}H]InsP, 16 $\pm$ 0.3%; [^{3}H]inositol, 78 $\pm$ 1.6%. The effect of TRH on the levels of ^{3}H-labelled inositol sugars is illustrated in Figure 6. TRH stimulated a rapid, transient increase in [^{3}H]InsP$_3$ to 410% of control at 15 s; the level declined after 15 s but was still above control after 5 min. The level of [^{3}H]InsP$_2$ was also increased by 15 s and attained its highest level of 450% of control at 30 s after TRH addition; its level declined after 30 s but was above control at 5 min. In contrast, [^{3}H]InsP was not elevated until 30 s after TRH and [^{3}H]inositol until 1 min after TRH addition. In four separate experiments, the effects of TRH on the levels of [^{3}H]inositol sugars after 30 s, expressed as percentages of unstimulated levels (means $\pm$ S.E.M.), were: [^{3}H]InsP$_3$, 246 $\pm$ 19%; [^{3}H]InsP$_2$, 316 $\pm$ 21%; [^{3}H]InsP, 138 $\pm$ 7%; and [^{3}H]inositol, 100 $\pm$ 3%. These results demonstrate that TRH stimulates inositol lipid metabolism, at least in part, by causing hydrolysis of PtdIns(4,5)P$_2$ by a phospholipase C and that the time course of InsP$_3$ accumulation is consistent with the notion that PtdIns(4,5)P$_2$ hydrolysis is the initial event in TRH stimulation of inositol lipid metabolism. Because there is no evidence in mammalian cells that the levels of InsP$_2$ or InsP can be increased by ligand stimulation of synthesis de novo, accumulation of InsP$_2$ and InsP during TRH stimulation of GH$_3$ cells may have been due to either hydrolysis by a phospholipase C of PtdIns4P and PtdIns, respectively, or dephosphorylation by a phosphatase of InsP$_3$ and InsP$_2$, respectively.

As stated above, it is generally agreed that an elevation of [Ca^{2+}]$_i$ serves to couple the interaction of many stimulants with plasma membrane receptors to the stimulation of a variety of cellular processes. Like TRH action in GH$_3$ cells, the elevation of [Ca^{2+}]$_i$ induced by stimulants may be caused, at least in part, by mobilization (or redistribution) of cellular calcium. Because in some of these cells, a very rapid effect after stimulant-receptor interaction is enhanced hydrolysis of PtdIns(4,5)P$_2$ to yield InsP$_3$, it was proposed that InsP$_3$ may mediate mobilization of cellular Ca^{2+} (29). Recently, this hypothesis was supported by observations that InsP$_3$ releases Ca^{2+} from a nonmitochondrial pool(s) in "leaky" rat pancreatic acinar cells (30) and in saponin-permeabilized rat (31) and guinea pig (32) hepatocytes. Prior to our studies, similar observations had not been made with regard to the mechanism of action of physiological secretagogues in endocrine cells. In parallel with our finding that TRH causes mobilization only from a nonmitochondrial pool(s) in intact GH$_3$ cells (33), we showed that InsP$_3$ causes rapid release of Ca^{2+} from a nonmitochondrial pool(s) in saponin-permeabilized GH$_3$ cells.

Saponin-permeabilized GH$_3$ cells were shown to accumulate Ca^{2+} in an ATP-dependent manner into mitochondrial and nonmitochondrial (uncoupler insensitive)

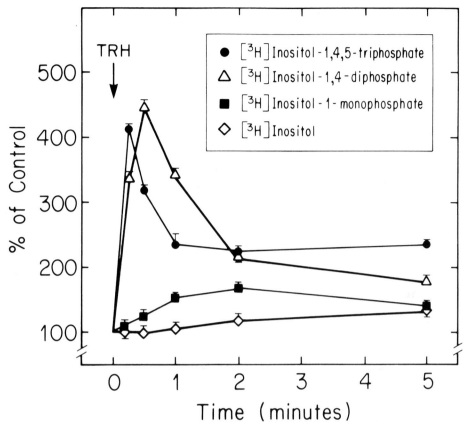

Figure 6. Effect of TRH on the levels of InsP₃ ([³H]Inositol-1,4,5-triphosphate), InsP₂ ([³H]Inositol-1,4-diphosphate), InsP ([³H]Inositol-1-monphosphate) and inositol ([³H]Inositol) in GH₃ cells. (Reproduced from Rebecchi and Gershengorn (24).)

pools. The nonmitochondrial pool exhibited a high affinity of Ca^{2+} and a small capacity. The mitochondrial pool had a lower affinity for Ca^{2+} but was not saturated under the conditions tested. Permeabilized cells buffered free Ca^{2+} to 129 ± 9.2 nM when incubated in a cytosol-like solution initially containing 200 to 1000 nM free Ca^{2+}, primarily by mitochondrial accumulation. This value is identical to the $[Ca^{2+}]_i$ measured in resting cells (4). InsP₃, but not other inositol sugars, caused release of calcium from the nonmitochondrial pool(s) in permeabilized cells; half-maximal effect occurred with approximately 1 uM InsP₃. The release of Ca^{2+} was followed by its reuptake, also into a nonmitochondrial pool(s). These data demonstrate that InsP₃ can mobilize calcium from a nonmitochondrial pool(s) in GH₃ cells.

In conclusion, I propose the following sequence of events for one pathway through which TRH may stimulate prolactin secretion: TRH interaction with its receptors on the plasma membrane activates the hydrolysis of PtdIns(4,5)P₂ to yield InsP₃, perhaps by directly stimulating a specific phospolipase C. InsP₃, in turn, interacts with a nonmitochondrial pool(s) of calcium, perhaps in the endoplasmic reticulum, to release Ca^{2+} and elevate $[Ca^{2+}]_i$ transiently. Cytoplasmic free Ca^{2+}, in an unknown manner, then activates the exocytotic process and leads to prolactin secretion.

REFERENCES

1. Tashjian AH Jr, Lomedico ME, Maina D. (1978): Biochem Biophys Res Commun 81:798
2. Gershengorn MC. (1982): Mol Cell Biochem 45:163
3. Douglas WW. (1968): Br J Pharmacol Chemother 34:451
4. Gershengorn MC, Thaw C. (1983): Endocrinology 113:1522
5. Snowdowne KW, Borle AB. (1984): Am J Physiol 246 (Endocrinol Metab 9):E198
6. Albert PR, Tashjian AH Jr. (1984): J Biol Chem 259:5827
7. Gershengorn MC, Hoffstein ST, Rebecchi MJ, Geras E, Rubin BG. (1981): J Clin Invest 67:1769
8. Gershengorn MC, Thaw C, Gerry RH. (1983): Cell Calcium 4:117
9. Tsien RY. (1980): Biochemistry. 19:2396
10. Tsien RY, Pozzan T, Rink TJ. (1982): J Cell Biol 94:325
11. Geras E, Rebecchi MJ, Gershengorn MC. (1982): Endocrinology 110:901
12. Caswell AH, Hutchinson JD. (1971): Biochem Biophys Res Commun 42:43
13. Hallett M, Schneider AS, Carbone E. (1972): J Membr Biol 10:31
14. Seeman P. (1972): Pharmacol Rev 24:583
15. Thaw C, Wittlin SD, Gershengorn MC. (1982): Endocrinology 111:2138
16. Michell RH. (1975): Biochim Biophys Acta 415:81
17. Michell RH, Kirk CJ, Jones LM, Downes CP, Creba JA. (1981): Philos Trans R Soc London Ser B 296:123
18. Hokin MR, Hokin LE. (1953): J Biol Chem 203:967
19. Berridge MJ. (1982): Cell Calcium 3:385
20. Rebecchi MJ, Monaco ME, Gershengorn MC. (1981): Biochem Biophys Res Commun 101:124
21. Drummond AH, Macphee CH. (1981): Br J Pharmacol 74:967
22. Schlegel W, Roduit C, Zahnel G. (1981): FEBS Lett 134:40
23. Sutton CA, Martin TFJ. (1982): Endocrinology 110:1273
24. Rebecchi MJ, Kolesnick RN, Gershengorn MC. (1983): J Biol Chem 258:227
25. Rebecchi MJ, Gershengorn MC. (1983): Biochem J 216:287
26. Martin TFJ. (1983): J Biol Chem 258:14816
27. Macphee CH, Drummond AH. (1984): Mol Pharmacol 25:193
28. Drummond AH, Bushfield M, Macphee CH. (1984): Mol Pharmacol 25:201
29. Berridge MJ. (1983): Biochem J 212:849
30. Streb H, Irvine RF, Berridge MJ, Schulz I. (1983): Nature 306:67
31. Joseph SK, Thomas AP, Williams RJ, Irvine RF, Williamson JR. (1984): J Biol Chem 259:3077
32. Burgess GM, Godfrey PP, McKinney JS, Berridge MJ, Irvine RF, Putney JW Jr. (1984): Nature 309:63
33. Gershengorn MC, Geras E, Spina Purello V, Rebecchi MJ. (1984): J Biol Chem (in press)

Prolactin. Basic and clinical correlates
R.M. MacLeod, M.O. Thorner and U. Scapagnini (eds.),
Fidia Research Series, vol. I,
Liviana Press, Padova © 1985

Section III
Intracellular pituitary mechanisms
regulating prolactin release

DUAL INTRACELLULAR SIGNALING BY Ca^{2+} AND LIPIDS MEDIATES THE ACTIONS OF TRH

T.F.J. Martin

Dept. of Zoology, University of Wisconsin, Madison, Wisconsin

The cellular mechanism by which thyrotropin-releasing hormone (TRH) triggers the release of pituitary hormones has been the focus of much experimentation since the elucidation of the structure of this tripeptide hormone. Early efforts centered around implicating cyclic AMP in the pathway of stimulus-secretion coupling and the imprint of this work is still evident in physiology textbooks where TRH is listed as one of many hormones which activate adenylyl cyclase. In truth, a possible role for cyclic AMP as a messenger in TRH action remains controversial with substantial experimental support against (1,2) and some for (3) such a role. Nonetheless, the focus of much recent research has shifted toward possible roles for Ca^{2+} and lipids in transducing the TRH signal in pituitary cells. Increasing support for the role of these messengers has accumulated and will be the subject of this article. It must be borne in mind, however, that the nonavailability of specific TRH antagonists and the absence of biochemical information on the TRH receptor precludes any definitive statement about possible receptor subtypes such as have been identified for other small molecular weight agonists.

DUAL EFFECTS OF TRH ON PROTEIN PHOSPHORYLATION: MEDIATION BY Ca^{2+} AND LIPIDS

Our studies and those of a number of other laboratories have employed clonal, TRH-responsive, prolactin-secreting rat pituitary cells (GH$_3$cells). In order to identify potential second messengers for TRH, we initiated studies of protein phosphorylation in GH$_3$ cells. Cells were incubated with [^{32}P] orthophosphate and treated briefly with a variety of agents known to influence prolactin secretion. Subsequently, cultures were rapidly terminated and subcellular fractions were prepared. For most studies, a high-speed supernatant fraction was examined by two-dimensional isoelectric focussing-SDS polyacrylamide gel electrophoresis followed by autoradiography. In the initial studies (1), the actions of TRH were contrasted with those of VIP, cholera toxin, and cyclic

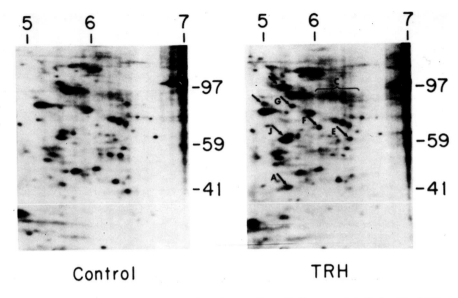

Figure 1. Effect of TRH on protein phosphorylation. Cells were labelled with [^{32}P] or-thophosphate for 60 min and treated with 1 uM TRH for 10 min. High speed supernatant fractions were analyzed by IEF/SDS PAGE as described in ref. 1. S97 indicated in Table I does not enter the IEF dimension.

AMP (cAMP) analogs, agents which mimic or elevate cyclic AMP levels. These studies showed a) that cAMP activated a number of protein phosphorylation events which TRH did not, and b) that TRH stimulated the phosphorylation of a number of proteins which cAMP did not. It was concluded that TRH activated a cAMP-independent pathway

Table I. *Effects of TRH on protein phosphorylation in GH$_3$ cells*

Protein designation	Effect of TRH	Ca^{2+} translocation	Lipid stimuli
S97	+	+	—
A	+	+	±
E	+	—	+
F	+	—	+
C	+	—	+
J	+	—	+
G	+	—	+

+ indicates stimulation, — no effect, ± marginal stimulation

of protein phosphorylation. The pattern of protein phosphorylation stimulated by TRH consisted of seven cytosolic phosphoproteins as shown in Figure 1 and Table I.

In order to evaluate a possible mediating role for Ca^{2+} in TRH action, similar studies (4) of protein phosphorylation were undertaken with agents which alter Ca^{2+} translocation (60 mM K^+, A23187, Ba^{2+}, 4AP, TEA, SVT, valinomycin, oligomycin-antimycin). Ca^{2+} translocation stimulated the phosphorylation of two proteins which corresponded to two of the seven identified by TRH stimulation (Table I). For one of these phosphoproteins (S97), increased phosphorylation in vitro was observed upon Ca^{2+} addition. In intact cells, TRH was found to exert an extremely rapid (< 15 s) and transient (~ 60 s) stimulatory effect, presumably the result of a rapid effect of the hormone in elevating cytosolic $[Ca^{2+}]$. Recent studies with the Ca^{2+} indicator quin 2 (5,6) or with aequorin (7) have confirmed the rapid elevation of cytosolic $[Ca^{2+}]$ by TRH. These studies suggested that Ca^{2+}-dependent protein kinase(s) and elevated cytosolic $[Ca^{2+}]$ constitute an effector system which accounts for two of seven phosphorylation events observed with TRH.

A third class of experiments ultimately allowed identification of the pathway which mediates TRH stimulation of the remaining five cytosolic proteins by a cAMP-independent, non-Ca^{2+}-activated pathway (8). These studies were motivated by the outcome of parallel studies which had identified a "phosphatidylinositol response" to TRH (9). During the course of protein phosphorylation studies it was observed that increased [^{32}P] labeling of PI and PA occurred upon TRH stimulation. Subsequent characterization of this response by our lab (9,10) and others (11-14) showed that the initial response to TRH consisted of a rapid phospholipase C-type hydrolysis of polyphosphoinositides as represented diagrammatically in Figure 2. Initial products of hydrolysis were found to consist of diacylglycerol (DG) and inositol triphosphate (IP$_3$).

Since the appearance of these molecules within the cells occurred within seconds of TRH addition, a possible second messenger role for either DG or IP$_3$ was possible. Increasing experimental support has implicated IP$_3$ as a second messenger for Ca^{2+} release from intracellular pools as promoted by agonists in other systems (15). A similar pathway may mediate TRH effects on Ca^{2+}. We have pursued a second messenger role for DG; the discovery of TRH stimulation of DG levels provided a plausible mechanism by which TRH stimulates the phosphorylation of five cytosolic proteins.

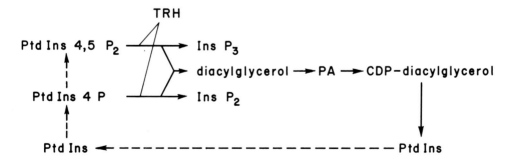

Figure 2. Effect of TRH on inositol phosphatide metabolism. Schematic summary of experimental results presented in ref. 10.

Nishizuka and co-workers had discovered and characterized a novel protein kinase (protein kinase C) which was dependent upon lipids for activity (16). An anionic phospholipid (such as PS) was required in the presence of Ca^{2+}. These workers found that DG markedly potentiated enzyme activity especially at low Ca^{2+} concentrations. Results similar to these for GH_3 protein kinase C will be reported elsewhere (8). Nishizuka and co-workers further suggested that DG generated in response to agonist stimulation might serve to couple receptor occupancy with intracellular protein phosphorylation. Support for this hypothesis for agonist stimulation of platelet secretion has been presented (17).

We examined this hypothesis in GH_3 cells by comparing the actions of TRH to a variety of agents which either increase cellular DG levels (phospholipase C), promote inositol phosphatide turnover (bombesin), mimic DG (phorbol esters), or alter lipid metabolism in a manner yet to be characterized (melittin, arachidonic acid). In each case these agents were found to stimulate a pattern of non-Ca^{2+}-activated protein phosphorylation which mimicked that of TRH (Table I)(8). Mimicry of TRH effects by the phorbol ester TPA was of particular interest since additional studies showed that TPA was a direct activator of GH_3 cell cytosolic protein kinase C. It should be noted that TRH stimulation of the phosphorylation of four (E,F,C,J) of these five cytosolic proteins is very evident by 15 s following TRH addition, a time by which maximal DG accumulation has occurred.

Further evidence that the TRH receptor interaction results in activation of protein kinase C has been obtained in studies in which the subcellular distribution of the enzyme was examined (18). GH_3 cells were treated with a number of different secretagogues and rapidly fractionated into cytosol and particulate fractions. Protein kinase C activity was measured in both fractions as a PS-stimulated histone kinase. In unstimulated cells, most (94%) of the enzyme was found in the cytosol fraction. Brief (1 min) treatment of the cells with the phorbol ester TPA resulted in a major decline in cytosolic protein kinase C with near quantitative (ca. 80%) recovery in the particulate fraction. Treatment of GH_3 cells with TRH resulted in a time-dependent and concentration-dependent shift in the distribution of protein kinase C as well. Within 15 s of TRH treatment, up to 50% of the enzyme activity disappeared from the cytosol, an effect that was maintained in the presence of TRH. There was an accompanying increase in membrane-associated protein kinase C activity. Protein kinase C redistribution occurred with an EC_{50} of approximately 20 nM for TRH. Other agents which appeared to activate protein kinase C-mediated protein phosphorylation in GH_3 cells produced a shift in enzyme distribution similar to that seen with TRH (phospholipase C, melittin, synthetic diglycerides). Other secretagogues which appeared to activate cells through either a Ca^{2+}-dependent (60 mM K^+ or Ba^{2+}) or a cAMP-dependent (VIP) pathway did not influence the subcellular distribution of protein kinase C. From these studies we conclude that TRH rapidly activates protein kinase C in GH_3 cells, presumably by virtue of hormone-receptor induced DG appearance resulting from inositol phosphatide hydrolysis. Additional studies will be required to distinguish whether cytosol-to-membrane translocation or membrane stabilization of protein kinase C underlies the shift in subcellular distribution. We presume, although it remains to be demonstrated, that translocation or stabilization occurs at the plasma membrane.

The studies outlined here and summarized in Table I and Figure 3 enabled us to account for TRH stimulation of seven cytosolic proteins as consisting of the activation of two pathways of protein phosphorylation (Fig. 3), one involving Ca^{2+}-dependent protein kinases and the other involving protein kinase C. These two cellular pathways appear to be distinct and independent. Whereas depolarization-induced Ca^{2+} influx activates the Ca^{2+}-dependent pathway, protein kinase C activation does not occur as judged by any of the criteria described above (4,8,18). In contrast, phorbol esters specifically activate the protein kinase C-mediated but not the Ca^{2+}-dependent pathway (4,8). Since TRH appears to activate both pathways, we conclude that cell activation by this hormone involves dual intracellular messengers, Ca^{2+} (possibly via IP_3) and DG. Independent determinations of rapid TRH effects on $^{45}Ca^{2+}$ fluxes (19-21), cytosolic $[Ca^{2+}]$ (4-7), and DG (10,12) accumulation are consistent with the view described here.

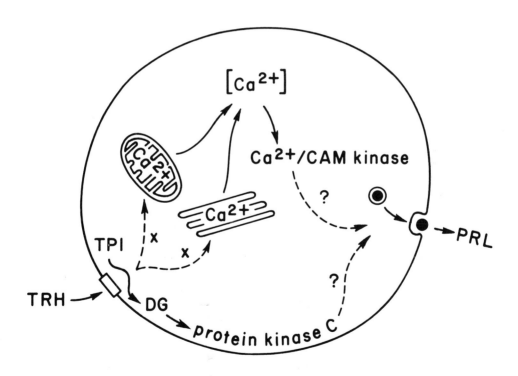

Figure 3. Schematic summary of TRH stimulation of protein phosphorylation. X designates a mediator for intracellular Ca^{2+} pool mobilization.

BIPHASIC EFFECTS OF TRH ON PROLACTIN SECRETION: POSSIBLE MEDIATION BY Ca²⁺ AND LIPIDS

The effector mechanism(s) responsible for regulating secretion is (are) unknown although it has been suggested that protein phosphorylation may play a role in this process. Studies of protein phosphorylation aid in the identification of second messengers of hormone action; however, until a phosphoprotein directly involved in exocytosis has been identified, such studies remain only suggestive of possible mechanisms underlying stimulus-secretion coupling. We initiated a series of indirect studies to determine whether independent Ca^{2+}- and DG-mediated pathways might be involved in the TRH stimulation of prolactin secretion in GH_3 cells (22,23).

As shown in Figure 4, TRH stimulation of prolactin secretion was found to exhibit virtually no latency with significant stimulation evident at 5 s following hormone addition. This can be contrasted with a 2 min latency seen with VIP (Fig. 5), a hormone that activates adenylyl cyclase in GH_3 cells. As is also evident from Figure 5,

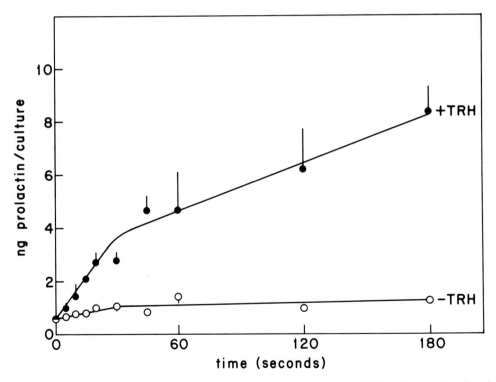

Figure 4. Effect of TRH on prolactin secretion. Monolayer cultures of GH_3 cells were incubated with (○) or without (●) 1 uM TRH for indicated times and medium prolactin content was determined by RIA. Stimulation by TRH was significant (P < .005) at all time points.

TRH stimulation of prolactin secretion was found to be biphasic. Phase I was immediate, burst-like and short-lived such that rates of secretion returned to near control by 1-3 min. Phase II consisted of a linear, sustained 2- to 4-fold elevated rate between 5 and 60 min. It should be stressed that these studies are completed within a time period during which only stored prolactin pools are being measured. Basal and TRH-stimulated (both phases I and II) prolactin secretion are completely uninfluenced during a 60-min incubation by the presence of high concentration of protein synthesis inhibitors. That is, although TRH is known to induce prolactin gene transcription and prolactin synthesis, such a stimulation constitutes a third phase response to TRH.

Additional studies have clearly distinguished the phase I and phase II secretory responses to TRH. These studies are summarized in Table II. Of interest are the distinctive requirements of phase I and II for extracellular Ca^{2+}. The phase I response was virtually completely insensitive to acutely removing Ca^{2+} or blocking its influx. However, the phase I response could be completely inhibited by preincubation for 30 min using these conditions. These studies indicate that the phase I response requires

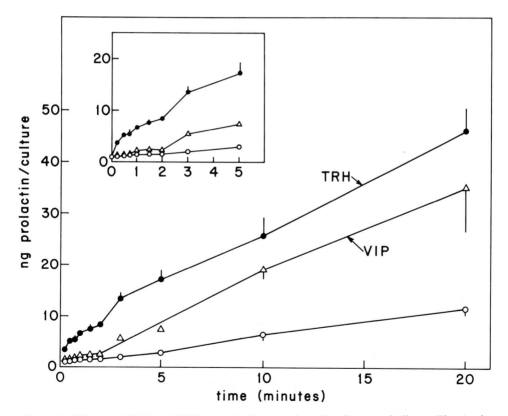

Figure 5. Effects of TRH and VIP on prolactin secretion. Details were similar to Fig. 4 using 1 uM TRH (●), 0.1 uM VIP (△) or no additions (○).

an intracellular Ca^{2+} pool. In contrast, phase II was partially inhibited by removing Ca^{2+} or blocking Ca^{2+} influx. We interpret these studies as indicating that Ca^{2+}, and probably Ca^{2+} influx, participate (along with some other effector) in the phase II response.

Table II. *Biphasic effects of TRH on prolactin secretion*

	Phase I	Phase II
EC_{50} for TRH	5 nM	1 nM
inhibition by EGTA	none	partial
inhibition by D600	none	partial
inhibition by EGTA preincubation	complete	partial
mimicry by other secretagogues	60 mM K^+, A23187, ionomycin, FCCP, CCCP, Ba^{2+}, 4 AP	TPA, melittin, phospholipase C, diglycerides

Further studies were directed at mimicking the kinetic features of phase I or phase II with secretagogues other than TRH. It was found that a wide variety of agents which altered Ca^{2+} translocation (see Table II) mimicked the phase I but not phase II response to TRH. These agents promoted a short-latency, burst-like, transitory secretory response qualitatively resembling phase I. The magnitude of the response seemed to bear a relationship to the likely magnitude and longevity of a cytoplasmic $[Ca^{2+}]$ rise. Although prolactin secretion with 60 mM K^+ was quantitatively greater than the phase I response to TRH (see Fig. 6), the response to K^+ could be adjusted to be quantitatively identical to the phase I response to TRH if Ca^{2+} channel blockers were added within 15 to 30 s of K^+ addition. We interpret this result as indicating that, when the cytoplasmic $[Ca^{2+}]$ rise to 60 mM K^+ is adjusted to more closely resemble that to TRH (4,5), the secretory responses become equivalent.

In contrast, agents found previously to activate protein kinase C-mediated protein phosphorylation (see Table II) promoted a secretory response which resembled the monotonically rising, sustained response characteristic of phase II. Additivity experiments also showed that the prolactin-releasing effects of TPA and phospholipase C at supraoptimal concentrations were nonadditive with the phase II response to TRH. In contrast, effects of VIP were additive. A comparison of the burst-like response to 60 mM K^+, the sustained response to TPA, and the biphasic response to TRH is shown in Figure 6.

These studies of biphasic secretion suggest that both pathways indicated in Figure 3 participate in regulating exocytosis in GH_3 cells. The phase I response to TRH may result from rapid, hormone-induced discharge of an intracellular Ca^{2+} pool, a resulting transient cytoplasmic $[Ca^{2+}]$ rise and a stimulatory effect of Ca^{2+} on exocytosis. In contrast, the phase II response to TRH may result from hormone-induced DG accumulation and protein kinase C activation. The partial Ca^{2+} dependency for phase II may result from a Ca^{2+} requirement for protein kinase C activation and may indicate a functional role for TRH-induced Ca^{2+} spiking. Although phase I and phase II may

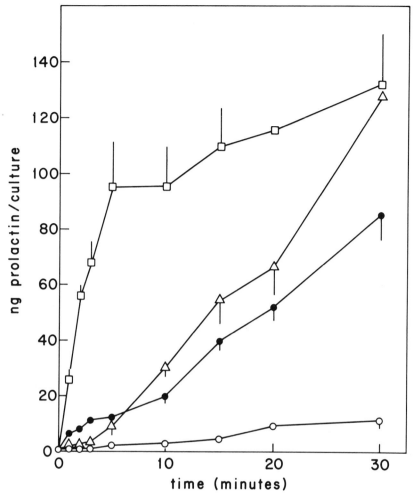

Figure 6. Comparison of secretory responses to 60 mM K+ (□), 1 uM TRH (●), 0.1 ug/ml TPA (△) or no additions (○).

appear to be temporally distinguishable, it is likely that both phases are initiated without latency but that the overall prolactin accumulation results from summation of the transient and sustained components.

EFFECTS OF Ca^{2+} AND LIPIDS ON PROLACTIN SECRETION IN PERMEABILIZED GH_3 CELLS

Baker and Knight (24) developed a permeabilized chromaffin cell preparation for directly examining effects of Ca^{2+} on exocytosis. We have used a similar approach to

explore the regulation of prolactin secretion in GH_3 cells (25). Cells were permeabilized by administering a series of voltage discharges to a cell suspension in a small capacitor
cell. 100% of the cells were rendered permeable to molecules smaller than 1000 daltons.
By titrating Ca^{2+} concentrations with Ca^{2+}-EGTA buffers, Ca^{2+}-dependent prolactin secretion can be demonstrated. Most preparations exhibit a Ca^{2+} sensitivity such
that 0.3-1 uM is half-maximally effective (Table III). Secretion in intact cells is
uninfluenced by this range of Ca^{2+} concentrations.

Table III. *Effects of Ca^{2+} on prolactin secretion in permeable and intact GH_3 cells*

[Ca^{2+}]	Prolactin release (% control)	
	Permeable cells	Intact cells
22 nM	100	100
68 nM	108	—
140 nM	113	—
350 nM	130	—
710 nM	162	107
2.0 uM	237	—
7.1 uM	294	—
18 uM	294	80

Recently, we have found that exposing permeabilized cells to synthetic diglycerides
or to phorbol esters can have either of two consequences: a) the Ca^{2+} sensitivity of
secretion appears to be shifted to the left (e.g., from EC_{50} = 0.3-1 uM to EC_{50} = 0.2
uM); b) a secretory response to these agents can be observed at extremely low Ca^{2+}
concentrations. TRH treatment of cells prior to permeabilization alters Ca^{2+}-
dependent secretion in a manner similar to direct diglyceride or phorbol ester treatment.

Although preliminary, these studies indicate that Ca^{2+} per se is a direct activator
of exocytosis in GH_3 cells as has been inferred previously from indirect studies. In addition, it appears that diglycerides are capable of directly activating exocytotic events.
What remains unclear at present is the nature of the Ca^{2+} and diglyceride receptor(s)
which mediate regulation of secretion. It is uncertain whether Ca^{2+} and diglyceride interact with a common component (e.g., protein kinase C) or whether these messengers
interact with distinct components which can independently influence aspects of exocytosis.

SUMMARY

TRH has been found to exert a rapid stimulatory effect on the breakdown of
polyphosphatidylinositides and to cause rapid Ca^{2+} mobilization. As a result, there is
rapid (< 15 s) activation of Ca^{2+}-dependent protein kinase(s) through an increase in
cytosolic Ca^{2+} and of protein kinase C probably through elevation of diacylglycerol
levels. Activation of these two independent pathways can account for altered patterns

of protein phosphorylation in GH_3 cells. It appears that effector mechanisms analogous to these may underlie biphasic effects of TRH on prolactin secretion with phase I and II mediated respectively by Ca^{2+} and by diacylglycerol (possibly in conjunction with Ca^{2+}). Direct stimulatory effects of these messengers on prolactin secretion have been demonstrated in permeabilized GH_3 cells.

ACKNOWLEDGMENTS

The author acknowledges the contributions of D.S. Drust, J.A. Kowalchyk, and S.A. Ronning to the studies reported here which were funded by the NSF and USPHS (AM 25861).

REFERENCES

1. Drust DS, Sutton CA, Martin TFJ. (1982): J Biol Chem 257:3306
2. Gershengorn MC, Rebecchi MJ, Geras E, Arevalo CO. (1980): Endocrinology 107:665
3. Gautvik KM, Gordeladze JO, Jahnsen T, Haug E, Hansson V, Lystad E. (1983): J Biol Chem 258:10304
4. Drust DS, Martin TFJ. (1982): J Biol Chem 257:7566
5. Gershengorn MC, Thaw C. (1983): Endocrinology 113:1522
6. Albert PR, Tashjian AH Jr. (1984): J Biol Chem 259:5827
7. Snowdowne KW, Borle AB. (1984): Am J Physiol 246:E198
8. Drust DS, Martin TFJ, submitted
9. Sutton CA, Martin TFJ. (1982): Endocrinology 110:1273
10. Martin TFJ. (1983): J Biol Chem 258:14816
11. Rebecchi MJ, Monaco ME, Gershengorn MC. (1981): Biochem Biophys Res Commun 101:124
12. Rebecchi MJ, Kolesnick RN, Gershengorn MC. (1983): J Biol Chem 258:227
13. Schlegel W, Roduit C, Zahnd G. (1981): FEBS Lett 134:47
14. Macphee CH, Drummond AH. (1984): Mol Pharm 25:193
15. Streb H, Irvine RF, Berridge MJ, Schultz I. (1983): Nature 306:67
16. Kikkawa U, Takai Y, Minakuchi R, Inohara S, Nishizuka Y. (1982): J Biol Chem 257:13341
17. Kaibuchi K, Takai Y, Sawamura M, Hashijima M, Fujikura T, Nishizuka Y. (1983): J Biol Chem 258:6701
18. Drust DS, Martin TFJ, in preparation
19. Ronning SA, Heatley GA, Martin TFJ. (1982): Proc Natl Acad Sci USA 79:6294
20. Gershengorn MC. (1982): Mol Cell Biochem 45:163
21. Tan KN, Tashjian AH Jr. (1981): J Biol Chem 256:8994
22. Martin TFJ, Kowalchyk JA. (1984): Endocrinology, in press
23. Martin TFJ, Kowalchyk JA. (1984): Endocrinology, in press
24. Knight DE, Baker PF. (1982): J Membrane Biol 68:107
25. Ronning SA, Martin TFJ, in preparation

Prolactin. Basic and clinical correlates
R.M. MacLeod, M.O. Thorner and U. Scapagnini (eds.),
Fidia Research Series, vol. I,
Liviana Press, Padova © 1985

Section III
Intracellular pituitary mechanisms
regulating prolactin release

CALCIUM MEDIATED INACTIVATION OF CALCIUM CONDUCTANCE IN A PROLACTIN SECRETING CELL LINE

B. Dufy, B. Dupuy, D. Georgescauld, and J.L. Barker

Laboratoire Neurophysiologie, Université de Bordeaux II,
Centre de Recherche Paul Pascal, C.N.R.S., Talence, France,
and Laboratory of Neurology, NINCDS, Bethesda, Maryland

The central role of Ca^{2+} ions in stimulus-secretion coupling is well recognized. In pituitary cells, as in other endocrine cells, the mean concentration of resting free Ca^{2+} ions is low, showing that most of the intracellular Ca^{2+} is bound. The transmission of specific signals across the membrane of the cell may trigger intracellular reactions leading to an increase in intracellular concentration of free Ca^{2+} through release from bound stores (1,2). Also, there are data available showing that pituitary cells are excitable and able to display action potentials with a prominent Ca^{2+} component (4,5); the transmembrane influx of Ca^{2+} ions through action potentials could be an effective way to provide the cell with the Ca^{2+} required for exocytosis (3,4,6).

In this study we have examined the role of intracellular divalent cation accumulation in the regulation of divalent cation entry in clonal pituitary cells. The results indicate that Ca^{2+} but not Ba^{2+} intracellular accumulation quickly inactivates voltage-dependent Ca^{2+} conductance and that this inactivation can be triggered by TRH in both Ca^{2+}- and Ba^{2+}-containing media. Therefore we suggest that intracellular Ca^{2+} accumulation, arising from extra- and/or intracellular sources, regulates extracellular Ca^{2+} entry.

GH_3/B_6 cells, originally obtained from Tixier-Vidal et al. (College de France, Paris), were maintained in a CO_2 buffered medium (F10) supplemented with 15% horse serum and 2.5% fetal calf serum according to methods previously described (3,5,7). Electrophysiological recordings were conducted on low-passage (10-16) cells 5-10 days after replating. The cells were studied at room temperature (23 ± 1 C) in medium containing (in mM): 142.6 NaCl, 5.6 KCl, 2.5 $CaCl_2$, 5 glucose, and 5 HEPES (pH 7.4). In some experiments the $(Ca^{2+})_0$ was raised to 10 mM since this often stabilized the recording. All of the data considered in the present study were derived from recordings lasting more than 30 min. Intracellular recordings were made with a single microelectrode filled with either 3 M KCl, 3 M CsCl, 1.5-3 M K^+-citrate, 0.7 M K_2SO_4, 3 M

CsCl + 45 mM EGTA, or 3 M KCl + 45 mM EGTA (tip resistances: 50-90 megohms). The cells were current- or voltage- clamped using a high-frequency switching circuit (DAGAN 8100). Ion changes or peptide additions in the vicinity of the recorded cells were accomplished by low pressure applications from closely positioned pipettes having tip diameters of 3-5 microns (7).

The relaxation (decay) of the inward current is masked by the presence of simultaneously developing outward currents attributed to an efflux of K^+ ions. In the experiments described in this study, the K^+ currents were minimized by loading the cell with cesium using CsCl (3 M) microelectrodes. The effectiveness of cellular Cs loading is illustrated by the firing of large prolonged (2-10 sec) Ca^{2+} spikes. Presumably, intracellular Cs^+ ions block outwardly directed currents in these cells, thus leaving inwardly directed current responses in relative isolation (Fig. 1). Under these recording conditions, Ca^{2+} current inactivation was measured with a double pulse method.

The inward current elicited by a test voltage clamp depolarization (Fig. 2A "control") was depressed following inward current evoked by a conditioning depolarization (Fig. 2). Application of this twin-step depolarizing command protocol led to a marked depression or elimination of the inward current response elicited during the second

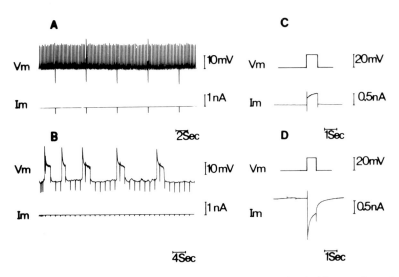

Figure 1. Comparison of voltage (Vm) and current (Im) traces obtained with recording micropipettes respectively filled with 3 M KCl and 3 M CsCl solutions. In A and C the pipettes were filled with KCl whereas CsCl was used in B and D. A and B represent current clamp recordings. B, loading the cell with Cs ions led to the firing of large prolonged action potentials (compare with action potential firing obtained with a KCl electrode (A)). Under voltage clamp conditions (Vh = -60 mV depolarizing step 20 mV) current traces (Im) obtained with KCl electrodes (C) showed a large outward current which was suppressed when CsCl electrodes (D) were used leaving a large inward current.

step (Fig. 2A "inactivation"). Since the inward current responses were dependent on $(Ca^{2+})_o$ (not shown) and were blocked by 10 mM Co^{2+} (Fig. 2A: "Co^{2+}") we tentatively conclude that these responses are calcium currents (I_{Ca}). I-V curves obtained in the presence of Co^{2+} were similar, if not identical, to those constructed for responses obtained during the second step (not shown, but compare the current response evoked during the second step with that elicited during Co^{2+} application).

For a constant conditioning-test interval in the double step depolarizing command protocol, the conditioning commands were only effective in depressing subsequent current responses when the cell was initially depolarized to potentials that evoked detectable inward currents. The potential dependency of the suppression is plotted in Figure 2B and corresponds to the potential range for generating active I_{Ca}s. By subtracting the leakage component of the current response (that remaining after elimination of all active currents) from the inward current response, the peak amplitude of I_{Ca} and the charge movement (I_{Ca} x time, or Q_{Ca}) can be determined. Figure 2C shows that Q_{Ca} evoked during the second step is inversely proportional to Q_{Ca} generated during the first step.

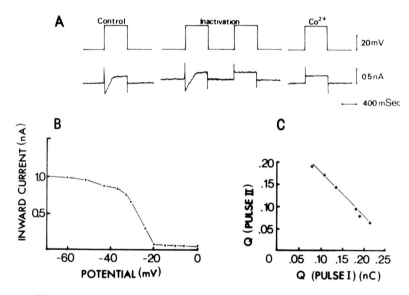

Figure 2. Ca^{2+} entry inactivates Ca^{2+} conductance in GH_3/B_6 cells. Intracellular recordings were made with CsCl-filled microelectrodes in a Ca^{2+}-containing medium. A. The cell was held at - 70 mV and stepped to - 40 mV for 0.5 sec, evoking an inward current response that relaxed in 200 msec ("control" trace). Application of a twin step depolarizing command protocol led to the elimination of the inward current response during the second step ("inactivation"). The remaining current response evoked during the second step is identical to that observed during Co^{2+} application ("Co^{2+}"). B. Inward current during the second step for a constant interval between the step. Depression of the inward current response occurs at - 40 mV and is complete by - 20 mV. C. The charge (Q) associated with second step is inversely proportional to the charge developed during the first step.

Similar double step experiments were conducted with the normal complement of Ca^{2+} ions being replaced by Ba^{2+} ions. Under these conditions the relaxation of the inward current response evoked during a depolarization command was much slower compared to that recorded in Ca^{2+}-containing medium (Fig. 3A) and the suppression of inward current in a double-step protocol was markedly less (Fig. 3B). Comparison of recovery from the suppression in Ba^{2+}- and Ca^{2+}-containing solutions revealed that recovery from complete inactivation was about five-fold slower in the latter medium (Fig. 3C).

The failure of Ba^{2+} to inactivate inward current strongly supports the hypothesis that inactivation of Ca channels results from the accumulation of intracellular Ca^{2+} ions. To further test this hypothesis microelectrodes filled with K^+-citrate, K^+-sulfate, or EGTA (45 mM) were also used in order to buffer intracellular Ca^{2+} ions. Recovery was equally rapid when the cells were recorded in Ca^{2+}-containing medium using K_2SO_4 or K^+-citrate microelectrodes or when EGTA (45 mM) was added to the solution used to fill the 3 M CsCl microelectrodes (Fig. 4). On the other hand addition of 10 mM $CaCl_2$ to the 3 M KCl or 3 M CsCl electrodes suppressed action potentials in current clamp conditions and all inward currents in voltage clamp conditions (not shown).

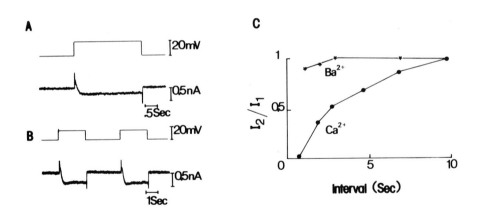

Figure 3. Ba^{2+} entry does not significantly inactivate Ba^{2+} conductance. Intracellular recordings were made with 3 M KCl microelectrodes in bathing solutions containing 10 mM Ba^{2+} instead of 10 mM Ca^{2+}. A. The cell was held at - 50 mV and depolarized to - 35 mV for two seconds. B. Closely spaced twin pulses show no decrement in the current evoked during the second step. C. Comparison of current amplitude ratios as a function of the inter-pulse interval in Ca^{2+}- and Ba^{2+}-containing solutions. At a one second inter-pulse interval the amplitude of the current evoked during the second step is 90% of that elicited during the first step in Ba^{2+} but close to zero in Ca^{2+}. In Ba^{2+} recovery is complete in 2-3 seconds, but a full 10 seconds are required in Ca^{2+}.

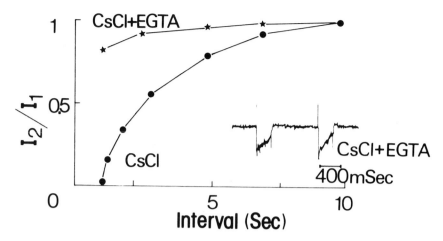

Figure 4. Comparison of current amplitude ratios as a function of interpulse interval for microelectrodes filled respectively with 3 M CsCl and 3 M CsCl + 45 mM EGTA. Inactivation is reduced when the cell is loaded with EGTA.

These results suggest that the accumulation of Ca^{2+} ions rapidly leads to depression of membrane conductance to Ca^{2+} ions and that this phenomenon is markedly attenuated when Ba^{2+} ions are the charge-carrying ions or when high concentrations of sulphate, citrate-ions, or EGTA are available to complex with intracellular Ca^{2+} ions. Ca^{2+} current decays during the pulse (Fig. 2A) and the inward tail current decreases in amplitude as the pulse is made longer (not shown) which suggests that the Ca^{2+} channels are indeed inactivated. We agree therefore with Matteson and Armstrong (8) who have recently reported that inactivation of the Ca^{2+} currents recorded in GH_3 cells under similar conditions is indeed due to inactivation of the conductance. However, since they were unable to alter the time course of recovery from inactivation with 50 mM EGTA delivered intracellularly through diffusion from a whole-cell patch electrode, they concluded, in contrast to results obtained in molluscan cells (9), that simple accumulation of Ca^{2+} ions was not the proximal mechanism leading to inactivation. Our results with EGTA (45 mM)filled micropipettes contrast with their data. As a tentative explanation, we suggest that the double pulse protocol addresses a slower component of Ca inactivation than that analyzed with the inward tail study. In molluscan neurons, the inactivation of calcium current has two components, a fast (with time constant of several milliseconds) and a slow (with time constant of several hundred milliseconds) (10,11). Moreover, it has been reported that the time course of recovery from inactivation of the Ca current is different from the single time constant inactivation of the Ca current observed during maintained depolarization (10). These two phenomena may therefore reflect different processes. Also, rapid changes in the level of $(Ca)_i$ (in terms of milliseconds) may not be efficiently buffered by pipettes containing EGTA in the whole cell patch clamp recordings.

Thyrotropin releasing hormone (TRH), that stimulates prolactin secretion from GH_3 cells (6), induces a complex sequence of changes in membrane excitability, the

182

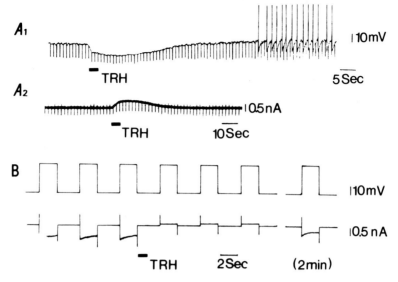

Figure 5. Thryrotropin releasing hormone (TRH: 50 nM) inactivates Ca^{2+} and Ba^{2+} conductance. Intracellular recordings were made with 3 M KCl-containing microelectrodes in medium containing 10 mM Ca^{2+} (A_1 and A_2) and 10 mM Ba^{2+} (B). A_1. TRH initially hyperpolarizes the cell by 10 mV; after the cell has recovered to its resting membrane potential, it spontaneously generates actions potentials. A_2. Under voltage clamp TRH (50 nM) induced a transient outwardly directed membrane current. B. Within several seconds, TRH (50 nM) completely suppresses all inward current responses obtained in Ba^{2+} (10 mM) bathing solution. Inward current responses return transiently, by two minutes though amplitudes are smaller.

first of which involves a transient increase in K^+ conductance (4) that appears to reflect release of intracellular Ca ions (1,2). We have examined the effects of TRH on inward currents evoked by depolarizing commands in Ca^{2+}- and Ba^{2+}-containing media. The results show that brief application of TRH induces a transient (15-30 sec) outward current associated with an increase in conductance at the level of the resting potential (Fig. 5A). During this transient period inward current response was eliminated in both Ca^{2+}- and Ba^{2+}-containing media (Fig. 5B). This data strongly suggests that Ca^{2+} ions released from intracellular stores by brief application of TRH can rapidly and reversibly inactivate voltage-dependent membrane conductance to Ba^{2+} and Ca^{2+} ions. Alternatively, the peptide might alter divalent cation conductance directly, but patch clamp analysis of Ca^{2+} channel activity with and without TRH will be necessary to consider this possibility further.

ACKNOWLEDGMENTS

This work was supported by grants from C.N.R.S. (A.T.P. Pharmacologie des recepteurs des neuromediateurs) Fondation pour la Recherche Medicale and Comité

Departemental de la Ligue Nationale de Lutte contre le Cancer (Dordogne). The authors are grateful to A.M. Courtes, S. Vitiello, D. Varoqueaux, N. Villaylek, and G. Gaurier for collaboration in various phases of these studies.

REFERENCES

1. Gershengorn MC, Thaw C. (1983): Endocrinology 113:1522
2. Ronning SA, Heatley GA, Martin TFJ. (1982): Proc Natl Acad Sci (USA) 79:6294
3. Dufy B, Vincent JD, Fleury H, Du Pasquier P, Gourdji J, Tixier-Vidal A. (1979): Science 204:509
4. Ozawa S, Kimura N. (1979): Proc Natl Acad Aci (USA) 76:6017
5. Dubinsky JM, Oxford GS. (1984): J Gen Physiol 83:309
6. Tan KN, Tashjian AH Jr. (1981): J Biol Chem 256:8994
7. Dufy B, Barker JL. (1982): Life Sci 30:1933
8. Natteson DR, Armstrong CH (1984): J Gen Physiol 83:371
9. Eckert R, Tilloston D. (1981): J Physiol (Lond) 314:265
10. Adams DS, Gage PW. (1979): J Physiol (Lond) 289:143
11. Kostyuk PG, Krishtal OA (1977): J Physiol (Lond) 270:545

Prolactin. Basic and clinical correlates
R.M. MacLeod, M.O. Thorner and U. Scapagnini (eds.),
Fidia Research Series, vol. I,
Liviana Press, Padova © 1985

Section III
Intracellular pituitary mechanisms
regulating prolactin release

MODULATION OF ANTERIOR PITUITARY ADENYLATE CYCLASE ACTIVITY AND PROLACTIN SECRETION BY MAITOTOXIN, A CALCIUM CHANNEL ACTIVATOR

G. Schettini, E.L. Hewlett, M.J. Cronin, K. Koike, I. S. Login, A.M. Judd, T. Yasumoto, and R. M. MacLeod

Depts. of Internal Medicine, Pharmacology, Neurology, and Physiology, University of Virginia, Charlottesville, VA, and Faculty of Agriculture, Tohoku University, Tsutsumi-dori, Sendai 980, Japan

The release of prolactin from the pituitary lactotroph is regulated by both stimulatory and inhibitory hormones (1). In response to these stimuli, changes in cell calcium (Ca^{2+}) metabolism, adenylate cyclase activity, and phospholipid turnover have been reported (2-4). *In vitro* release of prolactin is enhanced by an increase in Ca^{2+} concentration (5-6), whereas perifusion of pituitary cells with Ca^{2+}-free medium or the addition of Ca^{2+} channel blockers suppresses prolactin release (6). Depolarization of pituitary cells with K^+ increases $^{45}Ca^{2+}$ uptake and induces Ca^{2+}-dependent prolactin release (7). In addition Ca^{2+} ionophore A23187 and thyroliberin (TRH), which also increase $^{45}Ca^{2+}$ uptake, stimulate prolactin secretion from pituitary cells in culture (8-10). The involvement of cyclic AMP (cAMP) in the prolactin secretory process has been suggested because many compounds that change the cellular concentrations of cAMP also modify prolactin release (11-12). In addition, the inhibition of adenylate cyclase activity and cAMP accumulation with dopamine or its agonists, in prolactinomas (13) or normal pituitary tissue (14-15), is associated with suppression of prolactin release.

Calcium and cAMP have integrated actions to control cellular functions (16). Prolactin release induced by cAMP analogs or phosphodiesterase inhibitors requires the presence of Ca^{2+} (17-18). In the absence of Ca^{2+} these agents stimulate cAMP accumulation but not hormonal release (19). Moreover Ca^{2+} ionophore A23187 stimulates cAMP accumulation and prolactin release from primary culture of anterior pituitary cells (11). Therefore, increased Ca^{2+} mobilization and early activation of the pituitary cAMP system may act synergistically to stimulate the release of prolactin. Indeed in many cell types the action of Ca^{2+} is amplified by cAMP and, conversely, cAMP can modulate the intracellular Ca^{2+} status in certain circumstances (16).

Moreover Ca^{2+} serves as a regulator of cyclic nucleotide metabolism in some cellular systems, modulating both adenylate cyclase and phosphodiesterase activity (16).

The effectiveness of Ca^{2+} is often dependent upon the intracellular Ca^{2+}-binding protein calmodulin (CaM). Initially reported to be an activator of phosphodiesterase (20), CaM was shown to be a regulator of many other Ca^{2+}-dependent enzymes and to have a role in modulating many cellular processes (21). Furthermore CaM regulates Ca^{2+}-dependent adenylate cyclase activity in the brain (22) and in pancreatic islets (23). There is also evidence to suggest the involvement of CaM in the regulation of prolactin release and cAMP formation both in normal and clonal pituitary cells (11,24,25).

In the present study we investigated the role of Ca^{2+} and its interaction with the cAMP generating system in modulation of prolactin secretion. We then evaluated the involvement of CaM in the Ca^{2+} modulation of anterior pituitary adenylate cyclase activity. We used maitotoxin (MTX), a novel substance with Ca^{2+} channel activating properties.

STUDIES OF THE EFFECT OF MTX ON Ca^{2+} FLUX, cAMP ACCUMULATION, AND PROLACTIN SECRETION BY ANTERIOR PITUITARY CELLS

Recently Yasumoto et al. reported the extraction and partial purification of MTX from a marine dinoflagellate, *Gamdieridiscus toxicus* (26). MTX expresses properties of a potent Ca^{2+} channel activator. Indeed it increased $^{45}Ca^{2+}$ uptake and catecholamine release by pheochromocytoma cell line PC12h in a manner similar to that induced by K^+ depolarization (27). Both effects were reversed by the Ca^{2+} channel antagonist verapamil and manganese (27). Moreover, the MTX-stimulated catecholamine release was concentration-dependent, related to the extracellular Ca^{2+} levels but independent of sodium in the external medium (27). In contrast with the mechanism of action of Ca^{2+} ionophore A23187, MTX does not possess ionophoretic properties in mitochondrial membranes and liposomal preparation, indicating that MTX requires the integrity of the plasmalemma. Thus MTX appears to act through the activation of a Ca^{2+} channel (28).

In these studies we investigated the effect of MTX on Ca^{2+} flux, cAMP metabolism, and prolactin secretion by anterior pituitary cells. We determined the effect of MTX on Ca^{2+} exchange using the procedure described by Reeves (1975), Keppens et al. (1977) and Hirata et al. (1983) (29-31).

In dispersed anterior pituitary cells in suspension prepared as previously described (11), 40 ng MTX/ml induced an early and sustained activation of $^{45}Ca^{2+}$ exchange. MTX enhanced the amount of $^{45}Ca^{2+}$ associated with the cells within 30 sec, continuing for at least 30 min (Fig. 1).

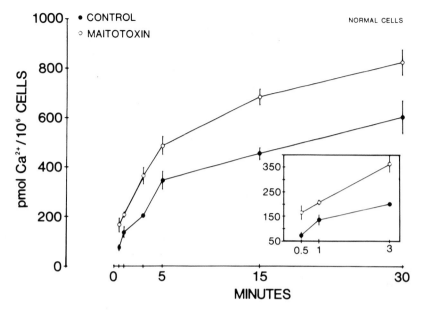

Figure 1. Effect of MTX on $^{45}Ca^{2+}$ exchange by dispersed anterior pituitary cells. Incubation of dispersed anterior pituitary cells with $^{45}Ca^{2+}$ in the presence of 40 ng/ml MTX for the indicated time caused an increase in the amount of $^{45}Ca^{2+}$ associated with the cells in comparison with untreated cells. The effect of MTX was evident at 30 sec (P < 0.05) and continued over the time course studied (P < 0.01).

Table 1. *Time course of the effect of MTX on cyclic AMP accumulation and pro-lactin release by primary culture of anterior pituitary cells*

A

| | cAMP pmol/well | | Prolactin ng/well | |
	Control	MTX 50 ng/ml	Control	MTX 50 ng/ml
30 sec.	1.5 ± 0.08	1.4 ± 0.02	516 ± 124	402 ± 32
1 min.	1.5 ± 0.04	1.2 ± 0.05	417 ± 22	433 ± 43
3 min.	0.98 ± 0.03	1.3 ± 0.05	—	1151 ± 58
10 min.	1.03 ± 0.06	1.34 ± 0.03	755 ± 245	3063 ± 124
30 min.	1.01 ± 0.05	1.34 ± 0.08	769 ± 43	6975 ± 241

B

| | cAMP pmol/well | | Prolactin ng/well | |
	Control	MTX 50 ng/ml	Control	MTX 50 ng/ml
30 sec.	4.07 ± 0.22	3.80 ± 0.4	240 ± 14	812 ± 115
1 min.	3.61 ± 0.13	4.43 ± 0.22	182 ± 24	1919 ± 222
3 min.	2.89 ± 0.01	5.53 ± 0.31	125 ± 12	3263 ± 162
10 min.	2.87 ± 0.11	4.20 ± 0.18	710 ± 75	9391 ± 580
30 min.	2.60 ± 0.14	—	852 ± 76	10922 ± 583

We also evaluated the effect of MTX on prolactin release and cAMP formation. The experiments were performed in primary culture of anterior pituitary cells pretreated or not with the phosphodiesterase inhibitor isobutylmethylxanthine (IBMX) 0.2 mM for 2 h. In the absence of IBMX, MTX 50 ng/ml significantly stimulated the release of prolactin at 3 min, an effect that continued to be observed for 30 min (Table 1A). While MTX did not increase cAMP levels in the absence of IBMX, it prevented the progressive time-related decrease in cAMP and there was a significant difference in pituitary cAMP content at 3, 10, and 30 min when compared to control cells (Table 1A).

In IBMX-treated cells, MTX produced a stimulation of both cAMP accumulation and prolactin release. The data in Table 1B show that prolactin release was significantly stimulated at 30 sec and cAMP accumulation was increased after 1 min of exposure to MTX. Because of these positive results we studied the effect of graded doses of MTX on cAMP accumulation and prolactin release in IBMX-treated cells. MTX progressively stimulated the accumulation of cAMP and the release of prolactin during 15 min of exposure (Fig. 2), with 1 or 5 ng MTX/ml ineffective to enhance either of the parameters, but 10 and 50 ng MTX/ml increasing both pituitary cAMP accumulation and prolactin release. These data are in keeping with our previous observation that Ca^{2+} ionophore A23187 stimulated both cAMP formation and prolactin release (11) and confirm our suggestion that Ca^{2+} and cAMP have an integrated role in regulating prolactin secretion.

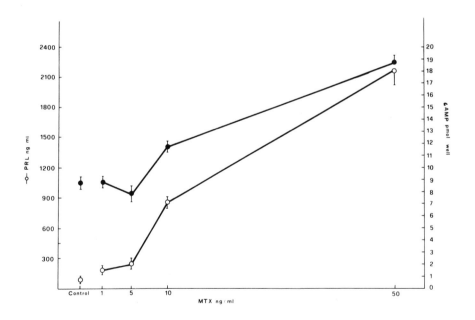

Figure 2. Effect of MTX on cAMP accumulation and prolactin release by primary culture of anterior pituitary cells. MTX progressively stimulated the accumulation of cAMP and the release of prolactin during 15 min of exposure for concentrations of 10 and 50 ng/ml.

We have just shown that MTX stimulates the accumulation of pituitary cAMP *in vitro*. Subsequently we studied whether MTX produces this effect by a direct action on anterior pituitary adenylate cyclase assayed as previously described (15). Hemipituitary glands were exposed for 10 min to 100 ng MTX/ml, then homogenized and their membranes assayed for adenylate cyclase. The data in Table 2 show that membranes prepared from MTX-pretreated glands have an increased adenylate cyclase

Table 2. *Effect of preincubation of anterior pituitary glands for 10 min with 100 ng MTX/ml on adenylate cyclase activity*

	pmol cAMP/mg protein/min
Control	32 ± 0.9
MTX 100 ng/ml	46.5 ± 3.1

activity as compared to non-treated membranes. The addition of MTX directly to the membrane preparation did not alter the enzyme activity, thus excluding a direct effect of the agent on the enzyme. These data show that the stimulatory effect of MTX on adenylate cyclase appears to be dependent on its Ca^{2+}-mobilizing property, requiring intact viable cells.

Ca^{2+}-CALMODULIN MODULATION OF ANTERIOR PITUITARY ADENYLATE CYCLASE ACTIVITY

The fact that enhanced pituitary adenylate cyclase activity is produced by MTX prompted us to investigate whether a Ca^{2+} signal is sufficient to produce this effect. A similar observation is reported in GH_3 cells (25), brain (22), and pancreatic islets (23) where Ca^{2+} has a biphasic action. However, the manner by which Ca^{2+} affects adenylate cyclase activity has not been determined. It might be possible that membranal CaM may represent a site for the action of Ca^{2+} on the enzyme. It is known that CaM modulates the Ca^{2+} regulation of adenylate cyclase activity in several cell types. We studied the effect of various concentrations of Ca^{2+} on pituitary adenylate cyclase activity. The data in Figure 3 show that increasing concentrations of Ca^{2+} up to 100 uM significantly stimulated anterior pituitary adenylate cyclase activity, whereas higher concentrations were either ineffective or inhibitory to the enzyme activity.

To study whether CaM affects anterior pituitary adenylate cyclase, we added CaM to anterior pituitary membrane preparations, both in the presence and absence of added Ca^{2+}. Membranes were prepared as previously described (15) or extensively washed with EGTA to reduce endogenous Ca^{2+} and CaM content (32). The addition of 10 ug CaM to membrane preparations not extensively washed with EGTA, both with and without exogenously added Ca^{2+}, caused a similar increase in anterior pituitary adenylate cyclase (data not presented). In contrast, when the membranes were extensively washed with EGTA to reduce the endogenous content of CaM, they showed a significantly lower basal enzymatic activity and less responsiveness to exogenous Ca^{2+} and CaM added alone. The addition of CaM was more effective in enhancing pituitary

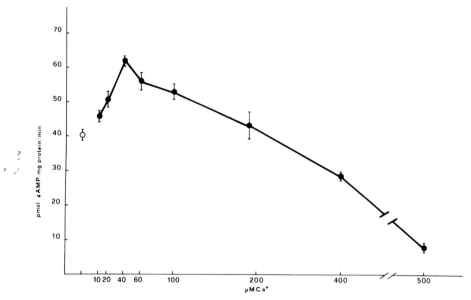

Figure 3. Effect of increasing concentrations of CaCl₂ on anterior pituitary adenylate cyclase activity.

adenylate cyclase in the presence of Ca^{2+} than without the cation (Table 3). In keeping with similar observations in pituitary GH_3 cells, brain, and pancreatic islets, we propose that Ca^{2+} and CaM are important modulators of anterior pituitary adenylate cyclase activity.

Table 3. *Effect of calmodulin (CaM) on anterior pituitary adenylate cyclase activity*

| | pmol cAMP/mg protein/min | |
	Agent alone	Agent plus 40 uM CaCl₂
Control	42.3 ± 0.5	51.5 ± 3.2
CaM 10 ug	49.2 ± 2.1	66.6 ± 1.8
CaM 20 ug	51.1 ± 0.6	81.8 ± 1.4

CONCLUSIONS

The data presented in this study demonstrate that MTX, a Ca^{2+} channel activator, stimulates pituitary Ca^{2+} exchange, adenylate cyclase activity, cAMP formation, and prolactin release. Moreover, anterior pituitary adenylate cyclase appears to be regulated by Ca^{2+} and CaM.

In conclusion our data indicate that the roles of Ca^{2+} and cAMP are integrated and constitutive in the control of prolactin secretion. The binding of Ca^{2+} to CaM stimulates adenylate cyclase and therefore increases cAMP formation that along with Ca^{2+} participates in the process of prolactin release.

ACKNOWLEDGMENTS

We gratefully acknowledge the skillful technical assistance of Carlos Valdenegro, Suzanne O'Dell, Catherine Harcus, and Gwen Baber and the valuable editorial assistance of Linda Day Evans and Susan Adams.

G.S. is a recipient of PHS Fogarty Center Fellowship 1 FO5 TWO 3627-01. R.M.M. is funded by USPHS Grant CA-07535 from the National Cancer Institute, I.S.L. is a recipient of a Teacher Investigator Development Award and is funded by NINCDS 5 KO7 NS00454 and BRSA 5 S07 RR05431. A.M.J. is a recipient of USPHS fellowship (F-32-CA-07137). M.J.C. is funded by RCDA 1 K04 NS 500601 and NS 18409.

REFERENCES

1. MacLeod RM, Scapagnini U (eds). (1980): Central and Peripheral Regulation of Prolactin Function. Raven Press, New York
2. Moriarty CM. (1978): Life Sci 23:185
3. Labrie F, Borgeat P, Drouvin J, Legace V, Giguere J, Raymond J, Godbout M, Massieotte J, Ferland L, Barden N, Beaulieu M, Cote J, Lepine J, Meunier H, Veilleux R. (1982): Handbook of Experimental Pharmacol 58:525
4. Canonico PL, MacLeod RM. (1983) In: Muller EE, MacLeod RM (eds) Neuroendocrine Perspectives. Elsevier/North Holland Biomedical Press, Amsterdam, vol 2:123
5. MacLeod RM, Fontham EH. (1980): Endocrinology 86:863
6. Thorner MO, Hackett JT, Murad F, MacLeod RM. (1980): Neuroendocrinology 31:390
7. Milligan JV, Kraicer J. (1971) Endocrinology 89:766
8. Gershengorn MC. (1980) J Biol Chem 255:1801
9. Tam SW, Dannies PS. (1980): J Biol Chem 255:6595
10. Tan KN, Tashjian AH Jr. (1981): J Biol Chem 256:8994
11. Schettini G, Cronin MJ, MacLeod RM. (1983): Endocrinology 112:1801
12. Swennen L, Denef C. 1982 Endocrinology 111:398
13. De Camilli P, Macconi D, Spada A. (1979): Nature 278:252
14. Giannattasio G, De Ferrari ME, Spada A. (1981): Life Sci 28:1605
15. Onali P, Schwartz JP, Costa E. (1981); Proc Natl Acad Sci USA 78:6531
16. Rasmussen H. (1981): Calcium and cAMP as Synarchic Messengers, John Wiley and Sons, New York
17. Lemay A, Labrie F. (1972): FEBS Lett 20:7
18. Tam SW, Dannies PS. (1981): Endocrinology 109, 403
19. Spence JW, Sheppard, MS, Kraicer J. (1980): Endocrinology 106:764
20. Cheung WY. (1970): Biochem Biophys Res Commun 38:533
21. Cheung WY. (1980): Science 207:19
22. Brostrom CO, Huang YC, Breckenridge BM, Wolff DJ. (1975): Proc Natl Acad Sci USA 72:64
23. Valverde I, Vandermeers A, Anjaneyulu R, Malaisse WJ. (1979): Science 206:225

24. Schettini G, Judd AM, MacLeod RM. (1983): Endocrinology 112:64
25. Brostrom MA, Brostrom LA, Brostrom CO. (1982): Biochim Biophys Acta 721:227
26. Yasumoto T, Nakajima I, Oshima Y, Bagnis R. (1979) In: Taylor DL, Seliger H (eds) Toxic Dinoflagellate Blooms. Elsevier/North-Holland, Amsterdam, p 65
27. Takahashi M, Ohizumi Y, Yasumoto T. (1982): J Biol Chem 257:7287
28. Takahashi M, Tatsumi M, Ohizumi Y, Yasamoto T. (1983): J Biol Chem 258:10944
29. Reeves JP. (1975): J Biol Chem 250:9413
30. Keppens S, Vandenheede JR, De Wulf H. (1977): Biochim Biophys Acta 496:448
31. Hirata M, Suematsu E, Koga T. (1983): Mol Pharmacol 23:78
32. Geagy M, Treisman G. (1981): Mol Pharmacol 19:256

Prolactin. Basic and clinical correlates
R.M. MacLeod, M.O. Thorner and U. Scapagnini (eds.),
Fidia Research Series, vol. I,
Liviana Press, Padova © 1985

Section III
Intracellular pituitary mechanisms
regulating prolactin release

ELECTROPHYSIOLOGICAL EFFECTS OF DOPAMINE ON PROLACTINOMA CELLS

J.M. Israel, P. Jaquet*, and J.D. Vincent

Inserm U. 176, 33077 Bordeaux-Cedex. *Laboratoire de Médécine Experimentale 13015 Marseille-Cedex, France.

It is generally accepted that an increase in internal calcium ($[Ca^{2+}]i$) is the "critical" event which leads to release of the hormone prolactin (1). Among mechanisms which have been proposed to account for the $[Ca^{2+}]i$ increase, activation of voltage-dependent calcium channels located in the plasmic membrane (2) has been investigated. Since calcium action potentials were recorded in anterior pituitary cells (3-6) it has been suggested that the necessary increase of cytosolic calcium could result from the spiking activity. Several authors have attempted to show that electrical activity of anterior pituitary cells could be modified by substances which influence prolactin release. Dopamine and gamma-aminobutyric acid, which decrease prolactin release, also inhibited the firing activity of pituitary cells (7-9). Thyroliberin (TRH) and estrogen are known to increase prolactin secretion and these substances triggered the firing of cells (4-6). Unfortunately, little is known about the detailed mechanism by which these substances act. If potassium ions seem to be implicated in the electrophysiological effect of TRH (6) we know of nothing that has been published on the membrane effects of dopamine. Recently, Douglas and Taraskevich (10) have proposed a possible calcium-blocking effect of dopamine on action potentials recorded from rat pars-distalis cells. We thus have been interested in taking a closer look at the mechanisms involved in modulation of prolactin release by dopamine.

For this study we used cells from human adenomas which had been characterized clinically as prolactin-secreting tumors, the secretion of which was modulated by bromocriptine. The cells were dissociated using an enzymatic treatment and then placed in coated Petri dishes (35 mm) and grown in Dulbecco's modified Eagle medium (DMEM). The cells were maintained in a CO_2 (6%) incubator at 37 C for a minimum of ten days before the electro-physiological experiments were performed. Electrical activity was recorded through a bridge amplifier using a single intracellular microelectrode for voltage recording and to pass current through the membrane so as to vary the potential of the cell.

During the experimental procedure, the cells were in a medium of DMEM buffered with Hepes to pH 7.5 and maintained at 36 C.

Under these conditions, the cells were relatively flat and it was difficult to impale them without causing some damage to the membrane. Nevertheless 50 to 70% of the cells tested gave data which could be interpreted.

The electrophysiological characteristics of these cells did not differ from those recorded in other types of human pituitary cells (11). They had a strong input mem-

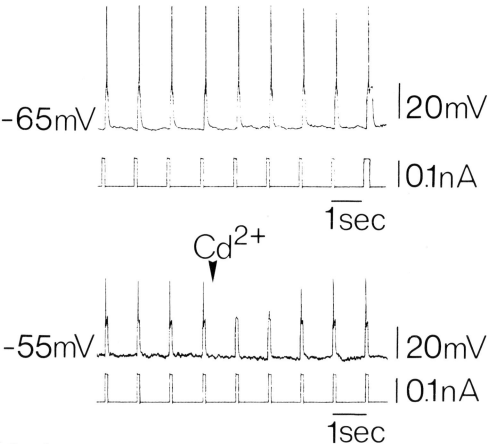

Figure 1.

Top: Electrical activity (upper trace) recorded from a human tumoral prolactin-secreting cell (resting potential: -65 mV) triggered by small depolarizing current pulses of O.1 nA, 120 msec duration, and frequency 1 Hz (lower trace). The action potential consisted in a brief response of 10 msec duration and 50 mV in amplitude.

Bottom: Ionic characteristics of the action potential: Cadmium (10 mM in the delivery pipette) was ejected for 100 msec close to the cell tested. It did not induce a modification of the resting potential of the cell but totally inhibited the action potential. This effect was reversible.

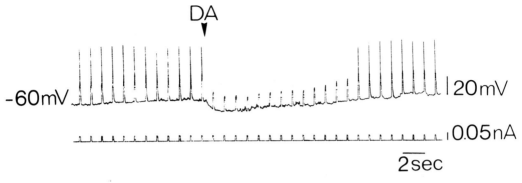

Figure 2. Effects of dopamine (DA) on the electrophysiological properties of human tumoral prolactin secreting cells. Action potentials were triggered by small depolarizing pulses (0.05nA; 100 msec; frequency: 1 Hz). When dopamine was ejected from the delivery pipette (dopamine: 0.1 nM; ejection time: 50 msec), the resting potential of the cell (-60 mV) was hyperpolarized and this effect lasted several seconds. The dopamine-induced response was due to a decrease in the membrane input resistance, i.e., the membrane conductance was increased. During the hyperpolarization, the action potentials were abolished and were displayed again when the "critical potential" was reached.

brane resistance (200 to 500 microhms) and a resting potential varying from -40 to -60 mV. As the spontaneous activity was dependent on the value of the resting potential, only 20 to 30% of the cells studied displayed spontaneous action potentials. Cells which were not spontaneously active elicited action potentials when a slight depolarization was induced by a depolarizing transmembrane current.

There were no differences between the characteristics of spontaneous and triggered action potentials. The amplitude was 40 to 50 mV with an average duration of 10 msec. These values are within the range of those found in rat tumoral pituitary cells (5-8) or in normal rat growth hormone-secreting cells *in vitro* (12).

In order to study the ionic properties of action potentials, we have used current blockers such as tetrodotoxin, which is known to block sodium current, and cobalt or manganese, which selectively inhibit calcium currents. Tetrodotoxin at high concentration (5 uM) had no effect on the amplitude or the duration of the spike, although cobalt and manganese blocked the action potentials in a reversible manner. These results were not surprising and corroborate data reported for GH_3 cells (3-5) and normal mammotrophs (6). Other studies have mentioned two components for the action potential, that is, the current responsible for the depolarizing phase was both sodium- and calcium-dependent (13). This discrepancy may be due to different culture conditions.

We have tested the effect of dopamine on the resting potential and on spontaneous electrical activity of the cells. Dopamine was ejected close to the cell studied through a micropipette connected to a pneumatic system (pressure, 0.1 bar; ejection time: 50 to 100 msec). Even at low concentration (1 to 10 nM in the delivery pipette), dopamine was able to induce a strong hyperpolarizing response which was due to a decrease of the membrane resistance. This hyperpolarization was repeatable and its duration and

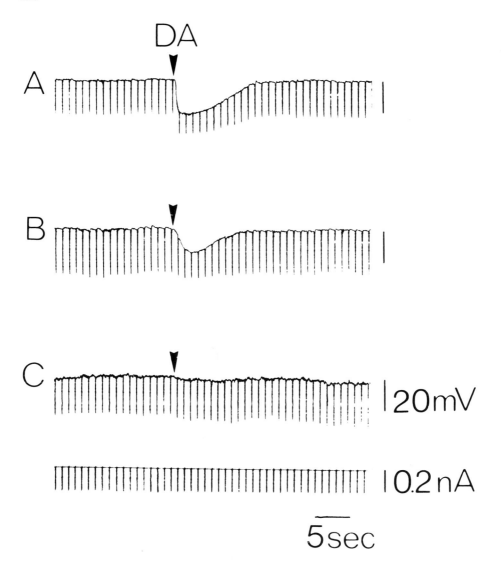

Figure 3. Blocking effect of haloperidol on the dopamine(DA)-induced response. The response to dopamine was recorded in normal medium (A) and in the presence of two concentrations of haloperidol. The rapid hyperpolarizing deflections of voltage were induced by small hyperpolarizing currents (lower trace: 0.2 nA; 120 msec; 1 Hz) and indicate the value of the input membrane resistance for both the resting potential and during the response induced by dopamine. At 0.1 nM (B) haloperidol reduced both the amplitude (by 40%) and duration of the dopamine-induced response, while at 0.1 uM (C) this response was almost completely blocked (resting potential of the cell: -55 mV).

amplitude were dependent on the dopamine concentration. We have recorded dopamine-induced responses with 10 fM dopamine ejected from the pipette, which indicates that the dopamine receptor is highly sensitive.

The dopamine-induced response was accompanied by an increase in the ionic conductance and modification of the response amplitude by varying the potential of the recorded cell can be used to indicate the ion or ions involved. This effect is due to the variation of the ionic "driving-force" which is a function of the cell potential. In consequence, when the cell was hyperpolarized, the response decreased in amplitude and reversed at -100 mV. This value strongly suggests the participation of potassium ions.

The response induced by dopamine was mimicked by bromocriptine. At 0.1 uM in the delivery pipette, bromocriptine induced the same hyperpolarizing response concomitant with a variation of the input membrane resistance and a reversal potential similar to that of the dopamine-induced response.

The response induced by dopamine was pharmacologically analyzed by studying drugs known to antagonize the effects of dopamine. All the antagonists used (haloperidol, domperidone, spiperone) blocked the response induced by dopamine. These results clearly indicate that the hyperpolarizing response induced by dopamine is mediated through a specific dopaminergic receptor located in the membrane of the cell.

This hyperpolarization may play a fundamental role in the stimulus secretion mechanism proposed by Douglas (17). The hyperpolarizing response to dopamine may lead to inhibition of prolactin release in two ways:

1) Without inhibiting factors, the voltage-dependent calcium channels are maximally activated, maintaining an elevated $[Ca^{2+}]_i$. The hyperpolarizing response induced by dopamine may inactivate the membrane calcium channels which in turn lead to a decrease of cytosolic calcium, and in consequence inhibits the hormone release.

2) The hyperpolarizing response induced by dopamine leads to the inhibition of action potentials. Some authors (10) have described a possible Ca^{2+}-blocking effect of dopamine similar to those of cobalt and manganese. This effect, which was reported for very high dopamine concentrations (0.1 mM), was never found in our experiments where the inhibitory effect of dopamine (0.1 to 10 nM) on firing was abolished by a slight depolarization of the membrane potential. However, the inhibition of calcium action potentials induced by dopamine led to the decrease of internal calcium and at least to the decrease of calcium-dependent hormone release.

In our case, the two mechanisms are possible and their effects may be cumulative. In conclusion, dopamine may exert its inhibiting effect on prolactin release by the modulation of the electrical activity of the cell, through the interaction of dopamine with a "receptor-potassium channel" complex located in the cytoplasmic membrane.

REFERENCES

1. Thorner, MO, Hackett JT, Murad F, MacLeod RM. (1980): Neuroendocrinology 31:390
2. Reuter H. Nature (1983) 301:569
3. Kidokoro Y. (1975): Nature 258:741
4. Taraskevich PS, Douglas WW. (1977): Proc Natl Acad Sci USA 74:4064

5. Dufy B, Vincent JD, Fleury H, Du Pasquier P, Gourdji D, Tixier-Vidal A. (1979): Science 204:509
6. Ozawa S, Kimura N. (1979): Proc Natl Acad Sci USA 76:6017
7. Douglas WW, Taraskevich PS. (1978): J Physiol 285:171
8. Dufy B, Vincent JD, Fleury H, Du Pasquier P, Goudji D, Tixier-Vidal A. (1979): Nature 282:855
9. Israel JM, Dufy B, Gourdji D, Vincent JD. (1981): Life Sciences 29:351
10. Taraskevich PS, Douglas WW. (1982): J. Physiol 326:201
11. Dufy B, Israel JM, Zyzek E, Dufy-Barbe L, Guerin J, Fleury H, Vincent JD. (1982): Mol Cell Endocrinol 27:179
12. Israel JM, Denef C, Vincent JD. (1983): Neuroendocrinology 37:193
13. Biales B, Dichter M, Tischler A. (1977): Nature 267:172
14. Douglas WW. (1968): Br J Pharmacol 34:451

Prolactin. Basic and clinical correlates
R.M. MacLeod, M.O. Thorner and U. Scapagnini (eds.),
Fidia Research Series, vol. I,
Liviana Press, Padova © 1985

Section III
Intracellular pituitary mechanisms
regulating prolactin release

CALCIUM-MEDIATED INTRACELLULAR SIGNALLING IN THE CONTROL OF PROLACTIN SECRETION FROM RAT ANTERIOR PITUITARY CELLS

Barry L. Brown, John G. Baird, Lawrence A. Quilliam, Janet E. Merritt, and Pauline R. M. Dobson

Department of Human Metabolism and Clinical Biochemistry,
University of Sheffield Medical School, Sheffield, S10 2RX, UK

There is considerable evidence supporting the notion that calcium ions have a major role in the control of prolactin secretion (1-4). Thus, agents (such as ionophores and K^+) which increase the intracellular Ca^{2+} concentration are associated with an increase in prolactin secretion, and many calcium- and calmodulin-antagonists inhibit secretion (1,4-6). Moreover, thyrotropin-releasing hormone (TRH)-stimulated prolactin secretion has been associated with increases in the frequency of Ca^{2+}-dependent action potentials (7), Quin 2 fluorescence (8), and phosphoinositide turnover (9-13). Many studies concerned with putative intracellular mediators have employed GH_3 tumor cells. Use of these cells overcomes many of the drawbacks associated with the cellular heterogeneity of the anterior pituitary gland. Indeed, from these studies has come the hypothesis that TRH may enhance prolactin secretion by causing mobilization of intracellular Ca^{2+}, possibly through the mediation of agonist-dependent production of inositol-1,4,5-trisphosphate (IP_3) liberated from the breakdown of polyphosphoinositide (Gershengorn, this volume). However, these cells may not possess the same intracellular control mechanisms as normal cells. In addition a study of the mode of action of dopamine is precluded due to a lack of high affinity receptors (14,15). The aim of this paper is to review some of the studies on the role of calcium in the control of prolactin secretion for normal pituitary cells.

Extensive work on the effect of TRH on polyphosphoinositide turnover carried out using GH_3 cells (11-13) has shown that, within seconds, inositol trisphosphate is produced by TRH-induced phospholipase C action on phosphatidylinositol 4,5-bisphosphate (PIP_2). However, less is known of the situation in the normal anterior pituitary. Nevertheless, we and others (9,10) have shown that TRH stimulates the accumulation of total inositol phosphates in normal cells; similar results have been reported for GnRH (16,17).

Recently we have extended this study to include an investigation of the involvement of calcium in this process and an investigation of the effect of dopamine. Measurement of phosphoinositide hydrolysis was as outlined previously (10). Briefly, after 3 days in culture, pituitary cells were preincubated with [³H]-inositol for at least 24 hours to allow labelling of phosphoinositide to isotopic equilibrium. After this period, the medium was removed and the cells were preincubated in Krebs Ringer Bicarbonate (KRB) with or without 10 mM Li^{2+}, which has been shown to inhibit inositol-1-phosphatase action (18-20). Test solutions were applied for the desired period (usually 1 hour), after which an aliquot was withdrawn for prolactin radioimmunoassay. Incubations were terminated with cold methanol, then monolayers were scraped off. Chloroform and water were added to separate the phases into water and non-water soluble portions. The inositol phosphates were extracted with Dowex (formate form) and eluted with ammonium formate/formic acid.

We have shown (10) that decreasing the extracellular Ca^{2+} concentration below 50 uM lowered prolactin secretion markedly without affecting inositol phosphate accumulation in the presence or absence of TRH. In addition, VIP (10 nM) and K^+ (50 nM), which are thought to enhance prolactin secretion by increasing cyclic AMP levels and raising intracellular Ca^{2+} respectively, do not cause a significant increase in inositol phosphate accumulation, in the presence of Li^+ over 60 minutes (Fig. 1).

Of interest were the effects of the so-called calcium antagonists on both prolactin secretion and inositol phosphate production. Both the organic (flunarizine, cinnarizine, methoxyverapamil) and inorganic (Co^{2+}, Mn^{2+}, Zn^{2+}) calcium antagonists virtually abolished basal and TRH-stimulated prolactin secretion (4). However, while the organic calcium antagonists reduced inositol phosphate accumulation very slightly, the inorganic calcium antagonists inhibited inositol phosphate accumulation almost completely. Results obtained with GH_3 cells indicated that the initial effect of the bivalent cations appears to be the inhibition of IP_3 production, rather than of inositol bisphosphate (IP_2) (21).

Canonico and co-workers (22) reported that dopamine (500 nM) inhibited [³²P] incorporation into phosphatidylinositol (PI), but not other phospholipids. However, this dose of dopamine is relatively high (the half maximal effect of dopamine on prolactin secretion being approximately 1 nM) and since [³²P] labelling follows the secondary event, i.e. PI re-synthesis, it was of considerable interest to determine whether dopamine affected the production of inositol phosphates. However, even very high concentrations of dopamine had no effect on basal or TRH-stimulated inositol phosphate production (23). Moreover, no effect was observed when dopamine or the dopamine agonist, bromocriptine (both at 100 nM-1 mM) were added to anterior pituitary cells while they were being labelled with [³H]-inositol (data not shown).

We, and others, have shown that dopamine can reduce intracellular cyclic AMP levels in anterior pituitary cells (24,25). Furthermore, the results obtained by Cronin et al. (26) have shown that pertussis toxin, by catalysing the ADP ribosylation of the inhibitory (Ni) subunit of adenylate cyclase, prevents dopamine from exerting its inhibitory effects. This suggests that adenylate cyclase may mediate at least some of the inhibitory actions of dopamine on prolactin secretion. However, the possibility remains that both the Ca^{2+} and cyclic AMP systems may be involved or that regulation by protein kinase C or arachidonic acid metabolites may be important.

The other product of phosphoinositide hydrolysis, diacylglycerol, has been shown

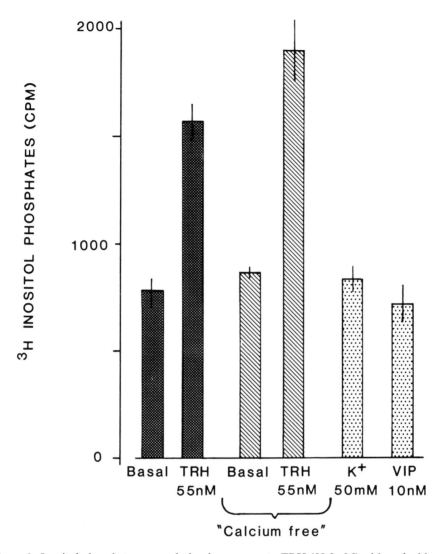

Figure 1. Inositol phosphate accumulation in response to TRH (55.0 nM) with and without extracellular calcium, K$^+$ (50 mM), and VIP (10 nM) in male rat anterior pituitary cells. Incubations were carried out for 60 minutes in KRB plus 10 mM Li$^+$. Each point is the mean of 3 determinations ± SEM.

(27) to activate a calcium- and phospholipid-dependent protein kinase (protein kinase C). We have recently studied endogenous phosphorylation, and the results have suggested that protein kinase C and its substrates are present in the anterior pituitary gland (28). We have, therefore, attempted to isolate this enzyme. Pituitaries (porcine) were homogenized in ice-cold Tris-buffer pH 7.5 containing sucrose (0.25 M), dithiothreitol

(5 mM), EDTA (2 mM), EGTA (2 mM), and PMSF (0.1 mM). A cytosolic extract, supplemented with cyclic AMP (1 uM), was applied to a DEAE-cellulose column and eluted by a 0-0.4 M KCl gradient. The active fractions were loaded onto a polyacrylamide gel-immobilized phosphatidylserine (PS) affinity column (CR Filburn, personal communication). Following washes with column buffer containing a) 1 mM $CaCl_2$, b) 0.1 mM $CaCl_2$, the enzyme was eluted with 2 mM EGTA. Fractions were stored at -20 C in 50% glycerol. Assays for PS-stimulatable enzyme activity were performed using histone and [^{32}P]-ATP as substrates. Protein kinase activity, eluted from the DEAE-cellulose column, was found to be CA^{2+} dependent and was stimulated by PS in a dose dependent manner (Fig. 2).

In summary (see Fig. 3), in contrast to the action of VIP, which involves activation of adenylate cyclase, TRH-stimulated prolactin secretion may be, at least in part, mediated by the extent of inositol phosphate and diacylglycerol production. It has, so far, not been possible, due to the heterogeneity of normal tissue, to monitor the individual inositol phosphates in response to stimulators and inhibitors. However, the results of total inositol phosphate accumulation are compatible with the notion that TRH may induce similar alterations in both normal and GH_3 cells. If this is so, the possibility exists that IP_3 is rapidly accumulated and may lead to mobilization of intracellular calcium (29). There is some evidence that the calmodulin/calcium complex

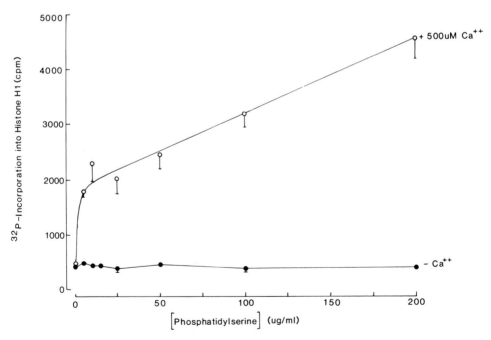

Figure 2. Phosphatidylserine dependence of ion exchange column purified protein kinase C in the presence and absence of calcium. Each point is the mean ± SEM of 3 determinations.

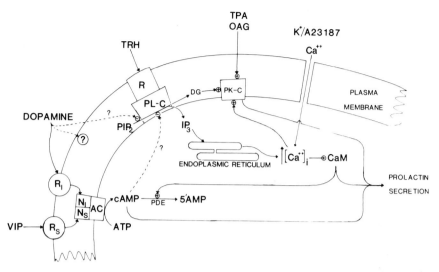

Figure 3. Schematic representation of possible intracellular events involved in the control of prolactin release from anterior pituitary cells. CaM = calmodulin; R, Rs, Ri = receptors; PL-C = phospholipase C; PK-C = protein kinase C; PDE = cyclic nucleotide phosphodiesterase; Ni, Ns = regulatory subunits of adenylate cyclase; DG = diacylglycerol; TPA = 12-0-tetradecanoyl phorbol-13-acetate; OAG = 1-oleoyl-2-acetyl glycerol; AC = adenylate cyclase.

may be involved in the secretory process (5,6). Moreover diacylglycerol, the other product of PI and polyphosphoinositide breakdown,may lead to activation of protein kinase C. This enzyme is clearly present in the normal pituitary as are its substrates. However, the function of these substrates remains to be determined.

While it is apparent that dopamine inhibits adenylate cyclase, possible additional effects seem likely. The cellular heterogeneity of the normal anterior pituitary gland and the lack of high affinity dopamine receptors in GH_3 cells are the major reasons underlying the lack of a clear picture of the mechanism of action of dopamine. The use of preparations of individual cell types, when they become available, should aid in the elucidation of the mode of action of dopamine and may also uncover additional regulatory events which are not apparent in GH_3 cells.

REFERENCES

1. Thorner MO, Hackett JT, Murad F, MacLeod RM. (1980): Neuroendocrinology 31:390
2. Gershengorn MC, Hoffstein ST, Rebecchi MJ, Geras E, Rubin EG. (1981): J Clin Invest 67:1769
3. Moriarty CM, Leuschen MP. (1981): Am J Physiol 240:E705
4. Merritt JE, Brown BL. (1984): J Endocrinol 101:319
5. Merritt JE, Tomlinson S, Brown BL. (1981): FEBS Lett 135:107

6. Schettini G, Judd AM, MacLeod RM. (1983): Endocrinol 112:64
7. Taraskevich PS, Douglas WW. (1977): Proc Nat Acad Sci USA 74:4046
8. Schofield JG. (1983): FEBS Lett 159:79
9. Leung PCK, Raymond U, Labrie F. (1982): Life Sci 31:3037
10. Baird JG, Dobson PRM, Wojcikiewicz RJH, Brown BL. (1983): Bioscience Reports 3:1091
11. Rebecchi MJ, Gershengorn MC. (1983): Biochem J 216:287
12. Macphee CH, Drummond AH. (1984): Mol Pharmacol 25:193
13. Martin TFJ. (1983): J Biol Chem 258:14816
14. Cronin MJ, Faure N, Martial JA, Weiner RI. (1980): Endocrinol 106:718
15. Gourdji D, Tougard C, Tixier-Vidal A. (1982): In: Ganong WF, Martini L (eds) Frontiers in Neuroendocrinology. Raven Press, New York, vol 7:317
16. Snyder GD, Bleasdale JE. (1982): Mol Cell Endocrinol 28:55
17. Raymond V, Leung PCK, Veilleux R, Lefevre G, Labrie F. (1984): Mol Cell Endocrinol 36:157
18. Sherman WR, Leavitt AL, Honchar MP, Hallcher LM, Phillips BE. (1981): J Neurochem 36:1947
19. Allison JH. (1978): In: Eisenberg F, Wells WW (eds) Cyclitols and Phosphoinositides. Academic Press, New York, p 507
20. Allison JH, Blisner ME. (1976): Biochim Biophys Res Commun 68:1332
21. Baird JG, Brown BL. (1984): Biochem Soc Trans (in press)
22. Canonico PL, Valdenegro CA, MacLeod RM. (1983): Endocrinol 113:7
23. Baird JG, Dobson PR, Brown BL (Submitted)
24. Barnes GD, Brown BL, Gard TG, Atkinson D, Ekins RP. (1978): Mol Cell Endocrinol 12:273
25. Ray KP, Wallis M. (1983): Mol Cell Endocrinol 27:139
26. Cronin MJ, Myers GA, MacLeod RM, Hewlett EL. (1983): Am J Physiol 244:E499
27. Nishizuka Y. (1983): Phil Trans R Soc Lond B 302:101
28. Merritt JE. (1983): PhD Thesis, University of Sheffield
29. Berridge MJ. (1984): Biochem J 220:345

Prolactin. Basic and clinical correlates
R.M. MacLeod, M.O. Thorner and U. Scapagnini (eds.),
Fidia Research Series, vol. I,
Liviana Press, Padova © 1985

Section III
Intracellular pituitary mechanisms
regulating prolactin release

DOPAMINE DECREASES PROLACTIN SECRETION INDUCED BY INCREASES IN CALCIUM MOBILIZATION IN THE 7315a PITUITARY TUMOR, BUT NOT THE MtTW15 PITUITARY TUMOR

A.M. Judd, K. Koike, G. Schettini, C.A. Valdenegro, E.L. Hewlett, T. Yasumoto, and R.M. MacLeod

Department of Internal Medicine, University of Virginia
School of Medicine, Charlottesville, Virginia

INTRODUCTION

The secretion of prolactin from anterior pituitary cells is modified by various agents, but dopamine appears to play a major role in controlling prolactin release *in vivo* (1). Dopamine may exert its effect on prolactin release by modifying the activity of various biochemical systems. Specifically, dopamine has been demonstrated to decrease phospholipid turnover (2,3), adenylate cyclase activity (4), the accumulation of intracellular cyclic AMP (5-7), and the release of arachidonic acid associated with TRH stimulation (unpublished observation). Calcium appears to be required for normal prolactin release since decreasing extracellular calcium or treating pituitary cells with calcium channel blockers markedly decreases prolactin release (8). In contrast, agents such as the calcium ionophore A23187 or maitotoxin, a calcium channel activator (9), markedly increase prolactin release from pituitary cells (10). Dopamine may exert some effects on calcium fluxes (8) although at least some of dopamine's action appears to be following calcium mobilization (6,11).

The MtTW15 and 7315a tumors are transplanted rat pituitary tumors that secrete prolactin and growth hormone and prolactin and ACTH respectively (12,13). These tumors were induced via long term treatment of rats with dimethylstilbestrol and trimethylaniline respectively (12,14). Both tumors possess dopamine receptors (15,16) although dopamine or its agonists do not decrease prolactin release from the tumors *in vivo* or *in vitro* (15,17). However, dopamine does decrease phospholipid metabolism in these tumors (3). We will present data on dopamine's effect on adenylate cyclase activity of the MtTW15 and 7315a tumor cells. We will, furthermore, describe the ef-

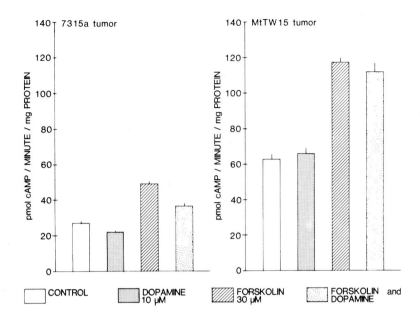

Figure 1. The effect of dopamine on basal and forskolin-stimulated adenylate cyclase activity of 7315a and MtTW15 tumors. Forskolin increases (p < 0.01) adenylate cyclase activity in both tumors. Dopamine decreases basal (p < 0.05) and forskolin-induced (p < 0.01) adenylate cyclase activity in the 7315a tumor, but has no effect on the MtTW15 tumor.

fects of altering cellular calcium balance on basal and dopamine-treated prolactin release from both tumors.

EFFECTS OF DOPAMINE ON TUMOR CELL
ADENYLATE CYCLASE ACTIVITY

In normal anterior pituitary cells, treatment with dopamine or its agonists decreases basal or stimulated adenylate cyclase activity (4,18). We have determined that the dopamine receptors present in 7315a but not in MtTW15 tumor cell membranes are coupled to adenylate cyclase. Tumor cell membranes were purified, then incubated with [^{32}P]-ATP, and adenylate cyclase activity determined by an established method (19,20). Using the 7315a tumor membranes, dopamine (10 uM) significantly (p < 0.05) decreased basal adenylate cyclase activity and blunted (p < 0.01) the increase of adenylate cyclase activity due to forskolin (Fig. 1), a direct activator of the catalytic subunit of adenylate cyclase (21). In contrast, dopamine affected neither basal nor forskolin-stimulated adenylate cyclase activity in the MtTW15 tumor membrane (Fig. 1). Therefore the MtTW15 tumor may be refractory to dopamine inhibition of prolactin release due to the dopamine receptor not being coupled to adenylate cyclase. However, another lesion must be postulated to explain the failure of dopamine to alter the release of prolactin by 7315a tumor cells.

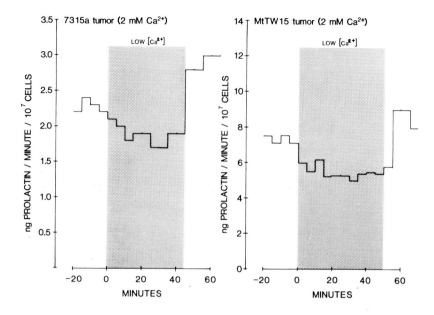

Figure 2. The effect of decreasing medium calcium concentration on perifused 7315a and MtTW15 tumor cell prolactin release.

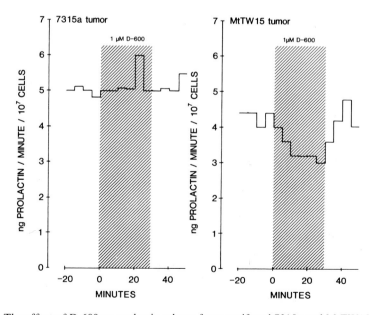

Figure 3. The effect of D-600 on prolactin release from perifused 7315a and MtTW15 tumor cells.

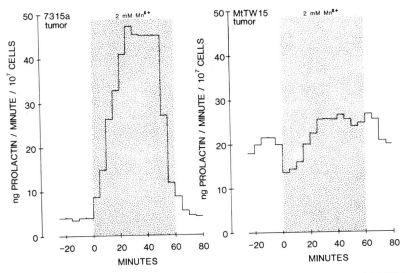

Figure 4. The effect of Mn²⁺ on prolactin release from perifused 7315a and MtTW15 tumor cells.

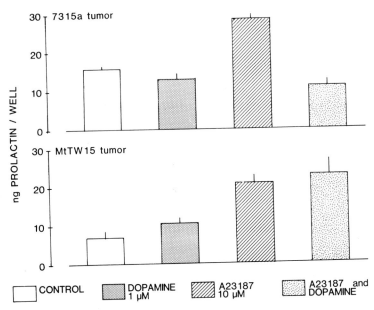

Figure 5. The effect of dopamine on ionophore A23187-induced prolactin release from primary cultures of 7315a and MtTW15 pituitary tumor cells. A23187 increased (p<0.01) prolactin release from both tumor cells. Dopamine decreased (p<0.01) A23187-induced prolactin release from 7315a tumor cells.

EFFECTS OF ALTERING CALCIUM BALANCE IN 7315a AND MtTW15 PITUITARY TUMOR RELEASE OF PROLACTIN

Decreasing extracellular calcium or treating with calcium channel blockers markedly decreases prolactin release from normal pituitary tissues (8). Since both tumors secrete 1/10 to 1/100 as much prolactin as normal pituitary cells (15,16), it was postulated that the tumor cells may handle calcium abnormally. In a series of experiments we have determined the effects of altering calcium balance on MtTW15 and 7315a tumor cell prolactin release. Tumor tissue was enzymatically dispersed with collagenase (22) and the cells placed in a standard perifusion apparatus as explained previously (8). Exposing these tumor cells to low Ca^{2+} medium decreases the release of prolactin about 20% (Fig. 2) while prolactin release is decreased by 70 to 80% in normal pituitary tissue (data not presented; ref. 8).

Similarly, D-600, an organic calcium channel blocker, has no effect on 7315a tumor prolactin release and a moderate effect on MtTW15 prolactin release (Fig. 3) but markedly decreases normal pituitary prolactin release (8). Paradoxically Mn^{2+}, which likewise blocks calcium channels, markedly stimulates prolactin release by 7315a tumor cells and in the MtTW15 tumor initially inhibits but later moderately stimulates prolactin release (Fig. 4).

These results taken together indicate that, unlike that of normal pituitary tissue, prolactin release from the 7315a tumor is marginally, if at all, dependent on extracellular calcium while the release of prolactin from MtTW15 tumors appears moderately dependent on extracellular calcium. The stimulation of prolactin by Mn^{2+} may be related to the ability of some ions to mimic the action of Ca^{2+} in such tumor cell lines as the GH_3 cell (23). Because the release of prolactin by tumor cells is 1 to 10% that by normal pituitary tissue (15,16) and prolactin release from the tumor cells is only moderately dependent on calcium, it appears likely that basal prolactin release by the tumor cells is so low that further suppression is not possible. This suppression of prolactin release may be related to a decreased influx of extracellular calcium since we have demonstrated that increasing extracellular calcium above 5 mM increases prolactin release from the tumor cells (data not presented). Recently basal prolactin release from GH_3 cells was likewise shown to be independent of extracellular Ca^{2+} concentration and GH_3 cell calcium influx was found to be low (24,25).

EFFECTS OF DOPAMINE ON IONOPHORE- AND MAITOTOXIN-INDUCED PROLACTIN RELEASE

Increasing calcium mobilization by the calcium ionophore A23187 or the calcium channel activator maitotoxin (9) stimulates prolactin release from normal pituitary tissues (6,10,11). We have used primary cultures of tumor cells to determine whether increasing calcium mobilization increases tumor cell prolactin release. MtTW15 and 7315a tumor cells were dispersed with collagenase, pipetted into 24-well plates (300,000 cells/well), and allowed to grow and attach to the plates for 5 to 7 days as described previously (7). On the day of an experiment the cells were washed extensively with serum free medium and incubated for 15 minutes with vehicle or drug. Ionophore A23187 (10 uM) significantly (p < 0.01) increased prolactin release from both the 7315a and the MtTW15 tumors (Fig. 5). We then treated the cells with dopamine to determine whether it would block A23187-induced prolactin release. Dopamine (10 uM), as reported previously (15,16), had no significant effect on basal prolactin release from either the MtTW15 or 7315a tumor cells. However, although dopamine did not affect A23187-induced prolactin release from the MtTW15 tumor it completely blocked (p < 0.01) A23187-induced prolactin release from the 7315a tumor (Fig. 5).

In subsequent experiments maitotoxin significantly (p < 0.01) increased prolactin release from both tumors, but dopamine blocked only maitotoxin-induced prolactin release from the 7315a tumor (Fig. 6).

CONCLUSIONS

Although dopamine inhibits prolactin release by normal pituitary cells the amine does not affect basal prolactin release by MtTW15 or 7315a pituitary tumor cells. Prolactin release from both tumors is only moderately dependent on extracellular calcium. However increasing calcium mobilization with calcium ionophore or maitotoxin increases prolactin release from both tumors. Therefore, at least under basal conditions, the tumor

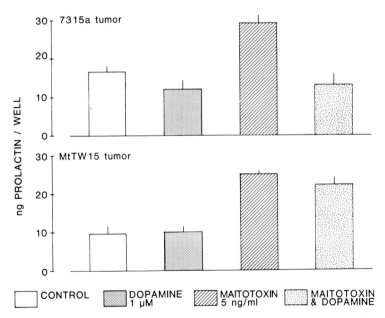

Figure 6. The effect of dopamine on maitotoxin-induced prolactin release from primary cultures of 7315a and MtTW15 pituitary tumor cells. Maitotoxin increased (p < 0.01) prolactin release from both tumor cells. Dopamine decreased (p < 0.01) maitotoxin-induced prolactin release from 7315a tumor cells.

cells may be refractory to dopamine inhibition of prolactin release due to a low prolactin release related to an abnormal calcium handling. In support of this hypothesis we demonstrated that dopamine blocks 7315a prolactin release induced by A23187 or maitotoxin. However, dopamine does not affect MtTW15 prolactin release induced by these agents. This difference may be related to the observation that dopamine inhibits 7315a tumor cell adenylate cyclase activity in a manner similar to that of normal pituitary cells but does not affect this activity in the MtTW15 tumor. These observations provide evidence that inhibition of adenylate cyclase activity may be requisite for dopamine inhibition of prolactin release induced by A23187 or maitotoxin. Furthermore, these observations indicate that the 7315a tumor may be a useful model for the study of the action of dopamine on prolactin release.

ACKNOWLEDGMENTS

We wish to thank Suzanne B. O'Dell and Margaret MacQueen for expert technical assistance during this study. Further thanks are expressed to Susan M. Adams for her expert editoral assistance. This study was supported by grant CA-07535 from the National Cancer Institute. AMJ is the recipient of NIH Postdoctoral Fellowship CA-07137

REFERENCES

1. MacLeod RM, Thorner MO, Login IS. (1980): Proceedings of the 28th International Congress of Physiological Sciences, Budapest p 81
2. Canonico PL, Valdenegro CA, MacLeod RM. (1982): Endocrinology 111:347
3. Canonico PL, Valdenegro CA, MacLeod RM. (1983): Endocrinology 113:7
4. Onali P, Schwartz JP, Costa E. (1981): Proc Natl Acad Sci USA 76:6531
5. Swennen L, Denef C. (1982): Endocrinology 111:398
6. Schettini G, Cronin MJ, MacLeod RM. (1983): Endocrinology 112:1801
7. Cronin MJ, Thorner MO. (1982): J Cyc Nucleotid Res 8(4):267
8. Thorner MO, Hackett JT, Murad F, MacLeod RM. (1980): Neuroendocrinology 31:390
9. Takahashi M, Tatsumi M, Ohizumi Y. (1983): J Biol Chem 258:10944
10. Schettini G, Koike K, Login IS, Judd AM, Cronin MJ, Yasumoto T, Mac Leod RM. Am J Physiol (Endo Metab), in press
11. Tam SW, Dannies PS. (1980): J Biol Chem 255:6595
12. Ueda G, Takizawa, Moy P, Marolla F, Furth J. (1968): Cancer Res 28:1963
13. MacLeod RM, Bass MB, Huang SC, Smith MC. (1968): Endocrinology 82:253
14. Bates RW, Garrison MM, Morris HP. (1966): Proc Soc Exp Biol Med 123:67
15. Cronin MJ, Valdenegro CA, Perkins SN, MacLeod RM. (1981): Endocrinology 109:2160
16. Cronin MJ, Keefer DA, Valdenegro CA, Dabney LG, MacLeod RM. (1982): J Endocrinol 94:347
17. Lamberts SWJ, MacLeod RM. (1979) Endocrinology 104:65
18. Giannattasio G, De Ferrari ME, Spada A. (1981): Life Sci 28:1605
19. Johnson RA, Walseth TF. (1979) Adv Cyc Nucleotide Res 10:135
20. Solomon Y, Loudos C, Rodbell M. (1974): Anal Biochem 58:541
21. Scannon K, Daly JW. (1981): J Biol Chem 256:9799

22. Connors JM, Wright KC, Judd AM, Liu C-M, Hedge GA. (1981): Hormone Res 14:1
23. Ozawa S, Kimura N. (1982): Am J Physiol 243:E68
24. Tan K-N, Tashjian AH Jr. (1984): J Biol Chem 259:427
25. Delbeke D, Scammell JG, Dannies PS. (1984): Endocrinology 114:1433

Prolactin. Basic and clinical correlates
R.M. MacLeod, M.O. Thorner and U. Scapagnini (eds.),
Fidia Research Series, vol. I,
Liviana Press, Padova © 1985

Section III
Intracellular pituitary mechanisms
regulating prolactin release

A POSSIBLE ROLE FOR DIACYLGLYCEROL IN REGULATING PROLACTIN RELEASE FROM ANTERIOR PITUITARY CELLS

K. Koike, A.M. Judd, T. Yasumoto, and R.M. MacLeod

Department of Internal Medicine, University of Virginia School of Medicine
Charlottesville, Virginia

The biochemical mechanism by which TRH stimulates and dopamine inhibits prolactin release from the anterior pituitary is not fully elucidated. Only recently have certain implicated processes, i.e., cyclic nucleotide involvement (1-6) and the Ca^{2+}-calmodulin system (6-10), been at least partially characterized. Phospholipid hydrolysis has been proposed as one of the earliest events associated with the activation of receptors in secretory cells (11-13). Likewise in prolactin secreting cells TRH is well recognized to enhance pituitary phosphatidylinositol (PI) metabolism while dopamine reduces this process (14-16). Diacylglycerol (DG), a metabolic product of phospholipase C-induced PI hydrolysis (15), is a direct activator of a Ca^{2+} - and phospholipid-dependent protein kinase (C-Kinase) (17-20). A study was designed to determine whether agents known to enhance C-Kinase activity are also involved in the mechanisms regulating prolactin release.

THE EFFECT OF PHORBOL ESTERS, SYNTHETIC DIACYLGLYCEROL, AND PHOSPHOLIPASE C ON PROLACTIN RELEASE

Phorbol esters directly activate protein kinase C (21,22) and therefore, we investigated the effect of 4 beta-phorbol 12 beta-myristate, 13-alpha acetate (PMA) on prolactin release. Primary cultures of anterior pituitary cells from female Sprague-Dawley rats were incubated for 15 minutes with PMA. PMA 0.1 uM and 50 uM significantly (p < 0.01) increased prolactin release (Fig. 1). In some tissue, it has been shown that Ca^{2+} ionophore A23187 enhances the effect of PMA (23-26), hence we examined the effect of A23187 and the calcium channel activator maitotoxin (27) on PMA-induced prolactin release. A23187 at 400 nM or maitotoxin at 2 ng/ml had no effect on prolactin release by themselves, however both of these agents significantly (p < 0.01) enhanced prolactin release induced by 0.1 uM and 50 uM PMA.

Synthetic DG, 1-oleoyl-2 acetyl-glycerol, exogenously added to intact platelets, intercalates into membranes and directly activates protein kinase C and thereby increases serotonin release from platelets (17). Therefore the effect on prolactin release of exogenously added synthetic DG (generous gift from Dr. J.T. Manson, Dept. of Biochemistry, University of Virginia) was examined. A 15 minute incubation of normal rat pituitary cells with synthetic DG at a concentration of 50 ng/ml significantly ($p < 0.01$) increased prolactin release (Fig. 2). Maitotoxin at 2 ng/ml markedly enhanced the DG-mediated prolactin release and shifted the concentration-response curve for DG-induced prolactin release to the left (i.e., DG. had a significant effect at a lower dose). Calcium ionophore A23187 (400 nM) caused a similar shift in the curve of DG-induced prolactin release (data not shown) and as shown in Figure 3 potentiated synthetic DG-induced prolactin release.

Exogenously added phospholipase C catalyzes PI hydrolysis and therefore releases endogenous DG (28). Therefore we examined the influence of exogenously added phospholipase C on prolactin release. As shown in Table 1, 100 mU/ml of phospholipase C significantly ($p < 0.01$) increased prolactin release after a 15 minute incubation and this effect was enhanced by 400 nM A23187.

Table I. *Influence of phospholipase C on prolactin release*

Treatment	Prolactin (ng/ml)
vehicle	651 ± 79
phospholipase C (10 mu/ml)	771 ± 90
phospholipase C (100 mu/ml)	1251 ± 78[a]
A23187 (400 nM)	840 ± 78
A23187 + phospholipase C (10 mu/ml)	1325 ± 64[ab]
A23187 + phospholipase C (100 mu/ml)	1851 ± 105[ab]

Values are expressed as mean ± SEM of 4 determinations per group
[a] $p < 0.01$ compared to vehicle or A23187 alone; [b] $p < 0.01$ compared to corresponding concentration of phospholipase C alone

Taken together, our results suggest that activation of protein kinase C and mobilization of Ca^{2+} ion may be synergistically involved in signal transduction for hormones such as TRH that induce phospholipid hydrolysis.

EFFECT OF DOPAMINE ON PHORBOL ESTER-, DIACYLGLYCEROL-, AND PHOSPHOLIPASE C-INDUCED PROLACTIN RELEASE

Dopamine inhibits PI turnover and prolactin release (16). We have investigated whether the dopamine inhibition of prolactin release is mediated by acting before or after protein kinase activation. As shown in Table II, 500 nM and 1 uM dopamine significantly reduced the prolactin release induced by 50 uM PMA. The stimulatory effect of synthetic DG on prolactin release was also reduced by co-incubation with 1

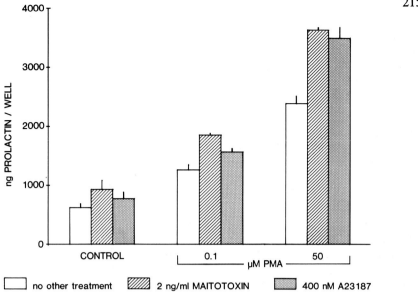

Figure 1. Effect of 15 minute incubation with PMA, A23187, or maitotoxin on prolactin release from primary cultures of anterior pituitary cells.

0.1 and 50 uM PMA significantly (p < 0.01) increased prolactin release. A23187 and maitotoxin significantly enhanced (p < 0.01) PMA-induced prolactin release. Values are expressed as mean ± SEM of 4 determinations per group.

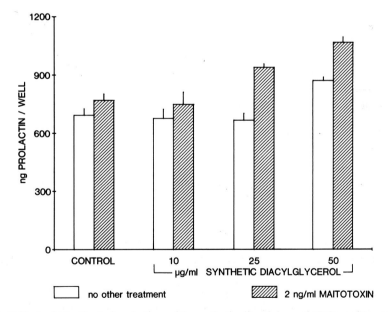

Figure 2. Effect of 15 minute incubation with synthetic diacylglycerol (DG) and/or maitotoxin on prolactin release from primary cultures of anterior pituitary cells. 50 ug/ml DG significantly (p < 0.01) increased prolactin release and maitotoxin significantly (p < 0.01) enhanced the effects at 25 and 50 ug/ml DG. Values are expressed as mean ± SEM of 4 determinations per group.

uM dopamine (Table III). Similarly, phospholipase C-mediated prolactin release is decreased by dopamine (data not presented). Since it was reported that PMA and DG are direct activators of protein kinase C (17-26), the inhibitory action of dopamine seems to be mediated at least at some step after activation of protein kinase C.

Table II. *Influence of dopamine on phorbol ester-induced prolactin release*

Treatment	Prolactin (ng/well)
vehicle	127 ± 7
dopamine (500 nM)	50 ± 10
dopamine (1 nM)	35 ± 7[a]
PMA (50 uM)	287 ± 59[a]
PMA (50 uM) + dopamine (500 nM)	174 ± 19[b]
PMA (50 uM) + dopamine (1 uM)	136 ± 13[b]

Values are expressed as mean ± SEM of 4 determinations per group
[a] $p < 0.01$ compared to vehicle; [b] $p < 0.01$ compared to PMA alone

Table III. *Influence of dopamine on synthetic diacylglycerol-induced prolactin release*

Treatment	Prolactin (ng/well)
vehicle	619 ± 79
dopamine (1 uM)	321 ± 56[b]
synthetic DG (50 ng/ml)	870 ± 18[a]
synthetic DG + dopamine	423 ± 27[c]

Values are expressed as mean ± SEM of 4 determinations per group
[a] $p < 0.05$ compared to vehicle; [b] $p < 0.01$ compared to vehicle; [c] $p < 0.01$ compared to synthetic DG alone

SUMMARY

Synthetic DG, PMA, and phospholipase C increase the release of prolactin from primary cultures of anterior pituitary cells. Increasing Ca^{2+} mobilization by treating cells with Ca^{2+} ionophore A23187 or calcium channel activator maitotoxin enhanced PMA-, synthetic DG- and phospholipase-induced prolactin release. The stimulatory effects of PMA, synthetic DG, and phospholipase C on prolactin release were reduced by co-incubation with dopamine. Therefore the secretagogue-induced hydrolysis of phospholipids to DG and the subsequent activation of protein kinase C may act in concert with small changes in cytoplasmic Ca^{2+} to mediate the secretagogue-induced increase in prolactin release. Dopamine may exert at least part of its inhibitory effect on prolactin release at a metabolic step distal to protein kinase C activation.

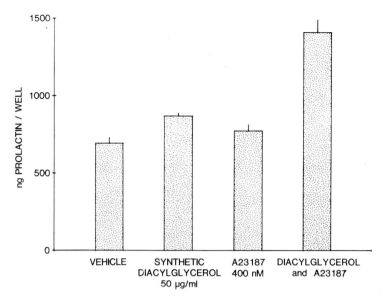

Figure 3. Effect of 15 minute incubation with 400 nM A23187 on synthetic diacylglycerol-induced prolactin release from anterior pituitary cells. 50 ug/ml DG significantly ($p < 0.01$) increased prolactin release. A23187 enhanced ($p < 0.01$) DG-induced prolactin release. Values are expressed as mean ± SEM of 4 determinations per group.

ACKNOWLEDGMENTS

Gratitude is expressed to Margaret V. MacQueen and Suzanne B. O'Dell for skillful technical assistance during the course of these experiments. Gratitude is expressed to Susan M. Adams for patience and skill in the preparation of this paper. This study was supported by Fellowship CA-07137 to AMJ and USPHS Research Grant CA-07535 from the National Cancer Institute to RMM.

REFERENCES

1. Naor Z, Snyder G, Fawcett CP, McCann SM. (1980): Endocrinology 106:1304
2. Swennen L, Denef C. (1982): Endocrinology 111:398
3. Barnes GD, Brown BL, Gard TG, Atkinson D, Ekins RP. (1978): Mol Cell Endocrinol 12:273
4. Onali P, Schwartz J, Costa E. (1981): Proc Natl Acad Sci USA 73:6531
5. Cronin MJ, Thorner MO., (1982): J. Cyclic Nucleotide Res 8 (4):267
6. Schettini G, Cronin MJ, MacLeod RM. (1983): Endocrinology 112:107
7. Merrit JE, Tomlinson S, Brown BL. (1981): FEBS Letters 135:107
8. Schettini G, Judd AM, MacLeod RM. (1983): Endocrinology 112:64
9. Gershengorn MC. (1982): Mol. Cell. Biochem 45:163
10. Gershengorn MC, Thaw C. (1983): Endocrinology 113:1522

11. Berridge MJ. (1981): Mol. Cell Endocrinol 24:115
12. Michell RH, Kirk CT. (1981): Trends Pharmacol Sci 7:86
13. Marshall PJ, Dixon JF, Hokin LB. (1980): Proc Natl Acad Sci USA 77:3292
14. Rebecchi MJ, Kolesnick RN, Gershengorn MC. (1983): J Biol Chem 258:227
15. Martin TFJ. (1983): J Biol Chem 258:14816
16. Canonico PL, Valdenegro CA, MacLeod RM. (1982): Endocrinology 111:347
17. Kaibuchi K, Takai Y, Sawamura M, Hoshijima M, Fujikura T, Nishizuka Y. (1983): J Biol Chem 258:6701
18. Kawahara Y, Takai Y, Minakachi R, Samo K, Nishizuka Y. (1980): Biochim Biophys Res Commun. 97:309
19. Ieyasu H, Takai Y, Kaibuchi K, Sawamura M, Nishizuka Y. (1980): Biochim Biophys Res Commun 108:1701
20. Sano K, Takai Y, Yamanishi J, Nishizuka Y. (1983): J Biol Chem 258:2010
21. Castagna M, Takai Y, Kaiguchi K, Samo K, Kikkawa U, Nishizuka Y. (1982): J Biol Chem 257:7847
22. Niedel JE, Kuhn LJ, Vandenbark GR. (1983): Proc Natl Acad Sci USA 80:36
23. Wang JL, McClain PA, Edelman GM. (1975): Proc Natl Acad Sci USA 72:1917
24. Schleiner RP, Gillespie E, Daiuta R, Lichtenstein LM. (1982): J Immunol 128:136
25. Goldstein IM, Hoffstein ST, Weissmann G. (1975): J Cell Biol 66:647
26. Virgi MAG, Steffes MW, Estensen RD. (1978): Endocrinology 102:706
27. Schettini G, Koike K, Login IS, Judd AM, Cronin MJ, Kasumoto T, MacLeod RM. Am J Physiol, in press
28. Rittenhouse SE. (1982): Cell Calcium 3:311

Prolactin. Basic and clinical correlates
R.M. MacLeod, M.O. Thorner and U. Scapagnini (eds.),
Fidia Research Series, vol. I,
Liviana Press, Padova © 1985

Section III
Intracellular pituitary mechanisms
regulating prolactin release

INHIBITORS OF ARACHIDONIC ACID RELEASE AND METABOLISM BLOCK BASAL AND cAMP-STIMULATED PROLACTIN RELEASE FROM GH$_3$ CELLS

Anna Marie Camoratto and Lindsey Grandison

Department of Physiology and Biophysics
UMDNJ-Rutgers Medical School
Piscataway, N.J. 08854 USA

INTRODUCTION

The intracellular processes which are activated by receptor ligands to stimulate prolactin release have not been fully elucidated. Previous studies have suggested that cAMP may play a modulatory role in secretion (1). More recently other second messengers have been identified. TRH, a receptor ligand which can induce prolactin release, has been shown to stimulate the turnover of polyphosphatidylinositol (2). As a result two intracellular signals are generated: a diglyceride, which may activate C kinase, and triphosphoinositol which can cause Ca mobilization from internal stores. In addition to these mechanisms we, as well as other groups, have implicated arachidonic acid as another possible intracellular modulator of prolactin secretion (3,4). Arachidonic acid can be released from membrane phospholipids by the action of phospholipase A2. This is the rate-limiting step in the generation of bioactive arachidonic acid metabolites. We observed that inhibitors of phospholipase A2 block basal prolactin secretion and in addition block receptor-ligand induced release. The stimulation of prolactin release by vasoactive intestinal peptide (VIP) was blocked by the phospholipase A2 inhibitor dibromoacetophenone (5). The mechanism of VIP action is thought to involve activation of adenylate cyclase and accumulation of cAMP. In order to clarify the steps at which arachidonic acid metabolites might be acting to influence prolactin release we investigated the involvement of arachidonic acid in cAMP-stimulated prolactin release. For this purpose the effects of inhibitors of arachidonic acid release and metabolism on cAMP-mediated prolactin release were examined.

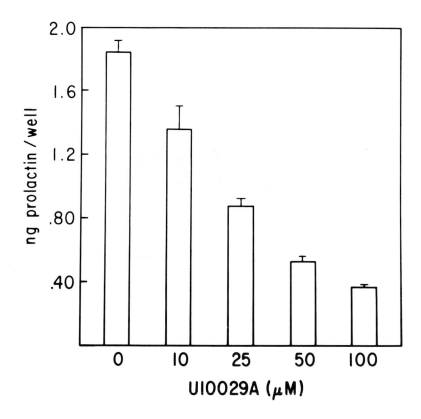

Figure 1. Effect of U10029A on basal prolactin release. Cells were incubated for four hours without or with U10029A. N = 5; p < 0.05 for control vs U10029A.

EFFECTS OF INHIBITION OF ARACHIDONIC ACID RELEASE ON PROLACTIN SECRETION

Addition of the phospholipase A2 inhibitor U10029A to cultures of GH_3 cells resulted in a dose-related decrease in prolactin secretion over the range 10-50 uM (Fig. 1). Incubation of the cells with a higher dose of the compound did not produce any further inhibition of release. The effect of U10029A on VIP-stimulated prolactin release was examined (Fig. 2). VIP produced a significant increase in prolactin release which could be blocked by a low dose of U10029A.

When forskolin was used instead of VIP to activate adenylate cyclase, stimulation of prolactin release was noted (Fig. 3). Following a 30 minute incubation the stimulation was dose-related over the range 0.1-10 uM. No further stimulation of release was elicited by a higher dose of forskolin. After 90 minutes of incubation, there was a greater percentage increase in prolactin release from cells exposed to the lowest dose of for-

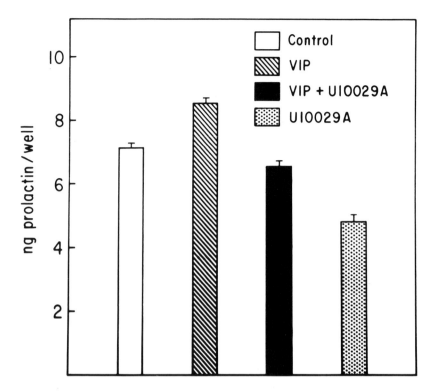

Figure 2. Effect of U10029A on VIP-stimulated prolactin release. Cells were incubated for three hours without or with 100 uM VIP in the absence or presence of 10 uM U10029A. N = 4; p < 0.05 for VIP versus control or VIP + U10029A, and U10029A vs control.

skolin; however, higher doses produced no greater stimulation than low doses at this time. The effects of a phospholipase A2 inhibitor on forskolin-induced prolactin release were next examined. Forskolin-induced prolactin release was prevented by 25 uM U10029A after 1.5 hours of incubation. After 3.0 hours, inhibition of forskolin-induced prolactin release was noted using both 10 and 25 uM U10029A (Fig. 4).

In order to determine whether U10029A was acting prior to or after the accumulation of cAMP, the effects of U10029A on cAMP-induced prolactin release were examined. Addition of 8-bromo-cAMP, a stable analog of cAMP, to the cells stimulated prolactin release (Fig. 5). The enhancement of secretion was blocked by a dose of U10029A which did not affect basal release.

EFFECTS OF INHIBITORS OF ARACHIDONIC ACID METABOLISM ON FORSKOLIN-INDUCED PROLACTIN SECRETION

To further establish the involvement of arachidonic acid in cAMP-induced prolactin release, the effects of inhibitors of arachidonic acid metabolism on forskolin-

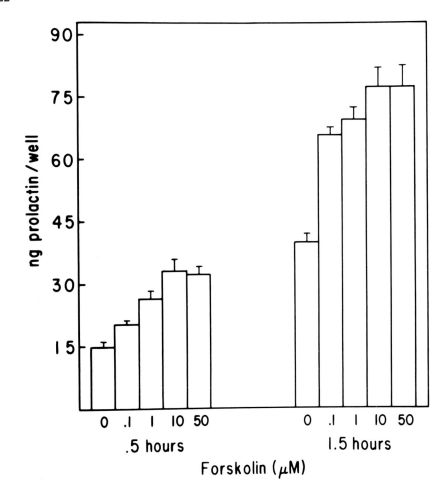

Figure 3. Effect of forskolin on basal prolactin release. Cells were incubated without or with various concentrations of forskolin and samples of the media were collected after 0.5 and 1.5 hrs. N = 7; p < 0.05 for forskolin vs control at 0.5 and 1.5 hrs.

induced release were examined. Eicosatetraynoic acid (ETYA), a competitive inhibitor of arachidonic acid, at low doses produced no (10 uM) or partial (25 uM) inhibition of forskolin-induced prolactin release (Fig. 6). Higher doses of ETYA (50 and 100 uM) completely blocked forskolin-induced release. BW755c (3-amino-1[m-trifluoromethyl-phenyl]-2-pyrazoline), an inhibitor of selected enzymes in the metabolism of arachidonic acid, was also used. BW755c at concentrations used in this experiment had no effect on basal prolactin secretion. BW755c at 116 uM partially blocked forskolin-induced prolactin release and at 224 uM completely blocked the action of forskolin (Fig. 7). Additional experiments (not shown here) demonstrated that BW755c at higher doses was effective in reducing basal prolactin levels. Another inhibitor of arachidonic acid

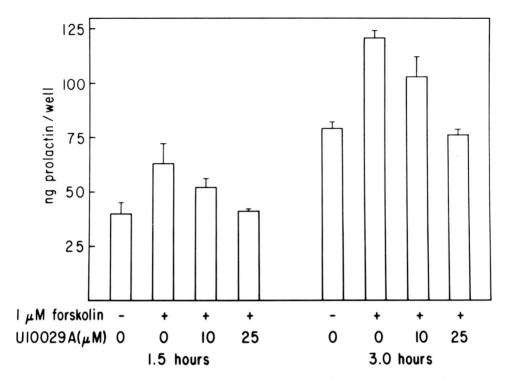

Figure 4. Effect of U10029A on forskolin-stimulated prolactin release. Cells were incubated without or with 1 uM forskolin in the absence or presence of U10029A. Samples of the media were collected after 1.5 and 3.0 hours of incubation. N = 6; p< 0.05 for forskolin vs control or forskolin + U10029A (25uM) at 1.5 hrs and forskolin vs control or forskolin + U10029A (10 and 25uM) at 3.0 hrs.

metabolism, nordihydroguaiaretic acid (NDGA), blocked forskolin-stimulated prolactin release (Fig. 8). Incubation of the cells with NDGA alone, at the concentration shown here, did not affect basal release. In other experiments higher concentrations of NDGA were observed to reduce basal prolactin secretion (data not shown).

DISCUSSION

These data provide support for the suggestion that arachidonic acid metabolites have a role as intracellular modulators of prolactin secretion. The phospholipase A2 inhibitor, U10029A, was effective in decreasing basal and cAMP-induced prolactin secretion. We have previously reported that in GH$_3$ cells basal and receptor ligand-induced prolactin release can be reduced by dibromoacetophenone (5). This phospholipase A2 inhibitor was also shown to reduce basal and stimulus-induced release of [^{3}H]-

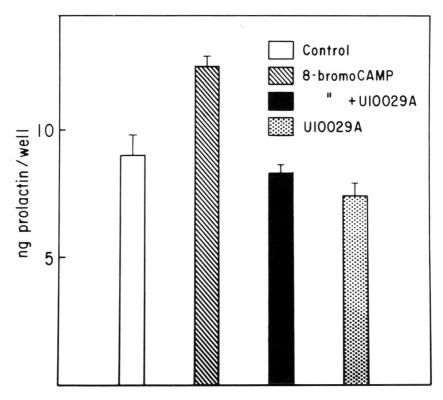

Figure 5. Effect of U10029A on 8-bromo-cAMP stimulated prolactin release. Cells were incubated without or with 3 mM 8-bromo-cAMP in the absence or presence of 1 uM U10029A for 0.5 hours. N = 4; p < 0.05 for 8-bromo-cAMP vs control or 8-bromo-cAMP + U10029A.

arachidonic acid from prelabeled GH$_3$ cells (Camoratto and Grandison, submitted). In primary cultures of bovine anterior pituitary cells the phospholipase A2 inhibitors quinacrine and dibromoacetophenone decreased basal and stimulus-induced prolactin release. The observation that inhibition of phospholipase A2 reduces prolactin secretion suggests that arachidonic acid is involved in modulating prolactin release.

Confirming previous reports we observed that VIP, forskolin, and 8-bromo-cAMP stimulated prolactin release. Since VIP and forskolin stimulate adenylate cyclase and 8-bromo-cAMP mimics cAMP, these observations indicate that cAMP can have a role as an intracellular modulator of prolactin release. The phospholipase A2 inhibitor U10029A blocked VIP- and forskolin-induced prolactin release suggesting that arachidonic acid may be involved in cAMP-induced prolactin release. The inhibition of 8-bromo-cAMP-induced prolactin secretion by an inhibitor of phospholipase A2 suggests that arachidonic acid acts at a step subsequent to accumulation of cAMP. These observations are consistent with a model in which cAMP initiates a process which ultimately causes the release of arachidonic acid and as a consequence prolactin secre-

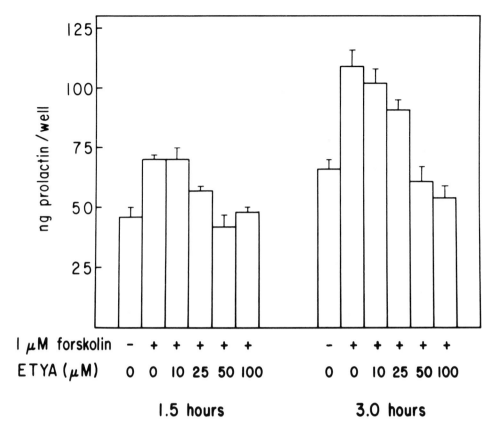

Figure 6. Effect of ETYA on forskolin-stimulated prolactin release. Cells were incubated without or with forskolin in the absence or presence of ETYA. Samples of the media were collected after 1.5 and 3 hrs of incubation. N = 4; p < 0.05 for forskolin vs control or forskolin + ETYA (25, 50 and 100uM).

tion is increased. Alternately, arachidonic acid metabolites may have a permissive role and thereby allow expression of cAMP action. Schettini et al. (6) have reported that inhibition of arachidonic acid release can prevent stimulus-induced accumulation of cAMP in primary cultures of rat anterior pituitary cells. Thus arachidonic acid metabolites may be acting at more than one step in the intracellular processes that lead to increased prolactin release. Although the mechanism remains unresolved, it is apparent that agents which interfere with arachidonic acid release or metabolism prevent cAMP-induced prolactin secretion.

The concentration of free arachidonic acid in the cell is very low or undetectable due to the rapid conversion of arachidonic acid to bioactive metabolites. In this study three inhibitors of arachidonic acid metabolism were used. ETYA blocks all metabolic pathways of arachidonic acid (7). BW755c inhibits the cyclooxygenase and lipoxygenase pathways (8). Its effects on other arachidonic acid metabolizing enzymes have not been

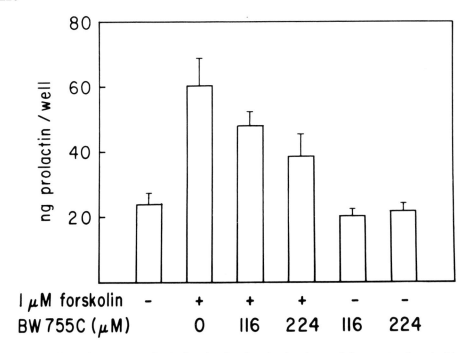

Figure 7. Effect of BW755c on forskolin-stimulated prolactin release. Cells were incubated without or with forskolin in the absence or presence of BW755c for 1.5 hours. N = 4; p < 0.05 for forskolin vs control or forskolin + BW755c.

pound can block the newly-described NADPH-dependent cytochrome P450 oxygenase pathway (10). The effectiveness of ETYA in blocking forskolin-induced prolactin release suggests that an arachidonic acid metabolite, rather than arachidonic acid itself, is necessary for secretion. An inhibitor of the cyclooxygenase pathway, indomethacin, has previously been shown to have no effect on prolactin release (3); thus cyclooxygenase products do not appear to be involved. Either the lipoxygenase or the NADPH-dependent cytochrome P450 oxygenase products may be active. The lack of specificity of NDGA and the unexamined action of BW755c on NADPH-dependent cytochrome P450 oxygenase preclude accurate identification of the arachidonic acid metabolite(s) involved in prolactin secretion.

SUMMARY

The effects of inhibitors of arachidonic acid release and metabolism were examined with respect to basal and stimulated prolactin release during short term incubation of GH_3 cells. The phospholipase A2 inhibitor U10029A reduced basal release and

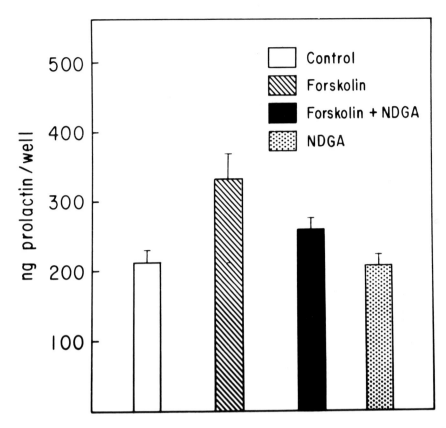

Figure 8. Effect of NDGA on forskolin-stimulated prolactin release. Cells were incubated without or with 1 uM forskolin in the absence or presence of 1 uM NDGA for three hours. N = 6; p < 0.05 for forskolin vs control or forskolin + NDGA.

examined. Lipoxygenases are also inhibited by NDGA (9) and at higher doses this compound can block the newly-described NADPH-dependent cytochrome P450 oxygenase pathway (10). The effectiveness of ETYA in blocking forskolin-induced prolactin release suggests that an arachidonic acid metabolite, rather than arachidonic acid itself, is necessary for secretion. An inhibitor of the cyclooxygenase pathway, indomethacin, has previously been shown to have no effect on prolactin release (3); thus cyclooxygenase products do not appear to be involved. Either the lipoxygenase or the NADPH-dependent cytochrome P450 oxygenase products may be active. The lack of specificity of NDGA and the unexamined action of BW755c on NADPH-dependent cytochrome P450 oxygenase preclude accurate identification of the arachidonic acid metabolite(s) involved in prolactin secretion.

SUMMARY

The effects of inhibitors of arachidonic acid release and metabolism were examined with respect to basal and stimulated prolactin release during short term incubation of GH_3 cells. The phospholipase A2 inhibitor U10029A reduced basal release and release induced by VIP, forskolin, and 8-bromo-cAMP. Inhibitors of arachidonic acid metabolism, ETYA, BW755c, and NDGA, blocked forskolin-induced prolactin release. These data provide further evidence that arachidonic acid may participate as an intracellular modulator of prolactin secretion. In addition this study suggests that arachidonic acid may in part exert its action at a step subsequent to the accumulation of cAMP.

ACKNOWLEDGMENTS

This study was supported in part by NIH grant AM 32827.

REFERENCES

1. Dannies P. (1982): Biochem Pharmacol 31:2845
2. Martin TFJ. (1983): J Biol Chem 258:14816
3. Grandison L. (1984): Endocrinology 114:1
4. Canonico PL, Schettini G, Valdenegro CA, MacLeod RM. (1983): Neuroendocrinology 37:212
5. Camoratto AM, Grandison L. (1983): Fed Proc 42:868
6. Schettini G, Cronin MJ, O'Dell SB, MacLeod RM. (1983): Fed Proc 42:299
7. Gibson KH. (1977): Chem Soc Rev 6:489
8. Higgs GA, Moncada S, Dave JR. (1978): Biochem Pharm 28:1959
9. Hamberg M. (1976): Biochim Biophys Acta 431:651
10. Snyder GD, Capdevila J, Chacos N, Manna S, Falck JR. (1983): Proc Natl Acad Sci USA 80:3504

Prolactin. Basic and clinical correlates
R.M. MacLeod, M.O. Thorner and U. Scapagnini (eds.),
Fidia Research Series, vol. I,
Liviana Press, Padova © 1985

Section III
Intracellular pituitary mechanisms
regulating prolactin release

SERINE PROTEASE INHIBITORS DECREASE *IN VITRO* PROLACTIN AND GROWTH HORMONE (GH) SECRETION OF RAT PITUITARIES

I. Nagy, G. B. Makara, Gy. Horvath, Gy. Rappay, M. Kurcz, and S. Bajusz

Heim Pal Pediatric Hospital, Institute of Experimental Medicine,
CHINOIN Pharmaceutical Works, Institute for Drug Research,
Budapest, Hungary

The proteases demonstrated in the anterior pituitary (1-6) might be involved in the processing, release, and degradation of the pituitary hormones. The role, if any, of proteases in hormone secretion might be demonstrated by pituitary enzyme activity changes accompanied by the endocrine function of the gland or by protease inhibitors. It has been shown recently that the serine/thiol protease inhibitor tripeptide aldehyde t-butyloxycarbonyl-DPhe-Pro-Arg-H (BOC-dPPA) is a potent inhibitor of the release of immunoreactive corticotrophin, beta endorphin (7), growth hormone (GH), and prolactin (8) in *in vitro* systems.

In the present experiments the effect of BOC-dPPA and other tripeptide aldehydes like DPhe-Pro-Arg-H (dPPA), BOC-DPhe-Leu-Lys-H (BOC-dPLL), and BOC-DPhe-Phe-Lys-H (BOC-dPPL) on the *in vitro* prolactin and GH secretion of the newly synthetized hormones were studied. These tripeptide aldehydes are known to inhibit trypsin and trypsin-like enzymes (9); the thrombin-catalyzed transformation of fibrinogen to fibrin is also inhibited by the Arg-aldehydes (9). The substances are non-toxic and do not interfere with the main metabolic pathways of the cellular metabolism at the concentration used (8).

Adult CFY rats were used as pituitary donors. Pituitary glands for cell cultures were dispersed with trypsin. After repeated washing of the cells they were suspended in TCM 199 supplemented with 10% new-born calf serum. One ml aliquots of the suspension containing $5-8 \times 10^5$ cells/ml were explanted into multiwell disposotrays and maintained as reported earlier (10). Freshly excised pituitary quarters were incubated in TCM 199 in a shaker bath and gassed with 95% O_2 and 5% CO_2. The tripeptide aldehydes were dissolved and mixed into the incubation medium. The newly synthetized prolactin and GH were measured on the base of the [^{3}H]-Leu incorporation into the hormones

(11). The radioactive proteins were isolated by polyacrylamide gel electrophoresis. Immunoreactive prolactin and GH content of the media and cell homogenates were assayed with antibodies obtained from the Rat Pituitary Hormone Distribution Program of the NIADDK. Total cell proteins were measured according to Lowry et al. (12).

EFFECT OF BOC-DPhe-Pro-Arg-H AND DPhe-Pro-Arg-H

During 8 hours incubation of pituitary quarters of male rats with 1.0 mM BOC-dPPA the release of [^{3}H]-prolactin was decreased by 24.7%, incubation with 3.0 mM resulted in 55.4% inhibition, and a slight accumulation of [^{3}H]-prolactin was detected in the tissue fragments (Fig. 1). The total newly synthesized [^{3}H]-prolactin (the sum of the released and retained hormone) was equal in every case (data not shown). A similar trend of changes was observed in iPRL (Fig. 1). The inhibition of prolactin release by BOC-dPPA was dose dependent and hormone biosynthesis was not disturbed. The GH output seemed to be less sensitive to the treatment. 1.0 mM BOC-dPPA had no influence. Statistically significant inhibition (50%) of the [^{3}H]-GH release occurred only in the presence of 3.0 mM BOC-dPPA (data not shown).

The effect of 1 mM BOC-dPPA on pituitary cell cultures has been also tested. The compound inhibited the release of [^{3}H]-prolactin after 4 hours by 60% and after 24 hours by 43%, the reduction of iPRL output was similar (Fig. 2). A modest (21.5%),

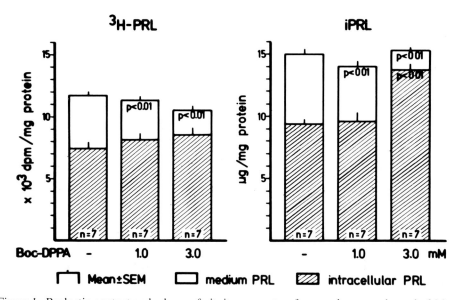

Figure 1. Prolactin content and release of pituitary quarters from male rats at the end of 8 hours incubation in the presence of 1.0 mM or 3.0 mM BOC-DPhe-Pro-Arg-H. The [^{3}H]-prolactin of media and tissue fragments is summarized on the left and the iPRL on the right panel of the figure. The open bars represent the radioactivity of the newly synthesized hormone or the immunoreactive hormone concentration in the media, the hatched bars that in the tissue.

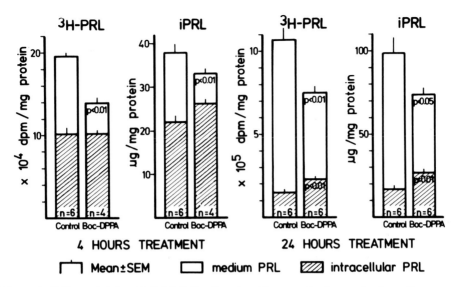

Figure 2. Effect of 1.0 mM BOC-DPhe-Pro-Arg-H on prolactin production of rat anterior pituitary cell cultures after 4 (left panel) and 24 hours (right panel) treatment. The open bars represent the radioactivity of the newly synthesized hormone or the immunoreactive hormone concentration in the media, the hatched bars that in the cells.

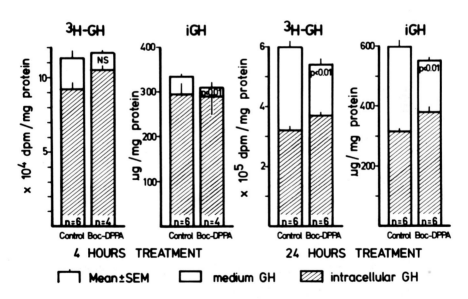

Figure 3. Effect of 1.0 mM BOC-DPhe-Pro-Arg-H on GH production of rat anterior pituitary cell cultures after 4 (left panel) and 24 hours (right panel) treatment. The open bars represent the radioactivity of the newly synthesized hormone or the immunoreactive hormone concentration in the media, the hatched bars that in the cells. NS = not significant.

but statistically significant decrease of the total [³H]-prolactin biosynthesis was observed only after 24 hours exposure. Four hours of BOC-dPPA treatment of cultures led to a significant decrease in iGH release, the fall of [³H]-GH release was statistically not significant; the total [³H]-GH and iGH was not affected (Fig. 3). After 24 hours the reduction of GH release became more explicit (Fig. 3), but no changes in the total [³H]-GH biosynthesis and iGH content occurred (data not shown).

The effect of 1.0 mM dPPA, a tripeptide aldehyde with nonprotected N-terminus, on prolactin and GH secretion was investigated in pituitary quarters. The [³H]-prolactin release was reduced by 40%, the iPRL by 20% after 8 hours incubation. The cellular [³H]-prolactin, iPRL, and the GH production was unchanged (data not shown).

EFFECT OF BOC-DPhe-Leu-Lys-H

Pituitary quarters from female rats were placed into TCM 199 containing 0.1, 0.31, or 1.0 mM BOC-dPLL and incubated for 4 hours. The lowest concentration of the Lys-aldehyde reduced [³H]-prolactin release by 27% and 0.31 mM by 45%, but only the latter diminution was statistically significant (Fig. 4). The total biosynthesis of the [³H]-prolactin was similar to that of the control pituitaries (Fig. 4). 1.0 mM of the drug resulted in a conspicuous fall of the [³H]-prolactin biosynthesis, and the release of the

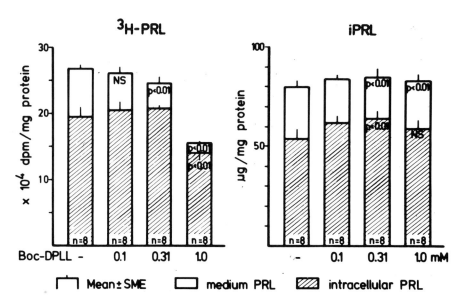

Figure 4. Prolactin production of pituitary quarters from female rats in the presence of different concentrations of BOC-DPhe-Leu-Lys-H after 4 hours incubation. The [³H]-prolactin of media and tissue fragments is summarized on the left, iPRL on the right panel of the figure. The open bars represent radioactivity of the newly synthesized hormone or the immunoreactive hormone concentration in the media, the hatched bars that in the tissue. NS = not significant.

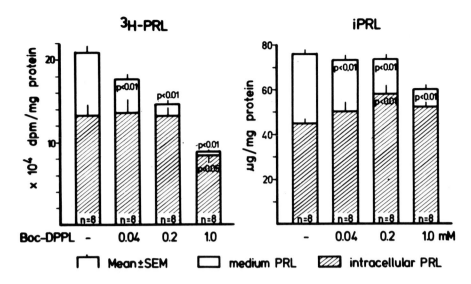

Figure 5. The effect of various concentrations of BOC-DPhe-Phe-Lys-H on [³H]-prolactin (left panel) and iPRL (right panel) production of anterior pituitary quarters from female rats after 4 hours incubation. The open bars represent radioactivity and immunoreactive hormone concentration in the media, the hatched bars that in the tissue. NS = not significant.

newly synthetized hormone was inhibited by the two highest concentrations, but the total amount of the immunoreactive hormone in the medium + cells was identical in each group (Fig. 4). While prolactin secretion was disturbed by BOC-dPLL, the production of GH was practically unaffected (data not shown).

EFFECT OF BOC-DPhe-Phe-Lys-H

BOC-dPPL was the most effective inhibitor of prolactin release of incubated pituitary quarters; 0.04 mM resulted in 47%, 0.2 mM 79%, and 1.0 mM in 94% diminution of [³H]-prolactin level in the incubation medium (Fig. 5). The total biosynthesis of the radioactive prolactin was not influenced by 0.04 mM BOC-dPPL (data not shown); the higher concentrations resulted in 26% and 56% decrease, respectively. The iPRL was also decreased in the medium by gradually increasing doses; the sum of the iPRL in the medium and cells decreased only in the presence of 1.0 mM BOC-dPPL (Fig. 5). BOC-dPPL seems to be also a selective inhibitor of prolactin secretion since [³H]-GH secretion was reduced by the tripeptide aldehyde only in 1.0 mM concentration (data not shown).

The experiments were designed to investigate the *in vitro* effect of various Arg- and Lys-aldehyde serine/thiol protease inhibitors on prolactin and GH biosynthesis and on the release of the newly synthetized hormones. The observations concur with earlier findings (7, 10) and provide clear evidence that serine/thiol protease inhibitors whose effect are time-, sequence-, and dose-dependent may decrease newly synthetized [³H]-prolactin and [³H]-GH release. The relative inhibiting potency of [³H]-prolactin release was BOC-dPPL > BOC-dPLL > BOC-dPPA > dPPA. The [³H]-GH release was less influenced by the tripeptide aldehydes than the release of the [³H]-prolactin. A pronounced [³H]-GH inhibiting effect of BOC-dPPA was achieved only by a higher dose (3.0 mM) or a longer exposure. Although 0.2 mM BOC-dPPL inhibited [³H]-prolactin release by 79%, it had no effect on the output of [³H]-GH, and the BOC-dPLL was completely selective in [³H]-prolactin release inhibition. That the sensitivity of the different cell types to the release inhibiting effect of the serine/thiol protease inhibitors is not identical is not surprising, since the ionic environment may also cause dissimilar release of prolactin and GH from the pituitary tissue (13) or from pituitary secretory granules (14). Another well documented difference in the function of lactotrophs and somatotrophs is that the major part of the *in vitro* synthetized prolactin is released while the "new" GH is retained by their producing cells (15).

The results suggest that the pituitary proteases are components of the prolactin and GH release regulating systems. Inhibitor sensitivity suggests that the target enzyme(s) of the inhibitors may belong to the family of serine, or perhaps the thiol proteases. Possible targets are the trypsin and trypsin-like enzymes present in the pituitary tissue (3,6) since their catalytic reaction is inhibited by dPPA, BOC-dPPA, BOC-dPLL, and BOC-dPPL (9 and our unpublished data). The dPPA and BOC-dPPA inhibit the transformation of fibrinogen (9) which may point to involvement of the plasminogen-plasmin system, which also occurs in the pituitary (3,16). However, the Lys-aldehydes used are weak inhibitors of this reaction (our unpublished data), which argues against the involvement of a plasminogen activator.

The cellular localization of the putative enzymes inhibited by the tested Arg- and Lys-aldehydes also needs further investigation. The proteolytic enzymes of the membrane of hormone producing cells may have a role in the release process (17,18) but proteases of the internal cell compartments (6, 19,20) may also be involved.

The hormone release-inhibiting effect of tripeptide aldehydes is not a consequence of toxic side effects of the drugs. It was well documented in previous metabolic studies that dPPA and BOC-dPPA have no cytotoxic effects (8). The present experiments proved that the tripeptide Arg- and Lys-aldehydes so far tested inhibited *in vitro* biosynthesis of [³H]-prolactin and [³H]-GH at most slightly in short term experiments, while the biosynthesis of the nonhormonal cellular proteins was undisturbed. In all cases the deficit of the radioactivity in the trichloracetic acid protein precipitates of the samples (data not shown) could be accounted for by the reduced radioactivity of the prolactin and GH.

In summary, exposure of anterior pituitary tissue or cell cultures to Arg- and Lys-aldehyde tripeptides known to inhibit various serine/thiol proteases resulted in a marked inhibition of the release of the de novo synthetized [³H]-prolactin and of the immunoreactive prolactin pool. The effect of the inhibitors on GH release was less marked and on the total biosynthesis of the two hormones it was slight or negligible. The data presented here support the hypothesis that limited proteolysis may be a component in the cellular regulatory mechanisms of prolactin and GH release, and the enzyme(s) may be serine/thiol protease(s).

ACKNOWLEDGMENTS

We thank the NIADDK and Dr. A. F. Parlow for the supply of RIA reagents, Dr. Zs. Acs for supervision of hormone determinations, Mr. G. Folly for statistical analysis of the data, and Mr. I. Csapo for photography. The skillful technical assistance of Ms. A. Deak, Zs. Vadasz, E. Vass, V. Garamvolgyi, I. Hejtejer, and Mr. F. Czemniczky is gratefully acknowledged.

REFERENCES

1. Adams E, Smith EL. (1951): J Biol Chem 191:651
2. Meyer RK, Clifton KH. (1956): Arch Biochem Biophys 62:108
3. Ellis S, Nuenke JM, Grindeland RE. (1968): Endocrinology 83:120
4. Doebber TW, Divor AR, Ellis S. (1978): Endocrinology 103:1794
5. Kenessey A, Paldi-Haris P, Makara GB, Graf L. (1979): Life Sci 25:437
6. Chertow BS. (1981): Endocr Rev 2:137
7. Barna I, Graf L, Makara GB, Rappay Gy. (1982): Neuropeptides 3:65
8. Rappay Gy, Nagy I, Makara GB, Horvath Gy, Karteszi M, Bacsy E, Stark E. (1984): Life Sci 33:337
9. Bajusz S, Barabas E, Tolnay B, Szell E, Bagdy D. (1978): Int J Peptide Protein Res 12:217
10. Rappay Gy, Nagy I, Makara GB, Bacsy E, Fazekas I, Karateszi M, Kurcz M. (1979): In Vitro 15:751
11. MacLeod RM, Lehmeyer JE. (1974): Endocrinology 94:1077
12. Lowry OH, Rosenbrough NJ, Farr AL, Randall RJ. (1951): J Biol Chem 193:265
13. MacLeod RM, Fontham EH. (1970): Endocrinology 86:863
14. Lorenson MY, Robson DL, Jacobs LS. (1983): J Biol Chem 258:8618
15. MacLeod RM, Abad A. (1968): Endocrinology 83:799
16. Albrechtsen OK. (1957): Brit J Haemat 3:284
17. Leblanc P, Patton E, L'Heritier A, Kordon C. (1980): Biochem Bioph Res Commun 96:1457
18. Almenoff J, Wilk S, Orlowski M. (1981): Biochem Bioph Res Commun 102:206
19. Perdue JF, McShan WH. (1962): J Cell Biol 15:159
20. Tesar JT, Koenig H, Hughes C. (1969): J Cell Biol 40:225

Prolactin. Basic and clinical correlates
R.M. MacLeod, M.O. Thorner and U. Scapagnini (eds.),
Fidia Research Series, vol. I,
Liviana Press, Padova © 1985

Section III
Intracellular pituitary mechanisms
regulating prolactin release

FROM BACTERIA TO BETAS:
IN QUEST OF THE SOUL OF THE MAMMOTROPH

M.J. Cronin, J.A. Anderson, S.N. Perkins, J. Weiss, D. Koritnik*, C. Bethea**, A.A. Weiss, W.S. Evans, A.D. Rogol, M.O. Thorner, and E.L. Hewlett

University of Virginia School of Medicine, Charlottesville, Va 22908
*Bowman Gray School of Medicine, Winston-Salem, NC 27103
**Oregon Regional Primate Center, Beaverton, OR 97006

INTRODUCTION

We have employed the anterior pituitary mammotroph as a model endocrine cell because of its unique tonic inhibition by the hypothalamus, because of the availability of clonal prolactin cells, and because this cell most often becomes deranged as an adenoma in the human pituitary. This triune circumstance has conspired to foster a productive research climate such that knowledge of the cell physiology of the mammotroph is well advanced.

In this overview, we shall describe our studies employing several new probes and techniques. First, the ability of a bacterial adenylate cyclase to produce markedly elevated levels of cAMP and prolactin release will be addressed. Then, the response of individual mammotrophs, identified with the reverse hemolytic plaque assay, will be shown in relation to enhanced cAMP levels. Finally, beta-adrenergic agonists, which activate the cAMP generating system in the anterior pituitary (unpublished observation), will be discussed in regard to the mammotroph and somatotroph.

EXTRACYTOPLASMIC ADENYLATE CYCLASE (ECAC)

The most convincing approach to proving that the activity of the adenylate cyclase molecule (as opposed to that of phosphodiesterase, etc.) can dictate the rate of prolactin release would be to show that reconstitution of active catalytic adenylate cyclase into prolactin cells increases exocytosis. Unfortunately, enriched preparations of eukaryotic adenylate cyclase are unstable, and reconstitution protocols have yet to be

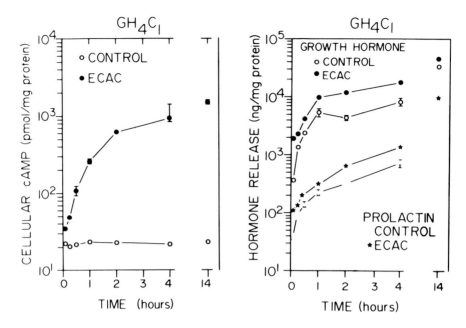

Figure 1. The response of GH4C1 clonal cells to extracytoplasmic adenylate cyclase (ECAC) is illustrated. The ECAC was extracted from *Bordetella pertussis* bacteria and applied to monolayer cultures of the clones for the times indicated. cAMP and protein were extracted from the cells and the medium content of prolactin and growth hormone was determined by RIA. Control wells (open symbols) received the ECAC vehicle. Notice the log scales (mean ± SEM).

fruitful. Until this capability is available, we have attempted an alternative approach using prokaryotic extracytoplasmic adenylate cyclase (ECAC), a calmodulin-dependent enzyme present primarily on the outer leaflet of *Bordetella pertussis* organisms and in their growth medium (1,2).

Bacterial extracts exhibiting marked adenylate cyclase enzymatic activity in cell-free protocols were applied to normal rat anterior pituitary cells as well as to prolactin-secreting clonal cell lines. In primary cultures of normal anterior pituitary cells, cAMP levels (max = 280 x basal) and prolactin release (max = 17 x basal) were enhanced by ECAC in a concentration-dependent manner over a 2 hour incubation period (data not shown). In Figure 1, the time course of ECAC activity is illustrated in GH4C1 clonal cells. At 5 minutes (the earliest time studied) there was a significant increase in both cAMP levels and hormone release compared to control conditions. In the continued presence of ECAC, cAMP continued to rise for hours and remained elevated at 14 hours. Likewise, the enhanced hormone release was maintained for much of this time course (Note the log scales.).

These effects appear to be reversible; washing out the ECAC and testing the cell's response to secretagogues a day later demonstrated no response difference from that of cells never exposed to ECAC. The ECAC effects are also calcium-dependent; nominally calcium-free medium prevented the elevation of cAMP levels and secretion patterns induced by ECAC in 2 mM calcium medium. Finally, the specificity of this approach was addressed with *Bordetella* transposon mutants that do not express the ECAC phenotype; extracts of these bacteria with protein contents identical to that of the wild-type bacterium had no impact on pituitary cell cAMP concentrations or hormone release.

HEMOLYTIC PLAQUE ASSAY FOR PRIMATE MAMMOTROPHS

Fontana and colleagues (3) introduced the reverse hemolytic plaque assay to mammalian endocrine cells. Neill and Frawley (4) showed the applicability of this technique to rat anterior pituitary cells. We were fortunate to acquire anterior pituitary tissue from *Macaca fascicularis* monkeys that had participated in a long-term study of steroid contraceptives. The tissue was enzymatically and mechanically dispersed to single cells and cultured for several days to allow recovery from the dispersion trauma. On the

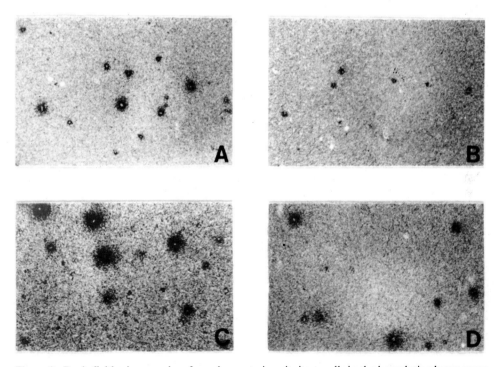

Figure 2. Dark-field micrographs of monkey anterior pituitary cells in the hemolytic plaque assay are shown surrounded by sheep red blood cells. A = vehicle treated; B = dopamine (10 uM) treated; C = forskolin (30 uM) treated; D = dopamine + forskolin treated. The quantitation of the population responses is listed in Table I. Notice the heterogeneity of plaques within a given treatment group.

day of a plaque assay, some cells were removed from the culture plastic and seeded into Cunningham chambers consisting of poly-1-lysine coated microscope slides. Then, either vehicle or 10 uM dopamine was added for 20 minutes at 37C. After the preincubation period, forskolin (30 uM), a direct stimulator of adenylate cyclase activity, forskolin + dopamine, dopamine alone, or vehicle was added to a series of chambers simultaneously with anti-human prolactin serum (1:50, #AFP C12081, courtesy of NIAMDD) and guinea pig complement. Plaques were allowed to develop for 30 minutes at 37 C; cells were then fixed with 2% glutaraldehyde. The coverslips were popped off and the cells were stained with methyl green pyronin and preserved. For quantitation purposes, the plaque areas (50 plaques/slide) were measured with a Zeiss videoplan and the proportion of cells forming plaques was determined (400-600 total cells/ treatment group) for 2 independent experiments.

Table I lists the data and Figure 2 illustrates typical low-power darkfield micrographs. We found that dopamine itself inhibited both the percentage of cells forming plaques and the average area of the population of plaques. Forskolin increased the size of the plaques, whereas dopamine antagonized this forskolin-induced change. There was a similar trend in the percentage of cells forming plaques.

Table I. *The Effect of Dopamine and Forskolin on Monkey Prolactin Cells*

	% Plaques	Area of Plaques (u^2)
Control	41 ± 1	2,290 ± 130
Dopamine	29 ± 1*	1,930 ± 110*
Forskolin	52 ± 5	3,450 ± 180*
Forskolin + Dopamine	45 ± 4.5	2,680 ± 140

* indicates groups that are different from control (mean ± SEM)

Thus, it is now possible to study prolactin release from single, living mammotrophs in the primate. Hormone release from these cells can be inhibited by dopamine and stimulated by enhanced cAMP levels, confirming and extending our earlier plaque assay observations of rat mammotrophs (5). The high percentage of cells releasing prolactin may reflect higher circulating prolactin values observed in monkeys treated with a contraceptive steroid. Alternatively, the dispersion and culture process may have selected for mammotrophs. A dramatic feature revealed by the plaque assay is the apparent heterogeneity of the population of prolactin cells. A major question now is whether this technology can be applied in a dynamic mode to address the hypothesis of mammotroph subpopulations.

BETA-ADRENERGIC AGONISTS AND PROLACTIN RELEASE

Denef and Baes observed that beta-adrenergic agonists evoke prolactin release from superfused aggregates made from rat anterior pituitary cells (6). Intrigued by these fin-

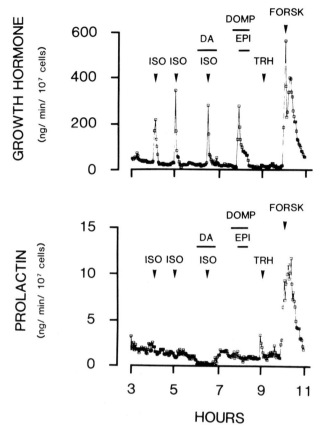

Figure 3. Hormone release by perifused, acutely dispersed rat anterior pituitary cells in response to various agents is illustrated. The two hormones were measured in the same eluate. The drugs were exposed for either 1 h (dopamine), 50 min (domperidone), 30 min (epinephrine), or 5 min (arrow) at the following concentrations: 1-isoproterenol (ISO), 100 uM; dopamine (DA), 10 uM; domperidone (DOM), 10 nM; epinephrine (EPI), 100 nM; thyrotropin releasing hormone (TRH), 10 nM; forskolin (FORSK), 3 uM. Beta-adrenergic activity was highly correlated with growth hormone release, while there was no effect on prolactin release. As a positive control, dopamine inhibition of prolactin release was antagonized by the dopaminergic antagonist domperidone. The enhanced cAMP levels induced by forskolin rapidly stimulated the release of both hormones as a final positive control.

dings, we used the beta-adrenergic radioligand [^{125}I]-iodocyanopindolol to measure receptors directly in porcine (7) and rat (8) anterior pituitary. We then attempted to confirm and extend the earlier report by investigating the prolactin response in a system similar to that used by Denef and Baes. We report here that beta-adrenergic agonists had no effect on prolactin secretion by acutely dispersed rat anterior pituitary cells.

In four independent experiments, up to 1 uM of the beta-adrenergic agonist 1-isoproterenol had no effect on prolactin secretion, whereas 1-epinephrine, 1-norepinephrine, and dopamine inhibited prolactin release (Fig. 3).

Epinephrine was unable to stimulate prolactin secretion even in the presence of domperidone, a dopaminergic antagonist; this concentration of domperidone did, however, block the inhibition of prolactin caused by epinephrine's activation of dopamine receptors. Forskolin and thyrotropin-releasing hormone consistently and rapidly stimulated prolactin secretion, thereby demonstrating that the mammotrophs could be activated by secretagogues. Human pancreas tumor growth hormone-releasing factor-40 (hpGRF) and somatostatin had no effect on prolactin release. In contrast to these negative findings with prolactin secretion, beta-adrenergic agonists (as well as forskolin and hpGRF) markedly stimulated growth hormone release from these same preparations (Fig. 3, as previously reported in ref. 9.

In their initial report, Denef and Baes (6) described beta-adrenergic stimulation of prolactin release from rat anterior pituitary cells that had been dispersed and then reassociated into spherical aggregates by constant gyratory shaking during 5 days in culture. In our system, which employs a similar perifusion device, the anterior pituitary cells were dispersed and immediately placed in the apparatus, thus affording a study of responsiveness of the cells within a few hours of removal from the animal. Using this model, we were unable to repeat Denef and Baes' observations on beta-adrenergic stimulation of prolactin release.

The possible reasons for this disparity in results raise interesting questions about the control of prolactin release at the level of the pituitary gland. One mundane explanation is that the enzyme treatment of the gland may acutely uncouple or destroy beta-adrenergic receptors which may then be reconstituted with time in culture. Such enzymatic inactivation would have to be selective for beta-adrenergic receptors residing on the mammotroph, however, because the mammotroph retains its responsivity to the inhibitory action of dopamine, and the somatotroph can clearly be stimulated by beta-adrenergic agonists. Another possibility is that the prolactin response to beta-adrenergic agonists does not exist *in vivo* but develops only *in vitro* in the extended absence of the normal internal milieu or as some other artifact of the culture conditions for aggregate formation.

More intriguing is the hypothesis that beta-adrenergic agonists act as prolactin secretagogues only in the presence of contacts or defined arrangements between the mammotroph and other cell types in the gland. Just such specialized cell junctions develop during culture in rotation-mediated aggregation (10); moreover, Denef and Andries (11) have demonstrated paracrine effects on prolactin secretion in this model (see also Denef, this volume). Any such contacts or close associations that exist between cells *in vivo* would obviously be disrupted in our acutely dispersed preparation. Further study of these possible interactions between various anterior pituitary cells may contribute to the understanding of the complex regulation of prolactin release in vivo.

CONCLUSION

A novel array of probes and technology has allowed us to further characterize the mammotroph. Within the constraints of these approaches, prolactin release from populations as well as from individual cells of the anterior pituitary is stimulated by agents which increase cAMP levels (e.g., ECAC, forskolin) and inhibited by dopamine. For the first time, we have demonstrated the feasibility of amplifying normal and clonal prolactin cell activity with a prokaryotic enzyme, ECAC. Thus, the endogenous and regulated adenylate cyclase system can now be effectively bypassed. In our modest pilot studies of primate anterior pituitary cells using the plaque assay, prolactin cells appear to respond to challenges much as we have observed in rat cells. We now look forward to critically assessing living primate mammotrophs with this powerful new technique. Finally, we have discovered that beta-adrenergic agonists are potent growth hormone secretagogues, but have no apparent effect on prolactin release in acutely dispersed anterior pituitary. Whether this latter effect exists *in vivo* is the crucial issue we must face before formally proposing this response as physiologically relevant.

ACKNOWLEDGMENTS

This work was supported by a DuPont Fellowship, RCDA 1K04NS00601, NS18409, AM32632, AM22125, AI18000, AI18482TMP, The Rockfeller and Pratt Foundations. Excellent technical help was rendered by G. Baber, C. Cassada, M. MacLeod, R. Malcolm, and G. Vandenhoff.

REFERENCES

1. Hewlett EL, Urban MA, Manclark CR, Wolff J. (1977): Pro Natl Acad Sci 73:1926
2. Wolff J, Cook GH, Goldhammer AR, Londos C, Hewlett EL. (1984): Adv Cyclic Nucleotide & Protein Phosphorylation Res 17:161
3. Fontana S, Tramontano D, Ambesi-Impiombato FS, Rossi G. (1982): Endocrinology 110:1790
4. Neill JD, Frawley LS. (1983): Endocrinology 112:1135
5. Anderson J, Keefer D, Yasumoto T, Cronin M. (1984): 7th Int Cong of Endocrinology (Quebec)
6. Denef C, Baes M. (1982): Endocrinology 111:356
7. Perkins SA, Davis AL, Cronin MJ. (1983): 65th Ann Meeting of the Endocrine Society, 161
8. Perkins SA, Evans WS, Thorner MO, Cronin MJ. (1984): 7th Int Cong Endocrinology, in press
9. Perkins SN, Evans WS, Thorner MO, Cronin MJ. (1983): Neuroendocrinology 37:473
10. Van der Schueren B, Denef C, Cassiman JJ. (1982): Endocrinology 110:513
11. Denef, C, Andries M. (1983): Endocrinology 112:813

Prolactin. Basic and clinical correlates
R.M. MacLeod, M.O. Thorner and U. Scapagnini (eds.),
Fidia Research Series, vol. I,
Liviana Press, Padova © 1985

Section III
Intracellular pituitary mechanisms
regulating prolactin release

NEUROTENSIN STIMULATES PHOSPHATIDYLINOSITOL BREAKDOWN IN RAT ANTERIOR PITUITARY GLANDS *IN VITRO*

Pier Luigi Canonico, Maria Angela Sortino, Carmela Speciale, Maria Concetta Morale and Umberto Scapagnini

Department of Pharmacology, University of Catania School of Medicine,
Catania, Italy.

Neurotensin is a naturally occurring tridecapeptide originally isolated from extract of bovine hypothalami by Carraway and Leeman (1). Several studies have implicated a role for neurotensin in the control of pituitary hormone secretion. In support of this role, neurotensin-containing cell bodies are found in the hypothalamus (2), particularly in the median eminence and the medial and lateral preoptic area (3).

In ovariectomized rats intracerebroventricular injection of neurotensin has been found to lower prolactin levels while intravenously the peptide showed an opposite effect, suggesting that neurotensin can act directly on the pituitary to stimulate the release of prolactin (reviewed in 4). Accordingly, neurotensin stimulates prolactin secretion from incubated rat hemipituitaries (5,6).

We will present some results concerning the possible intracellular mechanism(s) by which neurotensin stimulates prolactin release *in vitro*. In particular we have focused our attention on the possible involvement of the so-called "phosphatidylinositol effect" and of arachidonate metabolism in neurotensin's effect at the pituitary. Our data confirm and extend results previously obtained with neurotensin in other cellular systems.

THE "PHOSPHATIDYLINOSITOL EFFECT" AND PROLACTIN SECRETION

A modified turnover of specific membranal phospholipids, the inositol lipids, is one of the earliest postreceptor events in many secretory cells; it appears to be involved in the transmission of information and in the responsiveness of the cells (7,8). The increase in phosphatidylinositol turnover due to the stimulation of a specific phospholipase C, causes an increase of 1,2-diacylglycerol, inositol-1,2 cyclic phosphates, and phosphatidic acid, which have been shown to act as second messengers and/or ionophores (see 7,8 for reviews).

Changes in phosphatidylinositol turnover may activate the secretory process initiated by certain hypothalamic hypophysiotropic hormones. The involvement of phosphatidylinositol cycle has been proposed in the mechanisms controlling the release of luteinizing hormones (LH) induced by gonadotrophin-releasing hormone (GnRH) (9) and in that of growth hormone (GH) induced by human pancreatic GH-releasing factor (GRF) (10). Concerning prolactin secretion, we recently showed that dopamine, the primary prolactin inhibiting factor, decreases the incorporation of radio-labeled phosphate, an index of phosphatidylinositol turnover, into anterior pituitary phosphatidylinositol *in vitro* and *in vivo* (11). On the other hand the hypothalamic tripeptide thyrotropin-releasing hormone (TRH) and bombesin, two potent stimulators of prolactin secretion, rapidly increase [^{32}P] incorporation into phosphatidylinositol and phosphatidic acid in prolactin-secreting GH pituitary cells (12) and hemipituitary glands (13). Rebecchi et al. (14), using GH cells, showed that TRH stimulates the rapid and specific hydrolysis of phosphatidylinositol and its conversion to 1,2-diacylglycerol and phosphatidic acid. TRH and dopamine effects on phosphatidylinositol labeling do not seem to be protein synthesis- and/or calcium-dependent phenomena. Cycloheximide, a protein synthesis inhibitor, or calcium channel blockers such as Mn^{2+} or D600, do not modify the incorporation of radiolabeled phosphate into phosphatidylinositol either in basal conditions or in the presence of either dopamine or TRH (12,13).

NEUROTENSIN AND PHOSPHATIDYLINOSITOL HYDROLYSIS

As indicated above, neurotensin may be involved in the regulation of prolactin secretion, possibly by a direct effect on specific receptors located on the mammotroph. It has been previously reported that in slices prelabeled with [^{3}H]-inositol, neurotensin provokes phospholipase C hydrolysis of inositol phospholipids (determined by measuring [^{3}H]-inositol 1-phosphate formation in the presence of 10 mM Li$^+$) (15). On the other hand neurotensin has been reported to stimulate calcium uptake at pituitary level and this effect in anterior pituitary cells in culture is antagonized by dopamine (16). This is of extreme interest in view of the well known relationship between the changes in inositol lipid metabolism and changes in cellular Ca^{2+} homeostasis that may be important to the control of exocytosis in cells.

Therefore, we investigated the effect of neurotensin on phosphatidylinositol breakdown in anterior pituitary glands incubated *in vitro*. Hemipituitary glands from female rats were incubated for 150 min in Medium 199 containing 10 uCi/ml [^{3}H]-myoinositol. The glands were then washed and reincubated for 30 min or other times in fresh Medium 199 with or without neurotensin and/or other drugs. Phospholipids were extracted by the method of Folch et al. (17) slightly modified. In brief, the method consists of homogenizing (in a Potter-Elvehjem type homogenizer) the tissue with a 2:1 chloroform-methanol mixture and washing the extract by addition to it of 0.2 its volume of KCl. The solvent systems employed to separate phospholipids were chloroform:methanol:NH$_4$OH:water (60:30:1.75:3.25, v:v:v:v) and then chloroform:methanol:acetic acid:water (60:12:8:2.5, v:v:v:v). Phospholipids extracted showed radioactivity almost exclusively confined to inositol lipids. As shown in Figure 1, neurotensin stimulated phosphatidylinositol hydrolysis in a concentration-dependent manner. The effect was already significant at 100 nM and was maximal at 1-10 uM. At the same concentrations neurotensin stimulated prolactin release, without affecting the release of other anterior pituitary hormones (LH, FSH, GH). The effect of neurotensin was rapid (already present at 1 min), maximal at 2.5 min and still present after 30 min (Fig. 2). To determine the specificity of the increased phosphatidylinositol breakdown produced by neurotensin, other proteins and peptides were tested. Fraction V bovine serum albumin (BSA) and somatostatin did not modify phosphatidylinositol hydrolysis (Fig. 3), while TRH produced changes in the turnover of the phospholipid similar to neurotensin (data not shown).

In the last few years, several studies with synthetic analogs of neurotensin have been performed to investigate structure-activity correlations. It was shown that the last C-terminal residue of the peptide cannot be removed, amidated, or N-methylamidated without a complete loss of biological activity (18-20). Subsequently, shorter analogs with full binding and pharmacological activities and others more active than neurotensin itself were synthesized.

We investigated the effect of some neurotensin related peptides on phosphatidylinositol breakdown in anterior pituitary glands incubated *in vitro*. As shown in Figure 4, neurotensin (1-6)-hexapeptide did not affect phosphatidylinositol hydrolysis

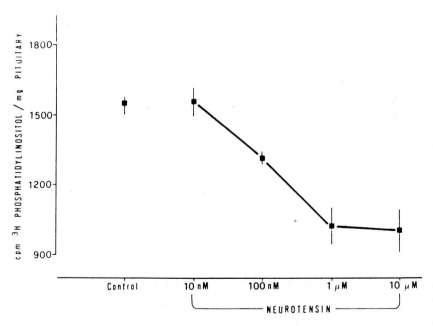

Figure 1. Effect of different neurotensin concentrations on phosphatidylinositol breakdown in hemipituitary glands incubated *in vitro*. Each value represents the mean ± SEM of 4 determinations for each group.

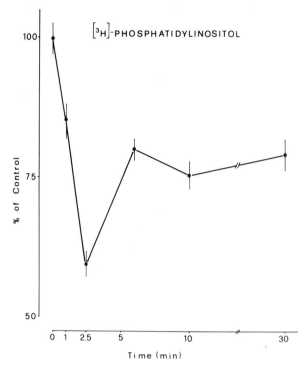

Figure 2. Time course of the effect of neurotensin on phosphatidylinositol breakdown in anterior pituitary glands incubated *in vitro*. Results are expressed as per cent of respective controls. Each value represents the mean ± SEM of 4 determinations per group.

for concentrations up to 5 uM. Conversely, Gln^4 neurotensin, an analog reported to be twice as active as neurotensin in corpus striatum and more active in other brain regions (19,21), significantly stimulated phosphatidylinositol breakdown already at a concentration of 50 nM. Acetyl neurotensin-(8-13), the shortest analog with the same binding and biological potency of neurotensin (21), produced stimulatory effects on phosphatidylinositol turnover similar to the natural peptide. These results indicate that a variety of neurotensin analogs also possess at the pituitary level a biological efficacy very similar to their ligand selectivity and relative potency in other cellular systems.

The increase of phosphatidylinositol breakdown produced by neurotensin did not appear to be dependent on protein synthesis or subsequent to Ca^{2+} mobilization, since 100 uM cycloheximide did not modify neurotensin-induced phosphatidylinositol hydrolysis and pre- and/or coincubation with EGTA or Mn^{2+} did not abolish the phosphatidylinositol response to the peptide (data not shown).

These results indicate that neurotensin has selective effects on phospholipid, in particular phosphatidylinositol, metabolism in the pituitary gland. The changes in phosphatidylinositol turnover can in turn produce specific intracellular events leading to the final event, the regulation of prolactin secretion.

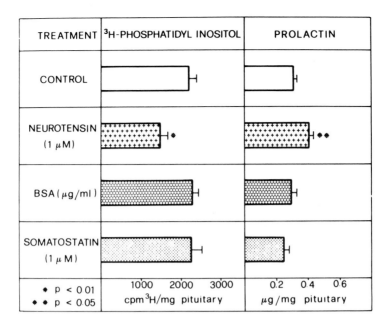

TREATMENT	³H-PHOSPHATIDYL INOSITOL	PROLACTIN
CONTROL		
NEUROTENSIN (1 μM)	*	**
BSA (μg/ml)		
SOMATOSTATIN (1 μM)		
* p < 0.01 ** p < 0.05	1000 2000 3000 cpm ³H/mg pituitary	0.2 0.4 0.6 μg/mg pituitary

Figure 3. Effect of neutrotensin, fraction V bovine serum albumin (BSA), and somatostatin on phosphatidylinositol breakdown and prolactin release from anterior pituitary glands incubated *in vitro*. Prolactin was determined with a double antibody RIA using materials and protocols supplied by the National Hormone and Pituitary Program. Results are expressed in terms of NIADDK rat prolactin RP-2 standard. Values represent the mean ± SEM of 4 determinations for each group.

NEUROTENSIN, ARACHIDONIC ACID METABOLISM AND PROLACTIN SECRETION: THE POSSIBLE INVOLVEMENT OF DIGLYCERIDE LIPASE

The "phosphatidylinositol response" is often accompanied by release and oxidation of arachidonate through the activity of specific lipases that cleave the fatty acid from membranal phospholipids (reviewed in 7,8). The role of arachidonate and/or its metabolites (i.e. prostaglandins, thromboxanes, leukotrienes, etc.) in the prolactin release process is still uncertain. We and others previously reported that phospholipase A_2 and phorbol myristate acetate, agents that increase intracellular arachidonate concentration, stimulate prolactin release from anterior pituitary cells perifused in columns (22) or in primary culture (23). Similarly, the polypeptide melittin, contained in bee venom, enhances phospholipase A_2 activity and dose-dependently stimulates prolactin release from primary cultures of dispersed bovine anterior pituitary cells (23). Conversely, quinacrine, p-bromophenacylbromide, and p-bromoacetophenone, antagonists of phospholipase A_2 activity, inhibit both basal and stimulated prolactin release *in vitro*

250

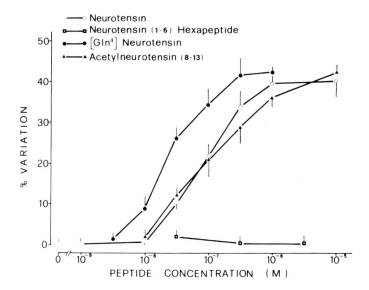

$[^3H]$ – PHOSPHATIDYLINOSITOL

Neurotensin
Neurotensin (1-6) Hexapeptide
$[Gln^4]$ Neurotensin
Acetylneurotensin (8-13)

% VARIATION

PEPTIDE CONCENTRATION (M)

Figure 4. Dose response curves of the effects of neurotensin, neurotensin (1-6)-hexapeptide, Gln⁴ neurotensin, and acetylneurotensin-(8-13) on phosphatidylinositol hydrolysis in hemipituitary glands *in vitro*. Results are expressed as per cent of corresponding control. Each value represents the ± SEM of 4 determinations per group.

(22,23). Moreover arachidonic acid itself (23,24), but not other fatty acids such as oleic or stearic acid (Canonico et al., unpublished observation), was found able to stimulate in a concentration-dependent manner prolactin release *in vitro*. All these results strongly suggest a role for an arachidonate metabolic pathway in the prolactin release process *in vitro*. It is unlikely that arachidonic acid acts directly, but instead it is more probable that one of its metabolites induces release of the hormone.

We investigated whether changes in the level of free or unesterified arachidonic acid may account for the effect of neurotensin at the level of the mammotroph. For this purpose pituitary glands were incubated for 150 min with 1 uCi/ml [³H]-arachidonic acid before neurotensin addition. The peptide caused a rapid increase in the level of free [³H]-arachidonic acid. To determine the concentration dependence of this effect, the level of free [³H]-arachidonic acid was measured in response to different concentrations of neurotensin at 2.5 min. Figure 5 shows the dose-response of neurotensin effect on free arachidonic acid levels. This increase in the concentration of the free fatty acid at the pituitary suggests that neurotensin may also stimulate prolactin release by stimulating the release (and therefore the availability) of arachidonic acid and/or its metabolites. Interestingly, recent studies by Kolesnick et al. (25) showed that TRH causes a similar rapid increase in the level of free arachidonic acid in mouse pituitary

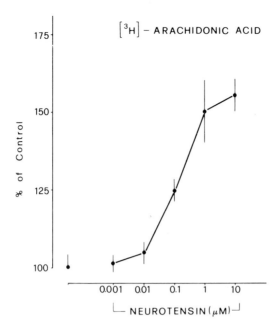

Figure 5. Dose response curve of the effect of neurotensin on free [³H]-arachidonic acid concentration in anterior pituitary glands incubated *in vitro*. Values are the mean ± SEM of 4 determinations for each group.

thyrotropic (TtT) cells. Moreover, in the isolated rat portal vein, neurotensin was found to elicit a dose-dependent contractile effect. This effect was abolished by inhibitors of phospholipase A_2 activity and of cyclooxgenase (26), suggesting that in other cellular systems the response to neurotensin may also be dependent upon the presence of a functional arachidonate pathway.

Recently, a specific diacylglycerol lipase which cleaves arachidonate directly from 1,2-diacylglycerol has been described in several tissues, including secretory cells (reviewed in 27, 28). It has been proposed that the combined activities of a phosphatidylinositol-specific phospholipase C, generating an arachidonate rich diacylglycerol (27), and of diacylglycerol lipase represent an alternative pathway for phospholipase A_2 to release arachidonate from membranal phospholipids (28). We have previously reported that the selective inhibitor of diacylglycerol lipase activity RHC 80267 (29) inhibits, in a concentration-dependent manner, basal prolactin release from pituitary cells in primary culture and from hemipituitary glands incubated *in vitro* (24,30). RHC 80267 also completely prevented the stimulatory effect of TRH and K+ on prolactin release (24,30). We investigated the possible involvement of this pathway in the mechanism(s) governing neurotensin stimulation of prolactin release *in vitro*. RHC 80267 (70 uM) reduced the concentration of free [³H]-arachidonic acid in the pituitary gland and completely

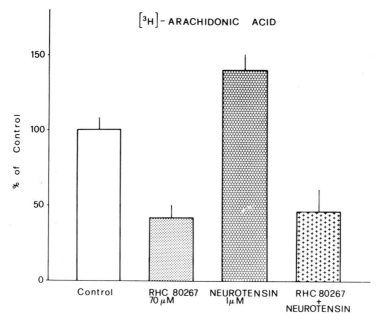

Figure 6. Effect of 70 uM RHC 80267 and 1 uM neurotensin on free [³H]-arachidonic acid concentration in anterior pituitary glands incubated *in vitro*. Values are expressed as mean ± SEM of 4 determinations for each group.

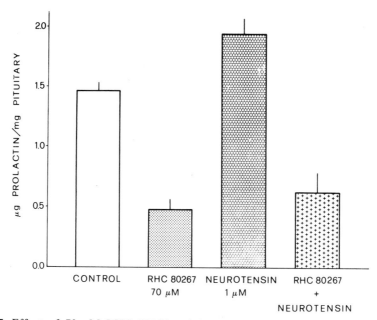

Figure 7. Effect of 70 uM RHC 80267 and 1 uM neurotensin on prolactin release from hemipituitary glands incubated *in vitro*. Values are the mean ± SEM of 4 determinations for each group.

counteracted the stimulatory effect of neurotensin on arachidonic acid metabolism (Fig. 6). This action was paralleled by complete inhibition of the stimulation of prolactin release produced by 1 uM neurotensin in anterior pituitary glands incubated *in vitro* (Fig. 7).

These results indicate that a diacylglycerol lipase pathway may link the "phosphatidylinositol effect", described in the pituitary for neurotensin as well as for other prolactin stimulating or inhibiting agents, to the production of arachidonate from mammotroph membranal phospholipids.

CONCLUSION

In conclusion, phospholipid metabolism, in particular that of phosphatidyl- inositol and arachidonate, seems to be an essential intracellular signal by which several prolactin stimulating or inhibiting factors, including neurotensin, influence the release of the hormone from the mammotroph. As a hypothetical model (Fig. 8) to explain the mechanism by which the hypothalamic peptide neurotensin stimulates prolactin release, we suggest that they increase phosphatidylinositol turnover; the diacylglycerol formed, may produce, through the activity of a diacylglycerol kinase, phosphatidic acid that is presumably recycled in part to phosphatidylinositol. However, part of the diacylglycerol produced from phosphatidylinositol may be cleaved by a specific diacylglycerol lipase to arachidonate. The fatty acid and/or its metabolites, as well as the phosphatidic acid formed may serve as calcium ionophores and activate

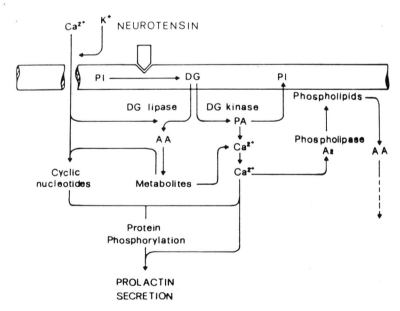

Figure 8. Schematic representation of possible intracellular events following the stimulation of specific membranal receptors by neurotensin at the mammotroph. PI = phosphatidylinositol; DG = 1,2-diacylglycerol; PA = phosphatidic acid; AA = arachidonic acid.

phospholipase A_2 that further liberates arachidonic acid from several membranal phospholipids. Consequently, all these intracellular regulators (arachidonate metabolites, calcium, etc.) of secretory mechanisms, directly or through the activation of other specific systems (i.e. protein phosphorylation), may affect prolactin release.

ACKNOWLEDGMENTS

We thank Ms. Norah Prestifilippo for her skillful editorial assistance and Mr. Stefano Maugeri for excellent technical help.

REFERENCES

1. Carraway R, Leeman SE. (1973): J Biol Chem 248:6854
2. Uhl GR, Snyder SH. (1976): Life Sci 19:1827
3. Kobayashi RM, Brown M, Vale W. (1977): Brain Res 126:584
4. McCann SM (1982): In: Muller EE, MacLeod RM. (eds) Neuroendocrine Perspectives. Elsevier Biomedical Press, Amsterdam, vol 1:1
5. Vijayan E, McCann SM. (1980): Endocrinology 105:64
6. Enjalbert A, Arancibia S, Priam M, Bluet-Pajot MT, Kordon C. (1982): Neuroendocrinology 34:95
7. Michell RH. (1975): Biochim Biophys Acta 415:81
8. Berridge BJ. (1981): Mol Cell Endocrinol 24:115
9. Snyder GD, Bleasdale JE. (1982): Mol Cell Endocrinol. 28:55
10. Canonico PL, Cronin MJ, Thorner MO, MacLeod RM. (1983): Am J Physiol 245:E587
11. Canonico PL, Valdenegro CA, MacLeod RM. (1983): Endocrinology 133:7
12. Sutton CA, Martin TFJ. (1982): Endocrinology 110:1273
13. Canonico PL, Bonetti AC, Scapagnini U, MacLeod RM. (1984): Biogenic Amines, in press
14. Rebecchi MJ, Kolesnick RM, Gershengorn MC. (1983): J Biol Chem 258:227
15. Downes CP. (1982): Cell Calcium 3:413
16. Memo M, Carboni E, Spano PF. (1983): V Joint Meeting Italian-Soviet Neuropharmacologists Abstract 13
17. Folch J, Lees M, Sloane Stanley GH. (1957): J Biol Chem 226:497
18. Granier C, Van Rietschoten J, Kitabgi P, Poustis C, Freychet P. (1982): Eur J Biochem 124:117
19. Folkers K, Chang D, Humphries C, Carraway R, Leeman R, Bowers CY. (1976): Proc Natl Acad Sci USA 73:3833
20. Rivier J, Lazarus LH, Perrin MH, Brown MR. (1977): J Med Chem 20:1409
21. Garcia-Sevilla JA, Magnusson T, Carlsson A, Leban J, Folkers K. (1978): Naunyn-Schmiedeberg's Arch Pharmacol 305:213
22. Canonico PL, Schettini G, Valdenegro CA, MacLeod RM. (1983): Neuroendocrinology 37:212
23. Grandison L. (1984): Endocrinology 114:1
24. Canonico PL, MacLeod RM. (1983): Soc Neurosci XIII Ann Meeting Abstract 208.19
25. Kolesnick R, Musacchio I, Thaw C, Gershengorn MC. (1984): Endocrinology 114:671
26. Rioux F, Quirion R, Leblanc MA, Regoli D, St-Pierre S. (1980): Life Sci 27:259
27. Prescott SM, Majerus PW. (1983): J Biol Chem 258:764.
28. Bell RL, Kennerly DA, Stanford N, Majerus PW. (1979): Proc Natl Acad Sci USA 76:3238
29. Sutherland CA, Amin D. (1982): J Biol Chem 257:14006
30. Canonico PL, Cronin MJ, Sortino MA, Speciale C, Scapagnini U, MacLeod RM. (1984): Proc Symposium Prolactin 1984, p 32

Prolactin. Basic and clinical correlates
R.M. MacLeod, M.O. Thorner and U. Scapagnini (eds.),
Fidia Research Series, vol. I,
Liviana Press, Padova © 1985

Section IV
Modification of prolactin
production by steroids

MODIFICATION OF PROLACTIN PRODUCTION BY STEROIDS: AN OVERVIEW

Alan D. Rogol and Claude Robyn

The subject of estrogen and progesterone regulation of prolactin biosynthesis continues to be an area of great interest and productivity. Dr. J. Gorski noted that estrogens stimulate gene transcription as measured by the incorporation of precursors into prolactin messenger RNA very early (less than one hour) in their time-course of action. The response was stable for 24 hours; however, there was a markedly different time-course for nuclear binding-peak within one hour followed by an exponential decline to control values by twelve hours. Since others have noted that in general, cytosine residues of DNA are hypo-methylated on active genes compared to inactive genes, these investigators studied the degree of methylation of DNA specific for prolactin in the liver and pituitary. Certain restriction sites near the prolactin genes were found to be hypo-methylated in the pituitary compared to liver. Further, DNase I digestion, which preferentially cleaves chromatin in the ''open'' or less condensed state, more effectively cleaved pituitary chromatin when compared to liver. They concluded that the transcribed region of the gene exists in an open configuration and that the cytosine residues in this portion of the gene are hypo-methylated and may be more susceptible to interaction with the estrogen receptor.

Laverriere et al. further investigated the state of methylation of DNA and the expression of prolactin and growth hormone genes by using the GH_3 CDL clone which has decreased prolactin secretion. High molecular weight DNA was obtained, digested with specific restriction enzymes, submitted to electrophoresis, blotted onto nitrocellulose, and hybridized with nick-translated rat prolactin or growth hormone probes. They found an inverse correlation of DNA methylation and rat prolactin and growth hormone gene expression. By using 5-azacytosine, a demethylating agent, the investigators showed increased prolactin gene expression. Taken together these papers show that rapid gene activation for prolactin is correlated to the degree of methylation of the expressed portions.

The hormonal regulation of prolactin secretion was considered in detail by other workers. Differences that are observed in primates and rodents have not always been emphasized. Bethea showed the estrogen dependence of prolactin secretion by primate pituitary cells in primary culture, using defined medium. Dopamine effectively suppressed prolactin secretion in the presence of estradiol throughout the 12 days of culture with essentially the same IC_{50}, approximately 10 nM. Camp and Barraclough have taken this analysis further by correlating steroid hormone receptor occupancy with the phasic release of LH and prolactin in the rat. They noted LH phasic release only at low estradiol concentrations but as the levels of estradiol and receptor occupancy in hypothalamic areas increased, phasic prolactin release occurred and was coupled to LH release. The addition of progesterone amplified the phasic release of the gonadotropins.

Further evidence for an interaction of estradiol and progesterone on prolactin release was noted by Deis and Alonso. Employing pseudopregnant rabbits they found that estradiol enhanced the prolactin secretory response to exogenous progesterone. However, this effect was not constant during the entire course of pseudopregnancy.

The next area of interest concerned the cellular effects of prolactin. Dr. Friesen reviewed evidence for the prolactin-mediated increase in the mammary gland and the rat lymphoma cell, Nb-2. Evidence for cell surface changes was presented within 1-2 hours after the addition of prolactin, followed in sequence by activation of ornithine decarboxylase, [³H]-thymidine incorporation, and an increased phosphorylation of 19,000 and 33,000 dalton proteins. As in many other systems divalent $F(ab')_2$ anti-prolactin receptor antibodies, that is, those that can cross-link the receptors, showed activity similar to prolactin itself. Evidence for a specific intracellular second messenger for prolactin bio-activity was presented. However, the nature of this activator is not presently known.

Further evidence for the direct effect of prolactin on mammary gland metabolism was presented by Falconer and Martyn. They presented evidence for a progressive inhibitory effect of pharmacologic doses of progesterone on hormone-stimulated fatty acid synthesis in pseudopregnant rabbits. In a similar system using mouse mammary explants, Rillema was able to show an effect of prolactin of phosphate uptake and incorporation into phospholipids. The increased activity of phosphate was noted in all fractions — organic, aqueous, and insoluble. Prolactin had a profound effect on phospholipid biosynthesis intiated 12 hours after exposure. Taken together with previous data these papers detail the intracellular events that occur concomitantly with milk formation.

Effects of prolactin on the immune system have been considered important. Spangelo and co-workers showed that concanavalin A - induced mitogenesis in immune spleen cells could be increased by prolactin, but only at low concentrations (0.1-10 nM). Higher concentrations were less effective but did not inhibit basal stimulation. There was however, no enhancement of B cell stimulation by lipopolysaccharide. Prolactin did affect antibody formation in spleen cells sensitized to sheep red blood cells in vitro. Increasing concentrations of prolactin significantly increased the numbers of placque forming cells. In the human, Russell and co-workers described specific prolactin receptors on B and T cells. They presented intriguing data for an interaction between prolactin binding and the binding of cyclosporine A. The binding of prolactin is enhanced at low concentrations of cyclosporine but inhibited at higher concentrations. A similar interaction was noted for the activation of ornithine decarboxylase. Thus, at concentrations of cyclosporine known to be immunosuppressive there is a specific competition for prolactin receptors in immunocompetent human cells. The consequences of this interaction in hyperprolactinemic patients are not yet known, but are an area of great interest.

Further effects of prolactin on tissues were noted by Chilton and Daniel who were able to show direct effects of prolactin on DNA synthesis and glandular differentiation in uterine endometrium of long term ovariectomized rabbits. Their studies showed that increased concentrations of uteroglobulin, progesterone receptor, and estrogen receptors followed prolactin treatment. The effects of prolactin were markedly enhanced by progesterone. Klemcke and co-workers showed that prolactin was necessary prepubertally for the development of hamster testicular prolactin receptors.

Use of prolactin receptors for site-directed chemotherapy against hormone sensitive tumors was the subject of a provocative paper by Blossey et al., who synthesized a prolactin-daunomycin conjugate. A cytotoxic effect was noted in cells with the prolactin receptor but not in those without. The effect was only partially inhibited by prolactin and is clearly dependent upon the internalization of the conjugate prolactin receptor complex. This strategy may serve well in some peptide hormone dependent cancers.

Finally Adler and co-workers presented evidence for a direct effect of prolactin on rat bone. Hypercalciuria was noted only in those rats rendered hyperprolactinemic. Urinary cyclic AMP was not changed. On histological sectioning of the leg bones decreased cortical mass and decreased calcium content were noted. Because urinary cAMP was not changed these effects were considered to be mediated by prolactin since any effect of parathyroid hormone would have been accompanied by increased urinary cyclic AMP concentrations.

Prolactin. Basic and clinical correlates
R.M. MacLeod, M.O. Thorner and U. Scapagnini (eds.),
Fidia Research Series, vol. I,
Liviana Press, Padova © 1985

Section IV
Modification of prolactin
production by steroids

ESTROGEN REGULATION OF PROLACTIN GENE TRANSCRIPTION AND CHROMATIN STRUCTURE

Jack Gorski, James Shull[*], James Weber[**], and Linda Durrin

Department of Biochemistry and Animal Science
University of Wisconsin, Madison, Wi.

INTRODUCTION

Prolactin is a complex hormone; complex in its biology, its regulation and even its gene structure. A variety of hormones regulate the pituitary gland's synthesis and release of prolactin. Among them, estrogens are a major regulator of prolactin biosynthesis in the rat and mouse. Our laboratory has focused on this aspect of prolactin regulation.

While the other regulators of prolactin production will be dealt with elsewhere in this volume, it is important to point out that several of these regulators also influence prolactin biosynthesis. For example, thyrotropin-releasing hormone (TRH) stimulates prolactin synthesis in cultured cells (1) and the concentration of prolactin mRNA measured by hybridization to prolactin cDNA (2). Two lines of evidence indicate that TRH regulates prolactin gene transcription. TRH induces increases in concentrations of nuclear precursors of prolactin mRNA (3) and increased transcription rate in TRH stimulated nuclei (4). Other stimulators of prolactin production include epidermal growth factor (5,6), vitamin D metabolites, such as $1,25(OH)_2 D_3$ (7) and androgens (8). Inhibitors of prolactin production include dopamine (9) which appears to reduce the concentration of prolactin mRNA (10,11). Prolactin production is also inhibited by platelet-derived growth factor (12), thyroxine (T_4) and triiodothyronine (T_3) (13), and glucocorticoids (14).

In the rat and mouse the ontogeny of prolactin synthesis appears to be estrogen dependent. Prolactin release and synthesis are relatively low in immature (1 to 21 days

---

[*] Present address: Department of Oncology, McArdle Labs, University of Wisconsin, Madison.
[**] Present address: Department of Immunology, Walter Reed Institute of Research, Washington, DC 20307.

old) males or females (15,16). At 4 and 8 days of age prolactin synthesis was not detectable by two-dimensional gel electrophoresis or immunoprecipitation, whereas growth hormone was a major synthetic product even before birth. In mice at 12 to 20 days of age prolactin synthesis was readily detectable, although quantitatively low compared to growth hormone. Injection of estrogen into 4 or 8 day old mice stimulated prolactin synthesis by several fold (15). In immature rats, 20 to 24 days old estrogen administration also markedly increased prolactin synthesis even though a basal level of prolactin synthesis was always present. Prolactin synthesis is much higher in cycling, pregnant, or lactating rats, indicating a general dependency on estrogens for optimal prolactin synthesis in these species.

We have studied the mechanisms of estrogen action on prolactin biosynthesis and believe that regulation of prolactin gene transcription is the site of estrogen action. Since other regulators in addition to estrogen appear to influence prolactin gene expression, an interesting model of biological regulation can be postulated. A discussion of our laboratory's current work on estrogen regulation of prolactin gene transcription and chromatin structure follows, with these complexities in mind.

Previously, we had shown that estrogen-induced prolactin mRNA concentration measured in *in vitro* translation assays (11) or in hybridization assays (17) could account for the increased prolactin synthesis due to estrogen. Increased synthesis or decreased turnover of mRNA pools, in turn, could account for the mRNA change that was observed. Hoffman et al. (18) showed that large prolactin mRNA precursors, which probably included the primary transcripts, could be detected only in tissue actively synthesizing prolactin. This suggested, but did not prove, estrogen was regulating prolactin gene expression at a transcriptional site. Recently, Maurer (19) and Shull and Gorski (20,21,22) have shown that *in vitro* nuclear transcription systems prepared from estrogen-treated animals showed higher rates of incorporation of precursor nucleotides into prolactin gene transcripts than did controls (Figure 1). The magnitude of the increase of 2 to 3 fold is similar to the increases in mRNA accumulation reported earlier if the increase in total RNA synthesis and cell number are taken into account. Growth hormone gene transcription was measured as a control and did not change significantly with estrogen treatment.

Two surprising findings of this study related to the time course shown in Figure 1 were: the extremely early response to estrogen (less than 1 hr) and the unexpected stability of the increase for 24 hours or longer after a single injection of the hormone. The rapidity of the response was surprising because prolactin mRNA accumulation and prolactin synthesis are not detectable until about 24 hours and do not peak until 3 to 7 days after hormone administration. However, these times would be appropriate if the turnover rate of prolactin mRNA was very slow (long half life). Turnover rates of prolactin mRNA have not been determined with great precision, but Stone et al. (11) showed that withdrawal of estrogen from estrogen-injected animals resulted in a slow decrease of prolactin mRNA activity. This suggests that this mRNA is relatively stable and turns over slowly.

The rapid effect of estrogen in stimulating transcription suggested that this was a "primary" effect of estrogen. Primary effects are defined as those responses to a hormone that are not mediated through the stimulation of protein synthesis. An exam-

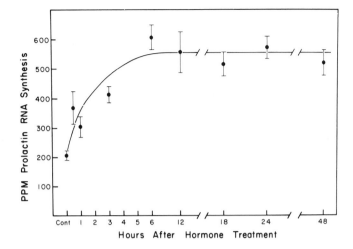

Figure 1. Stimulatory effect of 17 beta-estradiol on prolactin transcription. At the indicated times prior to sacrifice, male rats were injected IP with 10 ug of estradiol in sesame oil. Anterior pituitary nuclei were then prepared and prolactin transcription was assayed. Each data point represents the mean and standard error of the mean ($n = 3$) of prolactin RNA synthesis in nuclei pooled from 8-10 animals (Shull and Gorski, 1984).

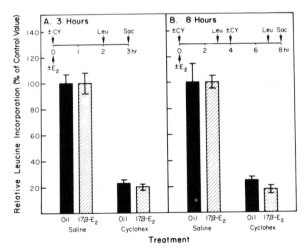

Figure 2. Inhibitory effects of cycloheximide on pituitary protein synthesis. A. Cycloheximide (or its saline vehicle) was injected 10 min prior to 17 beta-estradiol (or its oil vehicle). Two hours after hormone injection, [³H]-leucine was injected. B. Cycloheximide (or its saline vehicle) was injected 10 min prior to 17 beta-estradiol (or its oil vehicle) and again 4 h later. [³H]-leucine was injected 3 and 7 h following hormone treatment. At the indicated times, the animals were sacrificed and leucine incorporated into pituitary protein was measured as described (7). Each bar represents the mean and standard error of the mean of the relative level of leucine incorporation in individual pituitaries from a total of 5-8 animals (Shull and Gorski, 1984).

ple of a secondary effect is the estrogen stimulation of mammary gland growth via estrogen induction of prolactin synthesis in the pituitary.

We have determined that the early increase in transcription of the prolactin gene was a primary effect by using the protein synthesis inhibitor cycloheximide (22). Cycloheximide administration to 6 week old male rats decreases protein synthesis in pituitary tissue by about 80% (Figure 2). However, cycloheximide had no effect on the estrogen induced increase in prolactin gene transcription at either 3 h (Figure 3) or 8 h (Figure 4). Apparently estrogen has a primary effect on prolactin gene transcription which is not mediated via cycloheximide sensitive steps.

The second surprising finding in the time course studies was the stability of the estrogen induced transcription to a single administration of estrogen (Figure 1). We examined estrogen-receptor binding during the same time course of transcription measurement and observed the markedly different time course shown in Figure 5. As expected, estrogen bound to the nuclear form of the receptor increased rapidly to a peak at about 1 h after estrogen injection.

Thereafter, the estrogen bound to the nuclear receptor declined exponentially to near control levels by 12 h. Thus, the increased rate of transcription induced by estrogen appears not to be closely coupled to the nuclear form of the estrogen receptor. Subsequent studies have indicated that estrogen administration *in vivo* in addition to the primary stimulation, probably activates secondary responses which in turn influence prolactin gene transcription (21). This biphasic response includes an initial phase which is closely coupled to the estrogen-receptor complex (21).

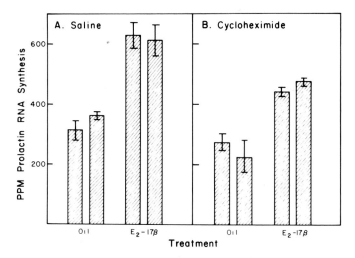

Figure 3. The induction of prolactin transcription by 17 beta-estradiol under conditions of inhibited pituitary protein synthesis: an examination at 3 hours. Sterile saline (A.) or cycloheximide (B.) was injected 10 min prior to 17 beta-estradiol or its sesame oil vehicle. The animals were sacrificed 3 h after hormone treatment and prolactin transcription was assayed as described in Experimental Procedures. Each data bar represents the mean and standard error (n = 3) for the assay of RNA synthesized by pituitary nuclei isolated from 8-10 animals (Shull and Gorski, 1984).

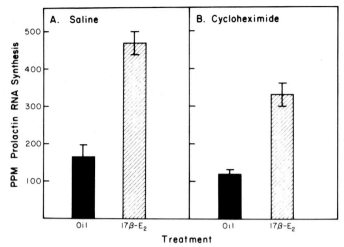

Figure 4. The induction of prolactin transcription by 17 beta-estradiol under conditions of inhibited pituitary protein synthesis: An examination at 8 hours. The animals were treated as described in Figure 2b. Upon sacrifice, prolactin transcription was assayed as described in Experimental Procedures. Each data bar represents the mean and standard error (n = 3) for the assay of RNA synthesized by nuclei isolated from 8-10 animals (Shull and Gorski, 1984).

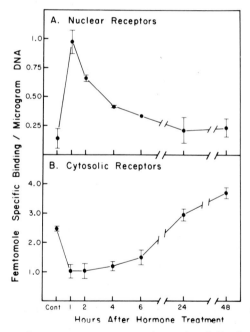

Figure 5. Time course of estrogen-receptor transformation following an injection of 17 beta-estradiol. The levels of transformed nuclear receptors and nontransformed cytosolic receptors were assayed at the indicated times following a single injection of 17 beta-estradiol (10 ug in sesame oil, IP). Each data point represents the mean and standard error of specific binding measurements in individual anterior pituitaries from 3-4 animals (Shull and Gorski, 1984).

PROLACTIN GENE STRUCTURE

The prolactin gene was first cloned by Chien and Thompson (23) who have generously shared their genomic clones with other investigators. The gene has 5 exons (DNA sequences coding for segments of the mature messenger RNA) and 4 introns (intervening sequences present in the gene and primary transcript but not present in the mature messenger RNA). The mRNA coding sequences present in cDNA have been sequenced by Gubbins et al. (24) and Maurer et al. (25). The overall organization of the prolactin gene is similar to the growth hormone gene. However, the intervening sequences of the prolactin gene are much larger, making this gene's overall size approximately 10 Kb, whereas the growth hormone gene is 2 Kb long.

Methylation of cytosine residues of CpG sequences in active genes is generally lower than in inactive genes. We determined the methylation patterns of the prolactin gene in pituitary as compared to liver tissue. We found that the cytosines in certain restriction nuclease cleavage sites were hypomethylated in DNA from pituitary and methylated in DNA from liver (Figure 6) (26). The hypomethylation was restricted to the region of the genome which is transcribed and both flanking regions of the gene contained methylated cytosines. When estrogen was withdrawn from Fischer 344 rats, the hyperplastic pituitaries regressed and prolactin synthesis decreased dramatically (27). However, estrogen withdrawal did not affect the hypomethylation of the prolactin gene, suggesting that there is a stable change in this gene in the pituitary (26). This observation is similar to those in a number of other genes in which the methylation patterns are correlated with the tissue's ability to express a particular gene, but not necessarily with the tissue's current activity. Chromatin structure also has been found to differ in active versus inactive genes. We have detected marked increases in the DNase I sensitivity of prolactin gene chromatin from pituitary tissue as compared to liver tissue (Figure 7). This nuclease sensitivity extends throughout the 35 Kb of DNA of the prolactin gene and its flanking sequences (Figure 6). The altered chromatin structure sug-

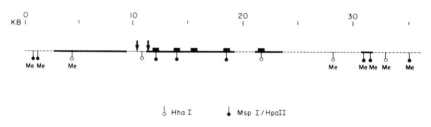

Figure 6. Summary of the methylation pattern, location of repetitive DNA sequences, and DNAse I hypersensitive sites associated with the prolactin gene domain in rat pituitary tumors. Translated regions of the prolactin gene are represented by filled boxes. Unique DNA sequences within and around the prolactin gene are represented by the solid line; regions of DNA containing repetitive sequences are represented by the dotted line2. Msp I/Hpa II and Hha I restriction sites are shown as solid and open circles, respectively. Sites which are methylated in pituitary tumors or control pituitaries of rats are indicated (Me). The two heavy arrows 5' to the first exon indicate the location of the hypersensitive sites observed in pituitary tumors (Durrin et al., 1984).

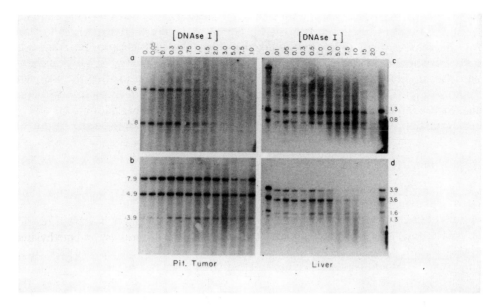

Figure 7. Tissue-specific DNAse I sensitivity of the prolactin and serum albumin gene chromatin in DES-induced pituitary tumors and in liver. Pituitary tumor or liver nuclei were digested 10 min with the concentrations of DNAse I shown at the top of the figure (ug/ml). Aliquots of purified DNA from pituitary tumor nuclei digests were restriction endonuclease cleaved with Msp I (a) or Hind III (b). Aliquots of purified DNA from the liver nuclei digests were restriction endonuclease cleaved with Eco RI (c and d). The DNA was fractioned by electrophoresis on 1 agarose gels and blotted onto nitrocellulose filters (Southern). The blots shown in panels a and c were hybridized to cloned genomic DNA fragments mapping within the coding region of the prolactin gene. Blots shown in panels b and d were hybridized to serum albumin cDNA. Sizes of restriction fragments (given in kb) were determined by running Hind III cleaved lambda DNA or Alu I cut pBR322 DNA in an adjacent lane. (Durrin et al., 1984).

gested by the DNase sensitivity is interpreted as being due to a more "open", or less condensed chromatin structure, which permits easier access to the DNA by the nuclease. The modified chromatin structure may extend even further than the approximately 35 Kb of genomic DNA available for making probes. The broad domain of modified chromatin structure is similar to previous reports of chromatin structure changes in the ovalbumin gene domain in which 100 Kb of DNA are present in a more open chromatin structure in oviduct tissue (28). The prolactin gene in liver tissue is not nuclease-sensitive; however, the serum albumin gene, which is expressed in liver, is DNase I sensitive in this tissue. In addition to the DNase I sensitive domain, selective regions of the prolactin gene's chromatin were hypersensitive to DNase I digestion (Figure 8). These two regions were in the 5' flanking regions approximately 100-200 bases and 1800-2000 bases upstream from the transcription initiation site (Figure 6). The more proximal site is in a highly conserved sequence where the rat and human prolactin genes have 90% base homology (29). Figure 6 summarizes the methylation and DNase I-sensitive and hypersensitive region of the prolactin gene region. Both the DNase I sensitive and hypersensitive regions were affected by withdrawal of estrogen even though prolactin gene transcription decreased. Chromatin structure, like methylation of the prolactin gene, appears to be closely linked with the differentiation of pituitary cells to a state where they can transcribe the prolactin gene. However, these changes in themselves do not bring about prolactin gene expression. It appears that the estrogen-receptor complex, and/or other regulators, are also necessary for transcription of this gene. Figure 9 illustrates our present conceptualization of the regulation of prolactin gene expression. It seems that developmental signals induce changes in the chromatin

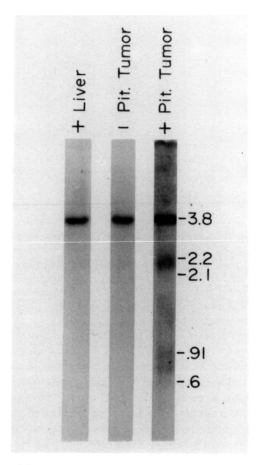

Figure 8. Localization of DNAse I hypersensitive sites near the prolactin gene. Nuclei were prepared from pituitary tumors or liver of F344 rats that had been treated 3 months with DES. After the nuclei were digested with 3 ug/ml DNAse I (lanes with +), DNA was purified and cut to completion with the restriction endonuclease Xba I. DNA was fractionated by electrophoresis on 1.5% agarose gels, transferred to nitrocellulose filters, and hybridized to probe E_2. The 3.8 kb band is the prolactin restriction fragment. In liver nuclei (lane 1) or pituitary tumor nuclei not treated with DNAse I (lane 2), no sub-bands are observed. In pituitary tumor chromatin treated with DNAse I (lane 3), two broad sub-bands are detected with sizes of approximately 2.2 kb and 0.8 kb (Durrin et al., 1984).

Estrogen-receptor Regulation of Prolactin Gene

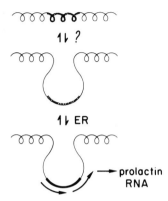

Figure 9. Model of developmental and estrogen regulation of prolactin gene transcription. Stage I involves the decondensation of tightly packed chromatin in the prolactin gene region. Unknown developmental factors regulate this process. Only limited transcription of the prolactin gene occurs. The second stage requires estrogen-receptors in some way to modify further the chromatin to permit optimal transcription rates.

structure of the prolactin gene that promote a more open configuration of the chromatin in this region of the genome. Accompanying these changes in chromatin structure is a change in the methylation of cytosines within the transcribed region of the gene. We have no evidence concerning cause and effect relationships between methylation and nuclease sensitivity. Neither do we have any evidence as to what the developmental signals are or when they occur.

With the altered chromatin structure in place, estrogen-receptor complexes can now cause further changes (not detectable by methods we have used to date) in the chromatin which then permit the access of the template to RNA polymerase and/or related factors which are necessary for transcription to begin. Preliminary evidence suggests that the estrogen-receptor complex in its transformed state in the nucleus is closely correlated with prolactin gene transcription. We believe that the mechanisms involved will eventually be discerned at the level of chromatin structure. A new model of estrogen interaction with target cells has suggested that the unoccupied estrogen receptor is targeted to the site of estrogen-receptor interaction (Figure 10) (30). If this is true then one might expect to find the unoccupied estrogen receptor associated at, or proximal to, the complex of DNA and protein that makes up the prolactin gene chromatin. However, at the present time there is no definitive evidence that the estrogen receptor directly binds to the DNA of the prolactin gene or its accompanying chromatin proteins. It is quite possible that the estrogen-receptor complex might cause some modification of a catalytic activity that in turn could influence the chromatin organization of the prolactin gene. Methodology is available which soon will permit the elucidation of these details of the mechanisms of estrogen regulation of prolactin gene expression.

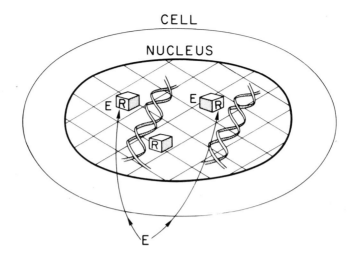

Figure 10. "New" model of estrogen receptor. R = receptor, E = estrogen, # = nuclear matrix or scaffold, ⚇ = DNA (Gorski et al., 1984).

ACKNOWLEDGMENTS

Supported in part by the College of Agricultural and Life Sciences, University of Wisconsin, Madison, WI 53706 and NIH grants HD08192 and CA18110, USPHS Fellowship 1F32 CA06730 and PF 1869 from the American Cancer Society (J.W.) and NIH Training Grant 5T32 HD07007 (J.S.).

REFERENCES

1. Dannies PS, Gautvik RM, Tashjian AH. (1976): Endocrinology 98:1147
2. Evans, GA, David DN, Rosenfeld MG. (1978): Proc Natl Acad Sci 75:1294
3. Potter E, Nicolaisen AK, Ong ES, Evans RM, Rosenfeld MG. (1981): Proc Natl Acad Sci 78:6662
4. Murdoch GH, Franco R, Evans RM, Rosenfeld MG. (1983): J Biol Chem 258:15329
5. Schonbrunn A, Krasnoff M, Westendorf JM, Tashjian AH Jr (1980): J Cell Biol 85:786
6. White BA, Bancroft FC. (1983): J Biol Chem 258:4618
7. Wark JD, Tashjian AH. (1982): Endocrinology 111:1755
8. MacLeod RM, Abad A, Eidson LL. (1969): Endocrinology 84:1475
9. Gibbs DM, Neill JD. (1978): Endocrinology 102:1895
10. Maurer RA. (1980): J Biol Chem 255:8092
11. Stone RT, Maurer RA, Gorski J. (1977): Biochemistry 16:4915
12. Sullivan NJ, Tashjian AH. (1983): Endocrinology 113:639
13. Maurer RA. (1982): Endocrinology 110:1507
14. Dannies PS, Tashjian AJ. (1973): J Biol Chem 248:6174
15. Slabaugh M, Lieberman ME, Rutledge J, Gorski J. (1982): Endocrinology 110:1489

16. Maurer RA, Gorski J. (1977): Endocrinology 101:76
17. Ryan R, Shupnik MA, Gorski J. (1979): Biochemistry 18:2044
18. Hoffman LM, Fritsch BK, Gorski J. (1981): J Biol Chem 256:2597
19. Maurer RA. (1982): J Biol Chem 257:2133
20. Shull JD, Gorski J. (1982): Endocrinology 110 (Suppl.):292
21. Shull JD, Gorski J. (1983): Fed Proc 42:206
22. Shull JD, Gorski J. (1984): Endocrinology 114:1550
23. Chien YH, Thompson ER. (1980): Proc Natl Acad Sci 77:4583
24. Gubbins EJ, Maurer RA, Lagrimini M, Erwin CR, Donelson JE. (1980): J Biol Chem 255:8655
25. Maurer RA, Erwin CR, Donelson JE. (1981): J Biol Chem 256:10524
26. Durrin LK, Weber JL, Gorski J. (1984): J Biol Chem (in press)
27. Wiklund J, Wertz N, Gorski J. (1981): Endocrinology 109:1700
28. Lawson GM, Knoll BJ, March CJ, Woo SLC, Tsai MJ, O'Malley BW. (1982): J Biol Chem 257:1501
29. Truong AT, Duez C, Belayew A, Renard A, Pictet R, Bell GI, Martial JA. (1984): EMBO J 3:429
30. Gorski J, Welshons W, Sakai D. Mol Cell Endocrinol (in press)

Prolactin. Basic and clinical correlates
R.M. MacLeod, M.O. Thorner and U. Scapagnini (eds.),
Fidia Research Series, vol. I,
Liviana Press, Padova © 1985

Section IV
Modification of prolactin
production by steroids

DNA METHYLATION AND EXPRESSION OF PROLACTIN AND GROWTH HORMONE GENES IN A RAT PITUITARY STRAIN SELECTED ON STEROID-DEPLETED MEDIUM

J.N. Laverrière*, M. Muller+, C. Tougard*, N. Buisson*, A. Tixier-Vidal*, J.A. Martial+ and D. Gourdji*

*Groupe de Neuroendocrinologie Cellulaire,
Collège de France, 75231 Paris Cedex 05, France, +Laboratoire de Genie
Génétique, Université de Liège, 4000 Sart Tilman, Belgium.

The family of "GH" rat pituitary tumor-derived cell lines provides an invaluable model for investigating the secretion of the rat polypeptide hormones prolactin and growth hormone (rGH) (1,2). These cell lines offer a homogeneous population of cells and multiple strains which differ in relative prolactin to rGH secretion ratios. Moreover, for a given strain, the secretion rate of both prolactin and rGH is highly dependent on the hormones and other factors supplied by the culture media. In this respect earlier reports from this laboratory (3,4) have shown that growing GH_3 or GH_3B_6 cells which actively secrete prolactin in a medium supplemented with charcoal-dextran stripped sera (CD medium, 75-99% depleted in total estrogen concentration), decreased prolactin secretion. The extent, as well as the reversibility, of the phenomenon was found dependent on the duration of culture in CD-medium. When GH_3B_6 cells were cultured for one week in this medium the inhibition reached approximately 60% as compared to control, and could be partially (3) or totally (4) prevented by adding 17 beta-estradiol. After use of serial subcultures for several months in CD-medium, prolactin secretion was lowered by more than 99% from the initial level. This could be reversed neither by using 17 beta-estradiol nor by growing back the cells in complete sera-supplemented medium. Thus a stable variant cell line called GH_3 CDL, which secretes minute amounts of prolactin as well as of rGH (Table 1), was established. The mechanisms by which the initial, reversible, and estrogen-dependent phenomenon was amplified and turned into an estrogen- independent state were investigated. During the past few years, a number of observations have indicated that DNA methylation could be involved in the inhibition of specific gene transcription (5, 6). We have attempted to determine whether this mechanism is implicated in the decreased expression of prolactin and rGH genes in GH_3 CDL cells.

Hence, we first compared the state of DNA methylation within prolactin and rGH genes in GH_3 CDL and GH_3B_6 cells, using as a control normal rat pituitary gland where both genes are actively expressed. For this purpose we have used Hpa II/Msp I restriction enzymes, which both cleave the sequence 5' CCGG 3'. Hpa II, however, cleaves the sequence only if the internal cytosine is unmethylated, whereas Msp I cuts the sequence whether the internal cytosine is methylated or not. In a second step, we investigated the effects of a demethylating agent, 5-azacytidine (5-azaC), with the final aim to correlate the drug-altered state of methylation with change of gene expression.

Table I *Level of prolactin and rGH production by GH_3B_6 and GH_3 CDL cells*

	Culture in N Medium (in days)	prolactin secreted in ug/mg cell prot/48h	rGH secreted in ug/mg cell prot/48h
GH_3B_6	permanent	40.0 ± 1.0	7.5 ± 1.3
	0	0.6 ± 0.01	not determined
GH_3 CDL	20	0.14 ± 0.03	0.035 ± 0.005
	40	0.29 ± 0.06	0.054 ± 0.005
	50	0.29 ± 0.10	0.042 ± 0.010

GH_3B_6 cells subcloned (2) from the GH_3 strain (1) are routinely cultured in N medium: Ham's F10 supplemented with horse (15%) and fetal calf sera (2.5%) as described (2). GH_3 CDL cells are routinely maintained in CD medium: Ham's F10 supplemented with horse (15%) and fetal calf sera (2.5%) twice extracted with charcoal-dextran, in which they secrete minute amounts of prolactin. For the present studies, GH_3 CDL cells were switched to N medium for the indicated durations. As shown, this did not significantly reverse the drastic attenuation of both prolactin and rGH secretion. Prolactin and rGH secreted in the medium were radioimmunoassayed as described (3). The results expressed as ug equivalent of NIAMDD-RPI standards are the mean ± SD of three independent determinations.

ANALYSIS OF THE STATE OF DNA METHYLATION

High molecular weight DNA was isolated from GH_3 CDL cells, GH_3B_6 cells, or the anterior pituitary, and digested with Hpa II and Msp I restriction enzymes. DNA restriction fragments were then separated by electrophoresis, blotted onto nitrocellulose, and hybridized with nick-translated prolactin (7) or rGH (8) probes.

Prolactin gene

Southern blotting analysis of Msp I digests hybridized with prolactin Hind IIIA probe (7) showed that the two major 1.64 and 4.56 Kb fragments expected from cleavage at the three Hpa II/Msp I sites within the prolactin gene (Fig. 1b) were detected in all DNA examined (Fig.1a, lanes M). Identical prolactin DNA-containing fragments were found in pituitary DNA digested by Hpa II (Fig. 1a, lane AH) indicating that the recognition sequences were also cleaved and thus were not methylated. In Hpa II digest of DNA isolated from GH_3B_6 cells (Fig. 1a, lane BH), only the 1.64 Kb fragment was conspicuous. This indicated that sites 1 and 2 were demethylated whereas site 3 was methylated. In Hpa II digest of DNA isolated from GH$_3$CDL cells (Fig. 1a, lane CH) both fragments were lacking, indicating that the three sites were methylated.

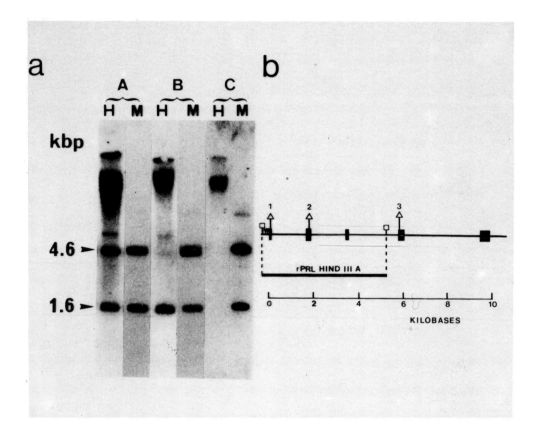

Figure 1. State of methylation of the prolactin gene

a - High molecular weight DNA isolated from the anterior pituitary (A), GH$_3$B$_6$ cells (B), and GH$_3$ CDL cells (C) (20 ug per lane) was digested with Hpa II (H) or Msp I (M) as indicated, subjected to electrophoresis on 0.8 - 1.0% agarose gel, blotted onto nitrocellulose and hybridized to nick-translated prolactin Hind III A probe (specific activity 0.5 - 2.109 cpm/ug) as described (26). Lambda DNA Hind III digest was used for molecular weight markers. Exposure to X-ray films was for 10 to 20 days with intensifying screens.

b - Structural organization of prolactin gene (7) :solid blocks represent exons. The location of the TATA box and Cap site are indicated by arrows and restriction sites for Msp I or Mpa II (△) are numbered from the 5' end to the 3' end of the gene. The genomic probe (prolactin Hind III A) used to detect the restriction fragments of the prolactin gene spans the 5' part of the gene extending from the 5' Hind III site (□) to the Hind III site located in the middle of the gene.

rGH Gene

The Msp I profiles of DNA probed with rGH cDNA containing plasmid showed three fragments of 5.0, 0.5, and 0.4 Kb respectively in DNA isolated from GH_3B_6 and GH_3 CDL cells (Fig. 2a, lanes BM and CM). The two smallest fragments were those expected from the rat GH gene sequence (9) (Fig. 2b) and from the hybridization properties of the cDNA probe used (see legend Fig. 2). This probe cannot hybridize with the intron fragment located between sites 3 and 4. The 5 Kb fragment corresponds to a site (site 1) located about 3.4 Kb upstream from the 5' end of the gene and already detected by Moore and coworkers (10). After Hpa II digestion of DNA isolated from

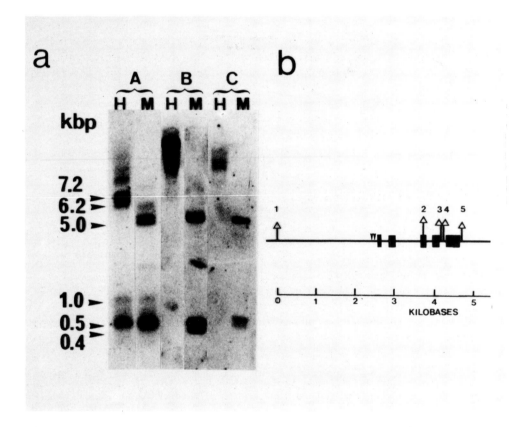

Figure 2. State of methylation of the rGH gene
a - DNA isolated from the anterior pituitary (A), GH_3B6 cells (B), and GH_3 CDL cells (C) was digested with Hpa II (H) or Msp I (M) as indicated and processed as described in the legend of Fig. 1 except that hybridization was carried out with rGH-cDNA (8): this probe hybridized with coding sequences only.
b - Structural organization of rGH gene (8): solid blocks represent exons. The location of the TATA box and Cap site are indicated by arrows. Restriction sites for Msp I or Hpa II (△) are numbered from 5' end to the 3' end of the gene (9).

GH$_3$B$_6$ cells (Fig. 2a, lane BH) or from GH$_3$ CDL cells (Fig. 2a, lane CH), large fragments of the genome containing the rGH remained intact, indicating that the five Hpa II/Msp I sites were fully methylated. In Msp I digests isolated from rat pituitary gland, the 0.4 Kb fragment was absent, while a 1.0 Kb band was detected together with fragments of molecular weights higher than 5 Kb. This could correspond to either allelic variations of the rGH gene or more probably to a methylation at the external cytosine that is inhibiting Msp I digestion. Pituitary DNA cut with Hpa II displays a restriction pattern roughly similar to that cut with Msp I, indicating a low level of methylation. As illustrated in Fig. 2a (lane AH) however, we have detected fragments of 7.2, 6.2, 1.0, and 0.5 Kb respectively. Such a complex pattern suggests a heterogeneous level of methylation for 5' CCGG 3' sites in the rGH gene and thus could reflect, as far as the rGH gene is concerned, a possible cellular and/or functional heterogeneity of the adult rat pituitary glandular cells (11).

Taken together, these findings suggested an inverse correlation between DNA methylation and prolactin and rGH gene expression. Moreover, DNA methylation appears to be the most probable mechanism accounting for the inhibition of prolactin and rGH gene expression in GH$_3$ CDL cells.

In order to obtain further evidence for a causal relationship between DNA methylation and the attenuated expression of both genes in GH$_3$ CDL cells, we used the nucleoside analog 5-azacytidine (5 azaC) that can partially demethylate DNA because of its potent inhibiting effect on DNA methyl- transferase (12).

EFFECT OF 5-AZACYTIDINE ON PROLACTIN AND GH GENES EXPRESSION

GH$_3$ CDL cells precultured for six days in normal serum supplemented medium (Table I) were exposed to 5, 10, or 50 uM 5-azaC for 60 hours, control dishes being carried out in parallel. In order to measure inheritable changes of DNA methylation, prolactin and rGH were assayed following three different durations elapsed after the end of 5-azaC treatment (4, 11 or 23 days, i.e. after an increasing number of cell divisions). As illustrated in Fig. 3, 5-azaC was found able to stimulate prolactin secretion by GH$_3$ CDL cells whatever the conditions but in a time and dose-dependent manner. Prolactin was drastically increased, i.e. by 14-fold or 25-fold above control when measured 11 or 23 days respectively, following the 5 uM 5-azaC treatment. Prolactin was stimulated to a far lower extent when measured four days after drug exposure. The lowest dose tested (5 uM) was found most potent. However, the actual stimulating effect of higher doses was most probably hampered by the cytotoxic effect of 5-azaC which increased in a dose-dependent manner from 30% at 5 uM to 70% at 50 uM. Complementary analysis at the cellular level by immunocytochemical detection, using a specific anti prolactin antiserum (13), showed that the number of immunoreactive prolactin cells increased from 4% in untreated cells to 60% in 5-azaC-ytidine treated cells (not illustrated). This favors the hypothesis that the increased production of prolactin occurred because the nucleotide analog uniformly increased prolactin gene expression in all cells rather than reversing a subpopulation from a low- to a high- expressing phenotype.

As shown in Figure 3, the action of 5-azaC on rGH secretion was markedly less efficient than on prolactin secretion. The maximal stimulation observed reached 5-fold above control 11 days after drug exposure. In addition it appeared that the 5-azaC-induced stimulation of rGH secretion was less dose-dependent and less persistent than that of prolactin secretion. These findings suggested that rGH was a weaker target for the demethylating agent than prolactin gene in GH_3 CDL cells. Consequently, in the following experiments, we have focused on the prolactin gene only.

COMPARATIVE EFFECTS OF 5-azaC ON PROLACTIN GENE DEMETHYLATION, PROLACTIN RNA LEVELS, AND INTRACELLULAR PROLACTIN CONTENT IN GH_3 CDL CELLS

For quantitating the effect of 5-azaC on DNA demethylation and to correlate it with gene expression we have examined in the same experiment the extent of prolactin gene demethylation, the level of prolactin mRNA, and the intracellular prolactin content. GH_3 CDL cells were treated with 5 uM 5-azaC or not for 48 hours and grown thereafter for 7 days in absence of the drug. At the end of this period they were collected and subjected to the three aforementioned analyses.

5-azaC-induced DNS demethylation

Msp I or Hpa II digests of DNA isolated from either 5-azaC-treated or control GH_3 CDL cells were fractionated by electrophoresis, blotted onto nitrocellulose, and hybridized with prolactin Hind III A probe (7). The autoradiograms of the Msp I digests (Fig. 4A, lanes M) displayed the same pattern as in Fig. 1a (lanes M). Three faint bands of 1.64, 4.56, and 7.0 Kb were clearly identified in the Hpa II digest of DNA isolated from treated cells; these bands were lacking in Hpa II digest of the DNA isolated from control cells. Two out of three bands (1.64 and 4.56 Kb) corresponded to the 5 azaC-induced demethylation of the three Hpa II sites located in the rat prolactin gene. The large 7.0 Kb fragment probably results from demethylation of only the two external sites. The extent of demethylation could be roughly estimated at 10%.

5-azaC-induced prolactin gene expression

Total RNA was isolated from control and treated cells of the same experiment and blotted onto nitrocellulose (14). The relative level of prolactin mRNA was quantitated by hybridization with nick-translated prolactin 800 cDNA plasmid (15). The results illustrated in Fig. 4B were that, concomitantly with the 5 azaC-induced demethylation of the prolactin gene, the relative level of prolactin mRNA was 2.5-fold stimulated as compared to control GH_3 CDL cells. This result is consistent with an increase in prolactin gene transcription.

The intracellular prolactin content was measured by radioimmunoassay as described (16). As illustrated in Fig. 4C the 5-azaC treatment elicited a 6.6-fold increase of the

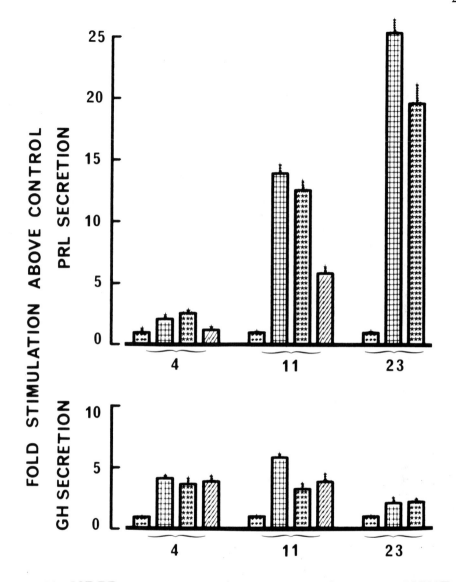

Figure 3. Effect of 5-azaC on prolactin and rGH secretion
GH₃ CDL cells cultured in N medium were untreated [·····] or treated with 5 uM - [======] ,10 uM - [·····] , or 50 uM - [\\\\\] 5-azaC for 60 hours and sub-cultured for 4, 11 or 23 days in absence of 5-azaC. Prolactin and rGH secreted in the medium were measured in the last 48 hours of the culture as described in legend of Table I. The results are expressed as fold-stimulation above the control, that are for prolactin and rGH respectively (in ug/mg cell prot/48h): 4 days, 0.19 ± 0.08 and 0.36 ± 0.03; 11 days, 0.26 ± 0.06 and 0.49 ± 0.06; 23 days, 0.14 ± 0.03 and 0.04 ± 0.005. Mean values ± SD (bars) of 3 independent determinations.

intracellular prolactin content. Altogether these findings strongly suggest a causal link among gene demethylation, specific mRNA level, and intracellular hormone content. However, in view of the increased rate of stimulation from one level to another, one cannot exclude the existence of some amplifying steps, namely at the translational level. Whether 5-azaC is involved or not in this latter process remains to be investigated.

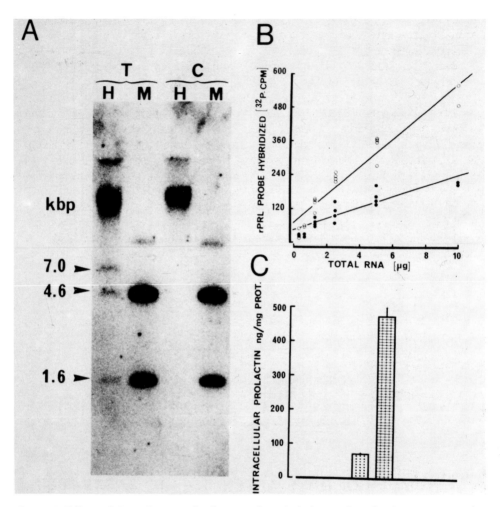

Figure 4. Effect of 5-azaC on prolactin gene demethylation and prolactin gene expression
A - High molecular weight DNA (20 ug per lane) isolated from GH_3 CDL cells treated (T) or not (C) by 5-azaC was digested either with Hpa II (H) or MspI (M) as indicated and processed as described in Fig. 1 legend.
B - Total RNA isolated from GH_3 CDL cells treated (O─O─O─O─O) or not (●─●─●─●─●) by 5-azaC were blotted onto nitrocellulose (14) and hybridized with nick-translated prolactin 800 cDNA plasmid (15). The extent of hybridization was determined by scintillation counting.
C - Intracellular prolactin was measured by radioimmunossay in cells treated - ▦▦▦ or not - [•••••••] by 5-azaC. Mean ± SD of 3 determinations.

The results of the present study support our premise that DNA methylation is implicated in the control of prolactin gene expression in GH₃ CDL cells. This is of particular interest in view of the procedure used for selecting this variant. Long-term culture in hormone depleted medium (CD medium, see above and 3, 4) induced a drastic inhibition of prolactin gene expression associated with prolactin gene methylation. Thus the presence of hormones, namely 17 beta-estradiol, might be required for preventing prolactin gene methylation and for preserving its high expression. Other examples of hormone-dependent demethylation events recently have been reported in the literature (17,18,19,20).

Particularly intriguing is how prolactin and rGH gene expression differ in level of activation following 5-azaC treatment. rGH gene was found less sensitive to demethylation than prolactin gene. An explanation of this phenomenon was provided by recording the potential CpG methylation sites (21) in both genes. As reported in Table II, these nucleotides are three-fold more abundant in rGH gene than in prolactin gene (7,22). The extent of methylation is therefore potentially greater in the rGH gene than in prolactin gene. Hence demethylation of a similar limited number of sites in both genes could result in a strong activation of the prolactin gene only. In agreement with the data are the results reported by Ivarie and Morris (24) showing that in the GH₃ cell line, successive exposures to methylating and demethylating agents preferentially modify the expression of prolactin gene. By contrast, Cherington and Tashjian (25) have shown that 5-azaC preferentially increased rGH gene expression in GH₄C₁ cells. Such discrepancy may result from a different state of DNA methylation of the prolac-

Table II *Frequency of CpG and GpC sites within and around the genes coding for rat (rPRL) and human (hPRL) prolactin and GH.*

Genes (# ref)	Total Sequences		5'Untranslated Sequences		Exons		Introns		3' Untranslated Sequences		Total Sequence % of C and G		
	CpG	GpC	CpG	GpC	CpG	GpC	CpG	GpC	CpG	GpC	C	G	C×G
rPRL (8)	0.9	3.5	0.8	2.7	1.3	4.6	0.8	3.4	0.7	2.7	19	19	3.7
hPRL (23)	1.5	3.5	1.0	1.7	3.7	6.7	1.2	3.3	0.8	2.6	20	17	3.4
rGH (9)	2.4	6.8	2.6	5.4	3.5	10.8	1.7	5.5	2.3	4.7	26	25	6.7
hGH (22)	2.5	6.8	2.0	5.7	3.8	8.4	2.2	6.5	1.7	6.5	28	28	7.7

The number of either dinucleotides CpG and GpC or nucleotides C and G was obtained from the referred published sequences. Their frequencies were expressed as the percent of either dinucleotides or nucleotides per number of bases in the region. The theoretical frequency (numbers in italics) of both CpG and GpC dinucleotides was calculated as the product of the frequencies of C and G nucleotides in each gene (column C x G). This comparative analysis shows that the disparity in the number of potential methylation sites in prolactin and rGH genes results from a deficiency in G and C contents of the prolactin gene. This unexpected difference is also noted in human genes. It may, likely, result from the larger size of introns of prolactin gene as compared to the GH gene. The spontaneous deamination of 5 methylcytosine to thymine, generating a transition mutation (21), yields a low frequency of CpG sequences in non-coding regions where selection would be less likely to occur than in coding regions (see columns introns versus exons and CpG versus GpC). In contrast, within the four genes sequence analyzed, the frequency of GpC sequences (numbers in italics) is close to their theoretical frequency (C x G column).

tin and the rGH genes in the two models (GH$_3$ versus GH$_4$C$_1$). Unfortunately there is still no information available concerning the pattern of gene methylation in GH$_4$C$_1$ cells. Other regulatory mechanisms are involved in the control of specific gene expression. In this respect, using different clonal tumor cell lines, we have recently obtained results which support the hypothesis that 5-azaC-insensitive mechanisms are superimposed on DNA methylation and participate in the inhibition of prolactin and rGH gene expression (Laverriere et al., manuscript in preparation). Involvement of such mechanisms in the hormonal control and differentiation of normal lactotrophs and somatotrophs of the rat pituitary gland could be considered.

ACKNOWLEDGMENTS

We thank D. Grouselle for RIA technical assistance and C. Pennarun and A. Bayon for illustrating and typing this manuscript. This work was supported by grants from the CNRS (E.R. 89) and MRI (contract no 83 V 0100).

REFERENCES

1. Tashjian AH Jr. (1979): Methods Enzymol 58:527
2. Gourdji D, Tougard C, Tixier-Vidal A. (1982): In: Ganong WF and Martini L (eds) Frontiers in Neuroendocrinology. Raven Press, New York, vol 27:317
3. Brunet N, Gourdji D, Moreau MF, Grouselle D, Bournaud F, Tixier-Vidal A. (1977): Ann Biol Anim Biochem Biophys 17:413
4. Brunet N, Gourdji D, Tixier-Vidal A. (1982): Mol Cell Endocrinol 18:123
5. Razin A, Riggs AD. (1980): Science 210:604
6. Navey-Many T, Cedar H. (1981): Proc Natl Acad Sci USA 78:4246
7. Cooke NE, Baxter JO. (1982): Nature 297:603
8. Seeburg PH, Shine J, Martial JA, Baxter JD, Goodman HM. (1977): Nature 270:486
9. Barta A, Richards RI, Baxter JD, Shine J. (1981): Proc Natl Acad Sci USA 78:4867
10. Moore DD, Walker MD, Diamond DJ, Conkling MA, Goodman HM. (1982): Recent Progress in Hormone Research 38:197
11. Tixier-Vidal A, Tougard C, Dufy B, Vincent JD. (1982): In: Muller EE and MacLeod RM (eds) Neuroendocrine Perspectives. Elsevier, Amsterdam, vol 2:211
12. Santi DV, Garrett CE, Barr PJ. (1983): Cell 33:9
13. Tougard C, Picart R, Tixier-Vidal A. (1982): Biol Cell 43:89
14. Thomas PS. (1980): Proc Natl Acad Sci USA 77:5201
15. Cooke NE, Coit D, Weiner RI, Baxter JD, Martial JA. (1980): J Biol Chem 255:6502
16. Morin A, Rosenbaum E, Tixier-Vidal A, Endocrinology, in press
17. Wilks AF, Cozens PJ, Mattay IW, Jost JP. (1982): Proc Natl Acad Sci USA 79:4252
18. Wilks AF, Seldran M, Jost JP. (1984): Nucleic Acids Res 12:1163
19. Mermod JJ, Bourgeois S, Defer N, Crepin M. (1983): Proc Natl Acad Sci USA 80:110
20. Clough DN, Morse BS, Kucherlapati RS, Davidson RL. (1984): Proc Natl Acad Sci USA 81:838
21. McClelland M, Ivarie R. (1982): Nucleic Acids Res 10:7865
22. Seeburg PH. (1982): DNA 1:239

23. Truong AT, Duez C, Belayew A, Renard A, Pictet R, Bell GI, Martial JA. (1984): EMBO J 3:449
24. Ivarie RD, Morris JA. (1982): Proc Natl Acad Sci USA 79:2967
25. Cherington PV, Tashjian AH Jr. (1983): Endocrinology 113:418
26. Maniatis T, Fritsch EF, Sambrook J. (1982): Molecular Cloning, a Laboratory manual. Cold Spring Harbor Laboratory, N. Y.

Prolactin. Basic and clinical correlates
R.M. MacLeod, M.O. Thorner and U. Scapagnini (eds.),
Fidia Research Series, vol. I,
Liviana Press, Padova © 1985

Section IV
Modification of prolactin
production by steroids

INTERACTION OF ESTRADIOL (E₂) AND DOPAMINE ON PROLACTIN SECRETION FROM PRIMATE PITUITARY CELLS CULTURED ON EXTRACELLULAR MATRIX AND IN SERUM-FREE MEDIUM

Cynthia L. Bethea

Reproductive Biology and Behavior, Oregon Regional Primate Research Center
Beaverton, Oregon 97006 and Department of Physiology,
Oregon Health Sciences University, Portland, Oregon 97201

In rodents and primates, the hypothalamus tonically inhibits prolactin secretion and cumulated evidence in both orders suggests that this inhibition is mediated by dopamine (1). In contrast, estrogen (E_2) is a rapid and potent stimulus for prolactin secretion in rodents (2), but much less effective in primates (3,4) unless hypothalamic inhibition is removed (5,6). Because E_2 rapidly elevates prolactin secretion in rodents, various parameters of E_2 and dopamine interaction on prolactin secretion have been examined. E_2 treatment decreases the sensitivity of dispersed rat pituitary cells to dopamine and dopamine agonists (7,8) although the mechanism of this action is unresolved (9-11). However, *in vivo* studies with humans and monkeys have demonstrated an increase in dopaminergic inhibition of prolactin secretion after E_2 treatment (12,13). This paper summarizes recent experiments with dispersed monkey pituitaries on extracellular matrix (ECM) and in serum-free medium (14,15) which were conducted to examine the inconsistencies between rodent and primate prolactin regulation by E_2 and dopamine at a cellular level.

The reagents, cell culture materials, and the procedure for dispersion of the primate pituitary are detailed in reference 14. The use of ECM for maintenance of human prolactin-secreting adenoma and pituitary cells has been previously described (16). Culture of the bovine corneal endothelial cells for the production of ECM was according to the method of Gospodarowicz et al. (17,18).

The dispersed pituitary cells were resuspended in either Ham's F12 containing 15% HS and 2.5% FCS (preliminary experiments) or a 1:1 mixture of DME and Ham's F12 (DME/F12) containing 10% FCS at a density of 2-4 x 10^5 cells/ml. The cells were plated in 24 or 48 well plates previously coated with ECM (1 ml/17 mm well; 0.5 ml/10 mm well) and allowed to attach overnight. The next morning, the plating medium (containing serum) was aspirated and replaced with serum-free medium. This was harvested and replenished every fourth day for prolactin analysis. When the cell yield from a dispersion permitted, two plates were seeded and the second plate was maintained in 10% charcoal-treated (C.T.) FCS (19). Drawing heavily from the studies of Sato and colleagues (20), a basic mixture of hormones and factors was added to DME/F12 which consisted of insulin (10 ug/ml = 1.7 uM), transferrin (10 ug/ml = 0.13uM), parathyroid hormone (0.5 ng/ml = 0.12 uM), thyroxine (19.5 pg/ml = 30 pM), fibroblastic growth factor (1 ng/ml, approx. 77 pM), selenium (4.29 ng/ml = 30 nM), cadmium (23.1 ng/ml = 30 nM), putrescine (88.2 ug/ml = 0.1 mM), ethanolamine (0.6 ug/ml = 10 uM), and a mixture of lipids consisting of oleic (0.5 ug/ml = 1.6 uM), lecithin (1.0 ug/ml = 1.3 uM), and cholesterol (1.95 ug/ml = 5 uM). Some cultures received only insulin, transferrin, selenium, and cadmium (ITSC).

In the experiments examining the effect of dopamine, the cells were plated in the inner 24 wells of 48 well plates previously coated with ECM and allowed to attach overnight. The next morning (Day 1), the plating medium was aspirated and replaced with serum-free DME/F12 containing only ITSC, plus and minus 10 nM E_2. On days 4, 8, and 12 after plating, the incubation medium was aspirated and the cells were exposed to dopamine in a dose-response fashion for 6 h in 250 ul of medium. DME/F12 with ITSC + E_2, was adjusted to 0.1 mM with ascorbate and with increasing concentrations of dopamine. On each plate there were 2 wells per group for each concentration of the dose-response curve. The mean prolactin concentration of the 2 wells was obtained and the percent change from the mean value of the control wells was calculated. The morphological appearance of the cultures was monitored by phase-contrast microscopy.

Medium prolactin concentrations were determined with a homologous human prolactin assay from NIAMDD that has been validated for use with monkey serum (21). All samples in an experiment were assayed within one assay, and the values are expressed in terms of human prolactin I-6 (E_2 exps.) and RP-1 (dopamine exps.). E_2 assays were performed as described by Resko et al. (22). Student's t-test was used for comparison of the E_2 treated and untreated cells and for point to point comparisons of the dopamine dose-response curves. Analysis of variance was used to compare overall secretion levels in E_2 treated and untreated cultures.

In 2 cultures from ovariectomized rhesus monkeys, prolactin concentrations in Ham's F12 plus 15% HS and 2.5% FCS increased and then declined on day 28 relative to the first sample. There was a slightly faster decline in prolactin with DME/F12 plus 1% FCS. Prolactin was as stable in DME/F12 and 1% FCS plus the basic hormone mix as in higher serum concentrations. Omitting the serum entirely caused lower prolactin levels on day 28, but the values were favorably comparable through day 24. In another culture of cells from an ovariectomized cynomolgus monkey, prolactin levels were stable in wells containing DME/F12 with only ITSC, and addition of the other factors had little effect. The combined means (ı SEM) for days 4 through 28 were 12.2 ± 0.3, 15.2 ± 0.3, 15.3 ± 0.4, 15.1 ± 0.3, 14.2 ± 0.3, 14.1 ± 0.6 and 13.5 ± 0.5 ug/ml suggesting a rise, stabilization, and then decline with time in culture.

In the presence of serum the undifferentiated cells had a fibroblast-like morphology and they overgrew the more granular, apparently hormone-secreting cells within 8 days

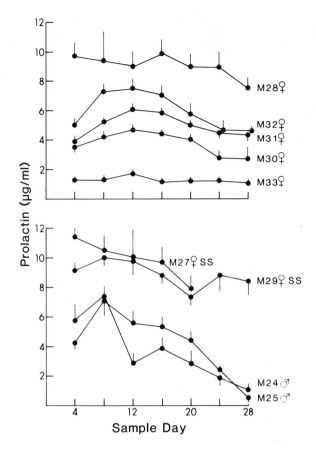

Figure 1. Medium prolactin levels in serum-free cultures of rhesus monkey pituitaries from males, females, and females with pituitary stalk-transections SS for 2 years. Reprinted with permission from Reference 14.

after plating. In serum-free medium the dividing cells had a rounder, compact shape and they appeared contact-inhibited at a lower density.

Prolactin secretion was then examined from cells obtained from animals in various physiological conditions. Pituitaries from rhesus males, females, and females with pituitary stalk-transections (SS) for at least 2 years were dispersed and plated overnight in DME/F12 plus 10% FCS. The next morning, the plating medium was replaced with DME/F12 plus the complete hormone mix and the cells were incubated for 28 days with medium changes every fourth day. The results of this survey are illustrated in Figure 1. The medium prolactin concentrations in the cultures from female animals (top panel) were stable over the 28 day period, with 4 out of the 5 cultures showing the previously observed rise and then slight decline in prolactin levels. The prolactin levels varied significantly from one culture to the next and were not correlated with the number of cells plated. In the bottom panel, the cells from the stalk-transected animals produced somewhat higher prolactin levels. Prolactin levels in the cultures of the male pituitaries also showed a rise after day 4, but then declined sooner than in the cultures of female pituitaries. Within each culture, comparison of the day 4 prolactin levels to each subsequent sample day yielded the percent change in hormone levels over time. The mean percent change of all the cultures as compared to day 4 was: $+26\%$ (day 8), $+17\%$ (day 12), $+11\%$ (day 16) -4% (day 20), -13% (day 24) and -24% (day 28).

The next series of experiments examined the effect of E_2 on prolactin production in cultures of male and female monkey pituitary cells. Each experiment was confined to one plate and the cells were maintained in either the complete hormone mix or ITSC, plus and minus 10 nM E_2. Upon termination the cells were harvested in 20 mM ammonium hydroxide.

Figure 2 illustrates the prolactin levels in 3 cultures of pituitaries from cynomolgus males (2 pituitaries pooled/culture) and in 2 cultures of pituitaries from rhesus females (1 pituitary/culture) maintained in DME/F12 plus the complete hormone mix, and in the presence or absence of E_2. The addition of E_2 maintained medium prolactin concentrations at a significantly higher level in all 5 cultures.

Figure 3 illustrates the medium prolactin concentrations in 2 cultures of pituitaries from rhesus males and in 3 cultures of pituitaries from rhesus females maintained in DME/F12 plus ITSC, and in the presence or absence of E_2. The medium prolactin

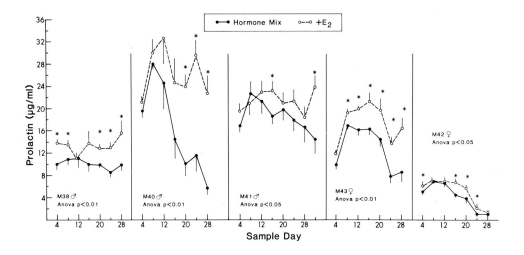

Figure 2. Medium prolactin levels in cultures of pituitaries from 6 male cynomolgus monkeys and from 2 female rhesus monkeys maintained in DME/F12 with the hormone mix, plus and minus 10 nM E_2. Each point represents the mean $\pm$ SEM and the asterisks designate the individual days which were significantly different ($p < 0.05$) with Student's t-test. Analysis of variance (ANOVA) was used to determine differences in overall prolactin production by control and E_2 treated cells. Reprinted with permission from Reference 14.

levels were significantly higher for 28 days in all cultures with E_2 addition. After day 28, E_2 was added to the control medium of the female pituitary cultures for an additional 4 days' incubation. M46 was a pregnant female (full term) with a large pituitary which yielded sufficient cells for 2 cultures. In the control medium, the prolactin levels did not initially increase as seen in other female cultures but gradually declined and then were relatively stable from day 12 through day 28. This seems consistent with the concept of steroid-supported prolactin synthesis during pregnancy in the in situ pituitary and then a 'de-induction' of that process in serum-free culture. In contrast, medium prolactin levels in the wells containing E_2 were significantly higher and exhibited little overall change from the initial sample.

Figure 4 illustrates the medium prolactin concentrations in 2 cultures of pituitaries from rhesus females maintained in DME/F12 plus 10% C.T. FCS, and in the presence or absence of E_2. RIA for E_2 after chromatography found 11 ± 3 pg/ml in the control medium versus 1487 ± 447 pg/ml in the medium to which E_2 was added. These were the only two cultures in which a comparison of prolactin levels in control and E_2 treated wells did not reveal significant statistical differences by analysis of variance.

Figure 5 compares the prolactin content of the cells maintained in the presence or absence of E_2 and terminated on day 28. Prolactin was significantly higher in 5 of these 7 cultures with E_2 treatment.

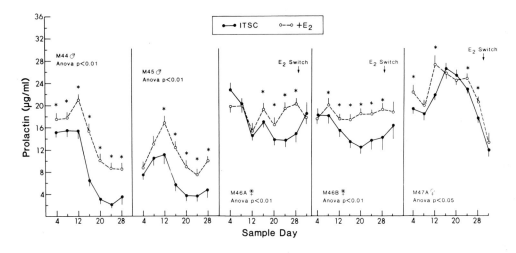

Figure 3. Medium prolactin levels in cultures of pituitaries from 2 male rhesus monkeys and in 2 cultures from 1 pituitary of a pregnant rhesus monkey and 1 culture of a pituitary from a normal female rhesus monkey. The cells were maintained on ECM in DME/F12 containing ITSC, plus and minus 10 nM E_2 through day 28, after which the control wells in the female cultures also had E_2 added for an additional 4 days. The representation of the data is as described in Figure 2. Reprinted with permission from Reference 14.

288

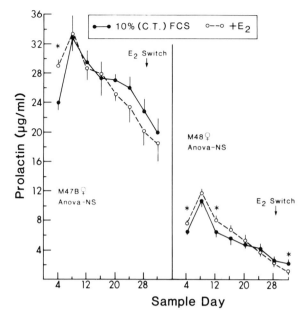

Figure 4. Medium prolactin levels in cultures of female rhesus pituitary cells incubated in DME/F12 containing 10% C.T. FCS, plus and minus 10 nm E_2 through day 28, after which E_2 was also added to the control wells for an additional 4 days. The representation of the data is as described in Figure 2. Reprinted with permission from Reference 14.

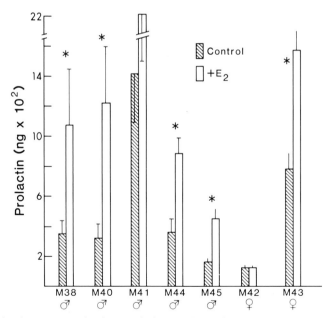

Figure 5. Prolactin content of primate pituitary cells maintained on ECM and in serum-free medium plus or minus 10 nM E_2 for 28 days. Reprinted with permission from Reference 14.

The next experiments examined the inhibitory effect of dopamine on prolactin secretion from cells maintained in the presence or absence of E_2 for 4, 8 and 12 days. Seven intact female rhesus monkeys, four ovariectomized (≥ 1 year) cynomolgus monkeys, and one intact male rhesus monkey were pituitary donors in these experiments.

Figure 6 illustrates the prolactin levels in the 6 hour dopamine challenges in 3 pituitary cultures from intact rhesus females. Prolactin generally increased after day

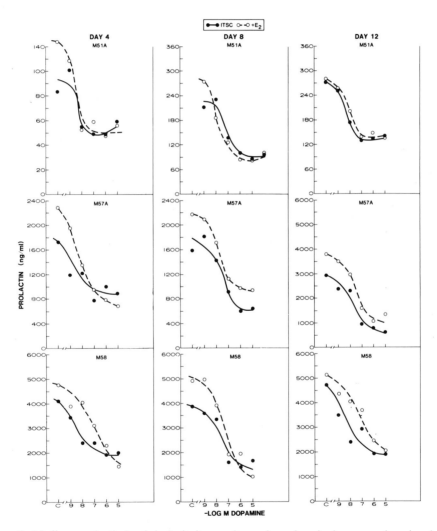

Figure 6. Medium prolactin levels in 3 pituitary cultures from female rhesus monkeys incubated in DME/F12 containing ITSC plus and minus 10 nM E_2 and then exposed to increasing concentrations of dopamine for 6 h after 4, 8 and 12 days in culture. Reprinted with permission from Reference 15.

290

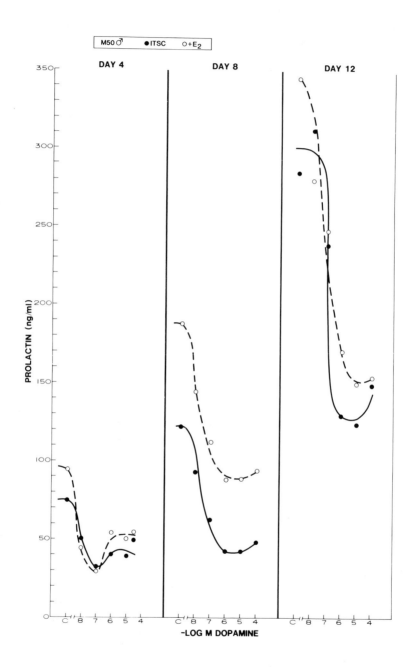

Figure 7. Medium prolactin levels in a pituitary culture from a male rhesus monkey treated as described in Fig. 6. Reprinted with permission from Reference 15.

4 and the difference in the scales on the ordinate should be noted. The prolactin levels were also higher in the E_2-treated wells which did not receive dopamine (controls designated point C) and were frequently higher throughout the entire dose-response. However, dopamine effectively suppressed prolactin secretion in the presence of E_2 for 4, 8, and 12 days and the IC_{50} (approx. 10 nM) did not vary.

Figure 7 illustrates the prolactin levels observed in the pituitary culture from the male rhesus monkey. Each dopamine challenge is drawn to the same scale to illustrate the overall changes occurring in prolactin secretion with time in culture. The control wells of the dose-response curve maintained with E_2 had significantly higher prolactin levels than those wells maintained in ITSC alone ($+25$, $+51$, and $+19\%$ on days 4, 8, and 12, respectively). Dopamine effectively inhibited prolactin secretion regardless of the overall level of secretion or the presence of E_2.

Figure 8 illustrates the mean percent inhibition (ι SEM) of prolactin in the 9 female cultures (intact and ovariectomized combined) in the presence and absence of E_2. On days 8 and 12 there is no difference in the dose-response inhibition of prolactin in the presence or absence of E_2. However, this representation of the data shows a significantly greater inhibition by dopamine after 4 days in the presence of E_2. This is apparently due to the poor response of the cells without E_2 at this time. There is an increase in the response of the cells in ITSC by day 8 in culture and little change in the E_2-treated cells.

The mean percent inhibition of prolactin in the four sister cultures maintained in 10% C.T. FCS is shown in Figure 9. On day 4 the E_2-treated cells exhibited a greater inhibition at the lower doses of dopamine similar to the cells in serum-free medium. However, by day 12, the inhibition response was lessened at the higher doses of dopamine, unlike the serum-free cultures.

Figure 10 compares the mean percent inhibition of prolactin secretion in each of the groups across time. In serum-free medium without E_2 there was a significant increase in inhibition from day 4 to day 8 at the two higher doses of dopamine. No significant differences were found in the dopaminergic inhibition with time when E_2 was added to the serum-free medium. Although E_2 seemed to decrease dopaminergic inhibition in the presence of serum by day 12, the variation among cultures was large and the differences across time were not significant.

E_2 RIA of incubation medium harvested on days 4 and 8 before the dopamine challenges in each culture registered less than blank (< 25 pg/ml) for the serum-free medium and 1654 ± 259 pg/ml for E_2-treated serum-free medium. The medium containing 10% C.T. FCS contained 73 ± 7 pg/ml and the medium containing serum with estrogen addition contained 1847 ± 310 pg/ml.

The studies described herein demonstrate that the use of ECM and a mixture of DME and F12 with insulin, transferrin, selenium, and cadmium maintains prolactin secretion for at least 12 days in cultures of pituitaries from male monkeys and for at least 20-25 days in cultures of pituitaries from female monkeys. Male and female pituitary cultures also show an increase in prolactin secretion and cell content when E_2 is added to this system. The primate cells were unresponsive to E_2 in 10% C.T. FCS, although E_2 stimulates prolactin secretion from rat pituitary cells in a similar paradigm (23). This may be related to the observation by West and Dannies that different batches of serum

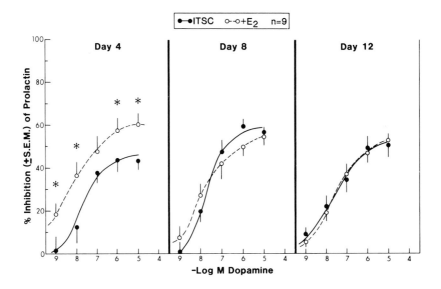

Figure 8. The mean percent inhibition of prolactin secretion caused by dopamine in the presence or absence of E_2 in 9 serum-free cultures of female monkey pituitaries (7 intact rhesus and 2 ovariectomized cynomolgus) after 4, 8 and 12 days in culture. The asterisks designate those points which are significantly different ($p < 0.05$) with Student's t-test. Reprinted with permission from Reference 15.

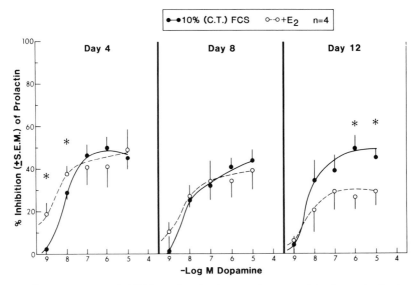

Figure 9. The mean percent inhibition of prolactin secretion caused by dopamine in the presence and absence of E_2 in 4 cultures of female monkey pituitaries in 10% C.T. FCS after 4, 8 and 12 days in culture. Reprinted with permission from Reference 15.

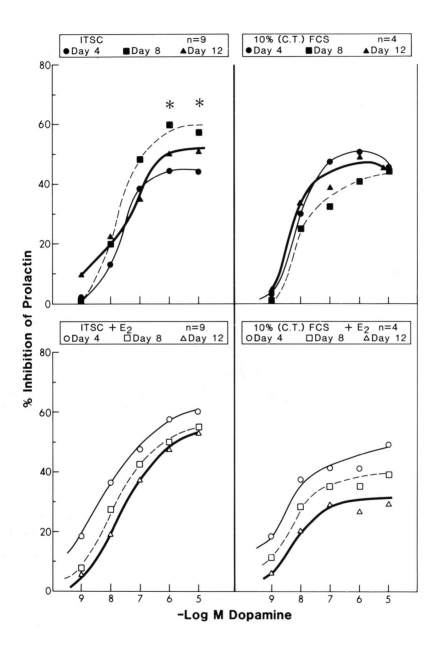

Figure 10. Comparison of the mean percent inhibition of prolactin secretion caused by dopamine in each of the treatment groups across time. Reprinted with permission from Reference 15.

caused a significant difference in estrogenic stimulation of prolactin production by primary cultures of male rat pituitary cells (8).

Previous studies which examined the effect of E_2 on prolactin secretion in monkeys with lesions in the medial basal hypothalamus (6) or with pituitary stalk-transections (7) concluded that E_2 more effectively stimulated prolactin secretion in the absence of hypothalamic inhibition. The results of the present study concur with these observations. However, since the E_2-induced increases in prolactin secretion in ovariec-tomized monkeys are modest (4,5) and since physiological increases in prolactin are correlated with increases in prolactin cell number (24) and/or require a long period of time as in pregnancy (25), the *in vivo* studies could not resolve whether E_2 induced in-creases in serum prolactin were due only to an increase in prolactin cell number, or were due also to a direct effect of E_2 on prolactin synthesis and release. Also, if the E_2 induced prolactin increases *in vivo* were due only to an increase in cell number, it was also possible that the mitosis or recruitment was mediated by other factors, as has been reported for E_2 supported growth of mammary, pituitary, and kidney tumor cells (26).

This study suggests that E_2 can act directly on primate pituitary prolactin process-ing and that the effects shown here do not require E_2-induced factors from other organs. Since previous studies *in vitro* have rarely shown E_2 to stimulate growth (27,28), it seems reasonable to speculate that the E_2-induced increases in prolactin pro-duction in this study of primate pituitary cultures are not due to increases in prolactin cell number. Also in the present study, 5 out of 7 cultures had a higher cell content of prolactin when estrogen was present. This observation is consistent with that of Milmore (5) who found a significant increase in the pituitary content of prolactin in ovariectomized monkeys with E_2 implants.

Dopamine tonically inhibits prolactin secretion and E_2 decreases the sensitivity of cultured rat pituitary cells to dopamine and agonists (8,9). In contrast, studies with humans and monkeys *in vivo* have shown an increase in dopaminergic inhibition of prolactin secretion after E_2 treatment (13,14), but examination of E_2 and dopamine interaction on primate prolactin secretion *in vitro* has been lacking.

This study demonstrates that E_2 does not decrease the inhibitory action of dopamine on female primate prolactin-secreting cells for at least 12 days in serum-free culture, and like the *in vivo* studies, suggests that there is initially a greater sensitivity of the prolactin cells to dopamine in the presence of E_2. This differential sensitivity was lost as the untreated cells exhibited an increase in inhibition with time in culture. This latter observation is consistent with *in vivo* reports of an increase in the dopamine sensitivity of the anterior pituitary following lesions of the medial basal hypothalamus in rats (29) or stalk-transection in monkeys (30). It is also possible that E_2 accelerated protein synthesis and thus facilitated membrane recovery from dispersion.

The male pituitary responded similarly with 1) an increase in prolactin secretion by day 8, 2) higher prolactin levels in the presence of E_2, and yet 3) no change in the effectiveness of dopamine to inhibit prolactin secretion regardless of significant changes in overall secretory activity or the presence of E_2.

An unexpected finding in this study was the difference in the response between serum-free cultures and cultures maintained in 10% C.T. FCS. The cells in charcoal-treated serum did not show any difference in dopamine sensitivity with time in culture and the addition of E_2 eventually decreased the maximal inhibition by dopamine. This is reminiscent of earlier experiments with dispersed rat pituitary cells which were conducted with charcoal-treated serum (8,9). However, it is unlikely that the presence of serum was responsible for the observed decrease in sensitivity in the rodent studies because the antidopaminergic effect of E_2 was also evident in a paradigm using quartered pituitaries and a short-term incubation (12). Nevertheless, this may warrant reexamination in serum-free medium.

Although the IC_{50} and percent inhibition of prolactin caused by dopamine was not decreased in the presence of E_2, in many cases the absolute levels of prolactin remained higher. This provides an indication of the means by which prolactin levels gradually increase in primates with high and sustained levels of E_2. That is, hypothalamic dopamine remains effective as E_2 increases prolactin synthesis and overall secretory activity. The eventual appearance of more prolactin-secreting cells may be due to E_2 directly or to E_2-stimulated growth factors (26). However, this primed population of cells will then secrete more prolactin in response to stimuli or removal of hypothalamic inhibition (4,7,31).

ACKNOWLEDGMENTS

Publication No. 1344 of the Oregon Regional Primate Research Center; supported by NICHHD Grant 17269 to CLB and NIH Grant RR-00163 for the Oregon Regional Primate Research Center.

REFERENCES

1. Weiner RI, Bethea CL. (1981): In: Jaffe RB (ed) Prolactin, Current Endocrinology Elsevier/North Holland, New York p 19
2. Neill JD. (1974): In: Knobil E, Sawyer WH (eds) Handbook of Physiology, Sect 7: Endocrinology. American Physiol Soc, Washington, DC, p 469.
3. Quadri SK, Oyama T, Spies HG. (1979): Endocrinology 104:1649
4. Millmore JE. (1978): Biol Reprod 19:593
5. Plant TM, Krey LC, Moossy J, McCormack JT, Hess DL, Knobil E. (1978): Endocrinology 102:52
6. Frawley LS, Neill JD. (1980): Biol Reprod 22:1089
7. West B, Dannies PS. (1980): Endocrinology 106:1108
8. Giguere V, Meunier H, Raymonde V, Labrie F. (1982): Endocrinology 111:857
9. DiPaolo T, Carmichael R, Labrie F, Raynaud J-P. (1979): Mol Cell Endocrinol 16:99
10. Heiman ML, Ben-Jonathan N. (1982): Endocrinology 111:1057
11. Gudelsky GA, Nansel DD, Porter JC. (1981): Endocrinology 108:440
12. Judd SJ, Rigg LA, Yen SSC. (1979): J Clin Endocrinol Metab 49:182
13. Neill JD, Frawley LS, Plotsky PM, Tindall GT. (1981): Endocrinology 108:489
14. Bethea CL. (1984): Endocrinology (in press)
15. Bethea CL. (1984): Endocrinology (in review)
16. Bethea CL, Ramsdell JS, Jaffe RB, Wilson CB, Weiner RI. (1982): J Clin Endocrinol Metab 54:893
17. Gospodarowicz D, Bialecki H, Greenberg G. (1978): J Biol Chem 253:3736

18. Gospodarowicz D, Mescher AL, Birdwell CR. (1977): Exp Eye Res 25:75
19. Horwitz KB, Kostlow ME, McGuire WL. (1975): Steroids 26:785
20. Barnes D, Sato G. (1980): Anal Biochem 102:255
21. Quadri SK, Spies HG. (1976): Biol Reprod 14:495
22. Resko JA, Ploem JG, Stadelman HL. (1975): Endocrinology 97:425
23. Liberman ME, Maurer RA, Claude P, Gorski J. (1982): Mol Cell Endocrinol 25:277
24. Pasteels JL, Gausset P, Danguy A, Ectors F, Nicoll CS, Varavudhi P. (1972): J Clin Endocrinol Metab 34:959
25. Weiss G, Butler WR, Hotchkiss J, Dierschke DJ, Knobil E. (1976): Proc Soc Exp Biol Med 151:113
26. Sirbasku DA. (1978): PNAS USA 75:3786
27. Antakly T, Pelletier G, Zeytinoglu F, Labrie F. (1980): J Cell Biol 86:377
28. Herbert DC, Ishikawa H, Masataka S, Rennels EG. (1978): Proc Soc Exp Biol Med 157:605
29. Cheung CY, Weiner RI. (1976): Endocrinology 99:914
30. Diefenbach WP, Carmel PW, Frantz AG, Ferin M. (1976): J Clin Endocrinol Metab 43:638
31. Quadri SK, Norman RL, Spies HG. (1977): Endocrinology 100:325

Prolactin. Basic and clinical correlates
R.M. MacLeod, M.O. Thorner and U. Scapagnini (eds.),
Fidia Research Series, vol. I,
Liviana Press, Padova © 1985

Section IV
Modification of prolactin
production by steroids

CORRELATION BETWEEN BRAIN AND PITUITARY ESTROGEN NUCLEAR AND PROGESTIN CYTOSOL RECEPTOR CONCENTRATIONS AND THE INDUCTION OF SPONTANEOUS PROLACTIN SURGES

Patricia Camp and Charles A. Barraclough

Department of Physiology, School of Medicine
University of Maryland, Baltimore, MD 21201

Prolactin surges accompany the increase in serum LH and FSH that occur on proestrous afternoon (1-6). These prolactin surges occur in the absence of such acutely applied stimuli as suckling, mating, stress, etc. and require estrogen to be expressed (7). In estrogenized-ovariectomized (OVX) rats, the phasic secretions of LH and prolactin also are coupled and their afternoon release patterns have diurnal rhythmicity (8). We recently reported that the surge release of LH depends upon adequate concentrations of estrogen bound to specific hypothalamic neuronal and pituitary nuclear receptors for minimal time periods (9,10). We also have correlated the effect of progressively increasing estrogen concentrations on specific estrogen hypothalamic and pituitary nuclear receptors (ERn) with synthesis of progestin cytosol receptors (PRc). We further related these receptor concentration changes to the ability of progesterone (P_4) to modify phasic LH secretion (9). Other studies analyzed the temporal relationships that exist between duration of estrogen receptor occupancy and diurnal LH surges. In these studies we examined how P_4 modifies LH release and the PRc concentrations required to elicit P_4-induced responses (10).

The present studies describe the prolactin responses obtained in these various steroid-treated groups. All of the forthcoming prolactin data are derived from the animals which provided information on changes in phasic LH secretion. Consequently, we are able to judge when LH and prolactin secretion are coupled and how varying the concentration and duration of steroid receptor occupancy affects phasic release of both gonadotropins. Since we already have considerable information on hypothalamic catecholamine dynamics in these animal models (11), we attempt in this discussion, to collate these observations into a unified picture of how the hypothalamus may regulate phasic LH and prolactin secretion.

EXPERIMENT 1: SERUM PROLACTIN CONCENTRATIONS IN RATS TREATED WITH VARIOUS DOSES OF E_2 ON DAY 0 AND WITH P_2 ON DAY 2

Seven day (day 0) ovariectomized (OVX) Sprague Dawley rats received a single Silastic capsule containing either 37.5 or 150 ug E_2/ml. Another group of rats received 3 capsules of 150 ug E_2. Two days later at 0900 h (day 2), two P_4 capsules (50 mg/ml in oil) were inserted s.c. into approximately one-half of the E_2-treated rats. Sequential blood samples were collected from these rats on day 2. The serum LH, E_2, and P_4 concentrations in these rats have been published previously (9). Also, changes in estrogen nuclear (ERn) and progestin cytosol (PRc) levels in preoptic area (POA), medial basal hypothalamus (MBH), corticomedial amygdala, and pituitary gland have been reported (9).

When Silastic capsules containing 37.5, 150, or 3 x 150 ug E_2/ml were inserted s.c. on day 0 they produced serum E_2 concentrations on day 2 of 6.3-7.6 (low), 12.3-19.2 (medium), and 27.8-37.6 (high) pg/ml respectively. Two P_4 capsules produced serum concentrations of 10-12 ng/ml. Control OVX serum values for E_2 were 3.8-4.2 pg/ml and 3.0 ng/ml for P_4.

The prolactin responses in these various animals are illustrated in Figure 1. Rats with low serum E_2 did not have prolactin surges on day 2, but as serum concentrations increased from medium to high values, prolactin surges occurred with peak values being significantly higher in rats with the high serum E_2 levels.

DOSE RESPONSE EFFECTS OF ESTROGEN ALONE OR WITH PROGESTERONE
ON SPONTANEOUS PROLACTIN SURGES IN OVX RATS

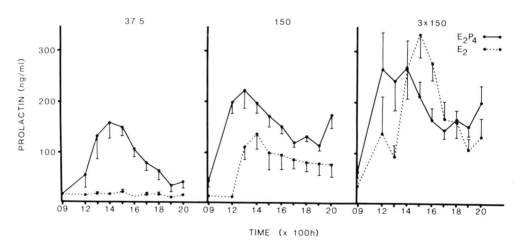

Figure 1. Spontaneous prolactin surges in E_2 or E_2P_2-treated OVX rats. Silastic capsules containing 37.5, 150 or 3 x 150 ug E_2/ml oil were placed 2 days earlier.

When P_4 was given, prolactin surges occurred in rats with low serum E_2 levels. As serum P_2 was progressively elevated to the medium range, P_4 significantly amplified and advanced, by one hour, the prolactin surge. At higher serum E_2 levels, P_4 no longer magnified or advanced the prolactin surge beyond that obtained with E_2 alone.

EXPERIMENT 2: TEMPORAL EFFECTS OF E_2 ON PROLACTIN SURGES; EFFECTS OF P_4

OVX rats received a Silastic capsule containing 150 ug E_2/ml. Two P_4 capsules were inserted into about 50% of these rats at 0900 h on days 0 to 4. Sequential blood samples were collected both on the day of insertion and the next day. Serum LH and

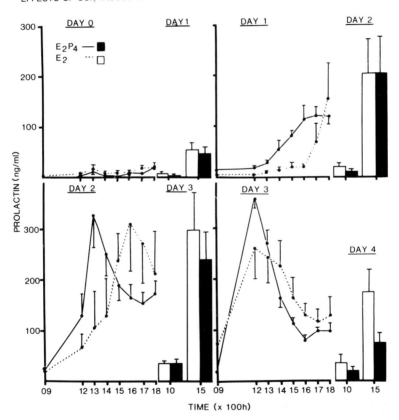

Figure 2. Temporal effects of estrogen on phasic prolactin release. Silastic capsules containing 150 ug E_2/ml oil were inserted at 0900 h, day 0. P_4 capsules were placed into separate groups of E_2-treated rats at 0900 h on days 0 to 4. Blood was sequentially collected on the day P_4 capsules were inserted and at 1000 and 1500 h on the following day.

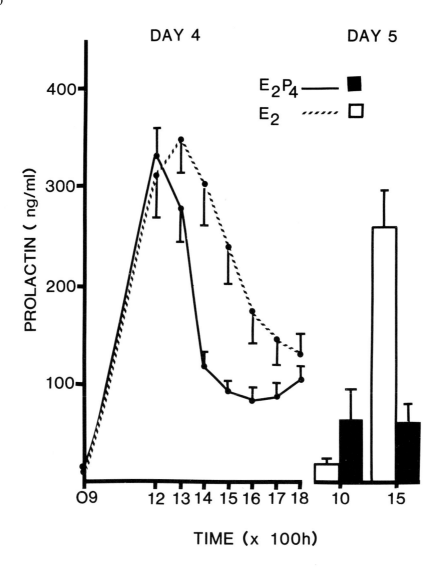

Figure 3. Prolactin responses in rats exposed to E_2 for 4 or 5 consecutive days of E_2. Day 5 rats which received P_4 on day 4 did not have an afternoon surge of prolactin.

steroid concentrations in these studies have been published previously (10). Hypothalamic and pituitary ERn and PRc concentrations in similarly treated rats also have been published (10).

The temporal effects of E_2 and P_4 on phasic prolactin release are illustrated in Figures 2 and 3. No prolactin surges occurred on day 0 and only small amounts of prolactin were released 24 h later. Two days of E_2 exposure resulted in significantly higher peak concentrations of prolactin in E_2-treated animals when compared to values obtained on days 0 or 1. Thereafter, although prolactin surged earlier in the afternoon (1200 h) between days 2-5, the peak concentrations were not significantly different.

P_4 had no effect on prolactin release on day 0 but advanced the time of prolactin release in day 1 rats. Thereafter, although a slight advancement in time (1 h) of prolactin release occurred on day 2, peak concentrations and patterns of release did not differ significantly from days 2 to 4. In contrast to the effects of P_4 on diurnal LH release, in which LH surges were extinguished on the day following P_4 treatment (10), diurnal prolactin surges continued in spite of P_4 exposure. Only after P_4 treatment of day 4 rats were afternoon surges of prolactin absent the following afternoon (day 5) (Fig. 3).

EXPERIMENT 3: EFFECTS OF TRH OR HALOPERIDOL ON PITUITARY PROLACTIN RELEASE IN E_2- OR E_2P_4-TREATED RATS

These studies were designed to test pituitary responsiveness to two drugs known to induce prolactin secretion. In both studies the E_2- or E_2P_4-treated animal model was the same as that described in Experiment 2. We studied pituitary responsiveness on days 3 or 5 since prolactin surges occur on day 3 but not on day 5 in rats treated 24 h earlier with P_4. Shown in Figure 4 are the prolactin responses elicited following the pulse injection of TRH (100 ug/rat). TRH produced a significant increase in serum prolactin within 2 min of administration and thereafter, prolactin remained elevated for the duration of the study. Prolactin serum concentrations were not significantly different between 2 and 60 min after TRH in E_2- or E_2P_4-treated rats nor were there any significant differences in prolactin levels in E_2- versus E_2P_4-treated rats on days 3 versus days 5. Equivalent amounts of prolactin were released on days 3 and 5 in both groups of steroid-treated rats. Haloperidol (1 mg/kg bw) produced a significant increase in serum prolactin within 15 min after treatment and thereafter, prolactin values remained elevated but were not significantly different from one another between 15-120 min. Further, the responses obtained in E_2- versus E_2P_4-treated rats did not differ on days 3 or 5 nor did the values obtained in either group differ when comparisons were made between the steroid-treated groups on day 3 versus day 5 (Figure 5).

DISCUSSION

In order for these prolactin data to provide meaningful information, they must be considered in the context of coupling and uncoupling of prolactin and LH release in these rats and associated changes in hypothalamic neuronal and pituitary steroid receptor concentrations. The changes in serum LH and in steroid receptor concentrations in these animals have been published recently (9,10).

Dose response correlations

While phasic LH release occurs in rats having low serum E_2 levels, prolactin surges are not observed until serum E_2 is elevated to the medium range. Thus, while the first

302

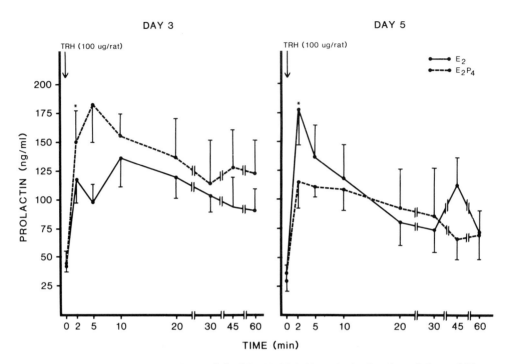

Figure 4. Pituitary prolactin release elicited by TRH (100 ug/rat) after 3 or 5 days of E_2 exposure. These responses were not significantly different from those which occurred in animals which received P_4 24 h earlier. Spontaneous prolactin surges occur in E_2P_4-treated rats on day 3 but not on day 5.

phasic release of LH correlates with the first significant rise in MBH and pituitary ERn concentrations, prolactin surges are not observed until POAERn levels increase. Thereafter, as hypothalamic and pituitary ERn concentrations rise to reach a plateau within the high serum E_2 range, peak serum prolactin levels parallel these receptor changes. In contrast, once LH surges occur in E_2-treated rats, the peak concentrations achieved are invariant in spite of increasing serum and hypothalamic and pituitary receptor levels (12).

E_2 acts directly (pituitary) and indirectly (hypothalamic) to alter pituitary gonadotropin secretion (LH, prolactin). In modulating LH release, estrogen affects numbers of LHRH receptors, the releasable pool size of LH and the phasic release of LHRH (13,14). The control of prolactin release is more complex as it involves both stimulatory (prolactin-releasing factor, PRF) and inhibitory (dopamine) controls. Dopamine inhibits prolactin secretion and prolactin is thought to feed back on tuberoin-

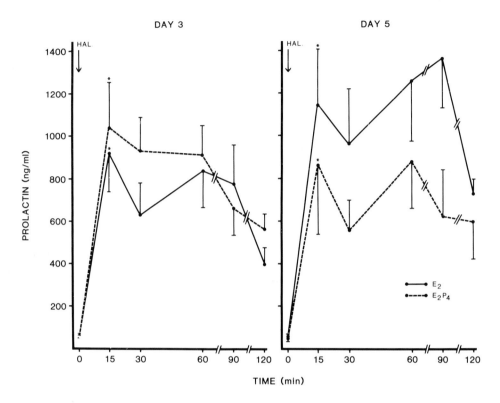

PROLACTIN RELEASE INDUCED BY HALOPERIDOL PULSE INJECTION
IN E_2 OR E_2P_4-TREATED OVARIECTOMIZED RATS

Figure 5. Pituitary prolactin release following the pulse injection of haloperidol (1 mg/kg bw) into rats exposed to 3 or 5 days of estrogen. The prolactin concentrations released did not differ with or between groups on either days 3 or 5.

fundibular neurons to regulate dopamine release and, ultimately, its own secretion. Estrogen modulates the release of dopamine into pituitary portal blood (15,16). Estrogen also directly stimulates lactotrophs to release prolactin (17,18) and desensitizes the anterior pituitary gland to the inhibitory action of dopamine (19,20). The secretion of LH in the absence of prolactin release in rats with low serum E_2 suggests that higher E_2 thresholds exist for activation of PRF (or inhibition of dopamine) versus LHRH release. Alternatively, differential pituitary cell responsiveness to varying estrogen concentrations also could account for the uncoupled secretion of LH and prolactin.

Distinct differences also were identified in the ability of P_4 to evoke or to amplify LH as compared to prolactin release. Only phasic prolactin release occurs in P_4-treated rats with low serum E_2. At these serum E_2 levels, prolactin synthesis is observed in MBH and pituitary but not preoptic area. Amplification of both LH and prolactin surges by P_4 occurs only after medium serum E_2 levels are attained and POA PRc induction occurs at these serum E_2 levels. We do not know whether pituitary responsiveness to a prolactin-releasing peptide (TRH, VIP etc.) is altered by the short exposure time to P_4 (3-4 h) but P_4 has no direct effect on pituitary responsiveness to LHRH (10). Consequently, P_4 amplification of LH surges is due to an increased release of LHRH and perhaps a similar increase in hypothalamic PRF also may occur.

Temporal effects of estrogen on prolactin and LH release

On day 0, neither LH nor prolactin surges occurred even though hypothalamic and pituitary ERn concentrations increased dramatically within 1 h of capsule insertion. After 24 h of E_2 exposure, phasic prolactin release was observed albeit in very reduced concentrations compared to those levels attained on days 2-5. In contrast, LH surges did not occur until at least 48 h of E_2 exposure. Again, this uncoupled release of prolactin versus LH could be due to estrogen modulating one or another of the components in the multi-control systems involved in prolactin secretion. Perhaps differential thresholds to serum E_2 concentrations and durations of E_2 exposure are required to activate the release of each hormone. By day 2, maximal LH and prolactin surges were obtained and thereafter, peak prolactin serum concentrations did not vary significantly for the next 3 days (to day 5). On the other hand, while diurnal phasic LH release occurs, peak LH concentrations are markedly reduced between days 2 and 4 (10). Bethea and Weiner (8) suggest that the hyperprolactinemia which develops with prolonged estrogen exposure (6-10 days) may account for suppression of the diurnal LH surge. In our studies, basal prolactin secretion was not elevated by the serum E_2 levels produced in these animals for 4-5 days. Consequently we favor the hypothesis proposed by DePaolo and Barraclough (21) that replenishment of the releasable LHRH pool may be more sluggish than restoration of the releasable LH pool. Earlier studies have shown that pituitary responsiveness to LHRH is similar after 2-4 days of E_2 esposure which suggests that less LHRH is released to discharge this stored LH. In contrast, once the mechanisms for phasic prolactin release are established, equivalent peak concentrations of this hormone are observed throughout the next 4-5 days.

Perhaps the most interesting differences between prolactin and LH release that we observed in these rats occurs after P_4 treatment. Regardless of the day on which it is given (days 1-4), P_4 always amplifies the LH surge. In contrast, no similar magnification of prolactin secretion occurs. On day 1, P_4 advances the time of prolactin release but the peak concentrations attained in E_2 versus E_2P_4-treated rats are not different. A second striking difference is the effect that P_4 has on phasic LH versus prolactin release 24 h after it is administered. P_4 consistently extinguishes diurnal LH rhythms within 24 h. In contrast, only after 4 days of E_2 exposure is P_4 effective in extinguishing prolactin surges (day 5). In earlier studies we performed an in depth analysis of the changes which occur in hypothalamic norepinephrine (NE) and dopamine turnover in day 3 rats exposed to P_4 on day 2 (22). Concomitant with the loss of phasic LH release on day 3, afternoon increases in NE do not occur, median eminence dopamine turnover rates are extremely high (22), portal blood dopamine is increased, and pituitary spiperone binding sites also are increased significantly (23). In spite of these changes, prolactin surges still occur. These observations argue strongly in favor of the existence and release of a PRF which seems capable of overriding inhibitory dopamine influences on pituitary prolactin secretion. We tested whether pituitary responsiveness differs in E_2- versus E_2P_4-treated rats on day 3 when phasic prolactin occurs or on day 5 when the diurnal rhythm is lost. The pituitary glands of animals injected with TRH on days 3 or 5 released the same concentrations of prolactin regardless of whether P_4 had been given 24 h earlier. The dopamine receptor antagonist, haloperidol, produced a greater prolactin response than TRH but neither day 3 or 5 rats nor E_2- versus E_2P_4-treated rats responded differently to the drug. Based on this information we conclude that the failure of day 5 rats (exposed to P_4 24 h earlier) to have prolactin surges is due to the failure of the hypothalamus to release PRF.

In conclusion, we believe that these studies provide interesting new information on how phasic prolactin and LH release may or may not be coupled depending upon the serum levels of E_2 and the duration of E_2 exposure. Further, they strongly support the concept that a PRF exists, which, when released spontaneously, evokes prolactin surges even from pituitary glands which are under the forces of dopamine inhibition (23).

REFERENCES

1. Kwa HG, Verhofstad F. (1969): Biochim Biophys Acta 133:186
2. Sar M, Meites J. (1969): Proc Soc Exp Biol Med 125:1018
3. Niswender GD, Chen CL, Midgley AR Jr, Ellis S. (1969): Proc Soc Exp Biol Med 130:793
4. Amenomori Y, Chen CL, Meites J. (1970): Endocrinology 86:506
5. Neill JD. (1970): Endocrinology 87:1192
6. Krieg RJ, Salisbury RL, MacLeod RM. (1983): In: Bhatnagar AS, The Anterior Pituitary Gland. Raven Press, New York, p 313
7. Neill JD, Freeman ME, Tillson SA. (1971): Endocrinology 89:1448
8. Bethea CL, Weiner RI. (1983): Proc Soc Exp Biol Med 172:65
9. Camp P, Barraclough CA. (1984): Neuroendocrinology (In Press)
10. Camp P, Akabori A, Barraclough CA. (1984): Neuroendocrinology (In Press)
11. Barraclough CA, Wise PM. (1982): Endocrine Rev 3:91
12. Wise PM, Camp-Grossman P, Barraclough CA. (1981): Biol Reprod 24:820
13. Clayton RN, Catt KJ. (1981): Endocrine Rev 2:186
14. Holt JD, Lasley BL, Wang CF, Yen SCC. (1977): J. Clin Endocrinol Metab 42:718
15. Cramer OM, Parker CR Jr, Porter JC. (1979): Endocrinology 104:419
16. Cramer OM, Parker CR Jr, Porter JC. (1979): Endocrinology 105:929
17. Nicoll CS, Meites J. (1962): Endocrinology 70:272
18. Ajika A, Krulich L, Fawcett CP, McCann SM. (1972): Neuroendocrinology 9:304
19. Raymond V, Beaulieu M. Labrie F, Boissier J. (1978): Science 200:1173
20. Gudelsky GA, Nansel DD, Porter JC. (1981): Endocrinology 108:440
21. DePaolo LV, Barraclough CA. (1979): Biol Reprod 20:1173
22. Rance N, Wise PM, Barraclough CA. (1981): Endocrinology 108:2194
23. Pilotte NS, Burt DR, Barraclough CA. (1984): Endocrinology (In Press)

Prolactin. Basic and clinical correlates
R.M. MacLeod, M.O. Thorner and U. Scapagnini (eds.),
Fidia Research Series, vol. I,
Liviana Press, Padova © 1985

Section IV
Modification of prolactin
production by steroids

THE ROLE OF ESTROGEN IN PROLACTIN RELEASE INDUCED BY PROGESTERONE IN PSEUDOPREGNANT RATS

R. P. Deis and Nia Alonso

Laboratorio de Reproduccion y Lactancia
LARLAC-CONICET, 5500 Mendoza, Argentina

A close relationship exists between the roles that the CNS and circulating levels of ovarian steroids play in the regulation of prolactin release. Estrogen (E) facilitates the release of prolactin and progesterone (Pg) has a dual effect; in certain experimental conditions it may inhibit or favour the release of prolactin (1). Cervical stimulation of the rat during proestrus or estrus induces pseudopregnancy which is associated with increased secretion of prolactin.

Luteal Pg is secreted in response to the luteotrophic action of prolactin. An active and phasic process of prolactin synthesis and release occurs in the first 12 h after cervical stimulation (2). Thereafter prolactin secretion continues as a twice daily surge, a nocturnal surge in the early morning, and a diurnal one in the late afternoon (3, 4). The diurnal surges need ovarian support (5, 6) and according to recent studies, are dependent on peripheral ovarian Pg (7). However, the maintenance of the nocturnal surges has been attributed to Pg action and the diurnal peak to the effect of the basal levels of estradiol (8). The present study describes the role of the ovarian hormones on the diurnal surge of prolactin during the first 9 days of pseudopregnancy.

Virgin female rats of the "Institute Strain" weighing between 180 and 250 g were used. During one week before vaginal stimulation the rats were checked for a 4-day estrous cycle. Vaginal stimulation was carried out for 1 min between 10:00 and 10:30 h on the first day of estrus with a glass rod connected to a dental drill. In our strain of rats, cervical stimulation induced pseudopregnancy in about 97% of the stimulated rats. The day following the stimulation was designed as Day 1 of pseudopregnancy. Bilateral ovariectomy was performed through dorso-lateral incisions under ether anaesthesia. Control, stimulated and operated rats were killed by decapitation, after which the blood was collected. Serum concentrations of prolactin were measured by RIA at two dose levels. The results are expressed in NIAMDD-rat prolactin RP-1 standard. All serum samples were assayed in a single assay so as to eliminate between assay variations. Student's t-test was used to assess the level of significance.

    In the present study we report the pattern of prolactin secretion measured at 17:00 and 18:00 h on selected days of the first 9 days of pseudopregnancy and compare it to that observed after progesterone treatment (Fig. 1). The steroid was administered s.c. at 10:00 h.

    On days 1, 2, 3, and 7 of pseudopregnancy, serum prolactin concentration was significantly higher at 18:00 h when compared to levels at 17:00 h (P < 0.02, P < 0.01, P < 0.01, and P < 0.001 respectively). There were no differences on day 5 but on days 6 and 9 of pseudopregnancy serum prolactin levels were significantly higher at 17:00 h (P < 0.05 and P < 0.005 respectively). The administration of Pg (10 mg) significantly increased serum prolactin values at 17:00 h as compared with control rats, on days 1, 2, 3, and 7 of pseudopregnancy (P < 0.05, P < 0.02, P < 0.02, and P < 0.005 respectively). Serum prolactin surges on days 5 and 6 of pseudopregnancy were significantly prevented by Pg (P < 0.02). On day 4, Pg did not modify prolactin level. Serum prolactin at 18:00 h was significantly elevated by Pg on days 6 and 9 (P < 0.02 and P < 0.05 respectively) and prevented on day 7 of pseudopregnancy (P < 0.02). The level of prolactin on days 1, 2, 3, and 5 was not modified by the treatment with Pg.

    The pattern of the diurnal prolactin surge obtained in the first nine days of pseudopregnancy agrees with the pattern described by several authors in pregnant and pseudopregnant rats (3, 4, 6). However it is interesting to note the significant differences in serum prolactin concentration between 17:00 and 18:00 h found on days 1, 2, 3, and 7 of pseudopregnancy. In the first 3 days, serum prolactin was higher at 18:00 h but on the following two days, serum prolactin values were similar at 17:00 and 18:00 h (the mean serum prolactin value at 18:00 h on day 4 was 212.1 ± 59.4, not mentioned in Fig. 1). It is difficult to explain the higher values of prolactin at 17:00 h as compared with values at 18:00 h on days 6 and 9 of pseudopregnancy while on day 7 the prolactin behavior was similar to that observed during the first 3 days of pseudopregnancy. An elevated level of circulating Pg seems to be necessary to maintain at least the diurnal surge of prolactin during the first 9 days of pseudopregnancy.

    In the first 5 days of pseudopregnancy, serum prolactin values at 18:00 h were higher or similar to those observed at 17:00 h. When the level of prolactin at 17:00 h was significantly lower, the administration of Pg elevated the values to those found in the untreated rats at 18:00 h. On the contrary, when the prolactin level at 17:00 h was similar or higher than at 18:00 h, the treatment with Pg lowered the level of prolactin significantly. Only on days 6 and 9 of pseudopregnancy, the serum prolactin values found at 18:00 h were smaller than at 17:00 h, and in these groups Pg was able to significantly increase serum prolactin to values similar to those measured at 17:00 h. It is evident then, that progesterone regulates the diurnal surge of prolactin. The time elapsed between the administration of Pg and the effect obtained on serum prolactin level might indicate the necessary delay for the steroid to exert its facilitatory effect on prolactin secretion. The presumably inhibitory effect of Pg observed when serum prolactin levels were already high may indicate that prolactin was already released some time before and was not to be considered as a real inhibitory effect of this ovarian steroid.

    The facilitatory role of Pg on prolactin release was postulated as early as 1937 by McKeown and Zuckerman (9), and later confirmed by Alloiteau and his group (10,11).

    In long term ovariectomized rats the nocturnal surge of prolactin can be induced by only one cervical stimulation but the prolactin diurnal surge is significantly attenuated

309

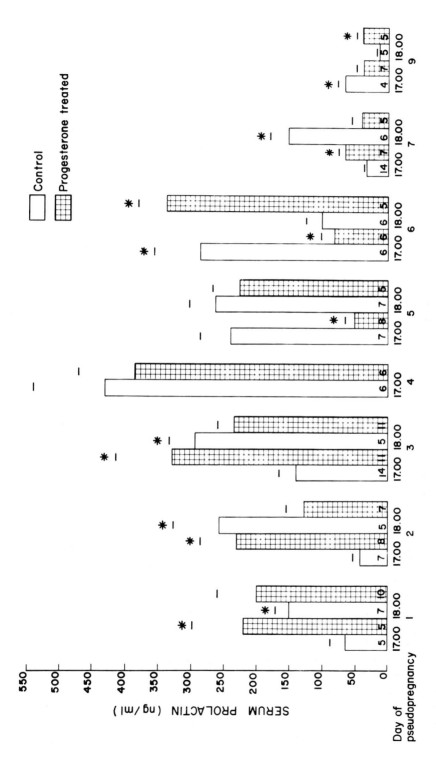

Figure 1. Effect of progesterone 10 mg injected (s.c.) at 10:00 h on serum prolactin concentration measured at 17:00 and 18:00 h respectively on different days of pseudopregnancy (numbers in columns are groups size and horizontal lines ± S.E.M.) (P values ranged from < 0.05 to < 0.001*).

(5). This correlates well with the suggestion that the circulating Pg might maintain this diurnal surge (7). However it has been recently shown that when ovariectomized rats are cervically stimulated twice, both the diurnal and nocturnal surge of prolactin are present (12). Nevertheless, the same authors (12) demonstrated that the maintenance of high Pg levels leads to a prolonged occurrence of prolactin surges in pseudopregnant rats.

In order to establish the role of estrogen on the release of prolactin induced by Pg in pseudopregnant rats, we selected two days of pseudopregnancy, days 3 and 9. Bilateral ovariectomy performed on day 2 of pseudopregnancy at 18:00 h or day 3 at 12:00 h was capable of blocking the 17:00 h surge of prolactin ($P < 0.001$) on day 3 (Figs. 2 and 3). A dose of 2 ug of estradiol benzoate injected after ovariectomy did not restore serum prolactin to control values. Progesterone (10 mg) injected to ovariectomized rats also had no effect. However, when a small dose of Pg (1 mg) was injected to ovariectomized estrogen primed rats, a significant increase of prolactin ($P < 0.001$) was observed on day 3 at 17:00 h. This facilitatory action of 1 mg of Pg on prolactin secretion was prevented ($P < 0.001$) when the rats were treated with sodium pentobarbitone (Nembutal 3,5 mg/100 g b.w.). This blocking effect of the anesthetic significantly increase serum prolactin to values similar to those measured at 17:00 h. It is evident then, that progesterone regulates the diurnal surge of prolactin. The time elapsed between aesthesic did not take place when injected to ovariectomized estrogen primed rats treated with 10 mg of Pg (Fig. 2).

Surprisingly, sham ovariectomy performed on day 2 of pseudopregnancy significantly ($P < 0.01$) reduced the levels of prolactin on day 3 at 17:00 h, while sham operation on day 3 at noon, did not affect serum prolactin measured 5 hours later (Fig. 3). A group of intact pseudopregnant rats was treated with the antiestrogen Tamoxifen to determine the role of estrogen on day 3 of pseudopregnancy. The administration of a single dose of Tamoxifen (50 ug/100 g b.w.) on day 1 or 2 of pseudopregnancy at 17:00 h did not modify the serum prolactin levels measured on day 3 at 17:00 h when compared with rats treated with the vehicle Tween 80. But when the antiestrogen was given 24 and 48 h before, a significant decrease of serum prolactin secretion was found on day 3 at 17:00 h ($P < 0.05$).

On the third day of pseudopregnancy a significant increase in serum estrogen takes place (13). Most probably this estrogen surge and the secretion that took place during the preceding cycle are responsible for the facilitatory action of Pg on the release of prolactin occurring at 17:00 or 18:00 h of the different days of pseudopregnancy. Results obtained in the ovariectomized pseudopregnant rats treated with estrogen and progesterone and the effect of Tamoxifen towards preventing release of prolactin support this postulation.

The inhibitory effect of sodium pentobarbitone on the release of prolactin induced by Pg (1 mg) on ovariectomized estrogen primed rats indicates the participation of central structures on the facilitatory effect of Pg. However, this inhibitory action could be overcome by increasing the dose of Pg to 10 mg. Most probably this effect may be attributed to a change in the sensitivity of the C.N.S. and pituitary to Pg induced by Nembutal.

On day 9 of pseudopregnancy serum prolactin levels at 17:00 and 18:00 h were much smaller than on the preceding days of pseudopregnancy (Fig. 1). A small but

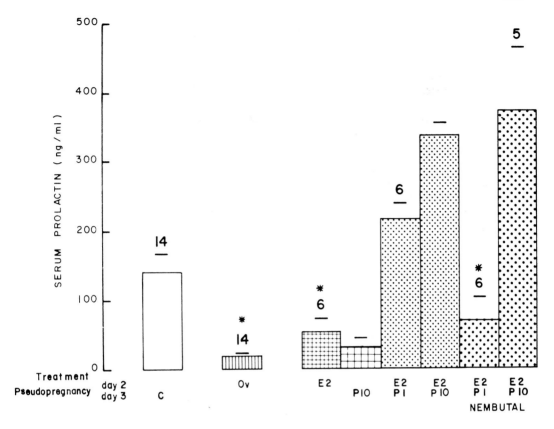

Figure 2. Effect of ovarian hormones on serum prolactin concentration on day 3 of pseudopregnancy (PS) at 17:00 h in rats ovariectomized the day before at 18:00 h. Estrogen 2 ug was injected at 17:00 h on day 2 of PS and progesterone on day 3 at 10:00 h. Sodium pentobarbitone (Nembutal) was injected at 13:00 h on day 3 of PS (numbers in columns are group sizes and horizontal lines ± S.E.M.) (P values ranged from < 0.05 to < 0.001*)

significant increase of prolactin secretion was obtained by Pg at 18:00 h but no change was noticed at 17:00 h. However the administration of E (2 ug) on day 8 at 17:00 h increased significantly serum prolactin (P < 0.005). When Pg (10 mg) was injected in estrogen primed rats, the release of prolactin was also significantly increased (P < 0.001) but was not different to the increase obtained in the group treated only with E on day 8 of pseudopregnancy (Fig. 4). Bilateral ovariectomy performed on day 8 did not modify serum prolactin concentration at 17:00 h of day 9 of pseudopregnancy. The administration of E (2 ug) immediately after ovariectomy was without effect on serum prolactin values measured next day at 17:00 h. This result contrasts with the facilitatory effect of E on prolactin secretion when it was injected on day 8 in intact pseudopregnant rats. Pg (1 mg or 10 mg) injected in ovariectomized-estrogen primed rats significantly increased the release of prolactin at 17:00 h (P < 0.05 and P < 0.005 respectively) when

312

compared to values obtained in ovariectomized rats with or without treatment with E. When Pg (10 mg) was injected to untreated ovariectomized rats at 10:00 h, serum prolactin concentration was not different from that measured in ovariectomized rats at 17:00 h on day of pseudopregnancy.

The results obtained in the group of rats studied on day 3 of pseudopregnancy showed a similar response to E and Pg compared to that already described on day 9 of pseudopregnancy. A marked lack of response to E or Pg when the steroids were injected independently was evident. The lower sensitivity of the C.N.S. and pituitary to the action of E on prolactin secretion contrasts with the effective action of E to induce prolactin release on proestrus afternoon in cyclic rats ovariectomized on diestrus day 2 and treated immediately after with a small dose of E (1 ug) (14). The failure of E to induce prolactin release in intact or ovariectomized pseudopregnant rats might be due to an effect of the previous increase of circulating Pg at the C.N.S. and pituitary level. It is known that Pg injection given 24 h before ovulation inhibits gonadotrophin release and prevents the ovulatory cycle from continuing (15, 16).

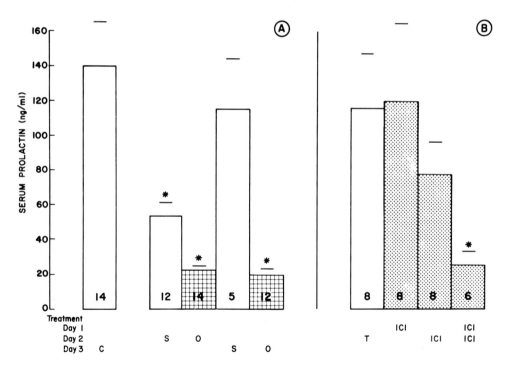

Figure 3. A. Serum prolactin concentration measured at 17:00 h on day 3 of pseudopregnancy (PS) in sham operated and ovariectomized rats. In one group the rats were operated on day 2 of PS at 17:00 h. In the other group operation was performed on day 3 of PS at 12:00 h.

B. Effect of Tween 80 (control group) or the antiestrogen Tamoxifen (50 ug/100 g b.w., ICI) administered at 17:00 h on day 1 or 2 of PS, on serum prolactin levels at 17:00 h of day 3 of PS. In another group Tamoxifen was injected 48 and 24 h before bleeding. (Numbers in columns are group sizes and horizontal lines ı S.E.M.) (P values ranged from < 0.05 to < 0.001*)

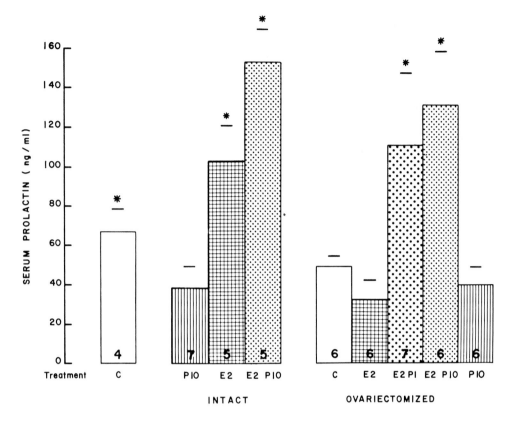

Figure 4. Effect of progesterone on estrogen primed intact or ovariectomized pseudopregnant rats on serum prolactin concentration measured at 17:00 h of day 9 of pseudopregnancy (PS). Ovariectomy was performed on day 8 of PS at 18:00 h. Estrogen 2 ug was injected on day 8 of PS at 18:00 h and progesterone 10 mg at 10:00 h on day 9 of PS. (Numbers in columns are group sizes and horizontal lines ± S.E.M.) (P values ranged from < 0.05 to < 0.001*).

It has been postulated that Pg action on the hypothalamus and pituitary might result in modifications of the estrogen receptor system (17). Recently it was shown that the ability of LHRH to stimulate LH secretion at proestrus is dependent on the sequence of ovarian steriods to which the hypothalamic- hypophyseal axis is exposed (18). Progesterone administered on diestrus day 2 is capable of preventing the modulatory effect of E on the hypothalamus and pituitary. If Pg is administered after a priming effect of E, then Pg potentiates the stimulatory action of LHRH on LH secretion. A similar sequence was obtained in the present studies on prolactin secretion during pseudopregnancy. It is evident that the sensitivity of the hypothalamic-hypophyseal axis to estrogen during pseudopregnancy is of a magnitude sufficient to facilitate the effect of Pg on the release of prolactin but not enough to allow a direct action of E on prolactin secretion.

The observations of the present study suggest a stimulatory feedback action of Pg on the release of prolactin. The presence of E seems to be a prerequisite for enhancement of the prolactin surge induced by Pg in pseudopregnant rats.

REFERENCES

1. Deis RP, Alonso N, Vermouth NT. (1973): Acta Physiol Latinoam 23:484
2. Alonso N, Deis RP. (1973/74): Neuroendocrinology 13:63
3. Butcher RL, Fugo NW, Collins WE. (1972): Endocrinology 90:1125
4. Freeman ME, Smith MS, Nazian SJ, Neill JD. (1974): Endocrinology 94:875
5. Smith MS, Neill JD. (1976): Endocrinology 98:324
6. de Greef WJ, Zeilmaker GH. (1976): Endocrinology 98:305
7. Takahashi M, Murakami N, Naito H, Suzuki Y. (1980): Biol Reprod 22:423
8. Freeman ME, Sterman JR. (1978): Endocrinology 102:1915
9. Mc Keown T, Zuckerman S. (1937): Proc R. Soc Series B 124:362
10. Alloiteau JJ, Vignal A. (1958): C R Acad Sci (Paris) 246:2804
11. Alloiteau JJ, Mayer G. (1967): Archs Anat microsc 56 (suppl 3-4):189
12. Gorospe WC, Freeman ME. (1981): Endocrinology 108:1293
13. Shaikh A, Abraham GE. (1969): Biol Reprod 1:378
14. Yokoyama A, Tomogane H, Ota K. (1971): Experientia 27:1221
15. Everett JW. (1944): Endocrinology 34:136
16. Caligaris L, Astrada JJ, Talleisnik S. (1971): Endocrinology 89:331
17. Reuter LA, Lisk RD. (1976): Nature 262:790
18. Prilusky J, Vermouth NT, Deis RP. (1984): J Steroid Biochem (in press)

Prolactin. Basic and clinical correlates
R.M. MacLeod, M.O. Thorner and U. Scapagnini (eds.),
Fidia Research Series, vol. I,
Liviana Press, Padova © 1985

Section V
Target cell function
and peripheral receptors
for prolactin

MECHANISM OF ACTION OF PROLACTIN
IN STIMULATING CELL GROWTH

Henry G. Friesen, Arieh Gertler, Ann Walker, and Harry Elsholtz

Department of Physiology, Faculty of Medicine, University of Manitoba
Winnipeg, Manitoba, Canada R3E OW3

Prolactin acts on a great variety of target tissues. Attempts have been made to catalog the wide ranging effects of prolactin into a coherent order (1). In mammals adequate lactation is essential for the survival of the species. Thus it is hardly surprising that the hormones and mechanisms involved in lactation have been extensively studied. The paramount importance of prolactin in this process is generally recognized. For adequate lactation to occur three distinct processes are involved: mammary growth, milk secretion, and milk removal.

Satisfactory lactation can only be expected when mammary glands have reached a proper state of development. Depending on the species this may involve growth and branching of ducts, lobuloalveolar development and growth of epithelial cells. Throughout postnatal life the growth of the mammary gland is regulated by mammogenic hormones from the anterior pituitary, ovary, and adrenal cortex. During pregnancy in many species the placenta also secretes hormones that promote mammary gland development.

The earlier evidence for pituitary involvement in mammary gland growth has been reviewed (2). Of particular significance was the finding that injection of ovarian hormones into hypophysectomized animals was without effect on mammary growth, in contrast to the effects produced in intact animals. Turner and his colleagues suggested that in addition to prolactin other specific mammogens in the pituitary may be responsible for mammary growth (3). This view was gradually abandoned as more evidence accumulated that prolactin and growth hormones might be the principal pituitary hormones involved. For example Talwalker and Meites (4) reported that lobuloalveolar development of the mammary glands could be produced in hypophysectomized-adrenalectomized- ovariectomized rats by injection of large doses of prolactin and GH in combination and to a lesser extent by prolactin alone, even in the absence of ovarian hormones.

316

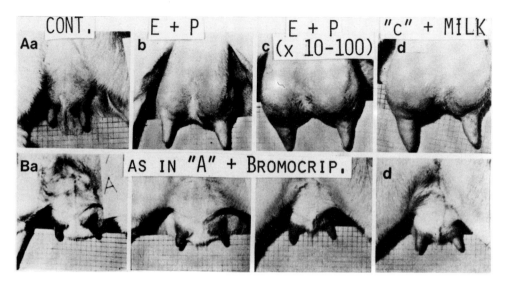

Figure 1. A. Photographs of the udder of a goat a) before steroid treatment; b) after 77 daily injections of estradiol benzoate (250 ug) and progesterone (60 mg); c) after changing the dose for a further 7 days to estradiol 2.5 mg/day, progesterone 6.25 mg/day, and (d) after subsequent twice daily milking for 10 days.

B. The udder of another goat treated as in A but in which the steroid and milking-induced release of prolactin was inhibited throughout most of the experiment by daily injection of bromocriptime (5 mg/day and 20 mg/day). Repoduced from Cowie et al. (5).

The effect of inhibiting prolactin secretion on estrogen-progesterone-mediated mammary gland growth has been examined in the goat (5) (Fig. 1) It is apparent when prolactin secretion is inhibited using bromocriptine that a major inhibition of steroid-induced mammary gland growth occurs. Experiments demonstrating stimulation by prolactin of mammary epithelial cell growth *in vitro* have been less convincing (6). Stimulation of [^{3}H]-thymidine uptake has been shown but few studies have demonstrated an increase in cell number following incubation with prolactin (7,8).

The growth promoting effect of prolactin also has been examined in relation to mammary tumors both *in vivo* and *in vitro*. In DMBA-induced rat mammary tumors prolactin is the major hormone regulating growth of the tumors. Again, demonstration that prolactin is a potent mitogen for mammary tumor cells *in vitro* is lacking.

Prolactin has a growth promoting effect on mammary tissue in some circumstances but it will also stimulate growth of other tissue. Splanchnomegaly of considerable degree is produced by injections of prolactin in pigeons. For example, a 2-fold increase in the size of the liver after administration of prolactin has been reported (9). In a chemically defined medium prolactin has been shown to be a significant growth factor for hepatoma cell growth (10) and rat hepatocyte proliferation (11). The latter was dependent on precisely defined culture conditions including a substrata of extracellular matrix derived from liver tissue.

A supportive role for pituitary factors in androgen-dependent prostate cell growth has been suggested by experiments in which prostatic atrophy is greater following hypophysectomy than that following orchiectomy. Prolactin has been the leading candidate for a role as the permissive growth factor. In primary cell culture of normal rat prostate epithelial cells in serum free medium evidence was obtained that prolactin, as well as unknown pituitary factors, has a direct mitogenic effect on the prostatic cells (12).

Very few of the studies in which prolactin has been proposed to stimulate cellular proliferation have focused on the mechanism of the hormone-induced mitogenesis. The majority of studies on the mechanism of action of prolactin have examined its role in stimulating milk secretion and more specifically, the stimulation of synthesis of milk constituents such as casein, alpha- lactalbumin, fat, etc. (13). The importance of the substrata on modulating the responses and influencing the mechanisms involved has been published (7,14).

The paucity of information on the mechanism of action by which prolactin stimulates growth relates in part to the relative difficulty of demonstrating clear cut *in vitro* effects on cell proliferation especially in the mammary glands. In normal mammary tissue additional problems are created by the degree of cellular heterogeneity and differential responsiveness to prolactin of cell types as well as the interaction of prolactin with other hormones on the response.

In 1980 we reported that a rat lymphoma cell line in suspension culture proliferated in a dose-dependent manner upon the addition of prolactin. Over a 3 day period, a 5- to 8-fold increase in cell number was found (15). We demonstrated that these lymphoma cells had prolactin receptors with a specificity similar to that observed in other target tissues for prolactin (16). There was parallelism between the specific binding of prolactin and stimulation of cell growth (Fig. 2). The ED_{50} for growth stimulation occurred at a concentration at which we detected approximately 20% receptor occupancy. Thus it appeared that as in many other systems examined, ''spare prolactin receptors'' for prolactin were found on the cell surface of the cells.

Additional evidence that the mitogenic effect of prolactin is mediated through prolactin receptors was demonstrated using antibodies generated against purified prolactin receptors from the rabbit mammary gland (16). Upon addition of antibodies to prolactin receptors to the culture medium one could stimulate lymphoma cell proliferation, thus mimicking the effects of prolactin. Divalent F(ab)2 fragments prepared from antibodies to prolactin receptors also stimulated Nb2 cell growth, while univalent F(ab) fragments were without effect, presumably because cross-linking of receptors is required to initiate prolactin effects (Fig. 3) (16).

Under appropriate conditions (i.e. with greater concentrations of anti- receptor antibodies) one could block the effects of prolactin on stimulating lymphoma cell growth. Similar results have been reported when the effects of antisera to prolactin receptors were studied on stimulation of casein or DNA synthesis in mammary gland explants (17). Thus stimulation of lymphoma cell proliferation and milk protein synthesis in mammary cells by prolactin is mediated by prolactin receptors. The fact that antibodies to prolactin receptors can mimic or substitute for prolactin demonstrates that appropriate activation of prolactin receptors is an adequate signal to trigger all the effects induced by prolactin in these two systems.

Clearly a better understanding of the structure and function of receptor as the in-

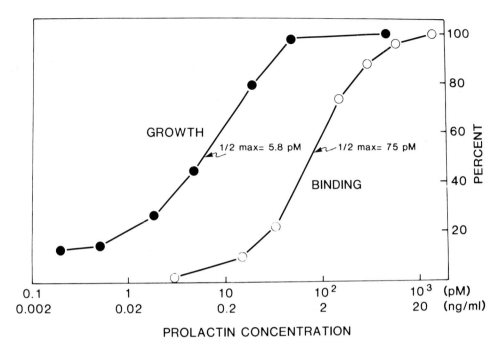

Figure 2. Comparison of the dose-dependent increase in cell number upon incubation of Nb2 cells with lactogenic hormone and extent of receptor occupancy. Reproduced from Shiu et al. (16).

itial mediator of the effect of prolactin is required. There are now several reports of the purification or characterization of prolactin receptors from rabbit mammary gland (18), rat and mouse liver (19,20), and ovaries (21). Antibodies to prolactin receptors from one species crossreact with prolactin receptors obtained from different tissues and/or different species indicating conservation of receptor structure (22). Cross-linking experiments have demonstrated that the hormone binding site of the prolactin receptor has a Mr of 40-45000 (23).

The control and regulation of prolactin receptors is complex and varies with age, sex, hormone status, nutrition, cell type, species, etc. Of the many factors which regulate prolactin receptors, one of particular interest identified recently is the rhythm of GH secretion. In males GH secretion is more pulsatile than in females. Experimentally, induction of prolactin receptors requires chronic stimulation of prolactin receptors by GH whereas pulsatile secretion of GH inhibits expression of prolactin receptors (24).

The intracellular distribution and recycling of receptors must also be taken into account. Employing quantitative EM radioautoradiography Posner and his colleagues have examined the endocytosis of peptide hormones by hepatocytes (25). They have concluded that internalization of hormone receptor complexes occurs rapidly with a defined vesicular traffic pattern directing the complexes to Golgi vesicles and lysosomes and subsequent recycling of the receptor. Unfortunately in these studies the marker

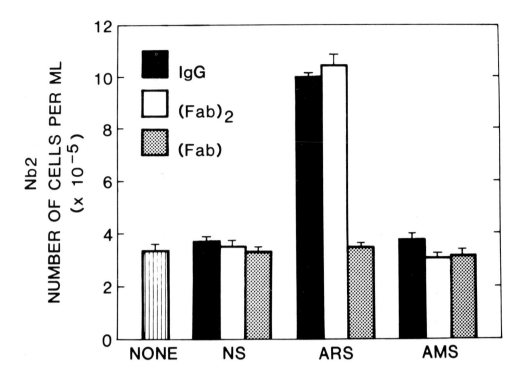

Figure 3. Stimulation of Nb2 cell growth by immunoglobulins (IgG) or (Fab)₂ fragments obtained from the antibodies generated against purified rabbit mammary gland prolactin receptors (ARS). The univalent (Fab) fragments failed to stimulate growth of cells perhaps because the univalent (Fab) fragments failed to initiate cross-linking of receptors. Neither IgG or any of the (Fab)2 or (Fab) fragments derived from normal guiena pig serum (NS) nor antisera generated against crude rabbit mammary membrane fragments (AMS) stimulated Nb2 cell growth. Reproduced from Shiu et al. (16).

which is identified is the [^{125}I]-labeled hormone and conclusions about the receptor have to be inferred indirectly. The role of the internalized receptor in mediating the effects of prolactin remains obscure. Since we know that antibodies to the receptor can substitute for prolactin in the induction of specific prolactin-like effects it seems that internalization of the hormone or fragments derived from prolactin is not required to mediate the action of prolactin. It may be however that the internalization is important for regulating the total receptor complement and compartmentalization in target cells.

In order to elucidate the cellular mechanisms which regulate or mediate prolactin-stimulated replication of the Nb2 lymphoma cells a series of studies on 'early' responses to prolactin was conducted. Upon exposure of the Nb2 cells to prolactin we observed progressive alteration of the lymphoma cell surface. The tightly compact cell with fine surface ruffles was gradually replaced by a cell with lengthening pseudopodia at 1 to

2 h. Subsequently an increase in ornithine decarboxylase was found at 6 to 8 h, followed by an increase in cell volume and finally an increase in [³H]-thymidine incorporation at 12 to 14 h was found prior to cell division.

The role of polyamines in prolactin-dependent growth was examined further (26). Ornithine decarboxylase (ODC) activity reached a maximum 6 to 8 h after addition of prolactin to stationary Nb2 cells, an effect reported previously by Richards et al (27). We found similar increases in ODC activity were also triggered under non-growth conditions, when high density cultures were transferred to fresh medium. These results suggested that rapid induction of ODC was not sufficient stimulus for triggering cell growth. On the other hand difluoromethyl-ornithine (DFMO, an ODC inhibitor) slowed the growth of Nb2 cells, indicating that polyamine synthesis was required for prolactin-stimulated cell proliferation. Thus, it seems that an increase in ODC is a necessary but not sufficient requirement for mediating cell growth. A similar conclusion was suggested by Rillema and Cameron (28) in relation to prolactin-stimulation of casein synthesis in mammary glands. Polyamines (spermidine, spermine) were more potent than diamines (putrescine, cadaverine) in restoring normal growth to DFMO-inhibited cultures.

In a second set of experiments, the effect of prolactin on cell protein phosphorylation was investigated. Two proteins, Mr 33,000 (pp33) and 19,000 (pp19), which became phosphorylated following prolactin stimulation were examined. The first, pp33, co-sedimented with the particulate cell fraction and was detectable only under reducing conditions when analyzed by SDS-polyacrylamide gel electrophoresis. It was most highly phosphorylated 1 to 3 h after prolactin stimulation. This phosphoprotein had a pI of 6.7 and associated with the ribosomal fraction suggesting that it was ribosomal protein S6. The 19K phosphoprotein appeared in the cytosol fraction and was unaffected by reducing agents. Maximal phosphorylation of pp19 occurred 7 to 9 h after prolactin stimulation. The identity of pp19 was not determined. A comparison of some of the characteristics of the two phosphorylated proteins is shown in Table 1. Prolactin stimulated the incorporation of ³⁵S-methionine into 33K and 19K proteins, suggesting that synthesis and phosphorylation of pp33 and pp19 could be regulated by prolactin. In Swiss 3T3 cells serum and epidermal growth factor activate a S6 (29) kinase causing up to 25-fold increase in the phosphorylation of 40S ribosomal protein S6. The phosphorylated form of S6, when associated with the 40S ribosomal subunits, confers upon the latter a selective advantage in entering polysomes. This suggests that S6 phosphorylation may increase the rate of protein synthesis by facilitating the initiation step in protein synthesis. Parenthetically, it is worth noting that prolactin increases protein synthesis within 3 h in the Nb2 cells.

Thirdly, the ability of anti-prolactin receptor antibodies to mimic prolactin stimulation of cell protein phosphorylation in Nb2 cells was tested. Divalent F(ab')₂ fragments stimulated [³²P] uptake and incorporation in a prolactin-like manner whereas monovalent Fab' fragments had no effect. However, if anti-Fab' antiserum was added to cells preincubated with anti-receptor Fab', phosphate uptake/incorporation was significantly (P < 0.01) stimulated. This supported an earlier study (16) suggesting that 'cross-linking' of prolactin receptors in the plasma membrane is important for hormone action.

The ability of Nb2 cells to retain a 'prolactin-like signal' following hormone withdrawal was examined. Cells exposed to prolactin for 10 min, then incubated without

Table 1. *Comparison of prolactin-responsive proteins pp33 and pp19*

	pp33	pp19
1. Subcellular Fraction	particulate (ribosomal)	soluble
2. Sensitive to 2-mercaptoethanol	+	—
3. Phosphorylated in non-stimulated cells	—	+
4. Inhibited by colcemid	+	+
5. Time of peak phosphorylation after prolactin exposure	1 - 3 h	7 - 9 h
6. Continual presence of prolactin necessary for phosphorylation	+	—
7. Isoelectric point	6.7	4.6, 5.7?
8. Possible identity	ribosomal protein S6	?

hormone and in the presence of anti-prolactin antiserum, were able to incorporate [^{32}P] at an enhanced rate for several hours. Therefore, in the Nb2 cells prolactin may act by triggering a sustained alteration in cell membrane structure or by generating an intracellular 'messenger' which stimulates protein phosphorylation. Several reports have demonstrated that upon exposure to prolactin, plasma membranes from target tissues generate a small molecular weight peptide which acts as a "second messenger" stimulating casein gene transcription in isolated mammary cell nuclei (30). However, concern has been expressed about the validity of the methodology employed in these studies and as yet these provocative studies have not been confirmed.

In further studies of prolactin-induced lymphoma cell growth we have found that tumor promoter 12-0-tetradecanoyl-phorbol-13-acetate (TPA) significantly enhanced the mitogenic activity of lactogenic hormones on Nb2-11C cells (a clone derived from Nb2 cells). At 125 pg/ml hGH with an optimal concentration of TPA (range 20-40 nM), 24-25 percent stimulation of cell doubling rates occurred (mean ± SEM 24.3 ± 1.2% at 20 nM, n = 15 and 25.1 ± 1.9% at 40 nM, n = 4). Half of this effect occurred when TPA concentrations of 1-2 nM were used. TPA alone had only a minimal effect on the proliferation of Nb2 cells.

The effect of addition of 20 nM TPA at different hGH concentrations is presented in Table 2. As shown, after 3 days in culture, TPA caused a significant increase in cell number at all seven concentrations of hGH although the relative effect was more pronounced at lower hormone concentrations. The SEM/average ratios were always less than 0.02 and the TPA effect was highly significant at all seven hormone concentrations ($p < 0.001$).

Calculation of the number of doublings was based on 5-6 determinations of the number of cells, through 3 days of the experiments, at each hormone concentration. Plotting the number of doublings versus time yielded straight lines ($r = 0.98$-1.00, $p < 0.01$), with the slopes equal to the doubling rate. It should be noted that these lines

Table 2. *The effect of TPA (20nM) on the number of cells, doubling rate, and time required for the first division of Nb2 cells after 24 h arrest in 10% horse serum.*

hGH (ng/ml)	TPA effect (treatment without TPA + 100) as percentage		
	Increase in cell no.[1]	Doubling rate[2]	Time required for 1st cell div[3]
0.031	152***	133***	76**
0.062	169***	129***	79**
0.125	171***	131***	86*
0.250	154***	120**	92*
0.500	125***	112*	97
1.000	120***	113**	116
2.000	124***	114*	103

* - $p < 0.05$; ** - $p < 0.01$; *** - $p < 0.001$

[1] The cell number in the control without hGH and TPA was 2.05×10^5 cells/ml; the maximal response in presence of 2.0 ng/ml hGH and TPA after 72 h of incubation was 1.34×10^6 cells/ml.

[2] The doubling rate varied from 0.13 doublings/24 h in treatment with 0.031 ng/ ml of hGH without TPA to 1.07 doublings/24 h with 2.0 ng/ml of hGH + 20 nM TPA.

[3] The minimal time (at 1-2 ng/ml of hGH) was 8.4 h and the maximal time (at 0.031 ng/ml of hGH without TPA) was 19.8 h.

did not start from the origin indicating the existence of a lag period prior to occurrence of the first division. Table 2 shows that TPA addition (20 nM) increased the doubling rate up to 30% and at lower hGH concentration significantly reduced the time required for the first division.

In order to achieve better understanding of the interaction between the effects of TPA and hGH the following experiments were carried out:

1. Exposure of the cells to TPA prior to addition of hGH.
2. Addition or withdrawal of TPA at various times of incubation.
3. Withdrawal of hGH in the presence or absence of TPA.
4. Flow cytometry through the first 22 h after addition of hGH, TPA or both.

It was found that pretreatment of the cells with 20 nM TPA for 24 h, in 10% horse serum had no effect on their further response to hGH. When TPA was removed by extensive washing and hGH or hGH + TPA was added, the doubling rate of the pretreated cells did not differ from those pretreated with 10% horse serum only.

Delayed addition of TPA to cells, one or two days after addition of the hGH, increased the doubling rate during the next 24 h up to the level found in cells treated with hGH and TPA throughout. On the other hand withdrawal of TPA from the cells after 22 h of exposure to 0.125 ng/ml of hGH and 20 nM TPA did not decrease the doubling rate through the next 20 h (22-42 h from the beginning of the experiment), as compared to the cells left in the presence of TPA. Such a decrease, however, occurred during the subsequent 30 h (42-72 h from the beginning of the experiment) in which the doubling rate decreased to the level found in cells cultured with hGH only.

Table 3. *Distribution of Nb2 cells in different phases of cell cycle after 14 h of incubation in presence of hGH with or without TPA.*

hGH (ng/ml)	TPA (20 nM)	Percent cells (av ± SD) in:			X^2
		G_0/G_1	S	$G_2 + M$	
0	—	80.8 ± 2.6	15.9 ± 5.2	3.3 ± 0.5	1.71 (NS)[1]
0	+	73.1 ± 3.2	21.5 ± 6.4	4.6 ± 0.2	
0.062	—	70.1 ± 3.8	26.9 ± 7.7	3.0 ± 0.1	19.45 (p<0.001)[1]
0.062	+	39.1 ± 6.4	53.6 ± 12.7	7.3 ± 0.4	
0.250	—	38.1 ± 4.2	52.5 ± 9.2	9.4 ± 0.2	22.68 (p<0.001)[1]
0.250	+	9.5 ± 3.8	74.7 ± 7.7	15.8 ± 0.5	

[1] For the difference in distribution in presence or absence of TPA.

Withdrawal of hGH gradually stopped cell proliferation and this effect was not influenced by the presence or absence of TPA.

Early effects of hGH and TPA additions (0, 62, 125 and 125 pg hGH/ml with or without 20 nM TPA) were studied through the first 22 h. Aliquots of cells were removed every 2 hours, fixed in 70% ethanol, stained for DNA with ethidium bromide, and the distribution of cells in the different phases of the cell cycle determined. Total cell counts were carried out in parallel.

The results obtained after 14 h of inculation are presented in Table 3. As can be seen, additions of hGH enhance the transition into the S and $G_2 + M$ phases in an obvious dose-dependent manner and this effect is dramatically increased in the presence of 20 nM of TPA, (p < 0.001). It should be noted that no increase in cell number occurred at this time.

In the controls without hGH the number of cells in G_0/G_1 phase remained constant and varied between 70-83% through 22 h. However, in presence of hGH 8-12 h after exposure to the hormone (depending on hormone dose and presence or absence of TPA) the transition to S phase started to appear.

Rate constants of G_0/G_1 - S transition were calculated by plotting the log of percentage of cells remaining in G_0/G_1 as a function of time through the descending period and multiplying the slope by -2.303. From the calculation it was possible to estimate the time of initiation of the descent, by extrapolating the linear curve to 82% (the average number of cells in G_0/G_1 through the first 8 h of the experiment).

These calculations (Table 4) clearly indicate the dependence of the initiation and the rate of G_0/G_1 - S transition on hGH and TPA. Addition of TPA also drastically decreased the number of cells that remained in the G_0/G_1 phase. (9.5 ± 3.8 vs 25.8 ± 4.5% in 0.250 ng/ml and 24.5 ± vs 43.8 ± 2.1% in 0.062 ng/ml of hGH; mean ± SD).

Thus, it seems that the enhancing effect of TPA results from: (1) increase of the G_0/G_1 - S transition rate, (2) decrease of the lag period required for entry into the S phase and (3) increase in the number of cells entering this transition.

It should be noted that not only TPA but also other phorbol diesters (4 beta-phorbol dibutyrate) enhanced the mitogenic activity of hGH and ovine prolactin (data not shown).

Preliminary experiments indicate that the enhancing effect of phorbol diesters did not result from changing the binding properties of the lactogenic hormones, since no significant differences in the total or non-specific binding of [^{125}I]-hGH in cells preincubated for 6 h with TPA were found.

Table 4. *The effect of hGH and TPA on G_0/G_1 S transition rate and on the time required for the initiation of the G_0/G_1 transition.*

Treatment hGH (ng/ml)	TPA (20 mM)	Time points used[1] for calculation (h)	Correlation[2] coefficient	Transition[3] rate (h^{-1})	Time required[4] for initiation (h)
0.250	—	10, 12, 14, 16	—0.99	0.166	9.1
0.250	+	8, 12, 14, 16	—0.97	0.352	8.4
0.062	—	12, 14, 16, 18	—0.94	0.085	11.2
0.062	+	10, 12, 14, 16	—0.99	0.195	10.0

[1] No increase in cell number occurred through this period
[2] Linear regression curve obtained by plotting the log of percentage of cells remaining in G_0/G_1 as a function of time at the indicated time points.
[3] (-slope) x 2.303
[4] Extrapolated to 82%.

Interestingly, an autonomous strain of Nb2 rat lymphoma node cells that does not require lactogenic hormones for proliferation in 10% horse serum supplemented medium did not respond to addition of TPA, although these cells bound ^{3}[H]-TPA in a manner similar to that of the dependent 11C clones.

Although the enhancing effect of TPA on lactogenic hormone-stimulated mitogenesis of Nb2-11C cells was clearly demonstrated, the mechanism of its action remains obscure. TPA and other phorbol diesters are potent tumor promotors (31) but the biochemical mechanism of action is only partially understood. It is suggested that TPA, which has a diacylglycerol-like structure, activates protein kinase C by formation of a quaternary complex composed of the enzyme, phospholipid, Ca^{2+}, and TPA (32). Activation of protein kinase C was demonstrated both *in vitro* and *in vivo* (33,34). It has also been reported that phorbol diesters increase the ratio of membrane associated/VS soluble form of this enzyme (35,36). Activation of protein kinase C may lead to phosphorylation of several cells proteins in the HL-60 promyelocytic leukemic cells (37) and 3T3 cells (38) and ribosomal protein S6 in Reuber H35 hepatoma cells (39). The latter finding is of particular interest in view of our observation (see above) that lactogenic hormones most likely stimulate phosphorylation of this protein in Nb2 cells. The most recent reports on the phosphorylation of diacylglycerol and phosphatidylinositol by virus transforming gene products (40,41) raises most interesting questions about interaction between the phosphatidyl-inositol cycle, phorbol diester effects, Ca^{2+} fluxes, and activity of protein kinase C. Whether the action of prolactin, human growth hormone, and other lactogenic hormones is mediated by any of those processes, however, awaits further investigation.

In summary, in one *in vitro* system, namely the Nb2 cell line, the role of prolactin as a growth factor has been examined. It is evident that TPA enhances the mitogenic response of prolactin while TPA has little effect by itself. This dependence between prolactin and other factors for full expression of prolactin effects is perhaps analogous to the requirement for the interaction of multiple hormones to produce mammary cell epithelial cell growth *in vivo*. In order to study the effect of prolactin on growth of mammary epithelial cells *in vitro* it will be desirable to develop experimental systems in which prolactin stimulation of growth is as marked and reproducible as in the Nb2 cells. Once this goal is achieved it should be possible to dissect the molecular and cellular mechanisms involved in prolactin-stimulated growth of mammary epithelial cells as well as of Nb2 lymphoma cells.

ACKNOWLEDGMENTS

We thank June McDougald for typing the manuscript. The research support from grants of the MRC Canada, USPHS-HD07843-12 and National Cancer Institute is gratefully acknowledged.

REFERENCES

1. Nicoll CS. (1964): Handbook of Physiology, Sec. 7, Endocrinology Vol. IV, part 2, Bethesda, Maryland, Am Physiol Soc, p 253
2. Folley SJ, Malpress FH. (1984): In: Pincus G, Thimann KV (eds) The Hormones. Academic Press, New York, p 695
3. Turner, CW. (1939): The Mammary Glands. In: Allen E, Danforth CH, Daisy EA (eds) Sex and Internal Secretions, ed 2. The Williams and Wilkins Co., Baltimore, p 740
4. Talwalker PK, Meites J. (1961): Proc Soc Exp Biol Med 107:880
5. Cowie AT, Forsyth IC, Hart IC. (1980): In: Hormonal Control of Lactation, Monographs on Endocrinology. Springer Verlag, p 122
6. Topper YJ, Freeman CS. (1980): Physiol Rev 60:1049
7. Nandi S, Kang J, Richards J, Guzman R. (1981): In: Pike MC, Siteri PK, Welsch CW (eds) Banbury Report: Hormones and Breast Cancer. p 445
8. Welsch CW. (1981): In: Pike MC, Siteri PK, Welsch CW (eds) Banbury Report: Hormones and Breast Cancer. p 299
9. Riddle, O, Bates RW. (1939): In: Allen E, Danforth CH, Daisy EA (eds) Sex and Internal Secretions, ed 2. The Williams and Wilkins Co., Baltimore, p 1088
10. Gatmaitan Z, Jefferson DM, Risiz Opazo N, Bienpica L, Arias JM, Dudas G, Leinwand LA, Reid LM. (1983): J Cell Biol 97:1179
11. Enat R, Jefferson DM, Risiz Opazo N, Gatmaitan Z, Leinwand LA, Reid LM. (1984): Proc Natl Acad Sci 81:1411
12. McKeehan WL, Adams PS, Rosser MP. Cancer Res 44:1998
13. Hobbs AA, Richards DA, Kessler DJ, Rosen JM. (1982): J Biol Chem 257:3598
14. Lee EYH, Parry G, Bissett. (1984): J Cell Biol 98:146
15. Tanaka T, Shiu RPC, Gout PW, Beer CT, Noble RL, Friesen HG. (1980): J Clin Endocrinol Metab 51:1058

16. Shiu RPC, Elsholtz HP, Tanaka T, Friesen HG, Gout PW, Beer CT, Noble RL. (1983): Endocrinology 113:159
17. Djiane J, Houdbine LM, Kelly PA. (1981): Proc Natl Acad Sci 78:7445
18. Shiu RPC, Freisen HG. (1974): J Biol Chem 249:7902
19. Krachenbuhi JP. (1983): J Biol Chem 258:305
20. Liscia DS, Vonderhaar BK. (1982): J Biol Chem 79:5930
21. Bonificiano S, Dufau M. (1984): J Biol Chem 259:4542
22. Shiu RPC, Friesen HG. (1976): Biochem J 157:619
23. Hughes JP, Simpson JSA, Friesen HG. (1983): Endocrinology 112:1980
24. Norstedt G, Palmiter R. (1984): Cell 36:805
25. Posner B, Khan MN, Bergeron JJM. (1982): Endocrine Rev 3:280
26. Elsholtz H, Shiu RPC, Friesen HG. (1984): Cancer Res, in press
27. Richards JF, Beer CT, Bourgeault C, Chan K, Gout PW. (1982): Mol Cell Endocrinol 26:41
28. Rillema JA, Cameron CM. (1983): Proc Soc Exp Biol Med 174:28
29. Novak-Hofer I, Thomas S. (1984): J Biol Chem 259:5995
30. Teyssot B, Houdebine LM, Dijane J. (1981): Proc Natl Acad Sci 78:6729
31. Blumberg PM. (1980): CRC Crit Rev Tox 8:153
32. Nishizuka Y. (1984): Nature (Lond) 308:693
33. Castagna M, Takai Y, Kaibuchi K, Sano K, Kiddawa V, Nishizuka Y. (1983): J Biol Chem 257:7847
34. Yamanishi J, Takai Y, Kaibuchi K, Sano K, Castagna M, Nishizuka Y. (1983): Biochem Biophys Res Commun 112:778
35. Kraft AS, Anderson WB. (1983): Nature (Lond) 301:621
36. Kraft AS, Anderson WB, Cooper HL, Sando JJ. (1982): J Biol Chem 257:13193
37. Feurstein N, Cooper HL. (1984): J Biol Chem 259:1782
38. Rosengurt K, Rodrigez-Pena M, Smith KA. (1983): Proc Natl Acad Sci (USA) 80:7244.
39. Trevillan JM, Kulkarni RK, Byus CV. (1984): J Biol Chem 259:897
40. Sugimoto Y, Whitman M, Cantley LC, Erikson RL. (1984): Proc Natl Acad Sci (USA) 81:2117
41. Macara IG, Marinetti GV, Balduzzi PC. (1984): Proc Natl Acad Sci (USA), in press

Prolactin. Basic and clinical correlates
R.M. MacLeod, M.O. Thorner and U. Scapagnini (eds.),
Fidia Research Series, vol. I,
Liviana Press, Padova © 1985

Section V
Target cell function
and peripheral receptors
for prolactin

INTERACTIONS BETWEEN PROLACTIN, INSULIN, CORTICOSTERONE, PROGESTERONE, AND 17 BETA-ESTRADIOL ON FATTY ACID SYNTHESIS IN EXPLANTS OF RABBIT MAMMARY GLAND IN CULTURE

I.R. Falconer and P. Martyn

Department of Biochemistry and Nutrition, University of New England
Armidale, NSW 2351, Australia

In the rabbit mammary gland during pregnancy, fatty acid synthesis is stimulated in a biphasic manner, initially from day 21 and secondly during the perinatal period (1). The medium-chain length fatty acids which are synthesized in the lactating gland form about 68 mole % of the fatty acids in rabbit milk triacylglycerol (2). The proportion of the medium-chain fatty acids synthesised is low during days 1-18 of pregnancy and increases appreciably at the time of the acceleration of fatty acid synthesis at days 19-21 (1). Close to parturition a decline in plasma progesterone concentration and a decrease in the ratio of progesterone and estrogen in blood occurs (3-5). Also close to parturition there is a surge of plasma prolactin (6) and an increase in the concentration of free glucocorticoids (3). In mammary explants obtained from 11-day pseudopregnant or mid-pregnant rabbits, cultured in the presence of insulin, corticosterone, and prolactin, fatty acid synthesis and the proportion of medium-chain length fatty acid increase markedly (7,8). It is well recognized that progesterone is essential for the growth of mammary alveolar structures but prevents the initiation of lactation in most mammals (3,9). In rabbits, lactose appears in the mammary gland in detectable amounts on day 24 of pregnancy. Injection of prolactin or cortisol during pregnancy stimulates lactogenesis, assessed by milk or lactose synthesis, whereas injection of progesterone (10 mg/day) prevents the initiation of these changes (10,11). In mammary explants from pseudopregnant rabbits, lactose synthesis (stimulated by prolactin) is inhibited in a dose-dependent manner at a range of 0.6 ng/ml-1.6 ug/ml of progesterone (12). In the present study we have examined, in mammary explants, the effect of a range of concentrations of progesterone on the rate of fatty acid synthesis when stimulated by prolactin, with varying concentrations of insulin, corticosterone, and 17 beta-estradiol. The effect of progesterone on the proportion of medium-chain length fatty acids was also examined.

PREPARATION AND CULTURE OF MAMMARY EXPLANTS

Rabbits were prepared as previously described (13). Explants of mammary alveoli were prepared by the method of Forsyth and Myres (14). Groups of 11 explants were cultured at 37 C in medium 199 containing 0.6 mM sodium acetate, 15 mM NaHCO$_3$-HEPES buffer (pH 7.4) polymyxin B sulphate and neomycin sulfate antibiotics (1-2 U/ml of medium) in an atmosphere of air. Sterile polythene vials were used for dilution of peptide hormone solutions from stock, in order to minimize possible loss of hormones due to adherence to glass. Viability of the mammary epithelial cells and alveolar integrity were confirmed by histological examination after staining with haematoxylin and eosin.

Fatty acid synthesis measurement and chain-length determination were essentially as described previously (15,16), as was the statistical treatment (13).

PROGESTERONE INHIBITION OF FATTY ACID SYNTHESIS

Table 1 shows that despite the low basal level of fatty acid synthesis in the gland on day 11 of pseudopregnancy, the proportion of medium-chain length fatty acids (C$_8$-C$_{12}$) produced was considerable. The presence of insulin, corticosterone and prolactin for 46 hours in culture stimulated fatty acid synthesis markedly without stimulating the proportion of medium-chain length fatty acids significantly. In the presence of progesterone (5 ug/ml) in addition to other lactogenic hormones, prolactin was ineffective in stimulating fatty acid synthesis. However progesterone did not alter the proportion of C$_8$-C$_{12}$ fatty acids.

Table 1. *Effects of progesterone on fatty acid synthesis and chain length in explants of mammary gland from pseudopregnant rabbits in organ culture*

Hours in culture	Hormones in culture	Fatty acid synthesis	
		nmol [1-^{14}C] acetate incorporated per h/mg explant	Moles % [1-^{14}C] acetate incorporated into C$_{8:0}$-C$_{12:0}$ fatty acids
0	NO HORMONE	0.6 ± 0.3	47.3 ± 3.3
46	I,C,P	4.4 ± 1.4	55.0 ± 3.4
46	I,C,P ± Pr	0.8 ± 0.3*	45.1 ± 7.8

* Significant reduction (P<0.01) due to progesterone
I - insulin, 5 ug/ml; C - corticosterone, 1 ug/ml; P - prolactin, 1 ug/ml
Pr - progesterone, 5 ug/ml.

In these experiments, a high proportion of medium-chain length fatty acid was synthesized by explants from mammary glands of 11-day pseudopregnant rabbits (Table 1) in contrast to an earlier report (8). This suggests the presence of active acyl-thioesterase II which specifically cleaves medium-chain length acyl moieties attached to fatty acid synthetase in the rabbit mammary gland (17). This synthesis of medium-chain length fatty acids may be a consequence of the high dose of chorionic gonadotropin used to induce pseudopregnancy, which could cause physiological precocity. Analogous to these rabbits, the mammary glands of rat and mouse have the capacity to synthesize a significant proportion of medium-chain length fatty acid during pregnancy, when the total synthesis of fatty acids is at a low basal rate (18,19).

EFFECT OF VARYING CONCENTRATIONS OF CORTICOSTERONE ON PROGESTERONE INHIBITION

The rate of fatty acid synthesis in mammary explants on day 11 of pseudopregnancy was very low at 0.07 ± 0.03 nmol/h/mg explant (mean ± S.E.M.; 9 replicates from 3 rabbits). When the explants from these rabbits were cultured for 46 hours in the presence of insulin (5 ug/ml) and corticosterone (1 ug/ml) fatty acid synthesis rose to 0.22 ± 0.09 nmol/h/mg explant (mean ± S.E.M.; 9 replicates from 3 rabbits). However, addition of prolactin (1 ug/ml) caused a marked stimulation (see Figure 1) which illustrates the results of three experiments with explants cultured at constant concentrations of prolactin and insulin (5 ug/ml), but varying concentrations of corticosterone and progesterone. Decreasing the concentration of corticosterone to 0.01 ug/ml did not significantly affect prolactin-stimulated fatty acid synthesis (Fig. 2). When progesterone was added in increasing dose a significant reduction was observed. Regression analysis showed a significant (P < 0.01) negative correlation between progesterone

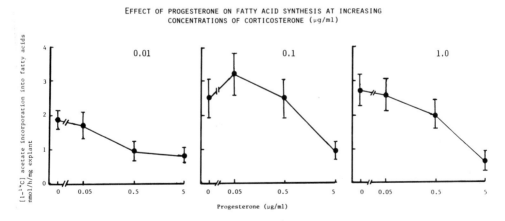

Figure 1. Effect of progesterone on fatty acid synthesis at increasing concentrations of corticosterone (ug/ml). Mammary explants from 11-day pseudopregnant rabbits were cultured for 44 hours in Medium 199 with insulin (5 ug/ml), prolactin (1 ug/ml), corticosterone, and progesterone. Groups of 10-11 explants were incubated at 37 C in Medium 199 containing 0.6 mM sodium [1-14C] acetate (10 uCi) and 5 mM glucose for 2 hours. Each value represents mean ± S.E.M. of 9 replications from 3 rabbits.

330

EFFECT OF PROGESTERONE ON FATTY ACID SYNTHESIS AT
INCREASING CONCENTRATIONS OF INSULIN (ug/ml)

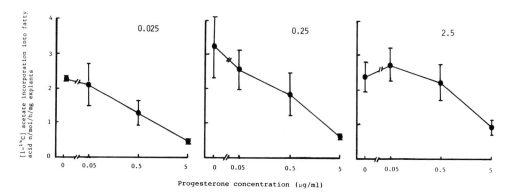

Figure 2. Effect of progesterone on fatty acid synthesis at increasing concentrations of insulin (ug/ml). Mammary explants from 11-day pseudopregnant rabbits were cultured for 44 hours in Medium 199 with insulin, prolactin (0.1 ug/ml), corticosterone (0.1 ug/ml), and progesterone and fatty acid synthesis was determined as described in Fig. 1 and the text. Each value represents mean ± S.E.M. of 9 replicates from 3 rabbits.

dose and fatty acid synthesis at all three different corticosterone concentrations. However at 0.1 and 1.0 ug/ml corticosterone concentration, only the highest concentration of progesterone showed an individually significant inhibition of fatty acid synthesis compared to incubation without progesterone (P< 0.01), whereas at the lower corticosterone concentration, 0.5 ug/ml progesterone was inhibitory (P < 0.01). Histological examination showed that these explants cultured in the presence of progesterone were viable and possessed alveolar integrity similar to the ones cultured in the absence of progesterone, other lactogenic hormones being present.

EFFECTS OF VARYING CONCENTRATIONS OF INSULIN ON PROGESTERONE INHIBITION

Without insulin, prolactin along with corticosterone failed to stimulate fatty acid synthesis in mammary explants from 11 day pseudopregnant rabbits cultured for 2 days. The rate of fatty acid synthesis was effectively basal at 0.28 ± 0.06 nmol/h/mg explant (mean ± S.E.M. of 9 replicates from 3 rabbits). In the presence of a range of concentrations (0.05, 0.5, 5.0 ug/ml) of progesterone in the absence of insulin, no significant changes in fatty acid synthesis were seen. As shown in Fig. 2 addition of insulin (0.025 ug/ml) at the start of the culture enabled prolactin to stimulate fatty acid synthesis markedly after 2 days. However a further increase in the concentration of insulin to 2.5 ug/ml did not effect a significant increase in prolactin stimulation. Similarly to the data in Figure 1, progesterone showed a consistent progressive inhibition of fatty acid synthesis stimulated by prolactin. Regression analysis of data presented in Figure 2 showed a significant ($P < 0.001$) negative correlation between progesterone dose and fatty acid synthesis at all insulin concentrations tested, with the steeper slopes for inhibition at the lower insulin concentrations.

Progesterone up to 5 ug/ml thus caused a progressive inhibition of milk fat synthesis in mammary explants in culture containing 0.025-2.5 ug/ml insulin and 0.01-1.0 ug/ml corticosterone. However these concentrations of progesterone are far removed from the level of the hormone in the pregnant rabbit, which was about 20 ng/ml (4). Injection of rats with progesterone at 5 mg/day elevated plasma progesterone concentrations above 0.5 ug/ml, which is closer to the concentrations which showed a direct inhibitory effect in the present study (20).

A low corticosterone (0.01 ug/ml) or low insulin (0.025 ug/ml) concentration was sufficient for prolactin to significantly stimulate fatty acid synthesis in organ culture and these hormone levels are close to the physiological range. The normal concentration of total plasma corticosterone in pregnant rabbits was 25 ng/ml (21) and the physiological range of insulin in rats at parturition was 2-5 ng/ml (22). At the lowest corticosterone and insulin concentrations used an increased sensitivity to the suppressive effects of progesterone was observed. A possible mechanism for this inhibition by pharmacological concentrations of progesterone is through competition for glucocorticoid receptors in the presence of low corticosterone concentrations, as shown in lactating rat mammary tissue (23).

Both the insulin and corticosterone concentrations in these experiments are well below those recently used in rabbit lobular cultures from mammary gland (24). These authors also used a range of concentrations of progesterone but found significant inhibition of fatty acid synthesis only at 20 ng/ml of progesterone in the presence of 25 ng/ml of prolactin (24).

Progesterone injected along with prolactin into pseudopregnant rabbits significantly reduced the stimulatory effect of prolactin on beta-casein gene transcription in mammary gland nuclei, but progesterone did not produce the same inhibitory effect when lactating rabbits were used instead (25). Culture of mammary explants from pseudopregnant rabbits for 24 hours with prolactin (0.1 ug/ml) and progesterone (1,5 ug/ml) showed no significant suppression of casein synthesis. Teyssot and Houdebine (25) suggest that steroid receptors might have decreased during culture, hence lowering the sensitivity to progesterone, but it is also reasonable to suggest that the culture was not continued long enough for the expression of a progesterone effect.

EFFECT OF 17 BETA-ESTRADIOL ON FATTY ACID SYNTHESIS

Figure 3 shows that fatty acid synthesis in mammary explants from 11 day pseudopregnant rabbits, cultured for 2 days in the presence of insulin (5 ug/ml), corticosterone (1 ug/ml) and prolactin (1 ug/ml), was not altered by the presence of a wide range of 17 beta-estradiol concentrations also in the medium (0.027-2700 ng/ml). Similarly the addition of 0.5 ug/ml of progesterone to the above hormonal combination was without any effect.

332

Our conclusion is that only pharmacological and not physiological concentrations of progesterone significantly suppressed prolactin-stimulation of milk-fat synthesis in explants of rabbit mammary gland. 17 beta-estradiol either alone or in combination with progestrone did not influence prolactin-stimulation at all. We also conclude that insulin is an obligatory hormone for the expression of prolactin stimulation in our experiments.

Effect of 17β-estradiol on fatty acid synthesis with (■) and without (▲) progesterone

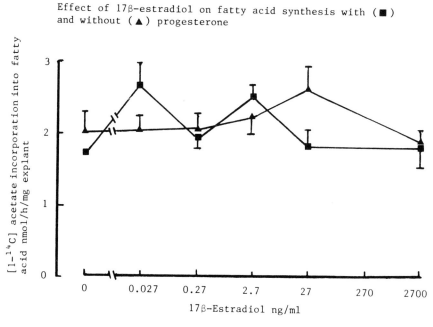

Figure 3. Effect of 17 beta-estradiol on fatty acid synthesis with (■) and without (▲) progesterone. Mammary explants from 11-day pseudopregnant rabbits were cultured for 44 hours in Medium 199 with insulin (5 ug/ml), prolactin (1 ug/ml) and corticosterone (1 ug/ml) and progesterone (0.5 ug/ml). At the end of culture the rate of fatty acid synthesis was determined as described in Fig 1. and the text. Each value represents mean ± S.E.M. of 9 replicates from 3 rabbits.

ACKNOWLEDGMENTS

This research was supported by a grant from NH & MRC of Australia. We greatly appreciate the statistical advice of Dr Vic Bofinger, the excellent histology by Mrs Angela Jones and the gift of ovine prolactin by NIAMDD, Maryland, USA. Mrs. Shirley Reynolds is thanked for typing the manuscript.

REFERENCES

1. Strong CR, Dils R. (1972): Biochem J 128:1303
2. Jones CS, Parker DS. (1981): Comp Biochem Physiol 69B:837
3. Denamur R. (1971): J Dairy Res 38:237
4. Challis RG, Davis J, Ryan KJ. (1973): Endocrinology 93:971
5. Quirk SM, Currie WB. (1984): Endocrinology 114:182
6. McNeilly AS, Friesen HG. (1978): Endocrinology 102:1548
7. Forsyth IA, Strong CR, Dils R. (1972): Biochem J 129:929
8. Strong CR, Forsyth I, Dils R. (1972): Biochem J 128:509
9. Kuhn NH (1971): In: Falconer IR (ed) Lactation. Butterworths, London, p 161
10. Meites J, Hopkins TF, Talwalker PK. (1963): Endocrinology 73:261
11. Assairi L, Delouis C, Gaye P, Houdebine LM, Ollivier-Bousquet M, Denamur R. (1974): Biochem J 144:245
12. Delouis C. (1975): Mod Probl Paediat 15:16
13. Martyn P, Falconer IR. (1984): Aust J Biol Sci 37:79
14. Forsyth IA, Myres RP. (1971): J Endocrinol 51:157
15. Falconer IR, Forsyth IA, Wilson BM, Dils R. (1978): Biochem J 172:509
16. Smith JV, Falconer IR. (1983): J Endocrinol 99:261
17. Knudsen J, Clark S, Dils R. 1976 Biochem J 160:683
18. Smith S, Ryan P. (1979): J Biol Chem 254:89
19. Bartley JC, McGrath H, Abraham S. (1971): Cancer Res 31:527
20. Elkarib AO, Garland HO, Green R. (1983): J Physiol 337:389
21. Gala RR, Westphal U (1967): Acta Endocrinol 55:47
22. Kuhn NJ (1977): In: Peaker M (ed) Comparative Aspects of Lactation. Academic Press, London, p 165
23. Quirk SJ, Gannell JE, Funder JW. (1983): Proc Endocrin Soc Aust 26:14
24. Carrington CA, Hosick HC, Forsyth IA, Dils R. (1983): J Endocrinol 97:157
25. Teyssot B, Houdebine LM. (1981): Eur J Biochem 114:597
26. Haslam SZ, Shyamala G. (1979): Biochem J 182:127

Prolactin. Basic and clinical correlates
R.M. MacLeod, M.O. Thorner and U. Scapagnini (eds.),
Fidia Research Series, vol. I,
Liviana Press, Padova © 1985

Section V
Target cell function
and peripheral receptors
for prolactin

ACTIONS OF PROLACTIN ON [^{32}P]-PHOSPHATE UPTAKE AND INCORPORATION INTO PROTEINS AND PHOSPHOLIPIDS IN MOUSE MAMMARY GLAND EXPLANTS

James R. Rillema

Department of Physiology, Wayne State University School of Medicine
Detroit, MI 48201 U.S.A.

The initiation of milk secretion is a complex and integrated process involving the actions of several hormones. Of critical importance for initiating milk production in cultured mammary gland explants from 12-14 day pregnant rats or mice are the hormones insulin, cortisol, and prolactin (1). Prolactin in concert with insulin and cortisol has been shown to accelerate the production of all the primary carbohydrates, lipids, and proteins found in milk (2). In rat or mouse mammary explants that are initially cultured with insulin and cortisol for 24-72 hours, a sequence of biochemical perturbations is observed in response to prolactin. Among these is the onset of the prolactin stimulation of casein and triglyceride biosyntheses which occurs about 6-10 hours after exposing mammary tissues to prolactin in culture (3,4). Subsequent to their synthesis, the triglycerides along with smaller amounts of other lipid products form lipid globules in the cytoplasm of the alveolar epithelial cells. The lipid globules are then surrounded by apical plasma membranes and expelled into the alveolar lumen (5). During lactation there is, therefore, a substantial turnover of plasma membrane in the alveolar epithelial cells. Associated with this turnover is an accelerated rate of synthesis of the phospholipids contained in membrane structures (6). The aim of these studies was to determine the time sequence whereby prolactin regulates the rate of [^{32}P]-phosphate incorporation into phospholipids in cultured mouse mammary gland explants.

Mammary explants from 12-14 day pregnant mice were initially prepared and cultured for 24-35 hours with 0.1 uM cortisol and 1 ug/ml insulin (3). Prolactin (1 ug/ml) was then added to certain of the cultures and incubations were continued for 2-24 hours. Tissues were pulse-labeled with 5 uCi/ml [^{32}P]-phosphate during the final 2 h of culture. (In preliminary studies the rate of [^{32}P]-phosphate incorporation into lipids was found to be linear with time for up to 6 hours.) After pulse-labeling, the tissues were homogenized and fractionated by the method of Bligh-Dyer (7) with the aqueous

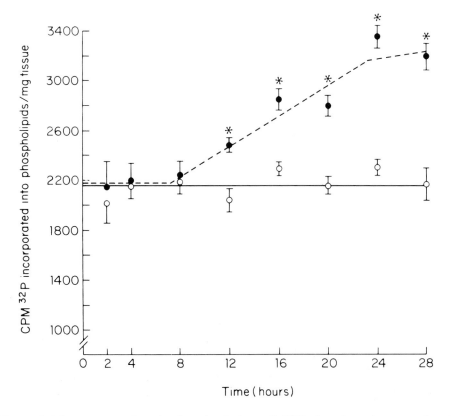

Figure 1. Time-course of prolactin stimulation of [^{32}P]-phosphate incorporation into phospholipids. Mammary explants were cultured for the times indicated in the absence (○) or presence (●) of 1 ug/ml prolactin. Tissues were pulse-labeled with 1 uCi/ml [^{32}P]-phosphate for the final 2 hours of culture. Radioactivity in the organic fraction of a Bligh-Dyer extraction was quantitated. Numbers represent the mean ± SE of 6 observations.

phase containing 2 M KCl buffered to pH 7.4 with 0.5 M phosphate. Radioactivity was then determined in the organic fraction (containing phospholipids), the aqueous fraction, and an insoluble fraction containing macromolecules. Figures 1-3 show that in all these fractions, prolactin effected a significant increase in radioactivity content; the onset of the prolactin responses was 8-12 hours after prolactin addition. Prolactin responses were observed with hormone concentrations of 2-5 ng/ml and above; maximal responses were observed with all prolactin concentrations between 25 and 1000 ng/ml (data not presented). Employing two-way thin layer chromatography (8), prolactin was found to enhance the rate of [^{32}P]-phosphate incorporation into the choline, ethanolamine, inositol, and serine phosphatide portions of the phospholipid fraction. In the Bligh-Dyer insoluble fraction, prolactin enhanced the rate of [^{32}P]-phosphate incorporation into both the phosphoprotein (including casein) and RNA portions of this fraction (data not presented).

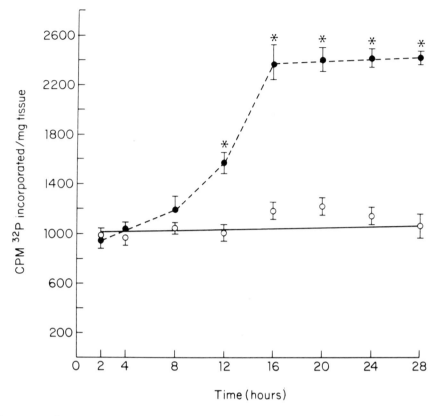

Figure 2. Time-course of prolactin stimulation of [^{32}P]-phosphate incorporation into macromolecules. Mammary explants were cultured for the times indicated in the absence (○) or presence (●) of 1 ug/ml prolactin. Tissues were pulse-labeled with 1 uCi/ml [^{32}P]-phosphate for the final 2 hours of culture. Radioactivity in the precipitate derived from a Bligh-Dyer extraction was then quantitated. Numbers respesent the mean ± S.E. of 6 observations.

The fact that prolactin enhanced the rate of [^{32}P]-phosphate accumulation in the aqueous portion of the Bligh-Dyer extracts suggests that prolactin enhances the rate of phosphate transport into the mammary alveolar cells. It is not known, however, whether this reflects a direct membrane transport activation by prolactin, or whether it is indirectly caused by the prolactin stimulation of phosphorylation reactions which then creates a more favorable gradient for phosphate transport into the alveolar cells. In either case, the increased accumulation of [^{32}P]-phosphate into the explants makes it likely that the specific activity of [^{32}P]-phosphate and other precursor pools is increased in response to prolactin. The enhanced rate of [^{32}P]-phosphate incorporation into phospholipids and phosphoproteins in response to prolactin could thus reflect entirely or in part the altered specific activity of the precursor pools rather than a real effect on the synthesis of these substances. Regarding the phospholipids, this would appear not to be the case since prolactin stimulates the rates of [³H]-choline and [³H]-inositol incorporation into their respective phospholipids without affecting the rate of transport of these precursors into the mammary cells (data not presented).

Regarding the phosphoproteins, however, the magnitude of the prolactin stimulation of [³²P]-phosphate incorporation does appear to be influenced by the enhanced rate of uptake of [³²P]-phosphate. When mammary explants from midpregnant mice (Table 1) or rabbits (Table 2) are exposed to prolactin and subsequently pulse-labeled with [³H]-leucine, the onset of the prolactin stimulation of [³H]-leucine incorporation into the phosphoprotein (casein) fraction (3) is 8-12 hours after addition of prolactin to the culture medium. Since prolactin has no effect on [³H]-leucine transport into cultured mouse mammary tissues (3), the prolactin stimulation of [³H]-leucine incor-

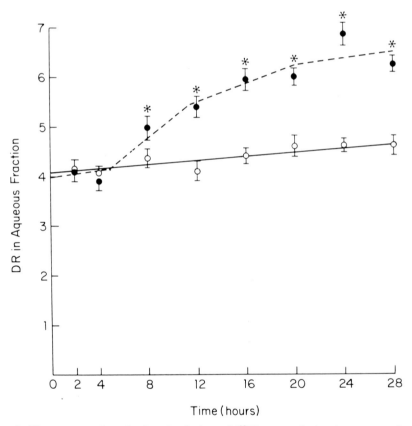

Figure 3. Time-course of prolactin stimulation of [³²P] accumulation in aqueous fraction of Bligh-Dyer extract. Mammary explants were cultured for the times indicated in the absence (○) or presence (●) of 1 ug/ml prolactin. Tissues were pulse-labeled with 1 uCi/ml [³²P]-phosphate for the final 2 hours of culture. Numbers represent the mean distribution ratios (D.R.) ± S.E. of 6 observations.

poration into phosphoproteins likely represents a real effect of prolactin on phosphoprotein synthesis. The magnitude of the prolactin stimulation of [³H]-leucine incorporation into the casein-enriched phosphoprotein fraction is between a 50 and 100% increase; this is typical and representative of the magnitude of this prolactin response which we have observed in our laboratory over the past decade (3). When determining the rate of [³²P]-phosphate incorporation into the phosphoprotein fraction, however, many laboratories, including ours (Fig. 3), have observed a 2-4 fold stimulation in response to prolactin. The difference in the magnitude of response when employing [³²P]-phosphate as compared with [³H]-leucine could be explained by the stimulation of phosphate transport into the prolactin-treated cells and a consequently increased specific activity of [³²P]-phosphate pools of those cells. Only a portion of the prolactin-stimulated incorporation of [³²P]-phosphate into the phosphoprotein fraction would then appear to represent a real effect of prolactin on phosphoprotein biosynthesis.

Table 1. *Time-course of prolactin stimulation of [³H]-leucine incorporation into phosphoproteins in mouse mammary gland explants.* *

Incubation Time (hours)	[³H]-leucine incorporation into phosphoproteins (dpm/mg wet tissue weight)		
	Control	Prolactin	P
4	381 ± 24**	319 ± 12	NS
6	340 ± 24	361 ± 10	NS
8	323 ± 17	356 ± 27	NS
10	383 ± 15	492 ± 38	< .05
12	380 ± 27	578 ± 29	< .05
18	388 ± 19	525 ± 17	< .05

* Explants were cultured for 4-18 hours in the presence of 1 ug/ml prolactin. [³H]-leucine (0.5 uCi/ml) was present for the final 2 hours of culture.
** Mean ± S.E. of 6 observations.

The most important feature of the present studies which contributes to our knowledge of how lactational processes are regulated is the observation that prolactin has a profound effect on phospholipid biosynthesis which is initiated about 12 hours after exposing cultured mouse mammary tissues to prolactin. In earlier studies with cultured mouse mammary tissues it was shown that the onset of the prolactin actions on casein and lipid biosynthesis occurs some 6-10 hours after exposing these tissues to prolactin (3,4). Lactose biosynthesis and the activities of the enzymes involved in lactose biosynthesis are stimulated subsequent to 12 hours after adding prolactin to cultured mouse (9) and rabbit (10) mammary gland explants. In view of the endomembrane flow associated with the transport and secretion of casein, triglycerides, and perhaps lactose from mammary cells, it makes intuitive sense that the onset of the prolactin stimulation of phospholipid synthesis should occur in concert with, or immediately subsequent to, the onset of the stimulation of milk product formation (Fig. 4). The biochemical mechanisms by which prolactin activates the processes associated with milk

Table 2. *Time-course of prolactin stimulation of [³H]-leucine incorporation into phosphoproteins in rabbit mammary gland explants.**

Incubation Time (hours)	[³H]-leucine incorporation into phosphoproteins (dpm/mg wet tissue weight)		P
	Control	Prolactin	
4	376 ± 27**	427 ± 20	NS
8	421 ± 21	382 ± 21	NS
12	381 ± 26	491 ± 29	< .05
16	347 ± 21	544 ± 53	< .05
20	349 ± 18	535 ± 40	< .05

* Explants were cultured for 4-20 hours with 1 ug/ml prolactin. [³H]-leucine (0.5 uCi/ml) was present for the final 2 hours of culture.
** Mean ± S.E. of 6 observations.

product formation are not totally understood. It is known that ongoing polyamine and RNA synthesis are essential for prolactin to express its action on milk product formation (2). Prolactin effects an enhanced rate of synthesis of both polyamines and total RNA some 4-6 hours after exposing mouse mammary tissues to prolactin (3,11). Prolactin also stimulates the activity of ornithine decarboxylase (ODC) within one hour after exposing cultured mammary tissues to prolactin; ODC is generally believed to be rate-limiting for polyamine biosynthesis in tissues. On a time sequence basis, these events are therefore in accord with the onset of the prolactin action on milk product forma-

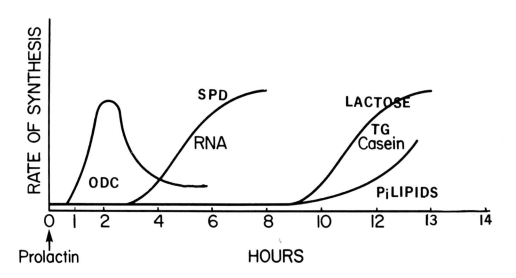

Figure 4. Sequence of prolactin actions on cultured mouse mammary gland explants. ODC = ornithine decarboxylase. SPD = spermidine. TG = triglycerides. P$_i$LIPIDS = phospholipids.

tion. Prolactin has also been shown to enhance the rate of casein mRNA formation by 2-4 fold within 1 hour after exposing rat mammary gland explants to prolactin (12). Temporally, this response occurs several hours prior to the onset of the enhanced rate of casein synthesis and it seems obvious that prolactin actions other than that on casein mRNA formation are rate-limiting for the onset of the enhanced rate of casein biosynthesis. Finally, several years ago Turkington et al. (13) reported that prolactin has a very early (30 min) action on enhancing cyclic AMP-dependent protein kinase activity and cyclic AMP binding in cultured mouse mammary gland explants. Whether these effects are of primary importance, however, for the subsequent actions of prolactin on milk product formation remains to be determined.

REFERENCES

1. Topper YJ. (1970): Rec Prog Horm Res 26:287
2. Rillema JA. (1980): Fed Proc 39:127
3. Rillema JA. (1973): Endocrinology 92:1673
4. Cameron CM, Linebaugh BE, Rillema JA. (1983): Endocrinology 112:1007
5. Keenan TW, Franke WW, Mather IH, Moore DJ. (1978): In: Larson BL (ed) Lactation. Academic Press, New York, vol 4:405
6. Kinsella JE, Infunte JP. (1978). In: Larson BL (ed) Lactation. Academic Press, New York, vol 4:476
7. Bligh EG, Dyer WJ. (1959): Can J Biochem Physiol 37:911
8. Abdel-Latiff AA, Yau SJ, Smith JP. (1974): J Neurochem 22:383
9. Turkington RW, Brew K, Vanaman TC, Hill RL. (1968): J Biol Chem 243:3382
10. Delouis C, Denamur R. (1972): J Endocrinol 52:311
11. Rillema JA, Linebaugh BE, Mulder JA. (1977): Endocrinology 100:529
12. Guyette WA, Matusik RJ, Rosen JM. (1979): Cell 17:1013
13. Turkington RW, Majunder GC, Kadohama N, MacIndoe JH, Frantz WL. (1972): Rec Prog Horm Res 28:417

Prolactin. Basic and clinical correlates
R.M. MacLeod, M.O. Thorner and U. Scapagnini (eds.),
Fidia Research Series, vol. I,
Liviana Press, Padova © 1985

Section V
Target cell function
and peripheral receptors
for prolactin

EVIDENCE THAT PROLACTIN
IS AN IMMUNOMODULATORY HORMONE

Bryan L. Spangelo, Nicholas R. Hall, and Allan L. Goldstein

Department of Biochemistry, The George Washington University
School of Medicine, Washington, D. C. 20037

A role for prolactin in regulating the immune system is suggested by a variety of data. Whether this regulation is facilitative or inhibitory appears to depend upon the concentration of prolactin used in the experimental model. In reporting prolactin suppression of leukocyte chemotaxis, Harris et al. (1) noted that only high levels of prolactin could inhibit leukocyte motility. By preincubating cells in prolactin at concentrations ranging from 10 to 2000 ng/ml, *in vitro* studies showed that at 1000 ng/ml prolactin, 4 out of 12 normal donor leukocytes had significantly depressed motility. At the highest concentration of 2000 ng/ml, the cells from 4 out of 8 subjects also showed decreased chemotaxis. The only statistically significant differences were noted when suppression occurred and doses less than 1000 ng/ml were ineffective. In a related study the comparative chemotactic data generated using cells from 3 patients with prolactin-secreting pituitary tumors revealed that one patient had significant enhancement of chemotaxis while another showed a significant decrease. The cells from a third patient exhibited normal motility. It appears therefore that reduced leukocyte chemotaxis can be correlated with abnormally high levels of prolactin.

Kelly and Dineen (2) reported that castrated male rats when treated with prolactin did not reject intestinal hookworms as quickly as control animals. The data were interpreted to support the hypothesis that prolactin (given twice daily at 1 mg/animal) affected the immuno-specific component (antibody and lymphocytes) of the immune response. Karmali et al. (3) described changes in lymphocyte responses to phytohemagglutinin (PHA) when cells were incubated in the presence of prolactin. Using a dose of PHA which produced submaximal stimulation, cells were incubated in the presence of 15 or 75 ng/ml of ovine prolactin. The lower dose did not effect lymphocyte responses to PHA but the higher dose produced consistently lowered counts (60.3% ± 9.3, percent of control). The 15 ng/ml dose was considered as being comparable to normal plasma-prolactin concentration while the 75 ng/ml concentration was pharmacological. It was concluded that prolactin could mediate the suppression of lymphocyte transformation during pregnancy, liver failure, certain cancers, and other situations during which prolactin is abnormlly elevated. The effect of bromocrptine on thymus growth in neonatal mice was also examined (3). It was reported that animals injected with this prolactin suppressing drug had a lowered organ size in proportion to body weight except for the thymus which was larger. Treated animals had a thymus-body weight ratio of .068 ± .001 while controls had a .046 ± .0055 ratio. These results are consistent with those generated using functional assays in that prolactin appears to exert an inhibitory influence over the thymus. Interestingly, these effects by prolactin on the immune system may not be unidirectional. It has been shown that congenitally athymic mice have abnormally low blood prolactin levels which can be normalized by thymic implantation at birth (4). Taken together these data suggest a complex interrelationship between prolactin and the thymus during ontogeny.

The underlying theme of the work discussed thus far is that elevated prolactin levels seem to mediate a suppression of the immune system. The situation with normal levels of prolactin appears to be much different. Berczi et al. (5) showed that hypophysectomized rats did not develop contact dermatitis in response to dinitrochlorobenzene (DNCB). However, treatment with prolactin (20 ug/day for 5 days) during DNCB challenge completely normalized the response. The contact dermatitis reaction is a delayed type hypersensitivity reaction involving T-cells and macrophages. Antibody production to sheep red blood cells (SRBC) in hypophysectomized rats was also found to be diminished (6). Daily treatment with prolactin was reported to reconstitute antibody production to SRBC. In general, lactogenic and growth hormone preparations were found to reconstitute both contact sensitivity and antibody production in hypophysectomized rats (7). These studies therefore point to an enhancement of both antibody production and cell-mediated immunity by prolactin. Our data also suggest a stimulatory role for prolactin via a direct effect upon the cells of the immune system (8).

As noted earlier, Karmali et al. (3) reported that lymphocytes stimulated with a submaximal dose of PHA (a T-cell mitogen) were not only unresponsive to 15 ng/ml prolactin, but were actually inhibited by 75 ng/ml prolactin. Using another T-cell mitogen, concanavalin-A (con-A), we have found an apparent stimulation of mitogenesis. Mitogen assays were performed according to the procedure of Thurman et al. (9). As shown in Table 1, bovine prolactin caused a significant enhancement of con-A-induced mitogenesis in murine spleen cells between 1 and .001 uM prolactin.

Table 1. *Prolactin enhances con-A induced mitogenesis*

Prolactin Concentration	con-A (0.125 ug/well) cpm	% change	P
0	94448 ± 7182	—	—
1 uM	125352 ± 3765	+ 32.7	<0.01
100 nM	144619 ± 4066	+ 53.1	<0.005
10 nM	137960 ± 5811	+ 46.1	<0.005
1 nM	138598 ± 4570	+ 46.7	<0.005
0.1 nM	100999 ± 5248	+ 6.9	NS

Table. 2 *Prolactin enhances con-A but not LPS induced mitogenesis*

Prolactin Concentration	con-A (0.125 ug/well)			LPS (5 ug/well)		
	cpm	% change	P	cpm	% change	P
0	94594 ± 2129	—	—	42561 ± 1132	—	—
100 nM	112500 ± 5691	+ 18.9	<0.025	44162 ± 541	+ 3.76	NS
10 nM	106264 ± 248	+ 12.3	<0.005	39023 ± 2003	—8.31	NS
1 nM	111137 ± 3881	+ 17.5	<0.025	44140 ± 712	+ 3.71	NS
0.1 nM	102528 ± 3802	+ 8.4	NS	41806 ± 1974	—1.77	NS
0.01 nM	89737 ± 1347	— 5.1	NS	45785 ± 2124	+ 7.58	NS

Because con-A is a T-cell mitogen, prolactin may specifically activate a sub-population of this cell type. Cells stimulated by the B-cell mitogen lipopolysaccharide (LPS) were not affected by prolactin (Table 2). In both experiments (Tables 1 and 2) the effect of prolactin on con-A-induced mitogenesis was dose dependent and occurred in a physiological range. Since prolactin by itself is not mitogenic (not shown), these experiments suggest a direct effect of prolactin upon activated lymphocytes.

The results of these experiments appear to contradict the previously discussed studies using PHA (3). This apparent discrepancy may be due to the activation level of the cells being evaluated. In the present studies with con-A we chose to use multiple doses of con-A in demonstrating stimulation with prolactin. We have subsequently pooled data (N = 6) at one dose of prolactin (1 nM) and have plotted percent changes versus con-A response (i.e, baseline). As shown in figure 1, prolactin enhaced proliferation of con-A stimulated cells only in a rather narrow range of initial stimulation. It can be seen that when spleen cells were stimulated by con-A so that tritiated thymidine incorporation was in the range of 60 to 120×10^3 cpm they were further stimulated by prolactin. Cells that were optimally stimulated by con-A ($>140 \times 10^3$ cpm) were not affected by prolactin (Fig. 1). In the baseline range of $0-40 \times 10^3$ cpm, con-A-stimulated cells were actually inhibited by 1 nM prolactin. Since the PHA dose used by Karmali et al. was sub-optimal their baseline stimulation may have been in this range.

The stimulatory effects of prolactin upon mitogenesis may be due in part to activation of cyclic nucleotides. Hadden et al. (10) have described changes in cyclic nucleotide levels in human peripheral blood lymphocytes by con-A and a succinylated derivative. Con-A was found to induce maximal proliferation between 25 and 50 ug/ml, but at higher concentrations there was progressively less proliferation. Succinylated con-A on the other hand gave comparable stimulation at 50 ug/ml to con-A but at higher concentrations this derivative maintained maximal stimulation. Measurements of cyclic nucleotide levels showed that both con-A and its derivative caused early increases in cyclic GMP levels in lymphocytes. However, succinylated con-A had no effect on cyclic AMP levels while con-A caused increases in cyclic AMP at higher concentrations. It was concluded that cyclic GMP is involved in the induction of the proliferative response while cyclic AMP may be responsible for a decrease in mitogenesis observed with high doses of con-A. Since prolactin enhanced con-A induced mitogenesis at suboptimal levels of activation (Fig.1), the mechanism involved may be increased levels of cyclic GMP. Several studies have been performed showing that in general cyclic GMP may promote

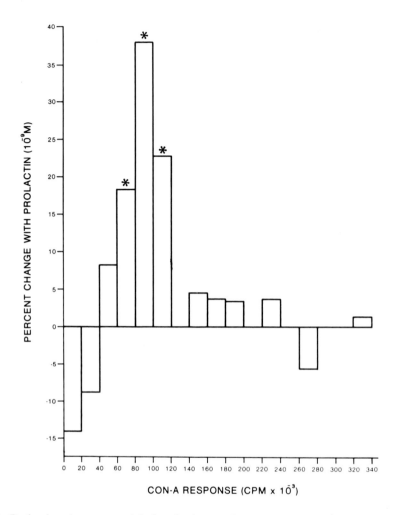

Figure 1. Prolactin enhances con-A-induced mitogenesis only at suboptimal levels of activation. Percent changes were calculated and plotted against the baseline response from individual experiments. (* Indicates that all data points found in this range were statistically significant in the individual experiments.)

lactogenesis while cyclic AMP is inhibitory. These studies indicate that cyclic GMP may mediate some of the stimulatory actions of prolactin in the mammary gland, but that cyclic AMP seems to inhibit the prolactin responses (11). In summary we have shown that bovine prolactin can enhance con-A induced mitogenesis of murine spleen cells and that this effect is observed in a restricted range of stimulation, suggesting that elevated cyclic GMP levels may in part mediate this effect.

Prolactin's activity in the mitogen assay suggested a direct effect upon lymphocytes. To further explore this possibility, prolactin's effect upon antibody production in primary immunization suspension cultures was determined. Spleen cells from C57BL6 male mice were sensitized to SRBC *in vitro* according to the procedure of Vann (12). Cultures were rocked and fed daily with a nutritive cocktail and prolactin was added to the cultures in the cocktail on days 0, 2, and 4. On day 5 plaque-forming cells (PFC) were determined by the method of Kappler (13). As shown in Table 3, prolactin caused a significant increase in the number of PFC from 100 nM to 1 pM. Studies are in progress to determine the optimal time for prolactin addition to the cultures. Also, interleukin-2 and thymosin alpha-1 concentrations will be measured in supernatants from these antigen sensitized cultures to determine whether prolactin effects their production. Preliminary evidence indicates that this may occur since immunoreactive thymosin alpha-1 was present in these supernatants (not shown). This *in vitro* enhancement of PFC reflects an increase in antibody production and together with the mitogen data demonstrates clearly that prolactin can be an immunopotentiating agent that apparently acts directly upon the cells of the immune system.

To test our hypothesis of direct interaction, experiments were designed to evaluate whether prolactin can specifically bind to splenic lymphocytes. The radio-receptor assay described by Lesniak et al. (14) was used. Since previous investigators had failed to detect prolactin receptors on resting lymphocytes (15) and since our mitogen data suggested an interaction with activated cells, we used spleen cells from animals previously sensitized to SRBC. Male C57BL6 mice were sacrificed 4 days after SRBC sensitization (0.2 ml of 10% SRBC, injected ip) and spleens were collected for the binding assay. To insure that an immune response had occurred, sera from all animals were tested for activity in the hemagglutination assay (not shown). As seen in the upper panel of Table 4, no specific binding by prolactin was detected from 15 to 240 minutes incubation time (36.4×10^6 cells/ml final concentration). As illustrated in the lower panel of Table 4, a second experiment using a range of cell concentrations (7.3 to 117×10^6 cells/ml) also resulted in no binding to spleen cells (2 hours incubation time). These two experiments indicate that prolactin does not bind specifically to antigen-stimulated spleen cells. Alternatively, the receptor assay may not be sensitive enough to detect specific receptors present in low concentration on the cell surface. Recently prolactin

Table 3. *Prolactin stimulates* in vitro *antibody production*

Prolactin Concentration	Direct PFC/culture (MEAN ± SE)	% change	P
0	49.3 ± 2.7	—	—
100 nM	65.5 ± 1.0	+ 32.9	<0.005
10 nM	69.8 ± 8.1	+ 41.6	<0.05
1 nM	73.0 ± 3.9	+ 48.1	<0.005
0.1 nM	74.0 ± 6.5	+ 50.1	<0.01
10 pM	80.0 ± 4.1	+ 62.3	<0.005
1 pM	72.5 ± 4.5	+ 47.1	<0.005
0.1 pM	60.0 ± 5.5	+ 21.7	NS

Table 4. *Prolactin does not specifically bind to antigen-stimulated cells*

	^{125}I-PRL (cpm)	^{125}I-PRL + bPRL (NSB) (cpm)	Specific Binding (%)
EXPERIMENT 1			
Time (Min.)			
15	820	935	< 0.1
30	1033	983	< 0.1
45	978	993	< 0.1
60	950	958	< 0.1
90	955	928	< 0.1
120	1180	1175	< 0.1
180	1470	1270	< 0.2
240	1535	1585	< 0.1
EXPERIMENT 2			
Cell Concentration (10^6 cells/ml)			
7.3	1373	1295	< 0.1
14.6	1135	1459	< 0.1
29.2	1318	1821	< 0.1
58.4	2165	2820	< 0.1
117.0	3505	4563	< 0.1

receptors were identified on human peripheral blood lymphocytes (16). These receptors were found to be present at a very low density (360/cell). Whether or not the receptor number changes during lymphocyte activation remains to be determined but the presence of a prolactin receptor on lymphocytes is certainly suggested by the results of our *in vitro* studies in which prolactin was added directly to lymphocytes.

The studies reviewed in this paper along with the data presented indicate the importance of prolactin in maintaining and stimulating the immune system. The well documented effects of steroid hormones on the immune system will need to be integrated with the data describing the actions of a polypeptide hormone whose influence on the immune system is just now coming to light.

REFERENCES

1. Harris RD, Kay NE, Seljeskog EL, Murray KJ, Douglas SD. (1979): J Neurosurg 50:462
2. Kelly JD, Dineen JK. (1973): Immunology 24:551
3. Karmali RA, Lauder I, Horrobin DF. (1974): Lancet 2:106 (Letter)
4. Pierpaoli W, Kopp HG, Bianchi E. (1976): Clin Exp Immunol 24:501
5. Berczi I, Nagy E, Asa SL, Kovacs K. (1983): Allergy 38:325
6. Berczi I, Nagy E, Kovacs K, Horvath E. (1981): Acta Endoctinologica 98:506
7. Nagy E, Berczi I, Friesen HG. (1983): Acta Endocrinologica 102:351

8. Spangelo BL, Hall NR, Goldstein AL, in preparation
9. Thurman GB, Ahmed A, Strong DM, Gershwin ME, Steinberg AD, Goldstein AL. (1975): Transplantation Proceedings 7:299
10. Hadden JW, Hadden EM, Sadlik JR, Coffey RG. (1976): Proc Natl Acad Sci USA 73:1717
11. Rillema JA. (1980): Federation Proceedings 39:2593
12. Vann DC. (1980): In: Mishell BB, Shiigi SM (eds) Selected Methods in Cellular Immunology. WH Freeman and Co, San Francisco p 60
13. Kappler JW. (1974): J Immunol 112:1271
14. Lesniak MA, Gorden P, Roth J, Gavin JR III. (1974): J Biol Chem 249:1661
15. Posner BI, Kelly PA, Shiu RPC, Friesen HG. (1974): Endocrinology 95:521
16. Russell DH, Matrisian L, Kibler R, Larson DF, Poulos B, Magun BE. (1984): Biochem Biophys Res Commun, in press

Prolactin. Basic and clinical correlates
R.M. MacLeod, M.O. Thorner and U. Scapagnini (eds.),
Fidia Research Series, vol. I,
Liviana Press, Padova © 1985

Section V
Target cell function
and peripheral receptors
for prolactin

INFLUENCE OF PROLACTIN ON DNA SYNTHESIS AND GLANDULAR DIFFERENTIATION IN RABBIT UTERINE ENDOMETRIUM

Beverly S. Chilton and Joseph C. Daniel, Jr.

Department of Anatomy, Medical University of South Carolina, Charleston, SC
and Department of Zoology, University of Tennessee, Knoxville, TN

In addition to its function as a mammotrophic, lactogenic, and luteotrophic factor, prolactin is also endometriotrophic. It acts directly on the mammalian uterus to enhance steroid binding and metabolism and to promote secretory activity and weight increase through progestational proliferation (1,2). The presence of high affinity binding sites for prolactin in the uteri of a variety of mammals (1,3,4,5) would seem to support this proposed endometriotrophic function.

A relationship between prolactin and steroid regulation of specific protein secretion by the rabbit uterus was recently reported by Daniel et al. (6). Long-term ovariectomized (LTOVX) rabbits (i.e. > 12 weeks) were injected with either prolactin or progesterone, or sequentially with both, and in some experimental groups with estradiol. Prolactin was given in phosphate buffered saline (PBS; pH 7.1) at 0.5-1.0 mg/24 h for 5 days, 3 mg progesterone/kg/24 h in corn oil was administered for 4 days, and estradiol was given for 3 days at 100 ug/kg/24 h. Controls consisted of estrous does, does 5 days pregnant or pseudopregnant, and LTOVX does injected with the carriers alone. Six h after the last injection the does were killed and uteri removed and flushed with PBS. Flushings were dialyzed and concentrated and the concentration of the protein uteroglobin (7,8) was determined by the immunodiffusion method of Oudin (9).

The uteri of does which have been ovariectomized for two to four weeks will secrete uteroglobin after administration of progesterone alone. By 12 weeks post-ovariectomy the uteri have atrophied and the endometria no longer secrete a normal pattern of proteins in response to exogenous ovarian steroid hormones, as shown by polyacrylamide gel electrophoresis (10). Administration of prolactin in sequence before progesterone to LTOVX does restored the capacity of their uteri to synthesize and secrete uteroglobin at a level equal to that found in intact does on the fifth day of pregnancy (Fig. 1A). Prolactin alone produced a significant increase in the concentrations of cytosol progesterone receptors (Fig. 1B) and estrogen receptors (Fig. 1C) to levels typical of estrous

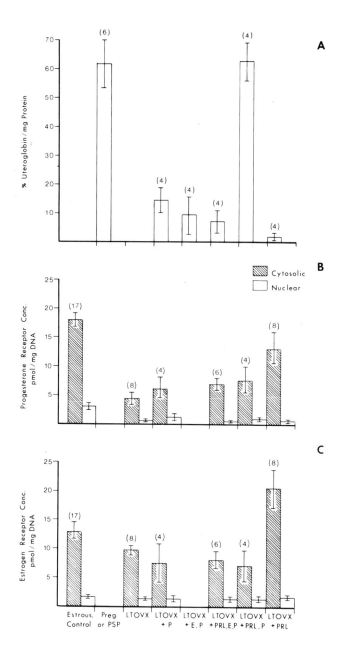

Figure 1. (A) Concentrations of uteroglobin secreted by the uteri of long-term ovariectomized (LTOVX) does treated with various combinations of progesterone (P), estradiol (E), and prolactin (PRL). Controls include values for estrous and 5-day pregnant or pseudopregnant (PSP) animals. Values are expressed as mean ± SEM. Concentrations of cytosol and nuclear progesterone (B) and estrogen (C) receptors are expressed as mean ± SEM. All values in parentheses represent the number of experimental animals per group.

does. None of the other treatments effected the same levels of response. The concentration of nuclear receptors remained low for all treatment categories (Fig. 1B,C). The addition of estradiol to the protocol, administered between prolactin and progesterone, blocked the uteroglobin response. This could have reflected the separation in time between the animals' receipt of prolactin and progesterone, or, what is more likely, the blockage of progesterone-induced uteroglobin by high concentrations of estrogen (11,12,13). As shown in Figure 1A, some uteroglobin was secreted in response to progesterone alone, but the secretory response was not as dramatic as with the prolactin, progesterone sequence. However, the administration of prolactin alone resulted in negligible uteroglobin secretion. Apparently, prolactin synergizes with progesterone in regulating uteroglobin production and affects the availability of cytosol estrogen and progesterone receptors.

Joseph and Mubako (14) reported that there is no significant increase in the wet weight of uteri of non-traumatized, ovariectomized rats receiving ovine prolactin. However, Ohno (2) demonstrated a prolactin-induced increase in uterine wet weight in ovariectomized immature rabbits and in 24-hr pseudopregnant rabbits. In addition, prolactin administration caused an accelerated progestational proliferation of the uterine endometrium in the 24-hr pseudopregnant rabbits. We elected to express any growth effect by a measure of DNA content. Initially, we calculated the endometrial mg DNA/g tissue ratio (Fig. 2A) for the following animal treatment groups: 1) prolactin (0.5 mg/24 h/5 days); 2) prolactin + progesterone (3 mg/kg/24 h for 4 days); 3) prolactin + estradiol (100 ug/kg/24 h for 3 days) + progesterone; 4) estradiol + progesterone; and 5) progesterone. As shown in Figure 2A, the value for LTOVX animals is lower than the value for estrous controls, and prolactin treatment caused no significant increase in the mg DNA/g tissue value compared with LTOVX animals. All other treatments resulted in values comparable to estrous controls.

Subsequent to these studies we evaluated the effect of all the different treatments on the rate of endometrial DNA synthesis. We measured DNA synthesis in isolated endometrial nuclei using an *in vitro* assay characterized by Wiklund and Gorski (15) and Stack and Gorski (16). In this assay, cell-free synthesis is catalyzed by DNA polymerase α and the rates of DNA synthesis are measured directly by using nucleoside triphosphates as the labeled precursors. Thus the uptake and phosphorylation steps are omitted. Also, because the endogenous nucleotide pools are washed out during nuclear isolation, endogenous nucleotide pools and resultant isotope dilutions do not influence the measurement of radiolabel incorporation. DNA synthesis, as measured by [^{3}H]TTP incorporation (30 C) in endometrial nuclei from estrous animals, was linear for up to 30 minutes. Consequently, DNA synthesis was measured for 10 minutes. Data are summarized in Figure 2B. Controls included the measurement of DNA synthesis by nuclei isolated from endometria of estrous animals, LTOVX animals, and LTOVX + estradiol (5 ug/12 h for 36 h). DNA synthesis values for estrous controls and LTOVX + estradiol were not significantly ($p > 0.05$) different (Fig. 2B), and nuclei from LTOVX animals incorporated only negligible amounts of the radiolabeled precursor. As shown in Figure 2B, prolactin administration to LTOVX animals resulted in a significant ($p < 0.01$) increase in the rate of DNA synthesis over LTOVX does, resulting in a value that was 40% of estrous controls. All other treatments resulted in values that ranged from 63-70% of estrous controls.

354

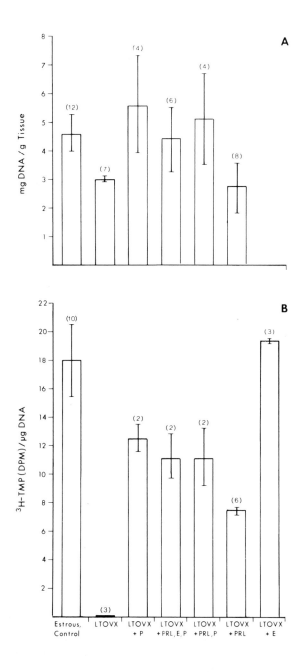

Figure 2. The effects of different hormone treatment regimes on the total mg DNA/g tissue (A), and on the rates of DNA synthesis in isolated endometrial nuclei (B). Values are expressed as mean ± SEM. All values in parentheses represent the number of experimental animals per treatment group.

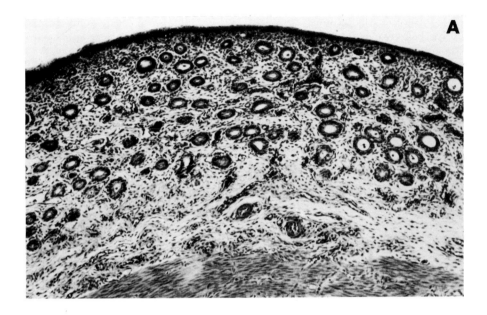

Figure 3. Endometrium from an estrous control rabbit (A). Note that the endometrial glands are simple tubular and the stroma is a vascularized, loose connective tissue. Endometrium from a doe 12 weeks after ovariectomy (B). Endometrial glands are minimal and the stroma appears prominent. X360.

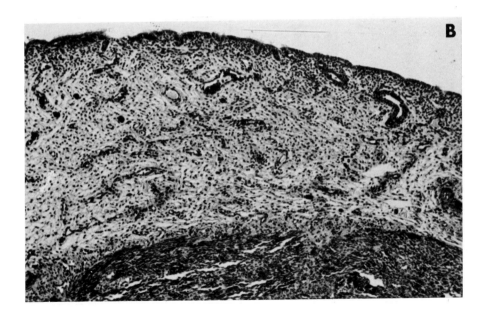

356

Because prolactin administration to LTOVX animals did result in an increase in DNA synthesis, we evaluated tissue sections for potential histological modifications. Whole uterine tissue was fixed in neutral buffered formalin, paraffin embedded, and sectioned (4-6 um). Sections were stained with hematoxylin and eosin. The uterine endometrium of estrous does is thrown into approximately six longitudinal mucosal ridges (17), yielding significant variability in the relative thickness of the uterine endometrium. A predominately non-ciliated, simple columnar epithelium borders the uterine lumen and the endometrium is punctuated with simple tubular glands (Fig. 3A). The endometrium appears to be thickest in the antimesometrial region of the uterus. Hoffman and Davies (17) have suggested that the extent of mucosal foldings and the degree of glandularity are altered by a recent pseudopregnancy or high levels of circulating estradiol. We used only virgin, estrous does in an effort to standardize our experimental animals. By 8 weeks post-ovariectomy, the rabbit uterus is about one-half the normal size (18) and by 12 weeks both endometrium and myometrium are thin and the cuboidal epithelium is flat, non-proliferating, and largely devoid of glandular structure (Fig. 3B). The stroma is thinner but appears prominent in a relative sense.

Figure 4 demonstrates that prolactin alone is capable of inducing new epithelial gland formation in the endometrium of LTOVX animals. Some of the glands have the elongated, coiled appearance of those characteristic of a progestational uterus. Preliminary ultrastructural studies revealed that 5 days after prolactin administration

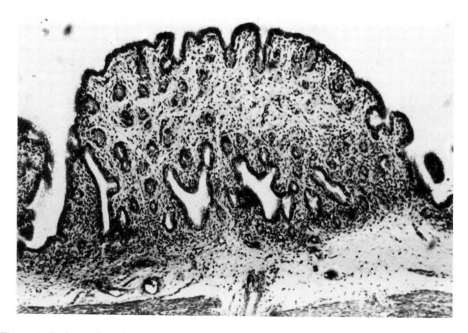

Figure 4. Endometrium from a LTOVX animal after exposure to prolactin for 5 days. Note the increase in glandular proliferation and the extension of the glands deep into the connective tissue. The increased mucosal surface area is also apparent. X360.

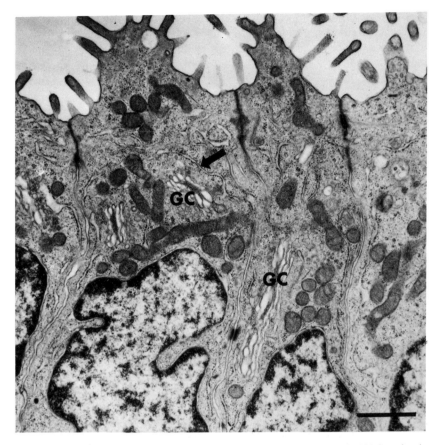

Figure 5. An electron micrograph of the uterine surface epithelium from a LTOVX animal treated with prolactin for 5 days. The apical protrusions contain numerous polysomes and mitochondria. Characteristic is the distribution of microvilli on the luminal surface. Note the small, pleomorphic mitochondria, dilated rough endoplasmic reticulum (arrow), and the well developed Golgi (GC) complexes. Nuclear chromatin is condensed. Bar 1 um, X15,750.

to LTOVX animals (Fig. 5), the surface and crypt epithelium of the uterus was composed of columnar cells with protrusions of the apical cytoplasm into the uterine lumen characteristic of secretory cells (19). The cellular cytoplasm contained an abundance of polysomes and some profiles of dilated rough endoplasmic reticulum. The Golgi complexes were hypertrophied, contained electron-opaque material, and were lateral rather than supranuclear in location. LTOVX controls are shown in Figure 6. The apparent reduction in the number of mitochondria, plus the absence of dome-like cytoplasmic protusions, and the presence of only a single Golgi profile suggest that these cells are quiescent.

Histologically there is pronounced variability in the individual animal response to prolactin, as well as an apparent graded responsiveness within each uterine horn. The

358

most significant glandular development was consistently found in the antimesometrial region of each uterine horn. This may be reflective of a differential tissue sensitivity to prolactin, not unlike the gradient of estrogen and progestrone receptors that has been reported along the length of human endometrium (20). Alternatively, steroids produced in the adrenal gland may support secretory activity after an initiating influence of prolactin. Radioimmunoassays of circulating steroids in rabbits ovariectomized for up to 11 months show that progesterone levels are maintained at 14-50% of those of estrous does and that estradiol levels are reduced by only 36% or less than estrous levels (21,22). These levels become severely reduced following adrenalectomy. It is important to note that even though prolactin administration alone initiated some endometrial gland formation in LTOVX animals, the synthesis and/or secretion of uteroglobin did not follow without exogenous progesterone, in our studies. Presumably then, adrenal progesterone is not sufficient to elicit a full response.

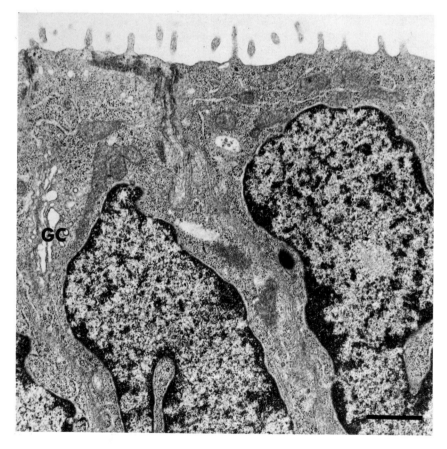

Figure 6. An electron micrograph of the uterine surface epithelium from a LTOVX control animal. Note the absence of apical protrusions and the sparse distribution of microvilli. Some profiles of rough endoplasmic reticulum are evident in these non-ciliated cells. Elements of a Golgi complex (GC) are apparent and the nuclear chromatin is condensed. Bar 1 um, X15,750.

We conclude that the complete endometrial response of proliferation and gland formation and specific protein synthesis and secretion in the rabbit, heretofore assigned to progesterone alone (or after estrogen priming), would now seem to result from a synergistic interplay of prolactin and progesterone.

ACKNOWLEDGMENTS

We would like to thank Ms. Amy E. Jetton, Mr. Christopher J. McAllister, and Ms. Kathryn T. Cowart for technical assistance, and Ms. Marion Hinson for secretarial assistance. This research was supported in part by the Medical University of South Carolina Biomedical Research Support Grant 1983-84.

REFERENCES

1. Williams GH, Hammond JM, Weisz J, Mortel R. (1978): Biol Reprod 18:697
2. Ohno Y. (1982): Acta Obst Gynaec Jap 34:252
3. Posner BI, Kelly PA, Shiu RPC, Friesen HG. (1974): Endocrinology 95:521
4. Tamaya T, Ohno Y, Ide N, Tsurusaki T, Okada H. (1980): Jap J Fert Ster 25:8
5. Rose J, Stormshak F, Adair J, Oldfield JE. (1983): Molec Cell Endocr 31:131
6. Daniel JC Jr, Jetton AE, Chilton BS. (1984): J Reprod Fert (in press)
7. Krishnan RS, Daniel JC Jr. (1967): Science 158:490
8. Beier HM. (1968): Biochim Biophys Acta 160:289
9. Oudin J. (1952): In: Corcoran AC (ed) Methods in Medical Research. Year Book Publishers, Chicago, p 335
10. Daniel JC Jr. (1980): In: Beato M (ed) Steroid Induced Uterine Proteins. Elsevier/North Holland Biomedical Press, Amsterdam, p 87
11. Loosefelt H, Fridlandski F, Savouret JF, Atger M, Milgrom E. (1981): J Biol Chem 256:3465
12. Janne OA. (1981): Acta Obstet Gynecol Scand Suppl 101:11
13. Kopu HT, Kokkonen EKT, Janne OA. (1981): Endocrinology 109:1479
14. Joseph MM, Mubaki HB. (1975): J Reprod Fert 45:413
15. Wiklund J, Gorski J. (1982): Endocrinology 111:1140
16. Stack G, Gorski J. (1983): Endocrinology 112:2142
17. Davies J, Hoffman LH. (1973): Am J Anat 137:423
18. Spencer RW, Daniel JC Jr. (1983): Theriogenology 20:571
19. Davies J, Hoffman LH. (1973): Am J Anat 142:335
20. Tsibris JCM, Fort FL, Cazenave CR, Cantor B, Bardawil WA, Notelovitz M, Spellacy WN. (1981): J Steroid Biochem 14:997
21. Chilton BS, Nicosia SV, Laufer MR. (1980): Biol Reprod 23:677
22. Overstrom EW, Black DL. (1980): Biol Reprod Suppl 22:134a

Prolactin. Basic and clinical correlates
R.M. MacLeod, M.O. Thorner and U. Scapagnini (eds.),
Fidia Research Series, vol. I,
Liviana Press, Padova © 1985

Section V
Target cell function
and peripheral receptors
for prolactin

INFLUENCE OF PROLACTIN
ON TESTICULAR PROLACTIN RECEPTORS
IN PREPUBERTAL HAMSTERS

H. G. Klemcke, K. S. Matt, and A. Bartke

Department of Obstetrics and Gynecology, The University of Texas
Health Science Center, San Antonio, Texas 78284

Prolactin plays a major role in the regulation of testicular function in rodents by its ability to enhance effects of luteinizing hormone (LH) on testosterone production (1-4). This effect of prolactin appears to be mediated by an increase in testicular LH receptors (5-8) and by an increase in testicular stores of cholesterol esters--steroidogenic precursors of testosterone (1). Recently, we have demonstrated that prolactin is also necessary to maintain its own testicular receptors in mature hamsters, and have obtained preliminary evidence that it may have a similar function in immature hamsters (9).

In developing male hamsters, serum prolactin concentrations increase dramatically, beginning at 16-19 days of age (10). In rats, this prolactin is required for normal testicular development (11-13), and in hamsters, reduced testicular growth and numbers of LH/hCG receptors are associated with pharmacological prevention of this prepubertal prolactin surge (14). The present study was conducted to ascertain whether alterations in testicular growth coincident with inhibition of the developmental increase in plasma prolactin are mediated in part by a modification in testicular prolactin receptors.

Syrian hamsters (LAK:LVG [SYR]) were bred in our own animal colony from Charles River Breeding Laboratories stock, and maintained from birth in a long photoperiod (14 h light:10 h darkness; lights on at 0700 h) at 22 ± 2 C. Animals received food and water ad libitum. Hamsters were divided into three treatment groups and, beginning at 14 days of age (day of birth designated as day 0), animals within each group received one of the following treatments: 1) sesame oil, 5 ul/10 g body weight; 2) 2-bromo-alpha-ergocriptine (CB-154; 39.3 ug in 5 ul sesame oil/10 g body weight); 3) CB-154 as above plus 16.67 ug ovine prolactin (NIH-P-S15) in 10 ul PBS (0.01 M sodium phosphate buffer containing 0.15 M NaCl, pH 9.0)/10 g body weight. Treatments were given once daily at 1000-1200 h for the next 17 days. On day 31, approximately 24 h after the last injection, hamsters were killed by decapitation and trunk blood collected (for measurement of LH, FSH, and prolactin concentrations in plasma).

362

Plasma LH and FSH were quantitated by double antibody radioimmunoassay techniques, as previously described (6,9). Plasma prolactin was measured using a homologous radioimmunoassay (15). Testes were removed, weighed, rapidly frozen in a dry ice-acetone mixture, and stored in an ultrafreezer at -70 C until assayed for prolactin receptors. Seminal vesicles were removed and weighed along with their secretions.

Testicular prolactin receptors were measured using iodinated ovine prolactin and a previously reported and validated procedure (9). The protein content of each experimental sample was measured in duplicate using a previously validated (16) modification of the Lowry procedure (17). Single classification analysis of variance was used to test for main effects, and the Student-Newman-Keuls test was used to test for significant differences among specific means. All data were examined for homogeneity of variance using Bartlett's test and for normality of distribution using the Kolmogorov-Smirnov test. Mathematical transformations were used where necessary. For all statistical tests, the 5% level of probability was considered significant.

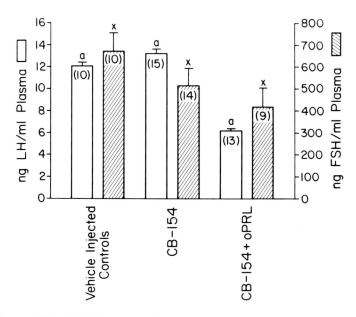

Figure 1. Plasma LH and FSH concentrations in prepubertal male hamsters maintained on a photoperiod consisting of 14 h light:10 h darkness (14L:10D). Beginning at 14 days of age and continuing for the next 17 days, hamsters received one of the following daily treatments: 1) sesame oil, 5 ul/10 g body weight; 2) CB-154, 39.3 ug in 5 ul sesame oil/10 g body weight; 3) CB-154 as above plus 16.67 ug ovine prolactin (NIH-P-S15)/10 g body weight. At 31 days of age, approximately 24 h after the last injection, the hamsters were killed by decapitation and blood was collected. Each bar represents the mean ± SEM. The number of hamsters in which each hormone was measured is indicated by the numbers within the bars. Data within a measured parameter which have different superscripts are significantly different (P < 0.05).

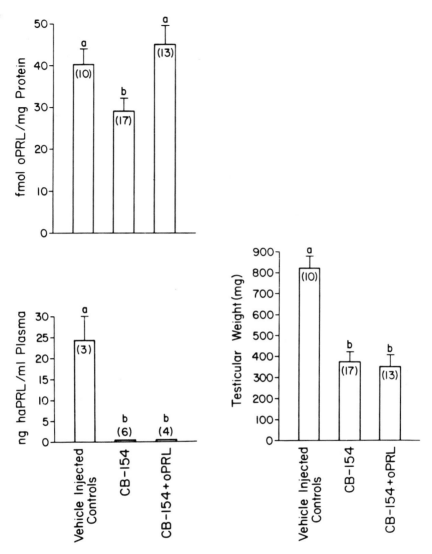

Figure 2. Plasma prolactin concentrations, testicular weights, and testicular prolactin receptor concentrations in prepubertal male hamsters maintained on a 14L:10D photoperiod and treated as described in Fig. 1. Each bar represents the mean ± SEM. The number of hamsters in which a given parameter was measured is indicated by the numbers within the bars. Data within a measured parameter which have different superscripts are significantly different (P <0.05).

As indicated in Figure 1, treatment with CB-154 or CB-154 plus ovine prolactin had no measurable effect on either plasma LH or FSH. However, there was a dramatic decrease in plasma prolactin (Fig. 2). Lowered plasma prolactin concentrations were accompanied by a dramatic 54% reduction in testicular weight, presumably due to a reduced rate of testicular growth. Also, growth of seminal vesicles was retarded ($P < 0.05$; 29 ± 4 vs. 63 ± 9 mg; mean $\pm$ SEM). Additionally, testes from CB-154-injected hamsters contained a diminished ($P < 0.05$) concentration of prolactin receptors. Injections of ovine prolactin had no measurable effect on testicular weight (Fig. 2), or on seminal vesicle weight (35 ± 3 mg), but did prevent the CB-154-induced reduction in prolactin receptor concentrations.

These data further substantiate that the prepubertal increase in prolactin is necessary for normal testicular development and indicate an involvement of testicular prolactin receptors in the maturational process. In bromocriptine- treated animals, reductions in testicular and seminal vesicle weights and in prolactin receptor concentrations occurred concomitantly with decreased plasma prolactin concentrations, whereas plasma FSH and LH concentrations were apparently unaffected by treatment. It is unlikely that effects of CB-154 represent direct effects on the tissues; more likely they reflect reductions in circulating prolactin (9). Moreover, prolactin injections were able to completely prevent this CB-154-induced reduction in prolactin receptor concentrations. One cannot disregard the possibility that some of the increased binding of labelled ovine prolactin to testicular receptor preparations may represent anti-ovine prolactin antibody contamination (9). However, we have previously demonstrated that treatment of adult male hamsters with injections of ovine prolactin does not lead to an increase in ovine prolactin binding to the heart, a non-target tissue (Klemcke, unpublished observations). Such data suggest that induced antibodies do not necessarily contaminate tissue receptor preparations, and argue against the potential significance of such a putative antibody contamination in the present study. Additionally, substantial supportive evidence obtained from our previous studies in pituitary engrafted hamsters (18,19) and in short photoperiod-housed hamsters injected with ovine prolactin for 3 days (Klemcke, unpublished observations) demonstrates the ability of prolactin to increase testicular prolactin receptors in the absence of increased circulating anti-prolactin antibodies.

The significant reduction in growth rate of the highly androgen-dependent seminal vesicles in CB-154-injected hamsters might indicate a reduction in plasma testosterone concentrations. However, androgen-independent effects of prolactin insufficiency (20) might also account for at least some of the alterations in seminal vesicle weights. The inability of injected ovine prolactin to reverse effects of CB-154 on testicular and seminal vesicle weights suggests the existence of a different--perhaps higher--threshold for stimulation by prolactin for these parameters. Hence, the dose and frequency of ovine prolactin administration were sufficient to stimulate a receptor increase, but for testicular and seminal vesicle weights, were inadequate to replace endogenous prolactin.

In summary, the data strongly suggest that prolactin exerts a significant influence on the prepubertal development of testicular prolactin receptors and indicate that suppression of plasma prolactin during the time period studied is incompatible with normal testicular development. The chain of cellular events initiated by a reduction in plasma prolactin might be envisioned to include a reduction in prolactin receptors which could lead to a reduced testicular sensitivity to circulating prolactin. This then would induce significant reductions in testicular LH receptors (9,14), which would be accompanied by decreased testicular sensitivity to circulating LH and ultimately culminate in reduced testosterone production, decreased spermatogenesis, and reduced testicular weight.

REFERENCES

1. Bartke A. (1971): J Endocrinol 49:317
2. Hafiez AA, Bartke A, Lloyd CW. (1972): J Endocrinol 53:223
3. Hafiez AA, Lloyd CW, Bartke A. (1972): J Endocrinol 52:327
4. Johnson DC. (1974): Proc Soc Exp Biol Med 145:610
5. Bex FJ, Bartke A. (1977): Endocrinology 100:1223
6. Bex F, Bartke A, Goldman BD, Dalterio S. (1978): Endocrinology 103:2069
7. Purvis K, Clausen OPF, Olsen A. (1979): Arch Androl 3:219
8. Morris PL, Saxena BB. (1980): Endocrinology 107:1639
9. Klemcke HG, Bartke A, Borer KT. (1984): Endocrinology 114:594
10. Vomachka AJ, Greenwald GS. (1979): Endocrinology 105:960
11. Negro-Vilar A, Saad WA, McCann SM. (1977): Endocrinology 100:729
12. de Jong RAP, van der Schoot P. (1979): Biol Reprod 21:1263
13. Baranao JLS, Legnani B. Chiauzzi VA, Bertini LM, Suescun MA, Calvo JC, Charreau EH, Calandra RS. (1981): Endocrinology 109:2188
14. Matt KS, Amador A, Stallings MH, Bartke A. 65th Annual Meeting of The Endocrine Society, San Antonio, TX, (1983): p 280 (Abstract 797)
15. Soares MG, Colosi P, Talamantes F. (1983): Proc Soc Exp Biol Med 172:379
16. Klemcke HG, Bartke A, Goldman BD. (1981): Biol Reprod 25:536
17. Markwell MK, Haas SM, Bieber LL, Tolbert NE. (1978): Anal Biochem 87:206
18. Klemcke HG, Bartke A, Amador A, Soares MJ, Talamantes F, Borer K. 65th Annual Meeting of The Endocrine Society, San Antonio, TX, (1983): p 281 (Abstract 804)
19. Klemcke HG, 17th Annual Meeting of The Society for the Study of Reproduction, Laramie, WY, (1984):, p 157 (Abstract 254)
20. Bartke A. (1980): Fed Proc 39:2577

Prolactin. Basic and clinical correlates
R.M. MacLeod, M.O. Thorner and U. Scapagnini (eds.),
Fidia Research Series, vol. I,
Liviana Press, Padova © 1985

Section V
Target cell function
and peripheral receptors
for prolactin

PROLACTIN-DAUNOMYCIN CONJUGATE INHIBITS *IN VITRO* GROWTH AND DNA SYNTHESIS IN CELLS CARRYING THE PROLACTIN RECEPTOR

H. C. Blossey, B. Gaier, Y. Zaltsman, and F. Kohen

Department of Hormone Research, The Weizmann Institute of Science
Rehovot 76100 Israel

It has been shown that a considerable number of tumors arising in endocrine regulated organs retain their ability to express hormone receptors and thus remain hormonally sensitive (1). During the past ten years the principles of endocrine tumor therapy, hormonal deprivation, or hormonal interference (2), have been established successfully with the use of steroid hormones, steroid hormone analogues, or other drugs that either interfere intracellularly with the receptor action or interfere with the regulation or synthesis of the appropriate steroid hormones (1).

Hormone action is highly specific and restricted to those cells containing the specific receptor. The question, therefore, arises as to whether the presence of hormone receptor sites may be exploited to provide a homing mechanism for chemotherapeutic agents suitably linked to the homologous hormone or a cognate ligand of high affinity for the receptor (3,4). A prerequisite of such a hormone-cytotoxic drug conjugate is that the chemical manipulation should not reduce either the cytotoxic activity of the drug or the binding affinity of the hormone to the receptor (4).

CONJUGATES OF HORMONES AND CYTOTOXIC DRUGS AS AN APPROACH TO SITE-DIRECTED CHEMOTHERAPY AGAINST HORMONE-SENSITIVE CANCER

Conjugates between steroid hormones and cytotoxic drugs have been described, but only a minor portion of these ligands showed a reasonable affinity to the appropriate hormone receptor (5). Hence a specific, receptor related toxicity of such a ligand has not yet been demonstrated unequivocally either *in vitro* (5) or *in vivo* (6).

The apparent limitations of this approach may be explained on the basis of the mechanism of steroid hormone action. Steroid hormones penetrate the cell membrane passively and biological recognition occurs inside the cell (7). By definition, the steroid hormone-cytotoxic drug ligand should have the same characteristics of penetrating the cell membrane. Due to the unimpaired toxicity of the drug moiety the conjugate might exert toxic effects within the cell regardless of whether there is a steroid hormone receptor or not.

On the other hand, the recognition of peptide hormones occurs on the cell surface. Here, the hormone transmits the signal for receptor activation, which includes the subsequent event, the internalization of the peptide hormone receptor complex in the form of clusters (reviewed in 4). Thus in contrast to steroid hormones, the uptake of a peptide hormone into the cell is dependent upon the homologous receptor. Consequently the cellular uptake of cytotoxic drugs covalently linked to peptide hormones under the same prerequisite, mentioned above, should be strictly dependent upon the presence of the cognate receptor.

It has been established that certain tumors express receptors to peptide hormones, e.g., breast cancers carry receptors for prolactin (8) and epidermal growth factor (EGF) (9) and melanomas express receptors for melanocyte stimulating hormone (MSH) (3). The receptor-mediated toxicity of a MSH-daunomycin conjugate (MSH-DAU) has been demonstrated for Cloudman S 91 melanoma cells *in vitro* (3). In the following paper we describe some of the characteristics of a prolactin-daunomycin (PRL-DAU) conjugate in various cell systems carrying the prolactin receptor.

CHARACTERIZATION OF A PROLACTIN-DAUNOMYCIN CONJUGATE IN CELL CULTURE

The reference system for the determination of prolactin receptors consisted of liver plasma membranes and granulosa cells in culture derived from immature rats pretreated with estradiol and pregnant mare serum gonadotropin (PMSG) (10). Compared to [^{125}I]-ovine prolactin, PRL-DAU had an almost unimpaired affinity to the prolactin receptor in both systems (11).

The minimal concentration of DAU for maximal toxicity in cultured granulosa cells was 4 uM (Table 1), and the addition of free prolactin did not modify this effect (data not shown). With respect to the DAU concentration present in the culture, PRL-DAU showed the same dose-related toxicity as DAU itself and this effect could be partially reduced by free prolactin (Table 1).

PRL-DAU at 5 uM inhibited [^{3}H]-thymidine incorporation in the granulosa cell system, but not in cells derived from androgen-dependent mouse mammary cancers (Shionogi 115) (Table 2) devoid of prolactin receptors. PRL-DAU at 50 uM inhibited DNA synthesis in cells derived from Shionogi 115 tumors, but the inhibition was considerably weaker than in rat granulosa cells. The reduction by free prolactin was just at the borderline of significance.

Plasma membranes derived from 9,10-dimethyl-1,2-benzanthracene (DMBA)- induced rat mammary cancers showed a wide spectrum of prolactin receptor concentrations (Fig. 1). The affinity of [^{125}I]-ovine prolactin to these prolactin receptors was comparable to the affinity of this ligand to the prolactin receptors in rat liver plasma membranes (Fig. 2). For cells in culture derived from a DMBA-induced rat mammary

Table 1. *Cytotoxic index (CI) of DAU and PRL-DAU for rat granulosa cells in culture.*

uM	DAU	PRL-DAU	PRL-DAU + PRL 4 uM
1	0.2	0.2	
2	0.7	0.7	
3	0.8	0.8	
4	1	1	0.5
6	1	1	
8	1	1	0.9

DAU and ovine prolactin were from Sigma. Granulosa cells were prepared and cultured as described (10). After two days in culture the medium was changed and the drugs added. After another two days in culture the CI was determined (3). In the PRL-DAU conjugate each mole of prolactin contained four moles of daunomycin; the given concentrations refer to the DAU moiety.

Table 2. *Inhibition of [³H]-thymidine incorporation (%)*

oPRL-DAU	rat granulosa cells	mouse mammary cancer (Shionogi 115)
	(in the presence of 2 uM free ovine prolactin)	
5 30 (10) p < 0.001	0	uM
50 uM	70 (45) p < 0.001	30 (20) p < 0.05

Cells were prepared and immediately incubated in Leibowitz L 15 medium, 5% fetal calf serum at 22 C for two hours in the presence of 200,000 cpm [³H]-thymidine (NEN, SPA 6 Ci/mmol). For further details see (12). The numbers reflect the mean of 12 wells; SE was $< 10\%$ according to Student's t-test.

cancer the minimal concentration of DAU for maximal toxicity was 2 uM (Table 3). Free prolactin did not modify this effect (data not shown).

Plasma membranes prepared from this tumor had a prolactinreceptor concentration of 18 fmol/mg protein. With respect to the DAU concentration present in the cell culture the minimal concentration of PRL-DAU for maximal toxicity was 4 uM (Table 3), and this effect could be reduced by free prolactin. As every tumor has its individual prolactin receptor concentration, further investigation is needed to evaluate the significance of different prolactin receptor concentrations for the sensitivity of the cells against PRL-DAU.

PEPTIDE HORMONE-DAUNOMYCIN CONJUGATES: MECHANISMS OF ACTION

The concept of using hormones as carriers for cytotoxic drugs in hormone-sensitive cancer has been described as an "approach to site-directed chemotherapy" (4). The

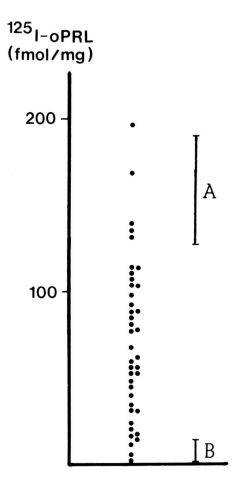

Figure 1. Prolactin receptor concentrations in plasma membranes of 40 DMBA-induced rat mammary cancers. Plasma membranes were prepared as described (13). Receptor determinations were carried out as one point assays in duplicates. [^{125}I]-ovine prolactin was prepared according to (14). The bars represent the range of prolactin receptor concentrations in rat liver plasma membranes (A) and granulosa cells in culture (B) according to (11).

feasibility of this approach has been demonstrated with a MSH-DAU conjugate in Cloudman S 91 melanoma cells (3) and could now be extended for a PRL-DAU ligand in rat granulosa cells as well as in cells derived from a DMBA-induced rat mammary cancer. Nevertheless there are still many open questions. As of now there is evidence only that the first and the last step in the course of PRL-DAU action are related to the prolactin receptor: it has been demonstrated that the recognition of the PRL-DAU ligand is clearly dependent upon and highly specific for the prolactin receptor (11); the last step in PRL-DAU action is the cytotoxic effect on the cell. This effect was reducible in the presence of free prolactin. This suggests that the free prolactin competed with the PRL-DAU ligand for prolactin receptor sites and thus reduced the uptake of the PRL-DAU conjugate by the cells.

Table 3. *Cytotoxic index of DAU and ovine PRL-DAU for cells in cultures derived from a DMBA-induced rat mammary cancer (tumor 79)*

uM	DAU	ovine PRL-DAU	ovine PRL-DAU + ovine PRL 20 uM
1	0.9	0.7	
2	1	0.8	
3	1	0.85	
4	1	1	0.7
6	1	1	
8	1	1	

Cells were prepared and cultured as described (15). After two days in culture the drugs were added. Medium was changed every two days and the drugs added. After 13 days in culture the CI was determined (3).

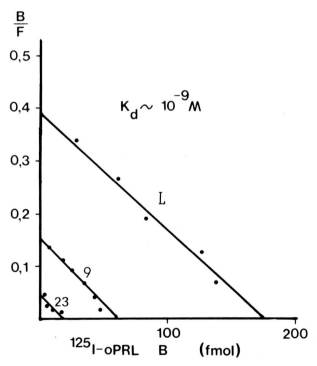

Figure 2. Scatchard analysis of prolactin receptors in plasma membranes of rat liver (L) and two DMBA-induced rat mammary cancers (ns. 9 and 23), representative for a medium and a low prolactin receptor concentration. The respective prolactin receptor concentrations were: L = 180 fmol/mg protein, 9 = 53 fmol/mg and 23 = 5 fmol/mg.

   With reference to the DAU moiety, the PRL-DAU conjugate showed toxicity for granulosa cells in the same range of concentrations as DAU itself. This suggests that in the range of PRL-DAU concentrations used, the cellular uptake of PRL-DAU is quantitatively identical to the uptake of DAU. By contrast, the toxicity of the conjugate in cells derived from a DMBA-induced mammary cancer was lower than the toxicity of DAU itself. This observation may be explained in different ways: the tumor cells had a low number of receptor sites and the action of PRL-DAU may be dependent on the prolactin receptor concentration; due to the transformation of the cells some of the prolactin receptors may have been inactive, a phenomenon which is well known for steroid hormone receptors in cancer cells (16); the tumor may have contained cells without a prolactin receptor or some of the tumor cells may have lost the prolactin receptor during the period of culture.

   For cells with non-detectable prolactin receptor concentrations, such as cells derived from androgen-dependent Shionogi 115 mouse mammary cancers, the PRL-DAU ligand was toxic only at a concentration equivalent to DAU 50 uM. This is more than tenfold the minimal concentration for maximal toxicity in rat granulosa and rat mammary cancer cells as described above. Although the purity of the PRL-DAU ligand was proven by thin layer chromatography, it cannot be ruled out that during the experiment the PRL-DAU conjugate was partially cleaved and DAU was set free from the ligand. On the other hand, the non-detectability of prolactin receptors in these tumors does not exclude the possibility of the presence of a small amount of functionally active receptors. It is known that although in normal mammary tissue the prolactin receptor concentration is at the borderline of detectability, this tissue is capable of responding to prolactin. On the basis of the extremely high concentration of PRL-DAU in this experiment and the non-reducible toxicity by free prolactin, we regard the toxicity of PRL-DAU for cells derived from Shionogi 115 mouse mammary cancers as unspecific. The mechanism of this toxicity may be based on the DAU-related interaction of PRL-DAU with the cell membrane. It has been demonstrated that adriamycin, a derivative of DAU, exerts cytotoxic effects without entering the cell (17).

   During the two days of incubation time of granulosa cells with DAU or PRL-DAU, no considerable difference in the time course of toxicity was observed. However, inhibition of DNA synthesis during two hours of incubation time was much slower with PRL-DAU than with DAU itself. This observation implies further evidence that PRL-DAU is taken up by the cell via time- dependent mechanisms probably involving internalization of the ligand at the cell surface, whereas DAU itself penetrates the cell membrane easily and reaches the nucleus within a few seconds (unpublished observation), thus leading to an immediate toxicity.

   The fate of the PRL-DAU ligand within the cell is not well understood. Binding experiments with MSH-DAU showed no interaction of the ligand with purified DNA whereas DAU itself was bound with high specificity (18). As the toxicity of MSH-DAU (3) and PRL-DAU is related to the respective receptors, it is reasonable to assume that both ligands undergo cleavage within the cell, and that the free DAU is responsible for the cytotoxic effects.

ACKNOWLEDGMENTS

This work was supported by the Schilling Foundation. H.C.B. is a research fellow of the Minerva and Minna James Heinemann Foundation. We are grateful to Mrs. M. Kopelowitz for skillful secretarial assistance.

REFERENCES

1. Iacobelli S, King RJB, Lindner HR, Lippman ME (eds). (1980): Hormones and Cancer, Raven Press, New York
2. Huggins C. (1965): Cancer Res 25:1163
3. Varga JM, Asato N, Lande S, Lerner AB. (1977): Nature 267:56
4. Lindner HR, Kohen F, Amsterdam A. (1980): In: Iacobelli S, King RJG, Lindner HR, Lippman ME (eds) Hormones and Cancer. Raven Press, NY, p 541
5. Muggia FM, Lippman ME, Heuson JC (eds). (1978): Reports from the Workshop on the Use of Steroids as Carriers of Cytotoxic Agents in Breast Cancer. Cancer Treatment Rep 62:1239
6. Hoff DDV, Rozencweig M, Slavik M, Muggia FM. (1977): J Urology 117:464
7. Martin PM, Sheridan PJ. (1982): J Ster Biochem 16:215
8. Shiu RPC. (1979): Cancer Res 39:4381
9. Osborne CK, Hamilton B, Nover M. (1982): J Clin Endocrinol Metab 55:86
10. Wang C, Hsueh AJW, Erickson GF. (1979): J Biol Chem 254:11330
11. Blossey HC, Gaier B, Kohen F. (1984): Proceedings of the 7th International Congress of Endocrinology, Abstract 2391
12. Weinstein Y. (1977): J Immunol 119:1223
13. Shiu RPC, Friesen HG. (1974): J Biol Chem 249:7902
14. Barkey RJ, Shani J, Amit T, Barzilai D. (1977): J Endocrinol 74:163
15. Costlow ME, Hample A. (1982): J Biol Chem 257:6971
16. NIH Consensus Developmental Conference (1980): Cancer 46:2759
17. Tritton TR, Yee G. (1982): Science 217:248
18. Wiesehahn G, Varga JM, Hearst JE. (1981): Nature 292:467

Prolactin. Basic and clinical correlates
R.M. MacLeod, M.O. Thorner and U. Scapagnini (eds.),
Fidia Research Series, vol. I,
Liviana Press, Padova © 1985

Section V
Target cell function
and peripheral receptors
for prolactin

PROLACTIN RECEPTORS ON RAT LYMPHOID TISSUES AND ON HUMAN T- AND B-LYMPHOCYTES: ANTAGONISM OF PROLACTIN BINDING BY CYCLOSPORINE

Diane Haddock Russell[1], Ruthann Kibler[2], Lynn Matrisian[3], Douglas F. Larson[1], Bonnie Poulos[2], and Bruce E. Magun[3]

Departments of Pharmacology[1], Molecular and Medical Microbiology[2], and Anatomy[3], University of Arizona, College of Medicine
Tucson, Arizona 85724

Prolactin may be the pituitary hormone of primary importance in the embryonic regulation of vertebrate growth, differentiation, and overall organization (1). Prolactin is coupled to altered macromolecular synthesis in a variety of mammalian tissues including spleen, thymus, kidney, liver, adrenals, heart, and reproductive tissues such as mammary gland and prostate (2-4). Administration of prolactin to rats induces ornithine decarboxylase (ODC), the rate-limiting enzyme in polyamine biosynthesis (5), and in certain tissues such as kidney, results in an elevated ribosomal RNA content (3).

Evidence suggests prolactin may have a physiological role in the regulation of humoral- and cell-mediated immune responses. Besedovsky and coworkers (6) have emphasized the parallel ontogeny in mammalian species of the immune and endocrine systems. For example, mice thymectomized near birth and congenitally thymusless mice with T-lymphocyte deficiencies displayed numerous endocrine disturbances, suggesting that the thymus is involved in the expression of the neuroendocrine system (7,8). Prolactin receptors have been identified for the first time on human T- and B-lymphocytes (9-11). These receptors may explain why antibody formation in response to sheep red blood cells and the development of dinitrochlorobenzene-induced contact dermatitis are impaired in hypox rats (12) and why immunocompetence can be restored by administration of prolactin, placental lactogen, or growth hormone. The administration of bromocriptine, which specifically decreases the release and thus the circulating level of prolactin, also suppresses antibody production and contact dermatitis, implicating prolactin as a physiological hormone in the regulation of immunocompetence (13). Immunocompetence again is restored by the administration of either prolactin or growth hormone.

Cyclosporine (CsA), a novel investigative immunosuppressive agent used in human organ transplant patients to inhibit rejection processes, blocked the prolactin-stimulated ODC activity in rat lymphoid tissues as well as in a variety of tissues with prolactin receptors including the kidney (3). The administration of CsA also rapidly elevated the serum prolactin level in rats to 4-fold of the control value within 1 h of injection. This elevation could be blocked by bromocriptine which decreases the serum prolactin level below control levels.

This paper reports the data obtained in this laboratory which substantiate the presence of prolactin receptors on lymphocytes and the effects of CsA to block prolactin action by altering both prolactin binding to these receptors and the subsequent increase in ODC activity.

Table 1. *Prolactin-stimulated ODC activity in intact and hypox rats: Effect of CsA*

		ODC (pmol/30 min/mg/protein)
Spleen		
	INTACT	
	PRL (22 mg/Kg BW)	66 ± 9*
	PRL/CsA (1.2 mg/Kg BW)	32 ± 3
	Vehicle	23 ± 5
	CsA/vehicle	24 ± 5
	HYPOX	
	PRL (22 mg/Kg BW)	816 ± 71*
	PRL/CsA (1.2 mg/Kg BW)	48 ± 9
	Vehicle	85 ± 20
	CsA/vehicle	52 ± 18
Thymus		
	INTACT	
	PRL (22 mg/Kg BW)	333 ± 27*
	PRL/CsA (1.2 mg/Kg BW)	172 ± 15
	Vehicle	182 ± 26
	CsA/vehicle	179 ± 13
	HYPOX	
	PRL (22 mg/Kg BW)	868 ± 123*
	PRL/CsA (1.2 mg/Kg BW)	556 ± 13
	Vehicle	473 ± 52
	CsA/vehicle	491 ± 48

*Data differ from vehicle controls (P < 0.001).

Vehicle-prolactin was dissolved in saline/0.05 N NaOH with the final pH adjusted to 7.5 with 0.1 N HCl. CsA was dissolved in 5% ethanol, sesame seed oil. All groups received both the saline and oil vehicle to correct for effects of the saline or oil vehicle on ODC activity. CsA was injected i.p. 15 min prior to administration of prolactin. ODC was measured 6 h after prolactin injection. Each value represents the mean ± SEM of at least 5 separate animals assayed in quadruplicate.

PROLACTIN-STIMULATED ORNITHINE DECARBOXYLASE ACTIVITY IN THE SPLEEN AND THYMUS OF INTACT AND HYPOPHYSECTOMIZED RATS: EFFECT OF CYCLOSPORINE

The basal activity of ODC was higher in spleen of hypophysectomized (hypox) rats than in intact rats (Table 1). In response to the administration of prolactin, ODC activity increased within 6 h to 860 pmol/30 min/mg protein in hypox rats compared to 66 in intact rats. A significant inhibition of ODC induction was demonstrated in both the intact and hypox rat spleen in response to CsA. In thymus, the basal activity of ODC again was higher in hypox rats (Table 1). However, in response to administration of prolactin, the elevation of ODC in thymus of both intact and hypox rats was approximately 2-fold. Administration of CsA completely blocked the ability of prolactin to induce ODC in the intact thymus and also significantly blocked the elevation in the thymus of hypox rats.

DEMONSTRATION OF PROLACTIN RECEPTORS IN SPLEEN AND THYMUS

Membrane fractions from spleen and thymus showed an average of 19% specific binding of $[^{125}I]$-prolactin. In the 3 preparations of each tissue assayed, the binding varied from 14 to 32% specific binding, and this binding was not affected by large excesses of cold growth hormone, insulin, or epidermal growth factor added to the incubation mixture. This percentage of specific binding was similar to that detected in human peripheral blood mononuclear cell (MNC) populations (9,11,14). This binding could be reduced to 1 to 4% specific binding by the addition of CsA to the assays.

EFFECT OF PROLACTIN ON RNA AND DNA CONTENT OF RAT THYMUS AND SPLEEN

In spleen, administration of prolactin resulted in a small but nonsignificant decrease in the RNA content as assessed 24 h after the injection of prolactin (Table 2). However, administration of prolactin daily X 2 and daily X 3 resulted in a significant decrease in RNA content of spleen. When prolactin was administered for 4 days the RNA content returned to normal suggesting there is a compensatory mechanism to return the RNA content toward control value. DNA content of the spleen was significantly depressed by 1, 2, or 3 injections of prolactin but, again, it returned to near normal control value when prolactin was administered daily for 4 days. In contrast to spleen, administration of prolactin resulted in a significant increase in RNA content of thymus in response to 1, 2 or 3 injections. Again, after 4 injections of prolactin, the RNA content returned toward normal value. DNA content of the thymus was decreased after 1 or 2 injections of prolactin and was not significantly different from controls after 3 or 4 injections of prolactin.

PROLACTIN RECEPTORS ON HUMAN PERIPHERAL
BLOOD MONONUCLEAR CELLS (MNC)

Since prolactin administration was capable of inducing ODC in rat spleen and thymus, lymphoid tissues with large populations of lymphocytes, we wondered whether we could demonstrate specific prolactin receptors on MNC. We found that [125I]-prolactin specifically bound to MNC at 37 C, reaching a plateau within 2 h of 24 pg bound/10^6 cells. The detection of specific binding at 4, 6, and 8 h demonstrated the same amount of specific binding detectable at 2 h. When [125I]-prolactin binding was performed at 4 C, the binding still plateaued within 2 h, but the specific [125I]-prolactin bound was 12 pg/10^6 cells. The saturation of specific [125I]-prolactin binding sites was measured as a function of the added concentration of [125I]-prolactin (Fig. 1). To insure equilibrium conditions, the binding assays were conducted at 4 C. Nonspecific binding was 40-50% of total [125I]-prolactin binding in all cases. The nonspecific binding in the presence of [125I]-prolactin plus excess cold prolactin was subtracted from binding in the presence of radiolabel alone to obtain the amount of specific binding. The insert to Figure 1 displays a Scatchard plot derived from specific [125I]-prolactin binding. Dissociation constant K_D app = 1.66 nM and the calculated receptor number was 360 per cell.

Table 2. *Effect of prolactin administration on RNA and DNA content of rat thymus and spleen*

	mg RNA/g wet wt.	mg DNA/g wet wt.
Spleen		
Control	5.97 ± 0.12	19.3 ± 1.34
Prolactin (22 mg/Kg BW)	5.48 ± 0.21	15.6 ± 0.73*
Prolactin, daily X 2	5.33 ± 0.18**	15.7 ± 0.81*
Prolactin, daily X 3	5.60 ± 0.07**	15.7 ± 0.72*
Prolactin, daily X 4	6.10 ± 0.29	18.3 ± 1.74
Thymus		
Control	5.08 ± 0.20	34.6 ± 1.99
Prolactin (22 mg/Kg BW)	5.42 ± 0.07**	30.9 ± 0.95**
Prolactin, daily X 2	5.51 ± 0.12**	31.2 ± 0.78**
Prolactin, daily X 3	5.43 ± 0.10**	33.1 ± 0.91
Prolactin, daily X 4	5.12 ± 0.07**	33.3 ± 1.1

* Data differ from control value ($P < 0.025$).
** Data differ from control value ($P < 0.05$).

Tissues were extracted 24 h after last injection. RNA content was determined by the method of Munro and Fleck (15) and DNA content by the method of Burton (16). Each value represents mean ± SEM of 10 separate animals.

EFFECTS OF CYCLOSPORINE ON SPECIFIC
[125I]-PROLACTIN BOUND TO MNC

CsA at concentrations between 0.1 nM and 10 nM increased the amount of prolactin bound to MNC about 4-fold when incubated at 37 C (Fig. 2). At concentrations of 1 and 10 uM CsA there was no detectable specific binding of [^{125}I]-prolactin. Interestingly, the ability of 10 nM CsA to enhance prolactin binding was abolished when the assays were conducted at 4 C. When tritiated CsA was incubated with MNC, and prolactin was added in increasing concentrations, it was found that 1 nM prolactin displaced more than 50% of the specific binding of tritiated CsA (1 nM) from MNC (Fig. 3). Specific binding of tritiated CsA was displaced totally at prolactin concentrations of 0.1, 1.0, and 10 uM. Figure 3 depicts a representative experiment which was performed 3 times with similar results. Growth hormone in similar experiments did not displace tritiated CsA.

EFFECTS OF A CYCLOSPORINE ANALOG
WITH NO KNOWN IMMUNOSUPPRESSIVE ACTION
ON PROLACTIN BINDING TO MNC

Cyclosporin H (CsH), an analog without the immunosuppressive action of CsA, was tested for its ability to alter prolactin binding to MNC (Table 3). CsA at 1 uM

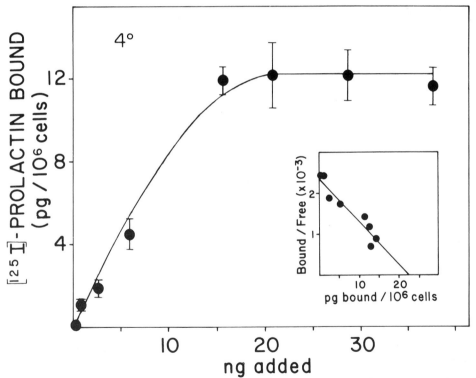

Figure 1. Specific [^{125}I]-prolactin binding to MNC at 4 C as a function of the concentration of radiolabeled prolactin. The assay was conducted as described in the text with the exceptions of a 6 h incubation period at each point and the addition of increasing amounts of radiolabeled prolactin. Results are the mean ± SEM of 6 determinations at each point. The insert displays a Scatchard plot derived from the specific radiolabeled prolactin binding data.

did not affect the amount of specific binding of prolactin whereas in the same experiment, the addition of 1 uM CsA was able to completely abolish any detectable specific binding of prolactin to MNC.

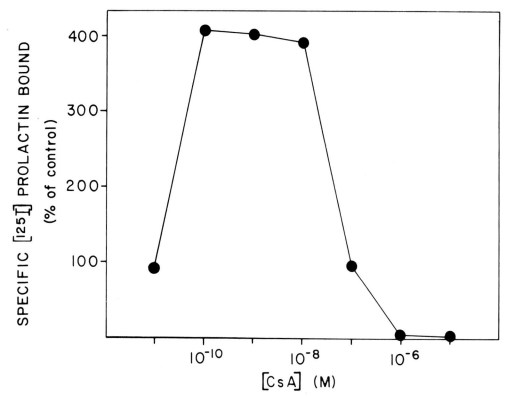

Figure 2. Effect of CsA concentration on specific binding of [125I]-prolactin to MNC. The assay was performed as described in the text with these alterations: 6 ng/assay of radiolabeled prolactin (ca. 100,000 cpm) was supplemented with unlabeled ovine prolactin to a final concentration of 1 nM. Cells were incubated for 4 h at 37 C. Nonspecific binding was determined by adding ovine prolactin to certain assays to a final concentration of 1 uM.

Table 3. *Prolactin binding to MNC in the presence of CsA or CsH*

	Specific Binding of PRL (pg/10^6 cells $\pm$ SE)
[125I]PRL (1 nM)	14.7 $\pm$ 2.0
[125I]PRL (1 nM) $\pm$ CsA (1 uM)	0
[125I]PRL (1 nM) $\pm$ CsH (1 uM)	14.3 $\pm$ 1.8

CsH was dissolved in ethanol at 40 mg/ml and diluted to the appropriate concentration with binding medium (11). Control cells in ethanol identically diluted were run to assure that ethanol did not affect [125I]-prolactin binding.

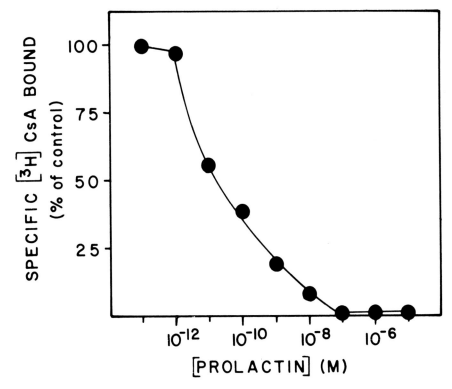

Figure 3. [³H]CsA (50,000 cpm/assay, 3 nM) was incubated with 2 x 10⁶ cells for 4 h under conditions described in the text except that the assay was conducted at 4 C. To assess nonspecific binding, cells were incubated with tritiated CsA plus 1 uM unlabeled CsA. Prolactin at concentrations between 0.1 pM to 10 uM was added at the initiation of certain assays to assess its ability to compete with tritiated CsA specific binding sites.

DEMONSTRATION OF THE SPECIFIC BINDING OF PROLACTIN TO HUMAN AND MOUSE CELL LINES

In order to determine whether prolactin receptors might be a general component of such cell lines, we measured prolactin specific binding to 4 cell lines in continuous culture. All cell lines tested had specific prolactin binding sites (Table 4). The highest amount of specific binding (91.1 pg/10⁶ cells) was detected for K562, human erythroleukemia cell line. Binding assays were performed on 2 x 10⁶ cells from populations grown for 3 days with cell densities of 5-10 x 10⁵ cells/ml.

EFFECT OF CYCLOSPORINE ON THE AMOUNT OF PROLACTIN BOUND TO T- AND B-LYMPHOCYTES ISOLATED FROM HUMAN SPLEEN

Previously we have reported the specific binding of [¹²⁵I]-prolactin to T- and B-cells fractionated from MNC (11). However, because it is difficult to obtain adequate numbers

Table 4. *Demonstration of specific binding of prolactin to human and mouse cell lines*

Cell Line	Origin	Specific Binding of PRL (pg/10^6 cells)
DAUDI	human (B-lymphoma)	46.1
K562	human (erythroleukemia)	91.1
EL-4	mouse (thymoma)	36.6
SP2/O-Ag14	mouse (plasmacytoma)	45.9

Table 5. *Effect of CsA on prolactin binding to T- and B-lymphocytes isolated from human spleen*

| | Specific Binding of PRL (pg/10^6 cells) | | | |
	T-Lymphocytes		B-Lymphocytes	
	Spleen 1*	Spleen 2	Spleen 1	Spleen 2
PRL (1 nM)	2.8	2.1	17.4	11.3
PRL (1 nM) + CsA (0.1 nM)	9.2	1.8	26.0	6.1
PRL (1 nM) + CsA (1 nM)	16.3	12.6	18.9	22.4
PRL (1 nM) + CsA (10 nM)	7.3	12.3	14.1	19.2
PRL (1 nM) + CsA (0.1 uM)	0.7	0.6	7.1	0.6
PRL (1 nM) + CsA (1.0 uM)	0.1	0	0	0.1

* Spleen 1 was from a 42-year-old female and spleen 2 from a 28-year-old male. Each value represents the mean of quadruplicate determinations. The SEM was 10% or less in all cases.

of B-lymphocytes from blood, we now have measured the amount of prolactin bound to T- and B-lymphocytes isolated from human spleen (Table 5). The T-lymphocytes isolated from 2 human spleens bound specifically 2.1 and 2.8 pg/10^6 cells prolactin whereas B-lymphocytes bound 11.3 and 17.4 pg/10^6 cells prolactin. Addition of 1 nM CsA elevated specific prolactin binding over 5-fold in T-lymphocytes from 2 separate human spleens. Inhibition of prolactin binding was detected at 0.1 and 1.0 uM in both T- and B-cell populations. The elevation of specific binding of prolactin to B-cells by 1 and 10 nM CsA was 2-fold or less in both cases.

The detection of the rapid induction of ODC in a variety of rat tissues in response to prolactin administration was suggestive of the widespread presence of prolactin receptors (3,17,18). The ability to induce ODC by prolactin in the same tissues after hypophysectomy constituted further evidence of a direct induction effect rather than a secondary effect of prolactin action. Tissues known to have prolactin receptors such as liver and kidney (19) demonstrated dose-dependent elevations in ODC activity within 6 h of prolactin administration (3). The relatively high ODC activity of rat kidney was abolished after hypophysectomy and restored by prolactin, suggesting that prolactin may be an important hormone in the maintenance of the high basal activity of ODC of rat kidney.

The ability of prolactin to alter ODC expression in the rat thymus and spleen suggested that T- and B-lymphocytes which are prevalent in these tissues might contain prolactin receptors and that prolactin could directly influence mitogenesis and/or the expression of lymphocyte gene products. Specific prolactin receptors were demonstrated in rat spleen and thymus. The prolactin binding assays conducted on membrane fractions from rat spleen and thymus demonstrated an average of 19% specific binding of [^{125}I]-prolactin. This binding was not affected by the addition of large excesses of cold bovine or ovine growth hormone, zinc-free insulin, or epidermal growth factor isolated from Rat-1 fibroblasts (submitted to Endocrinology). A similar percentage of specific binding of prolactin was detected in human peripheral blood MNC populations (9,11,14,20). Populations of T- and B-lymphocytes isolated from human spleen demonstrated prolactin receptors. Splenic B-cells bound 6 times as much prolactin as T-cells.

CsA, at concentrations known to be immunosuppressive, appears to be a specific competitor of prolactin receptors in spleen and thymus of rat, in human MNC, and in human spleen T- and B-lymphocytes. It recently has been reported that prolactin significantly enhanced the mitogenic potential of concanavalin A, a T-cell mitogen, on mouse splenic cell cultures but not lipopolysaccaride, a B-cell mitogen (21). This is intriguing in light of the ability of CsA to inhibit T-cell mitogenesis in response to plant lectin or transplantation antigens (22-24). Also, CsA does not suppress antibody responses to lipopolysaccaride in male mice (21).

In summary, prolactin receptors appear to be functional entities of T- and B-lymphocytes and to be specifically sensitive to CsA inhibition. Both specific binding of prolactin and induction of ODC are inhibited by CsA. An inactive analog of CsA with no immunosuppressive action, cyclosporin H, does not inhibit prolactin binding to MNC populations. It will be important to determine whether specific gene products of lymphocytes are regulated by prolactin.

REFERENCES

1. Riddle O. (1963): J Natl Cancer Inst 31:1039
2. Thomson MJ, Richards JF. (1978): Life Sci 22:337
3. Russell DH, Larson DF, Cardon SB, Copeland JG. (1984): Mol Cell Endocrinol 33:159
4. Bern HA, Nicoll CS. (1968): Recent Progr Hormone Res 24:681
5. Russell DH, Durie BGM. (1978): Polyamines as Markers of Normal and Malignant Growth. Raven Press, New York
6. Besedovsky H, Sorkin E. (1977): Clin Exp Immunol 27:1
7. Besedovsky HO, Sorkin E. (1974): Nature (Lond) 249:356
8. Pierpaoli W, Besedovsky HO. (1975): Clin Exp Immunol 20:323
9. Russell DH, Matrisian L, Kibler R, Larson D, Magun BE, Poulos B, Copeland JG. (1984): Fed Proc 43:818
10. Larson DF, Cardon SB, Copeland JG, Russell DH. (1984): Fed Proc 43:818
11. Russell DH, Matrisian L, Kibler R, Larson DF, Poulos B, Magun BE. (1984): Biochem Biophys Res Commun, in press
12. Nagy E, Berczi I, Friesen HG. (1983): Acta Endocrinol 102:351

13. Nagy E, Berczi I, Wren GE, Asa SL, Kovacs K. (1983): Immunopharmacology 6:231.
14. Russell DH, Larson DF, Matrisian L, Kibler R, Poulos B, Magun B, Copeland JG. (1984): Clin Pharmacol Ther 35:271
15. Munro HN, Fleck A. (1966): Meth Biochem Anal 14:113
16. Burton K. (1956): Biochem J 62:315
17. Richards JF. (1975): Biochem Biophys Res Commun 63:292
18. Thomson MJ, Richards JF. (1978): Life Sci 22:337
19. Dube D, Kelly PA, Pelletier G. (1980): Mol Cell Endocrinol 18:109
20. Russell DH, Kibler R, Larson DF, Poulos B, Magun BE. (1984): Fed Proc 43:1890
21. Spangelo BL, Hall NR, McGillis JP, Goldstein AL. (1984): Fed Proc 43:1610
22. Borel JF. (1983): Transplant Proc 15:2219
23. White DJG, Plumb AM, Pawelec G, Brons G. (1979): Transplantation 27:55
24. Ryffel B, Gotz U, Heuberger B. (1982): J Immunol 129:1978

Prolactin. Basic and clinical correlates
R.M. MacLeod, M.O. Thorner and U. Scapagnini (eds.),
Fidia Research Series, vol. I,
Liviana Press, Padova © 1985

Section V
Target cell function
and peripheral receptors
for prolactin

HYPERCALCIURIA AND BONE CHANGES IN MALE HYPERPROLACTINEMIC RATS

Robert A. Adler*, Martha Stauffer, Joseph Gutman, and Truls Brinck-Johnsen

Departments of Medicine and Pathology, Dartmouth Medical School,
Hanover, NH 03756

Premature osteoporosis may be an important complication of the galactorrhea-amenorrhea syndromes. Three groups of investigators have reported that women with prolactin-secreting pituitary tumors have evidence of bone mineral loss (1-3). The bone mineral deficit may persist after apparent cure of the prolactinoma (1), and it is unclear whether the osteopenia in prolactinoma patients is due to hyperprolactinemia per se, the associated hypogonadism, or some other factor (1-3). During normal lactation in the rat, calcium is mobilized from bone (4,5), and it has been postulated that prolactin is responsible for such a calcium-mobilizing action (6). However, there has been no direct demonstration of a prolactin effect on bone. We now report preliminary evidence of bone loss in hyperprolactinemic rats without hypogonadism.

From each of several litters of weanling Fischer rats, two males received 3 littermate anterior pituitary (AP) grafts under the kidney capsule. Two other males received muscle tissue grafts and served as controls. AP-grafted animals have normal growth hormone (7) and thyroid hormone (8) secretion. Although copulatory behavior is abnormal in hyperprolactinemic rats, male AP-grafted rats have basically normal gonadal function as manifested by normal testes weight and normal serum testosterone concentration (9). To compensate for the increased glucocorticoid secretion of AP-grafted rats, a subgroup of AP-grafted and muscle-implanted control rats were adrenalectomized at the time of grafting. All adrenalectomized animals received corticosterone pellets (Innovative Research of America) and drank 0.9% saline.

All surgery was performed soon after weaning, at age approximately 28 days and animals were maintained thereafter on a normal calcium diet for 7 to 9 weeks. Body

---

* Present address: Medical Service (111-P), Veterans Administration Hospital, Richmond, VA 23249.

growth rate was the same for all animals, including the adrenalectomized, corticosterone-replaced group. Approximately five weeks after pituitary or muscle implantation, the adrenalectomized rats were placed in individual metabolic cages for two 24-hour periods separated by one week. Urine was frozen for later assays. Urinary immunoreactive corticosterone (10) was within the normal range in AP-implanted and muscle-implanted adrenal- ectomized rats implanted with a corticosterone pellet one and two weeks before urine collection. Urinary calcium was determined by a modification of Gitelman's colorometric technique (11). Urinary cyclic AMP was determined by radioimmunoassay kit (Becton Dickinson). Values are reported as the average of two determinations. As shown in Table 1 below, urinary calcium was higher in the hyperprolactinemic rats, but urinary cyclic AMP excretion was similar.

Table 1. *Urinary excretion in hyperprolactinemic and control adrenalectomized, corticosterone-replaced rats*

	Calcium mg/100 gm BW 24 h	Cyclic AMP nmoles/100 gm BW 24 h
AP-implanted (n = 4)	34.9 ± 2.4*	88.0 ± 8.1
Muscle-implanted (n = 4)	22.1 ± 3.2	88.0 ± 6.6

* Different from muscle-implanted at $P < 0.02$.

At sacrifice (age approximately 11 weeks), all AP-implanted rats were found to have viable, well-vascularized pituitary grafts under the kidney capsule. Hind leg bones were rapidly removed and were placed in buffered neutral formalin for later histology. Tibiae from 11 hyperprolactinemic intact and 4 hyperprolactinemic adrenalectomized rats were compared with 10 muscle-implanted intact and 4 muscle-implanted adrenalectomized rats. Femora were studied from 7 AP-implanted (n = 4) and 6 control (n = 4) rats and from the adrenalectomized AP-implanted (n = 4) and control (n = 4) rats. One tibia from the latter subgroups was also frozen for later determination of bone calcium content.

Histological sections were made after decalcification of bones with EDTA, and cross sections from a standardized sampling site from the mid-tibial and mid-femoral diaphyses were stained with hematoxylin and eosin or toluidine blue.

In the tibiae of AP-implanted rats, an increase in vascular channels was seen (Figs. 1A, 2A). Similar-site cross-sections from control rats are shown in Figures 1B and 2B.

Although the endosteal surface was smooth in all sections, lining the endosteum of the bones of some AP-implanted rats there appeared to be hyperplastic osteoblasts with prominent golgi. In the non-adrenalectomized AP-implanted rats, there was no histological evidence of glucocorticoid excess, and the bone histology did not differ from that of adrenalectomized, corticosterone-replaced AP-implanted rats.

Bone area measurements were quantitated from images of the histological slides projected onto a GTCO digitizer by a camera lucida. Using an LED cursor connected to an IBM XT computer, bone cortical area was calculated by subtracting medullary cavity cross-sectional area from the total subperiosteal cross-sectional area. As shown in Table 2, bone area was decreased in femora from hyperprolactinemic rats.

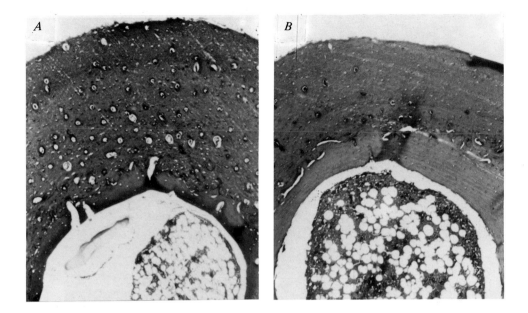

Figure 1A. Lower power view of the tibia from a hyperprolactinemic rat. Decalcified sections from the tibial diaphysis were made approximately 1 mm proximal to the fibula and were stained with toluidine blue.

Figure 1B. Lower power view of the tibia from a control rat, using methods as in Fig. 1A.

At sacrifice of the adrenalectomized, corticosterone-replaced subgroup, tibiae were weighed and then placed in 10% trichloroacetic acid (TCA) for 4 seven-day periods (12). The TCA was then assessed for calcium content per gram of bone tissue (11).

Table 2. *Mid-femoral bone cross-sectional area*

	Area (mm^2)
AP-implanted (n = 7)	3.06 ± 0.30*
(n = 7)	
Muscle-implanted	4.02 ± 0.20

* = Different from muscle-implanted group at P < 0.05.

Even in this small group of animals it was possible to demonstrate significantly less calcium in the bones of AP-grafted rats (114.7 ± 6.7 vs. 141.1 ± 8.0 mg/gram wet weight, P < 0.05).

Mattheij reported that AP-grafted rats have hypercalciuria (13). However, his animals were not adrenalectomized and therefore had glucocorticoid excess (10), which might lead to bone loss and hypercalciuria. However, we have now shown that adrenalectomized AP-grafted rats receiving physiologic replacement doses of corticosterone also

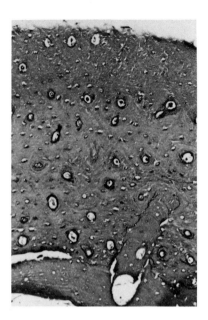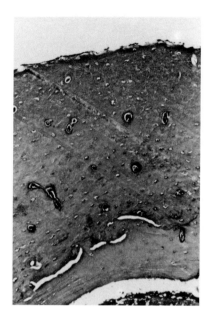

Figure 2. Higher power view of similar sections from A. AP-implanted rat and B. normoprolactinemic control rat.

have excess urinary calcium loss. The fact that urinary cyclic AMP was not elevated suggests that parathyroid hormone (PTH) was not involved in mobilization of bone calcium to produce the hypercalciuria, nor was there evidence to suggest decreased PTH secretion, causing hypercalciuria.

One possible cause of hypercalciuria is increased calcium absorption in the gut. Prolactin is claimed to increase gut absorption in Vitamin D-deficient rats (6), although non-adrenalectomized AP-grafted rats do not have increased gut calcium absorption (also in the absence of Vitamin D, 14). An alternative source of the excess urinary calcium is bone. Histological and morphometric analysis of bones from AP-implanted rats suggests decreased cortical bone. Furthermore, the calcium content of the bones from hyperprolactinemic rats was lower than that of controls. Thus, it is reasonable to assume that bone calcium contributes to the excess urinary loss of calcium.

The bone changes and hypercalciuria were observed in male hyperprolactinemic rats with essentially normal androgen secretion (9). Moreover, changes could be measured after only 7 to 9 weeks of hyperprolactin-emia in young rats. The histological alterations were similar in AP-grafted rats with and without adrenalectomy.

In summary the data suggest that excess secretion of prolactin itself can lead to osteopenia. Further studies will be necessary to prove the hypothesis that excess prolactin secretion per se is an important contributor to the osteoporosis noted in prolactinoma patients.

ACKNOWLEDGMENTS

The authors acknowledge the excellent assistance of Linda M. Dunnack, Louise Hawthorne, Michele Biron, Mary Grace Ceresia, and Kathleen Lemieux. We wish to thank Dr. Bill Roebuck for the use of the computerized area measurement system. This work was supported in part by grant S07RR05392 from the NIH.

REFERENCES

1. Schlecte JA, Sherman B, Martin R. (1983): J Clin Endocrinol Metab 56:1120
2. Klibanski A, Neer R, Beitins IZ, Ridgway EC, Zervas NT, McArthur JW. (1980): N Engl J Med 303:1511
3. Cann CE, Martin MC, Genant HK, Jaffe RB. (1984): JAMA 251:626
4. Rasmussen P. (1977): Calc Tiss Res 23:87
5. Ellinger GM, Duckworth J, Dalgarno AC. (1952): Brit J Nutr 6:235
6. Pahuja DH, Deluca HF. (1981): Science 214:1038
7. Adler RA, Herzberg VL, Sokol HW. (1983): Life Sci 32:2957
8. Adler RA. (1981): Endocrinology 108:543A
9. Svare B, Bartke A, Doherty P, Mason I, Michael SD, Smith MS. (1979): Biol Reprod 21:529
10. Adler RA, Brinck-Johnsen T, Herzberg V, Sokol HW. (1983): Endocrinology 112:773A
11. Gitelman HJ. (1967): Anal Biochem 18:521
12. Komarkova A, Zahor Z, Czabanova A. (1967): J Lab Clin Med 69:102
13. Mattheij JAM, Sterrenberg L, Swarts HJM. (1980): Life Sci 27:2031
14. Adler RA, MacLaughlin J, Holick MF. (1980): Clinical Research 28:383A

Prolactin. Basic and clinical correlates
R.M. MacLeod, M.O. Thorner and U. Scapagnini (eds.),
Fidia Research Series, vol. I,
Liviana Press, Padova © 1985

Section VI
Comparative aspects of
prolactin production and function

COMPARATIVE ASPECTS OF PROLACTIN PRODUCTION AND FUNCTION: AN OVERVIEW

Alan S. McNeilly

MRC Reproductive Biology Unit, Centre for Reproductive Biology,
Edinburgh EH3 9EW Scotland

The intriguing observations by Nicoll and his colleagues of the presence of a substance(s) in serum which augments, synergistically, the stimulatory action of prolactin in the pigeon crop sac assay is potentially very important. This material, christened 'synlactin' remains to be established but indirect evidence suggests that it may be an insulin-like growth factor (IGF). A similar effect of human serum acting synergistically to enhance the action of prolactin in promoting Nb2 lymphoma cell growth *in vitro* was described by Dr. Henry Freisen in an earlier presentation.

These observations may have considerable importance since they suggest that the biological activity of prolactin, at least in terms of mitogenesis, may be enhanced by factors which were hitherto unknown. The refinement of the bioassay systems should allow identification of the activity which is an essential next step. Certainly these results may clarify the discrepancy between some prolactin effects *in vivo* which cannot be adequately replicated *in vitro*.

The characterization of two distinct forms of prolactin in the pituitaries of cichlid fish, both of which exhibit salt-retaining activity but only one of which promotes length increase, offers an alternative way of enhancing the mitogenic activity of prolactin. Whether this is particular to the cichlid fish remains to be determined but Batten and colleagues have shown clear differences in immunological activities of prolactin between bony fish and both lower fishes and higher vertebrates.

In a series of elegant studies, Goldsmith has shown that plasma levels of prolactin are increased in birds incubating eggs and in periods of seasonal sexual inactivity. Whether prolactin is causally related to the suppression of sexual activity is not known although a reciprocal relationship between LH and prolactin has been clearly defined. The precise hypothalamic control of prolactin secretion in birds remains unclear. However, Goldsmith has recently shown that thyroidectomy prevents prolactin secretion in starlings while injections of thyroxine will stimulate prolactin release. Indeed thyroidectomized birds remain sexually mature indefinitely while maintained on long, stimulatory photoperiods.

Those observations provide the first clear linkage between prolactin and thyroid hormone secretion in any species. Even though TRH causes release of both prolactin and TSH in mammals and abnormal thyroid function is related to a disruption of reproduction, the interaction between these components is unclear. In the bird it remains to be established how thyroxine moderates prolactin secretion and, in turn, how photoperiod modifies thyroid function. However, the recognition and description of the interaction between the thyroid, prolactin, and reproductive function in birds is a major first step.

Prolactin. Basic and clinical correlates
R.M. MacLeod, M.O. Thorner and U. Scapagnini (eds.),
Fidia Research Series, vol. I,
Liviana Press, Padova © 1985

Section VI
Comparative aspects of
prolactin production and function

COMPARATIVE ASPECTS OF THE GROWTH-PROMOTING ACTIONS OF PROLACTIN ON ITS TARGET ORGANS: EVIDENCE FOR SYNERGISM WITH AN INSULIN-LIKE GROWTH FACTOR

Charles S. Nicoll, Thomas R. Anderson, Nora J. Hebert and Sharon M. Russell

Department of Physiology-Anatomy and Cancer Research Laboratory
University of California, Berkeley, CA 94720 USA

Prolactin has a wide variety of physiological actions among the vertebrates (1,2) and these effects of the hormone have been grouped into six categories (Table 1). Several of these actions involve stimulating growth of target organs in the different vertebrate groups (Table 2). It is generally assumed that the growth-promoting effects of the hormone on these organs involve a direct action on the cells that constitute them. Indeed, convincing evidence that prolactin directly stimulates mammary growth *in vivo* was obtained by Lyons and his colleagues soon after the hormone was purified (3,4).

Table 1. *General categories of prolactin's action*

1. Regulation of water and electrolyte balance	4. Reproductive actions
2. Control of growth and/or development	5. Effects on integumentary (ectodermal) structures
3. Metabolic effects	6. Interactions with steroid hormones

Table 2. *Some target organs that grow in response to prolactin*

Class	Organs
Mammals	Mammary gland, prostate, seminal vesicles
Birds	Crop-sac of pigeons and doves
Amphibians	Tail fin of larval anurans and of urodeles; gills, nuptial, cloacal pads
Fish	Seminal vesicles in some species, kidney

It is also well established that prolactin has a direct growth-promoting effect on the crop-sac of pigeons and doves (5,6). However, despite these positive *in vivo* results, there are numerous reports of the lack of a mitogenic effect of prolactin on mammary epithelium *in vitro* (7). Only a few studies have reported a direct stimulatory effect of prolactin on mammary cell division in culture (e.g. 8,9). In addition, we have made numerous attempts over the past 25 years to demonstrate an *in vitro* mitogenic effect of prolactin on the pigeon crop-sac and all of these efforts were without success (Nicoll, unpublished). Although prolactin stimulates growth of the amphibian tail fin *in vivo* (1,2,10,11) and it antagonizes thyroxine-induced regression of this structure, prolactin has only the latter effect *in vitro* (11). Thus, prolactin again fails to stimulate growth by a direct action on cells or tissue *in vitro*. These results suggest that a factor

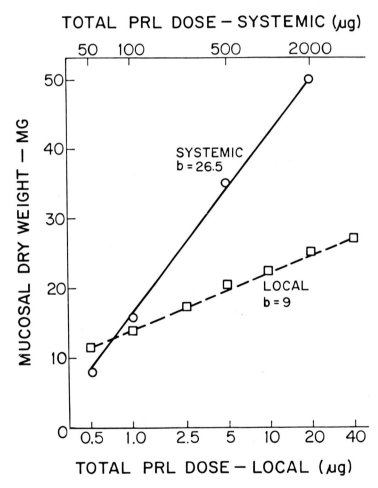

Figure 1. Dose-related effects of ovine prolactin on growth of the pigeon crop-sac mucosa. In the local assay the hormone was injected intradermally over one hemicrop so that it acted directly on the underlying responsive cells. In the systemic assay the hormone was injected in the loose skin between one of the legs and the lower abdomen. The dry weight of a 4 cm diameter disc of mucosal epithelium is the response index. Data from Nicoll (6,12).

or factors present *in vivo* is (are) missing from the *in vitro* experimental situations that have been tested.

Additional evidence suggesting that other factors are involved in the growth-promoting actions of prolactin on its target organs comes from comparisons of dose-response relationships of the hormone with the growth of the pigeon crop-sac mucosa. The crop-sac of birds is an expanded portion of the esophagus which is used to store food. In pigeons and doves the mucosal lining of this organ proliferates in response to prolactin. Clumps of dead epithelial cells are shed into the crop lumen and this "milk" is used to feed the young (1,5,6).

This response is used as a bioassay for prolactin, which can be injected at a site distant from the organ to induce a mucosal proliferation systemically (12) or the hormone can be injected into the skin overlying the crop to promote localized growth of the mucosal epithelium in the local microassay (5,6). When prolactin is injected subcutaneously at a site distant from the crop-sac a much steeper dose-response slope is obtained (12) than when the hormone is injected directly over the organ (6) by the local microassay procedure (Fig. 1). If the systemically-administered prolactin were acting in the same way as the locally-applied hormone, the slopes of the two dose-response relationships should be essentially the same, even though substantially more hormone is required to be effective systemically because it is diluted in the circulatory system. There are several possible explanations for this difference in slope. The systemically-administered hormone may be modified in the circulation to become more active, or it may have a longer half-life than it does locally. Alternatively, the higher doses of prolactin that are required for a systemic response may contain sufficient amounts of other pituitary hormones that act synergistically with prolactin (either directly or indirectly) to augment the response of the crop-sac to prolactin. The work of Bates *et al.* (13) gives credence to the latter suggestion. Another possibility is that the systemically-administered hormone may stimulate the production of a factor that acts synergistically with prolactin on the crop-sac mucosal epithelial cells.

In studying the basis for these discrepancies we have obtained evidence that the mitogenic action of prolactin on the pigeon crop-sac involves synergism with an insulin-like growth factor (IGF). Our experiments also revealed that an IGF and/or a hepatic factor may be involved in stimulating mammary growth.

RELATIONSHIP BETWEEN THE DRY WEIGHT AND THE DNA CONTENT OF THE CROP-SAC MUCOSA

In the local crop-sac assay procedure for prolactin the dry weight of a 4 cm diameter disc of mucosal epithelium is used to quantify the response (6). In order to verify that this measurement is a reliable index of growth of the cells, correlation and regression analyses were performed on previously recorded measurements (14) of the DNA content and dry weight of mucosal epithelial tissue samples. The results of these analyses are shown in Figure 2. Clearly, dry weight measurement is highly correlated with the DNA content of the mucosal epithelium. Hence, measuring mucosal dry weight is a reliable (although indirect) index of the cell number present in that tissue.

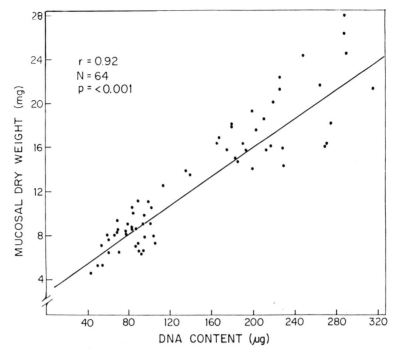

Figure 2. Relationship between the dry weight and the DNA content of 4 cm diameter discs of crop-sac mucosal epithelium. Data from Nicoll and Bern (14).

EFFECTS OF SYSTEMICALLY ADMINISTERED PITUITARY HORMONES AND EXTRACTS ON THE LOCAL RESPONSE OF CROP-SAC TO PROLACTIN INJECTION

Because of the difference in the dose-response slopes between locally-injected and systemically-administered prolactin (Fig. 1) experiments were conducted to determine whether factors present in pituitary extract, or any of the known pituitary hormones, either individually or in combination, could act synergistically with locally-injected pro-lactin when they were given systemically. The preparations were injected into the loose skin between one of the legs and the lower abdomen of pigeons according to the dose-schedule shown in Table 3. The doses used were selected on the following basis: Different amounts of the pituitary powder were injected systemically into pigeons to establish minimal stimulatory dose. The doses of the purified hormones were then determined from the amount of each that we would expect to be present in the pituitary

Table 3. *Doses of hormonal preparations used in systemic injections*

	Dose of preparation - ug/kg/day	
	Priming dose (day 1)	Maintenance dose (days 2-4)
Pituitary Powder	10,000	1,000
Prolactin	400	40
Growth Hormone	1,000	100
ACTH	24	2.4
LH, FSH, TSH	50	5

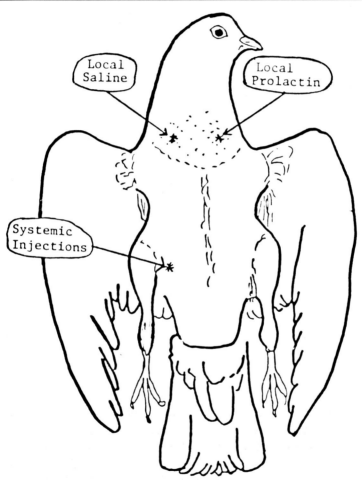

Figure 3. Diagram of the procedure used to study interactions between systemic treatments and the direct action of prolactin on the crop-sac. The systemically-injected materials were given subcutaneously in the loose skin between a leg and the lower abdomen. The saline treatment on the right side allows a measurement of the effects of the systemic treatment alone on the growth of the crop-sac mucosal epithelium. The prolactin-treated hemicrop allows assessment of possible interactions between the local prolactin and the systemic treatment.

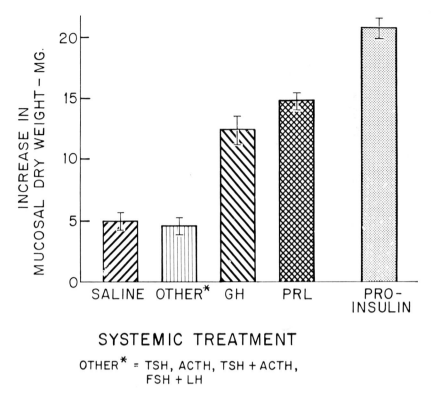

SYSTEMIC TREATMENT

OTHER* = TSH, ACTH, TSH + ACTH,
FSH + LH

Figure 4. Interaction between systemic treatments and local prolactin injections on the growth of the crop-sac mucosal epithelium. The responses of local injections of 1.0 ug of prolactin over one hemicrop are shown as the increase in mucosal dry weight over that of the saline-treated contralateral hemicrop.

powder based on data in the literature (15). A large "priming" dose was given on the first day and this was followed by smaller "maintenance" doses on the subsequent three days. During those three days, prolactin was injected locally twice daily over one side of the crop-sac of each pigeon and saline injections were given over the contralateral crop. This procedure is illustrated diagrammatically in Figure 3. It allows us to determine whether the systemic treatment alone had any effect on the crop-sac by measuring the mucosal dry wieght of the saline-injected side. In addition, we can determine, in the same pigeons, whether the systemic treatment affected the response to prolactin which was injected locally on the contralateral side.

The various hormone preparations caused little or no stimulation of the mucosa of the saline-injected side at the doses tested (15). In addition, the pituitary glycoprotein hormones (FSH, LH, TSH) and ACTH did not affect the response of the contralateral side to the locally-administered prolactin either individually or in different combinations (15 and Fig. 4). However, GH and prolactin significantly increased local response to prolactin. A crude pituitary extract was also highly effective in this test (15). These results suggest that the augmenting effects of the pituitary extract and of the prolactin and GH may be the result of stimulating of the production of some blood-borne factors. To test this possibility, the following experiment was conducted.

ANALYSIS OF SERUM FROM PIGEONS
FOR PROLACTIN-SYNERGISING ACTIVITY

Pigeons were injected with saline or ovine prolactin (10 mg/day for 3 days) and killed by decapitation. The blood was collected and the serum was separated and diluted to a concentration of 25% with physiological saline before being tested for crop-sac stimulating activity. The serum was also tested to determine whether it could augment the local response to a low dose of prolactin. The results of this experiment are shown in Figure 5. The serum from neither the saline-treated nor the prolactin-injected pigeons had significant direct crop-sac stimulating activity. In addition, the low dose of prolactin had minimal stimulatory activity. When the serum from saline-treated birds was combined with the low dose of prolactin, slight but significant augmentation of the

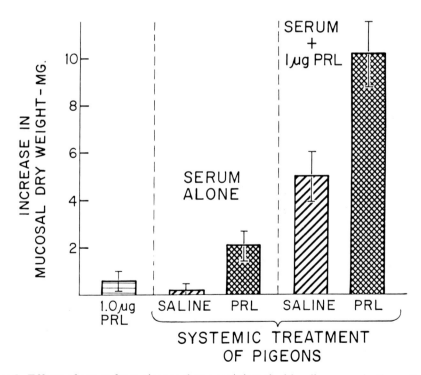

Figure 5. Effects of serum from pigeons that were injected with saline or prolactin on the local response of the pigeon crop-sac to 1.0 ug of ovine prolactin.

local prolactin response was observed. However, the serum from prolactin-treated birds showed a much greater augmentation of the local response to the hormone. These results indicate that serum from saline-injected pigeons contains a factor or factors that can act synergistically with prolactin to promote growth of the pigeon crop-sac mucosa. Injections of prolactin increase the serum concentration of this synergistic activity. Because the serum has no direct stimulatory activity by itself but shows prolactin synergising activity, we have called this activity synlactin (15,16).

ON THE NATURE OF THE CIRCULATING SYNLACTIN ACTIVITY

Prolactin and GH have similar effects on a variety of target organs (17). Since both hormones increased the responsiveness of the crop-sac to the locally-applied prolactin (Fig. 4), we considered some of their common actions that might be involved in this synergism. It has been reported that prolactin and GH increase the level of somatomedin

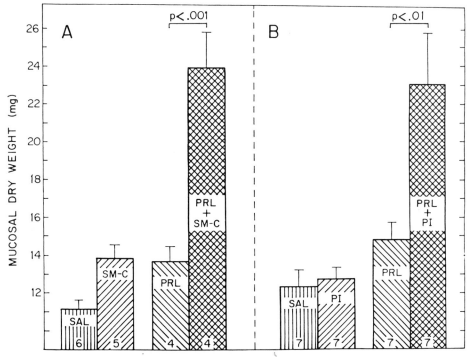

Figure 6. Effect of SM-C and proinsulin (PI) on the local response of the pigeon crop-sac to prolactin. Controlateral hemicrops were injected twice daily for two days with the indicated factors dissolved in physiological saline. The birds were killed on the third day of the experiment. In Expt. A, hemicrops were injected with a total dose of 8 ug of SM-C and 1.0 ug of prolactin, alone and in combination. In Expt. B, birds were treated with 10 ug of PI and 0.5 ug of prolactin. The number of pigeons in each group is shown within the bottom of each column. SAL = saline.

(SM) activity in the serum of hypophysectomized rats (18) and hypopituitary dwarf mice (19), and that they stimulate the secretion of SM activity by the perfused rat liver (20,21). Accordingly, it seemed worthwhile to investigate the possible involvement of IGFs as prolactin synergists. At this stage of our investigations purified preparations of SM were not available, but we could obtain ample quantities of proinsulin, which is a member of the IGF family of molecules (22).

When bovine proinsulin was injected systemically at a dose of 2 mg on day 1 and 0.2 mg on days 2-4, it was highly effective at synergising with locally-applied prolactin. (Fig. 4). These results indicate that the synergist that is present in the circulation of prolactin-treated pigeons (Fig. 5) and which is apparently stimulated by systemic injections of either prolactin or GH (Fig. 4) could be an IGF.

After completing the experiments with proinsulin, we obtained some highly purified human SM-C. It was tested along with the proinsulin for direct synergistic effects in the local crop-sac microassay. As shown in Figure 6, the SM-C itself had a slight stimulatory effect on the crop-sac epithelium and a low dose of prolactin stimulated a similar degree of growth. When the two hormones were combined, they showed a striking synergism. It would require at least a 10-fold increase in the dose of prolactin by itself to achieve the same degree of stimulation that was produced by prolactin plus SM-C. Similar results were obtained with proinsulin, although it did not stimulate mucosal growth by itself (Fig. 6).

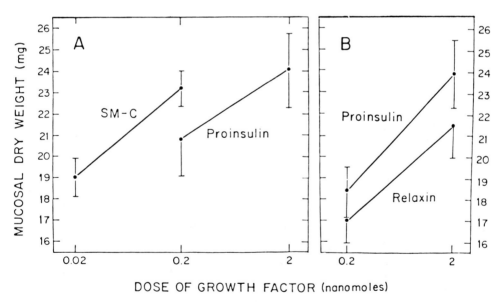

Figure 7. Comparisons of potencies of SM-C, relaxin, and PI as potentiators of the response of the pigeon crop-sac to prolactin. Hemicrops were treated with 0.5 ug of prolactin combined with the indicated doses of SM-C, relaxin, or PI. Responses to saline and to prolactin alone were 10.3 ± 1.0 and 16.0 ± 1.5 mg, respectively. Doses are shown in nanomoles to allow more meaningful comparisons to be made. We are assuming that the substances are of about equal purity. Each point represents data from 6-8 birds.

RELATIVE POTENCIES OF INSULIN-LIKE GROWTH FACTORS
AS PROLACTIN SYNERGISTS

Insulin, proinsulin, human SM-C, and relaxin (another member of the IGF family; (22) were tested at two doses for their ability to augment the crop-sac response to local injection of 1.0 ug of ovine prolactin. The proinsulin was used as a reference preparation. As is shown in Figure 7, SM-C was more potent than proinsulin whereas relaxin was less active. Insulin had almost no activity as a prolactin synergist in this system (data not shown). The relative potencies of these IGFs were as follows: SM-C = 436%, proinsulin = 100%, relaxin = 45%, and insulin = 1%. We also tested different preparations of multiplication-stimulating activity (MSA), which is the rat equivalent of SM-A or IGF II (23), and found that it was inactive as a prolactin synergist. These results indicate that the pigeon crop-sac receptor for IGF is unusual because in other systems proinsulin is usually much less active than insulin and relaxin generally has very little activity (24).

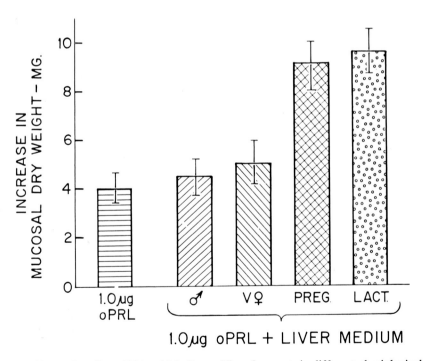

Figure 8. Effects of medium 199 in which slices of liver from rats in different physiological states were incubated on the local crop-sac response to 1.0 ug of ovine prolactin. V = virgin, PREG = pregnant and LACT = lactating. Each sample was assayed in 6 birds.

SECRETION OF SYNLACTIN ACTIVITY BY THE LIVER *IN VITRO*

The liver is a major source of IGFs in postnatal mammals (25). Accordingly, we investigated whether this organ from pigeons could secrete a prolactin synergist *in vitro*. In addition, we investigated whether the liver of mice and of rats in different physiological states could also secrete such a synergist. Liver tissue from these animals was cut into slices about 0.5 mm thick and incubated in medium 199 for 3-4 hours at a concentration of 50 mg of tissue/ml. The liver tissue was removed, the medium was centrifuged, and the supernatant was filtered through Whatman No. 1 paper. The medium was then diluted 1:5 with medium 199 and tested for crop-sac stimulating activity in the local assay (6). In addition, the medium samples were injected along with 1.0 ug ovine prolactin to test for prolactin-synergising activity. The medium in which slices of pigeon or rat liver were incubated had no prolactin-like activity when it was injected over the crop-sac alone (Table 4). In contrast, when medium containing secreted factors from the liver of pigeons, a mid-pregnant mouse, or a multiparous female rat was injected along with the low dose of prolactin, a striking synergism was obtained (Table 5).

Table 4. *Crop-stimulating activity of pigeon and rat liver medium alone*

Material Injected[1]	Response as % of Control
Saline	100 ± 5.0
1 ug oPRL	116 ± 6.5[2]
Pigeon liver medium	106 ± 7.8
Liver medium - prolactin or GH-treated rats	102 ± 5.7
Liver medium - pregnant rats	108 ± 8.0
Liver medium - lactating rats	106 ± 6.2

[1] Each group contained 8 pigeons

[2] $P < 0.05$

Table 5. *Prolactin synergising activity in medium from incubations of pigeon, mouse, and rat liver slices*

Material Injected	Crop-sac Response as % of Control
Saline	100 ± 0.6
1.0 ug oPRL	122 ± 7.4
Pigeon liver medium + 1.0 ug oPRL	172 ± 20.6
Pregnant mouse liver medium + 1.0 ug oPRL	160 ± 14.3
Female rat liver medium + 1.0 ug oPRL	186 ± 13.5

The ability of liver slices from rats in different physiological states to secrete this prolactin-synergising activity *in vitro* was then evaluated. For this experiment we used liver from young adult male and female rats, and from pregnant or lactating females. The results in Figure 8 show that liver medium from the male and virgin female rats had no prolactin-synergising activity. In contrast, liver from the pregnant and the lactating rats did secrete significant amounts of a prolactin synergist.

The liver of pregnant and lactating rats is exposed to high levels of placental lactogens and/or pituitary prolactin. Accordingly, it was of interest to determine whether prolactin could stimulate hepatic secretion of synlactin activity. Fifteen virgin female rats (2-month-old) were divided into 3 groups of 5 each and given twice daily subcutaneous injections of saline, bovine GH, or ovine prolactin. The two hormones were given at a dose of 1.0 ug/gm body weight/injection and the rats were treated for 7 days. On the eighth day they were killed and their livers sliced for incubation in medium 199. None of the hormone treatments caused the liver to secrete prolactin-like activity, as determined by the crop-sac assay (Table 4). Figure 9 shows that the medium in which liver slices from saline-treated virgins were incubated had no synlactin activity. Injections of GH into the females did not increase the ability of their livers to secrete prolactin-synergising activity *in vitro*, but prolactin treatment had a striking effect (Fig. 9).

MITOGENIC EFFECTS OF PROLACTIN, IGFS, AND HEPATIC FACTORS ON THE MAMMARY GLAND

Our findings that prolactin and IGFs act synergistically to promote growth of the crop-sac, and that the liver secretes synlactin activity, led us to investigate whether IGFs and/or liver factors might be involved in regulating the growth of other prolactin-responsive target organs. Accordingly, we investigated the mitogenic effects of IGFs, prolactin, and liver factors on rat mammary gland explants *in vitro*.

In order to conduct these studies, we developed a new mammary mitogenic assay. Other investigators have found it difficult to show mitogenic effects of prolactin on mammary explants from pregnant rats or mice *in vitro* (7). We reasoned that this difficulty was due to the fact that the pregnant glands are, in effect, "saturated" with endogenous mitogenic factors, including placental lactogens (26). Accordingly, rats that were 14-16 days pregnant were hysterectomized to eliminate some of these factors. Sixteen to eighteen hours later their mammary glands were removed and cut into explants, which were incubated in medium 199 for 6 hours. [3H]-labeled thymidine was present for the entire incubation period or was added during the last four hours of incubation. The mammary explants were then processed to isolate the DNA, which was counted for [3H] activity.

The effects of incubating mammary explants in medium in which liver slices had been previously incubated are shown in Figure 10. The medium containing products from male and virgin female liver slices had no mitogenic activity on the mammary explants. In contrast, medium from the incubation of liver slices from pregnant rats doubled [3H]-thymidine incorporation into DNA and liver medium from lactating females increased incorporation by about 50%. In this assay system, human SM-C and rat prolactin had mitogenic activity also, but bovine proinsulin was inactive (Fig. 11).

This mitogenic effect of the human SM-C is consistent with the recent results of Furlanetto and diCarlo who found that IGF-I stimulated growth of human mammary tumor cells *in vitro* (27). These results are of considerable significance because they indicate that hepatic factors may be involved in mammary growth.

Our results indicate that the growth-promoting effects of prolactin on the pigeon crop-sac involve both direct and indirect mechanisms. The direct effect appears to involve sensitization of the mucosal epithelial cells to the mitogenic action of a synergist (16). The indirect effect involves stimulation of the secretion of a synergist from some other source, which may be the liver.

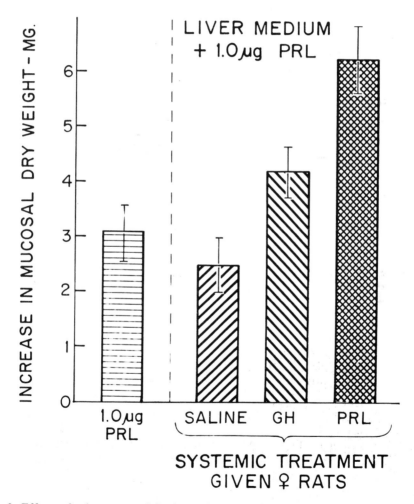

Figure 9. Effects of subcutaneous injections of saline, bGH, or ovine prolactin on the *in vitro* secretion of PRL-synergising activity by slices of virgin female rat liver. Each sample was assayed in 8 birds.

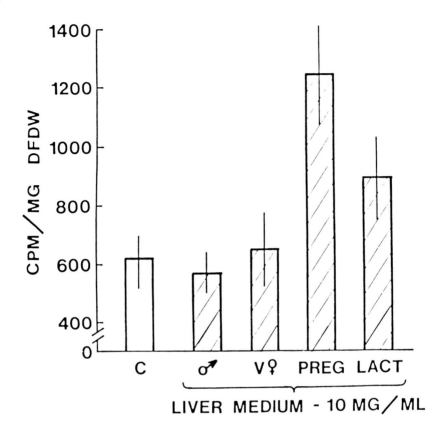

Figure 10. Effects of liver incubation medium at 10 mg tissue equivalent/ml on [³H]-thymidine incorporation into DNA of rat mammary gland explants incubated for 6 h *in vitro*. The medium was obtained from incubations of liver slices from male, virgin female (V), and pregnant (PREG) and lactating (LACT) rats. C = control. Each group consisted of 5 incubation flasks. The results are shown as CPM per mg defatted day weight (DFDW).

Several lines of evidence support the suggestion of an indirect effect. When prolactin was injected systemically at a dose that had little or no stimulatory effect on the crop-sac, the responsiveness of the organ to the direct mitogenic action of the hormone was greatly increased (Fig. 4). The systemically-administered prolactin also increased the serum level of a prolactin synergist (Fig. 5). Because systemically-injected proinsulin could mimic the augmenting effect of systemic prolactin the possibility arose that the synergistic activity in the serum of the prolactin-treated birds is due to an IGF. This suggestion was substantiated by the demonstration that several IGFs augmented the crop-sac response to prolactin when they were combined with the hormone and injected directly into the organ (Fig. 6). The results with liver incubation medium indicate that this organ is a source of the prolactin synergist (Table 5; Figs. 8-10) and that prolactin can stimulate hepatic secretion of this activity (Figs. 8-11).

Our results with the mammary gland explants also indicate that an IGF may be involved in the growth of this target organ of prolactin. Somatomedin-C and prolactin did have direct mitogenic effects on mammary explants *in vitro* (Fig. 11). More significantly, medium from incubation of liver from pregnant and lactating rats had mammogenic activity but liver medium from male and virgin female rats did not (Fig. 10). These results with liver medium in the mammary assay are consistent with our findings with the crop-sac. Only medium from incubates of liver from pregnant or lactating rats had significant synlactin activity (Fig. 8). It should be noted here that the synergist secreted by the liver is not prolactin itself; the liver incubation medium alone was inactive in the crop-sac assay (Table 4) and had no detectable prolactin activity in an RIA for rat prolactin (data not shown). Furthermore, it is unlikely that SM-C is responsible for this synergism, because analysis of similar medium samples in an RIA for human SM-C showed that the liver of virgin and pregnant females secretes similar amounts of that IGF (Russell and Nicoll, unpublished).

Our findings with the liver incubation medium samples are significant in relation to previous studies which were of undetermined physiological significance. Ovine and rat prolactin were reported to stimulate the secretion of bioactive SM (i.e., sulfate incorporation into cartilage) by perfused liver of male rats (20,21). Surprisingly, prolactin was 20 times more potent in this regard than was GH. Furthermore, prolactin injec-

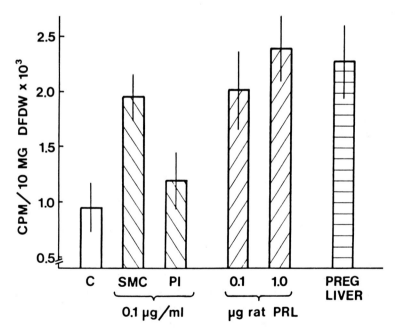

Figure 11. Effects of human somatomedin-C (SMC), bovine proinsulin (PI), rat prolactin and pregnant (PREG) rat liver incubation medium on [³H]-thymidine incorporation into DNA of rat mammary explants *in vitro*. See legend of Fig. 10.

408

tions restore the serum levels of bioactive SM (sulfation factor activity) in hypophysectomized rats (18). However, these prolactin treated rats do not grow! Thus, the SM
activity that is secreted by the liver in response to prolactin cannot be the same as the
SM that is involved in the promotion of somatic growth. Accordingly, the prolactin-
stimulated hepatic SM activity is probably involved in regulating other functions.

Our results presented here indicate that the prolactin-stimulated SM activity in rats
(18,20,21) may be related to the synlactin activity that we found in pigeons. The role
of this factor in rats and pigeons may be to stimulate the growth of prolactin-responsive
organs (i.e. the mammary gland and crop-sac, respectively) in concert with prolactin.
In view of the evidence that prolactin-dependent synlactin activity is secreted by the
liver, other data in the literature take on a new significance.

It has been reported that the hepatic receptors for prolactin increase during pregnancy in rats, (28,29) mice (30) and rabbits (31). Our results indicate that these receptors
could be concerned with synlactin secretion by the liver in response to prolactin. Thus,

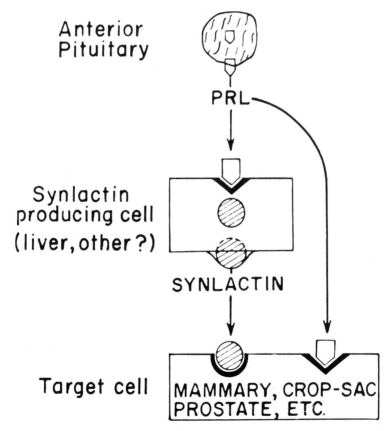

Figure 12. Schematic diagram of the synlactin hypothesis. Adapted from Laron's (34) diagram
of the somatomedin hypothesis.

during pregnancy when the plasma levels of lactogenic hormones are high (i.e. from the pituitary and/or from the placenta), the liver is presumably sensitized to prolactin, as evidenced by the increase in receptors for the hormone. If these receptors are involved in synlactin secretion, the condition of pregnancy would favor high circulating levels of the growth factor. The synlactin could then act in concert with prolactin and ovarian steroids to promote mammary growth. Anderson *et al.* (15) have suggested that a similar mechanism may operate to promote growth of the crop-sac of pigeons and doves during egg incubation when plasma prolactin levels are rising (32,33).

Our synlactin hypothesis is presented schematically in Figure 12, modified from Laron's (34) diagram of the somatomedin hypothesis. Obviously, the mechanism of prolactin's growth-promoting effects would appear to have much in common with that of GH. However, in the case of the latter hormone, an IGF is thought to mediate its growth-promoting effects [hence the term somatomedin (25)] but IGFs alone have little or no activity on the crop-sac (16): their mode of action appears to be primarily synergistic. Accordingly, we named the prolactin-synergising activity synlactin rather than lactomedin (16).

ACKNOWLEDGMENTS

Our research was supported by NSF grant PCM82-05383 and by funds from the Committee on Research of the University of California at Berkeley.

REFERENCES

1. Nicoll CS. (1974): In: Knobil E and Sawyer W (eds) Handbook of Physiology Section 7: Endocrinology, Vol 4:253
2. Clarke WC, Bern HA. (1980): Horm Prot Pept 8:106
3. Lyons WR, Li CH, Johnson RE. (1958): Rec Prog Horm Res 14:219
4. Lyons WR. (1942): Proc Soc Exp Biol Med 51:308
5. Lyons WR, Page E. (1935): Proc Soc Exp Biol Med 32:1049
6. Nicoll CS. (1967): Endocrinology 80:54
7. Elias JJ. (1980): Horm Prot Pept 8:37
8. Mukherjee AS, Washburn LL, Banerjee MR. (1973): Nature 246:159
9. Banerjee MR, Wood BG, Kinder DL. (1973): In Vitro 9:129
10. White B, Nicoll CS. (1981): In: Gilbert LI, Frieden E (eds) Metamorphosis: a Problem in Development. Plenum Press, New York, p 363
11. Derby A, Etkin W. (1968): J Exptl Zool 169:1
12. Nicoll CS. (1969): Acta Endocrinol 60:91
13. Bates RW, Miller RA, Garrison MM. (1962): Endocrinology 71:345
14. Nicoll CS, Bern HA. (1968): Gen Comp Endocrinol 11:5
15. Anderson TR, Pitts DS, Nicoll CS. (1984): Gen Comp Endocrinol 54:236
16. Anderson TR, Rodriguez J, Nicoll CS, Spencer EM. (1983): In: Spencer EM (ed) Insulin-like Growth Factors/Somatomedins. Walter de Gruyter and Co, Berlin, p 71
17. Nicoll CS. (1982): Persp Biol Med 25:369
18. Bala RM, Bohnet HG, Carter JN, Friesen HG. (1977): Can J Pharmacol 56:984

19. Holder AT, Wallis M. (1977): J Endocrinol 74:223
20. Francis MJO, Hill DJ. (1975): Nature 255:167
21. Hill DJ, Francis MJO, Milner RDG. (1977): J Endocrinol 75:137
22. Blundell TL, Bedarkar S, Rinderknecht E, Humbel RE. (1978): Proc Natl Acad Sci USA 75:180
23. Spencer EM, Ross M, Smith B. (1983): In: Spencer EM (ed) Insulin-like growth Factors/Somatomedins. Walter De Gruyter and Co, Berlin, p 81
24. King GL, Kahn CR. (1981): Nature 292:644
25. Daughaday WH. (1981): In: Daughaday WH (ed) Endocrine Control of Growth. Elsevier Press, New York, p 1
26. Robertson CE, Friesen HG. (1981): Endocrinology 108:2388
27. Furlanetto RW, DiCarlo JN. (1984): Cancer Res 44:2122
28. Kelly PA, Posner BI, Tsushima T, Friesen HG. (1974): Endocrinology 95:532
29. Sasaki N, Tanaka Y, Imai Y, Tsushima T, Matsuzaki F. (1982): Biochem 203:653
30. Sasaki N, Yasuo I, Tsushima T, Matsuzaki F. (1982): Acta Endocrinol 101:574
31. Fix JA, Leppert P, Moore WV. (1981): Horm Metab Res 13:508
32. Goldsmith AR, Edwards C, Koprucu M, Silver R. (1981): J Endocrinol 90:437
33. Cheng MF, Burke WH. (1983): Horm Behav 17:54
34. Laron Z. (1982): Israel J Med Sci 18:823

Prolactin. Basic and clinical correlates
R.M. MacLeod, M.O. Thorner and U. Scapagnini (eds.),
Fidia Research Series, vol. I,
Liviana Press, Padova © 1985

Section VI
Comparative aspects of
prolactin production and function

PROLACTIN IN AVIAN REPRODUCTION: INCUBATION AND THE CONTROL OF SEASONAL BREEDING

A. R. Goldsmith

AFRC Research Group on Photoperiodism & Reproduction, Department of Zoology,
University of Bristol, Bristol BS8 1UG, U.K.

Among the many physiological processes involving prolactin in vertebrates the hormone appears to be an important component of the reproductive cycle in birds. There are major changes in its production and secretion during the nesting sequence and high prolactin concentrations occur during incubation. Also, prolactin secretion changes seasonally independently of incubation and is important in the broader context of photoperiodism. Here we will discuss current knowledge of the factors which initiate prolactin secretion and will assess the hormone's functions in avian reproduction.

PROLACTIN AND INCUBATION

It is now well established that a high rate of prolactin secretion occurs during the incubation phase of avian breeding cycles. Plasma concentrations of the hormone have been measured in a wide range of birds and much of the data are summarized in a recent review (1). Shown here, as an example, is the case of the domesticated canary (Fig. 1) in which females, during incubation, have levels some ten-fold higher than during nest building. Levels increase significantly in many birds during egg laying (2-6) but incubation is the major stimulus for prolactin secretion. In turkeys (3) and ducks (7), for instance, birds that had ceased laying and had begun incubating had much higher prolactin concentrations than females which continued to lay.

Contact with the eggs in the nest seems to be an important factor for many birds in maintaining high prolactin secretion during incubation, and typically there is a marked decline in plasma concentrations of prolactin if an incubating bird is separated from her nest (4,8-10). There is an equally rapid rise in circulating levels of the hormone when the eggs are returned and incubation is resumed (8,10). Species may differ, however, in their requirements for a stimulus for prolactin secretion. Male ring doves will continue to secrete prolactin if they are separated from their nests but are allowed to see their incubating partners through a transparent partition (11).

412

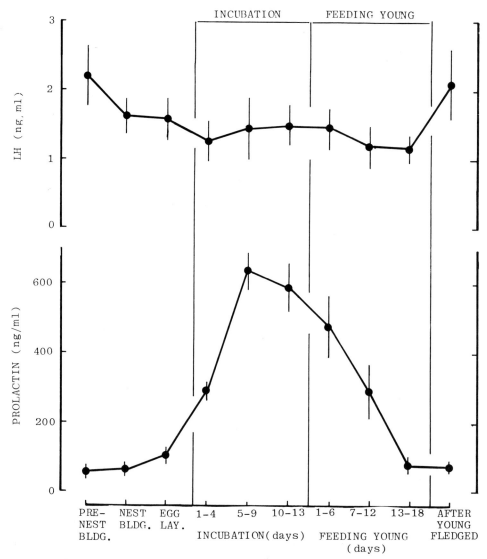

Figure 1. Plasma concentrations of LH and prolactin (mean ± sem) in female canaries during the breeding cycle, including nest building, egg laying, incubation, and feeding young.

While all species studied to date have high plasma prolactin concentrations during incubation, there are differences in parental secretory patterns after the young hatch which appear to be related to differences in the type of parental care shown. In precocial species where the young leave their nest immediately after hatching, parental prolactin output declines markedly as the young become semi-independent and levels remain low during the "chick-rearing" period (6,12,13). Clearly, the newly hatched young do not usually provide a sufficient stimulus for prolactin secretion. In turkeys replacement of eggs with poults caused a rapid decline in prolactin levels despite continued nest occupation by the hen (14). On the other hand, in birds with altricial young, in other words born naked and brooded in the nest by their parents for some days or weeks after hatching, prolactin levels in the parents decline more slowly (15,16). For example, in free living pied flycatchers, newly hatched young provide a positive stimulus for prolactin release, causing a secondary rise in prolactin concentration in the female parent after levels had begun to fall as a result of experimentally delaying the hatching date (17).

Pigeons and doves are familiar birds but they have an unusual characteristic in that they feed their young on regurgitated mucosal lining from the crop sac, a classic prolactin-dependent tissue. Plasma prolactin levels thus remain high after the end of incubation while the crop 'milk' is being produced (18,19). The presence of young in the nest is essential to maintain this response and there is evidence that regurgitation of crop 'milk' in itself stimulates a consequent short-term release of prolactin into the circulation (20).

Apart from the maintenance of the crop sac in the unique case of the Columbiformes, the functions of prolactin in birds during the phases of incubation and parental care are unclear. A role for the hormone in facilitating incubation behavior is often involved but direct evidence for this is equivocal (1,21). There is, however, increasing circumstantial evidence for a role of prolactin in suppressing reproductive development. Onset of incubation is usually accompanied by reduced secretion rates of gonadotrophin and reduced plasma levels of gonadal steriods (1), as illustrated for the canary in Figure 1. Disruption of incubation by removal of the eggs leads to a rise in plasma LH within 1 day in ducks (22), canaries (10), and doves (23,24). The rapid inverse changes in prolactin and LH after disruption and subsequent re-initiation of incubation in canaries are shown in Figure 2. The existence of an inverse relationship between these hormones does not, in itself, indicate a direct interaction between them, and the numerous examples of 'antigonadal' effects of exogenous (mammalian) prolactin in birds are usually attributed to actions at the level of the ovary or testis (reviewed in 1). In one study, however, the injection of anti-prolactin antiserum into incubating bantam hens caused a rise in plasma LH (5).

Analysis of the role of prolactin in avian reproduction should not be limited to the context of incubation. In many birds there is a significant increase in prolactin concentrations in the pituitary gland (25) and in the circulation (3,26,27) after photostimulation and, as outlined in the next section, data obtained from one photoperiodic species, the European starling, suggest that the hormone may be involved in the control of seasonal breeding.

PROLACTIN AND THE CONTROL OF SEASONAL BREEDING

In wild starlings the surge in prolactin secretion seen during incubation appears to be superimposed upon an underlying photoperiodically controlled pattern of prolactin release. Experimental manipulation of nests in a wild starling population in Cam-

414

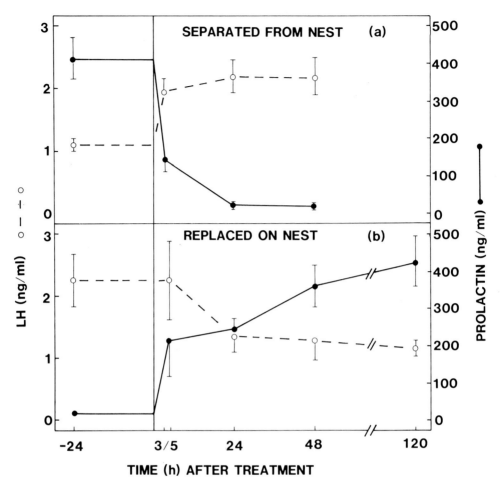

Figure 2. Plasma concentrations (mean ± sem) of prolactin (●) and LH (○) in female canaries after disruption and re-initiation of incubation behavior. (a) Birds were bled 3, 24 and 48 h after being separated from their nests, and hormone levels compared with those on the day before separation when the birds were incubating normally. (b) Birds which had been taken from their nests during incubation were replaced and bled 5, 24, 48 and 120 h after re-initiation of incubation. Hormone levels were compared with those on the day before replacement when the birds were in isolation.

bridgeshire allowed blood samples to be collected from birds at the same stage of breeding activity (either nest building, incubating, or feeding young) but at different times of the year, and, secondly, from birds at different phases of the breeding cycle but on the same calendar date (A. Dawson and A.R. Goldsmith, unpublished data). The latter set of samples showed, as expected, that birds incubating eggs or feeding young had higher levels of prolactin than those still engaged in nest building, but it was also clear that prolactin levels increased markedly during the breeding season, even in birds which were forced to prolong nest building activity for several weeks and which were not allowed to accumulate a clutch and begin incubating. Furthermore, both male and female starlings kept in aviaries show a clear rise in prolactin secretion during the spring months even though no nesting attempts are possible (28) and under controlled laboratory conditions this rise in prolactin can be reliably induced by exposure to long photoperiods (26,29,30).

   In captive male starlings held initially on short (8 h) days and then exposed to a simulated annual increase in daylength, LH levels begin to increase as the photoperiod reaches about 11.5 h, stimulating testicular maturation (26, Fig. 3). Plasma levels of prolactin increase some time later when daylengths have reached 14.5 h, rising to peak concentrations at the time of the reduction in LH and testicular regression. (Starlings are typical of most temperate zone birds in that they show spontaneous gonadal regression after prolonged exposure to long photoperiods, a condition known as photorefractoriness.) Prolactin levels also increase if birds are transferred to long photoperiods of fixed duration, and the rate of increase varies with the length of the photoperiod in a quantitative manner (29). Some comparisons are shown in Figure 4; transfer from 8 to 18 h daylengths causes a significant increase in prolactin within 3 weeks, peak concentrations being reached after 4 weeks, while transfer to 13 h causes a slower increase

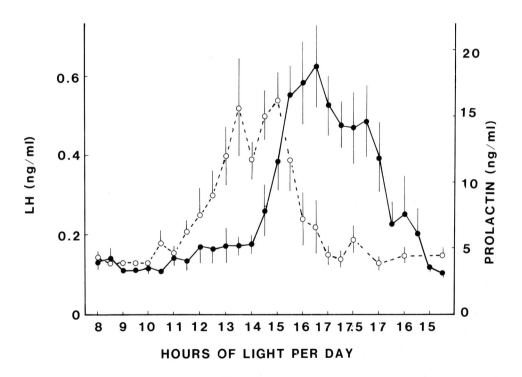

Figure 3. Plasma concentrations (mean ± sem) of prolactin (●) and LH (○) in male starlings exposed to a simulated annual change in photoperiod. The daylength was increased at the rate of 0.5 h per week, maintained at 17.5 h for three weeks and then decreased by 0.5 h per week.

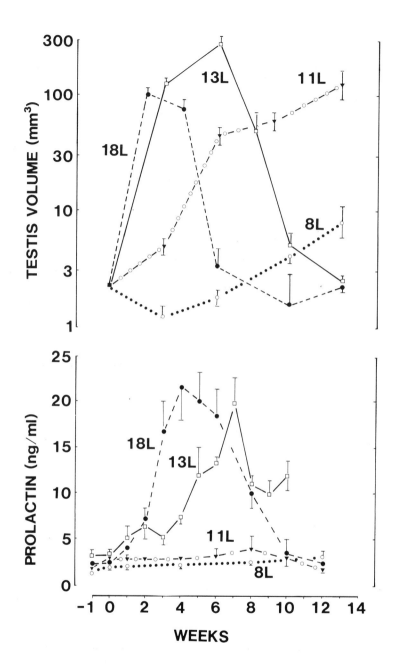

Figure 4. Mean (± sem) testicular width (note log scale) and plasma prolactin concentration in four groups of male starlings which were transferred from 8 h daily photoperiods to 11, 13, or 18 h photoperiods, or maintained on 8 h.

and a peak at 7 weeks. On 12.5 h daylengths the increase is slower still (26) while photoperiods below 12 h do not permit or cause prolactin release and levels stay low if birds are kept on 11 h or 8 h (Fig. 4). High prolactin levels subsequently decline gradually in starlings kept on long days for an extended period, but transfer to short days significantly accelerates the decrease, concentrations then falling rapidly to basal values (31).

Prolactin secretion is thus controlled photoperiodically in the starling, but what is the function of this hormone? In seasonally breeding rodents long-day induced prolactin release appears to contribute to sexual maturation, stimulating testicular gonadotrophin receptors and possibly also pituitary FSH secretion (32,33). There is no evidence that this is true in birds; reports do exist of gonado-stimulatory effects of ovine prolactin but most studies of the effects of exogenous prolactin indicate a suppressive effect on testicular function (1). In starlings, measurements of endogenous prolactin in the circulation do indicate an increase during the testicular growth phase when very long photoperiods are used (29,34) but the accelerated sexual maturation on 18 h compared with 13 h daylengths can be adequately accounted for by direct photoperiodically-induced FSH secretion (29). In fact, high prolactin concentrations are clearly not essential for testicular growth since maximal gonadal development is reached on 13 h before a marked increase in its concentration (Fig. 4). Birds maintained on 11 h days develop fully mature gonads, albeit rather slowly, but never exhibit high prolactin secretion (29, 34,35 and Fig. 4) and, as indicated below, suppression of prolactin secretion (by thyroidectomy) does not prevent testicular growth (36). Rather, evidence is now accumulating to indicate that prolactin plays a part, in contrast, in switching off the reproductive system induced by long days, i.e. the development of photorefractoriness.

The fundamental characteristics of reproductive refractoriness in starlings and similar birds have been summarized in recent reviews (37,38) but a brief account will be useful here. After a period of exposure to long photoperiods the gonads spontaneously regress, not due to exhaustion or incapacity of the gonads or the pituitary gland to respond to appropriate stimulation, but because a fundamental change has occurred at a "higher" level. For instance, the hypothalamic GnRH content is markedly reduced in refractory birds (A. Dawson and B.K. Follett, unpublished data). Gonadal regression is followed by a post-nuptial moult of the plumage and other events such as physiological and behavioral preparation for migration to the wintering grounds. Under experimental conditions the reproductive system remains suppressed as long as birds are maintained on long days but exposure of photorefractory starlings to short days for 4-6 weeks allows re-acquisition of photosensitivity; GnRH content of the hypothalamus again becomes high and subsequent photostimulation causes rapid gonadal maturation. Our present hypothesis concerning refractoriness envisages that long days may have two independent effects. They stimulate gonadotrophin secretion, so causing gonadal growth, but separately they cause the build-up in an as yet undefined "inhibitory process". Eventually this comes to override the stimulatory effects of long days and causes photorefractoriness and the spontaneous regression of the gonads (37,38). The physiological basis of this condition has proved difficult to elucidate but we do know that it is independent of any feedback inhibition from gonadal steroids (see below), and several observations in starlings now indicate a link with prolactin secretion.

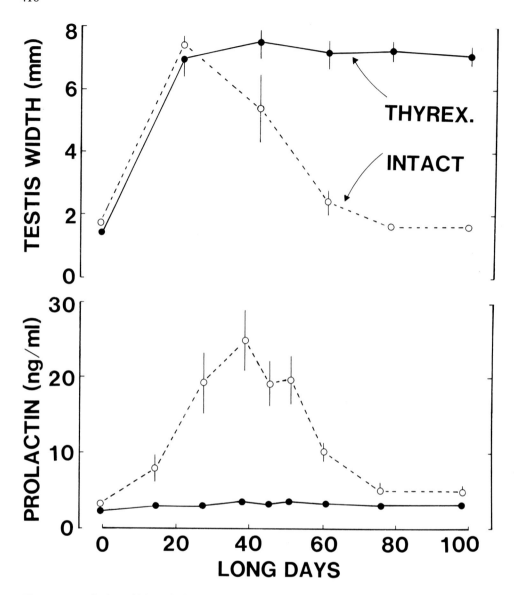

Figure 5. Testicular width and plasma prolactin concentration (mean ± sem) in intact (○) and thyroidectomized (●) male starlings after exposure to long (18h) photoperiods. Note that thyroidectomized starlings do not show an increase in plasma prolactin and do not become photorefractory.

This last point is demonstrated by the temporal correlations shown in Figure 4. The rate at which photorefractoriness develops on long days is proportional to the length of the photoperiod, thus testicular regression occurs in 4-6 weeks on 18 h daylengths but only after 8-10 weeks of exposure to 13 h days, and this is correlated with the delayed prolactin increase on 13 h. More importantly, although birds held on 11 h photoperiods reach full testicular maturity, this photoperiod is below the threshold required to trigger prolactin secretion and such birds never become photorefractory (29, 39). The physiological mechanisms leading to subsequent testicular regression and photorefractoriness must actually be initiated during the first 14 days of exposure to long (18 h) days, since birds photostimulated for this duration and subsequently transferred to 11 h become refractory a few weeks later; the testes regress and moulting occurs (31). This photoperiodic paradigm also causes a significant increase in plasma prolactin whereas

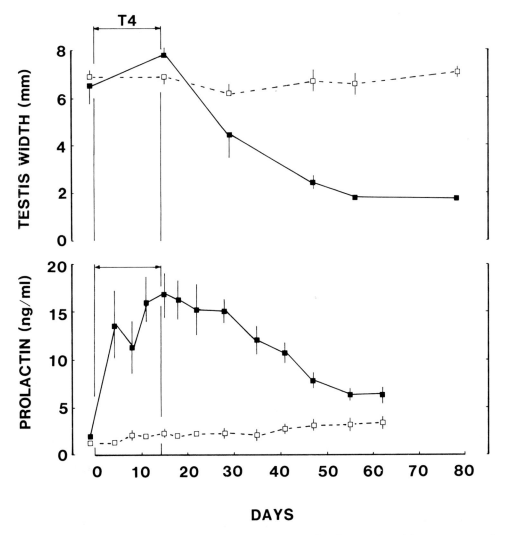

Figure 6. Testicular width and plasma prolactin concentration (mean ± sem) in two groups of thyroidectomized starlings kept on long (18h) daylengths. One group (●) received thyroxine (T4) in their drinking water for 14 days while the other group (○) remained as controls.

shorter periods of exposure to 18 h fail to stimulate prolactin release and full sexual maturity is sustained.

Another series of experiments showed that prolactin is associated not with testicular regression per se but only with long-day induced photorefractoriness (34). Sexually mature starlings transferred from 11 h to shorter (6 h) days do show a rather slow gonadal regression, but there is no increase in prolactin and such birds at the stage of full gonadal regression are not refractory; they do not moult and always remain responsive to photostimulation. Another important point is that onset of photorefractoriness on long days can occur in the absence of gonadal steroids and is not dependent upon the increase in gonadotrophin secretion which normally precedes it (28,30). Thus castrated male and female starlings, and also birds chronically implanted with a high dose of testosterone, become photorefractory and show a rise in prolactin on long days identical with that in control birds (28,30). In this respect the starling differs somewhat from some mammals in which gonadal steroids, particularly estradiol, stimulate prolactin secretion, as also appears to be the case in the domestic turkey (27).

Is prolactin a causal agent in the central mechanism of photorefractoriness (i.e. the termination of GnRH production and secretion) or does the hormone mediate one of the associated events such as testicular regression or the initiation of moulting? It is not yet possible to provide a definitive answer to this question. One obvious approach would be to suppress prolactin secretion by pharmacological means, as has proved valuable in mammalian studies by using bromocriptine. Unfortunately, although advances have been made in analyzing the hypothalamic control of prolactin secretion in birds (40-44) a specific pharmacological method of chronically suppressing its secretion has not yet been demonstrated. The alternative of injecting mammalian prolactin into starlings has so far proved inconclusive (A.R. Goldsmith and T.J. Nicholls, unpublished data). Treatment with ovine prolactin for 35 days caused testicular regression and even initiated a moult of the flight feathers but the testes redeveloped on long days after cessation of treatment, indicating that the hypothalamo-pituitary axis was not fully refractory. It is possible, though, that a foreign (in this case, ovine) prolactin is unable to activate the appropriate receptors or even to cross the blood-brain barrier. Unfortunately, bird prolactin is not available in sufficient quantities for physiological experiments. There is, however, an entirely different and rather surprising discovery that has extended the investigation of the role of prolactin in seasonality. This is that thyroidectomized starlings do not secrete prolactin, nor do they become photorefractory.

THE THYROID GLANDS AND PROLACTIN RELEASE

Thyroidectomy is reported to have a range of effects on avian reproductive cycles including both stimulatory and inhibitory influences on photoperiodically-induced testicular growth (45-47). The effects of thyroidectomy on gonadal function differ not only among species but may also vary according to the stage of the cycle at which the operation is performed (48,49). Starlings thyroidectomized while photosensitive and held on short days show normal testicular growth when subsequently photostimulated, but testicular regression does not occur and the gonads remain active indefinitely on long days (49). Thyroidectomized starlings kept under natural daylengths do show testicular regression under the decreasing daylengths of autumn and winter (50 and A. Dawson, unpublished data), but the spontaneous gonadal collapse in early summer indicative of photorefractoriness does not occur. To exclude the possibility that the presence of mature testes may be misleading, in that changes at the highest levels of the reproductive system may nevertheless have occurred, and that the testes are maintained, perhaps, by high TSH concentrations following thyroidectomy, tests of gonadal activity have recently been followed up by measurements of pituitary gonadotrophin concentrations and of hypothalamic GnRH content (36 and A. Dawson and B.K. Follett, unpublished data). Both remain high after thyroidectomy indicating that the operation

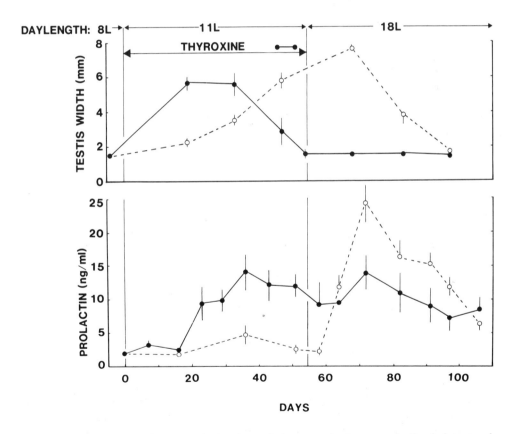

Figure 7. Effect of thyroxine on testicular size and plasma prolactin concentration in intact male starlings. Photosensitive birds were transferred from short (8 h) daylengths to 11 h daylengths for 54 days, and one group (●) received thyroxine in their drinking water throughout this time while another group (○) remained as controls. After cessation of thyroxine treatment both groups were transferred to 18 h photoperiods.

has indeed genuinely prevented the development of photorefractoriness at the highest levels. Two other physiological characteristics of refractoriness are also absent in thyroidectomized starlings: no moulting of the flight feathers occurs and there is no secretion of prolactin (36,49, Fig. 5). An interesting point is that starlings thyroidectomized after 4 weeks of long (17 h) days, when they are already sexually mature and after, as we now know, prolactin secretion rate has already begun to increase, become refractory at the same time as intact controls (49). This is another indication of the point made earlier that photorefractoriness is actually triggered some time before testicular regression can be observed.

Replacement of thyroxine in photostimulated, thyroidectomized starlings has the predicted effect of restoring the capacity to become photorefractory (Fig. 6). Testicular involution does not occur as an immediate response to thyroxine but a course of treatment lasting 14 days was followed by testicular regression some 14-28 days later, a time course of response comparable to that seen after photostimulation of normal, intact starlings with 18 h daylengths. Most importantly, the cessation of thyroxine treatment was not followed by testicular redevelopment; thyroxine did not simply cause gonadal regression but the reproductive system was afterwards refractory to long days. The thyroxine treatment also caused a rise in prolactin beginning before testicular regression (Fig. 6), with an amplitude and duration similar to that caused by exposure of intact starlings to long days (Fig. 4) and moulting of the flight feathers which began after the testes had reached minimal size.

Two questions now arise from these observations: First, is the activation of the thyroid glands the specific and ultimate cause of photorefractoriness, the start of a chain of events initiated under long days which leads eventually to a spontaneous reduction in hypothalamo-pituitary-gonadal activity? Alternatively, is the presence of a normally functioning thyroid gland simply an essential part of the metabolic background in which the processes leading to reproductive refractoriness and also prolactin secretion occur? The second question concerns the role of prolactin.

Data supporting a causal rather than permissive role for thyroxine come from experiments in which a hyperthyroid state is induced in intact starlings. A course of thyroxine administration lasting 35 days given to sexually mature starlings on 11 h photoperiods induced all the characteristics of photorefractoriness, i.e., complete testicular collapse, feather moult, unresponsiveness to subsequent long day stimulation after withdrawal of thyroxine, and a surge in prolactin secretion (35). An even more spectacular result is shown in Figure 7. Thyroxine administered to sexually immature birds on 11 h caused, initially, rapid testicular maturation, followed by regression, moulting, and refractoriness to long days. Thus the treatment appeared to have induced a complete reproductive cycle, including the customary prolactin release, in the time taken for the control birds to complete a slow testicular growth phase on the marginally stimulatory photoperiod used in this experiment. After the testes of the thyroxine-treated birds had fully regressed and moulting had begun, the treatment was stopped and the birds transferred to 18 h photoperiods to test their response (Fig. 7). The gonads remained fully regressed, indicating that the birds had indeed been rendered fully photorefractory. The control birds, meanwhile, showed the expected response to the increase in photoperiod: the testes remained mature for some days but then regressed as photorefractoriness was induced, preceded, of course, by an increase in plasma prolactin.

How does thyroxine cause photorefractoriness? Is it a direct effect of thyroxine (or triiodothyronine) or is the response mediated through thyroxine-induced prolactin secretion? In a recent, as yet incomplete, study injections of prolactin caused rapid testicular regression in long-day thyroidectomized starlings -- a regression which was faster and more complete than that induced by prolactin in intact birds on 11 h photoperiods (A.R. Goldsmith, unpublished data). Perhaps thyroidectomized birds fail to become refractory because they are unable to produce their own prolactin; this conjecture remains to be confirmed. We are also as yet unsure how thyroidectomy abolishes prolactin secretion. There is no direct evidence that thyroxine or triiodothyronine directly stimulate prolactin release from the pituitary gland, but an effect through alteration of TRH levels must also be considered. TRH has been shown to cause a short-term release of prolactin from chicken and turkey pituitary glands *in vitro* and *in vivo* (42,51,52). A final point is that thyroidectomized starlings not only fail to secrete prolactin but show a much-reduced synthesis; thyroidectomized starlings on long days do not show the massive increase in pituitary prolactin content characteristic of intact birds (A. Dawson and A. R. Goldsmith, unpublished data).

The last few years have seen a substantial increase in information on changes in prolactin secretion in avian breeding cycles. The long-suspected association of prolactin with incubation has been substantiated in a wide variety of species although its function in this context is still very much an open question. The photoperiodic control of prolactin release, a phenomenon seen also in sheep and cattle (53-55), is becoming an increasing focus of attention, while its dependence upon the thyroid axis, so dramatically emphasized in starlings, requires urgent investigation in other species. Sorting out the functions of avian prolactin is likely to take some time, there being such a range of potential target tissues already specified in birds and in other vertebrates, but the results reported in the preceding pages surely identify prolactin as an important if not indispensable component of the reproductive process.

REFERENCES

1. Goldsmith AR. (1983): In: Balthazart J, Prove E, Gilles R (eds) Hormones and Behaviour in Higher Vertebrates. Springer-Verlag, Berlin, p 375
2. Etches RJ, Garbutt A, Middleton AL. (1979): Can J Zool 57:1624
3. Burke WH, Dennison PT. (1980): Gen Comp Endocrinol 41:92
4. Proudman JA, Opel H. (1981): Biol Reprod 25:573
5. Lea RW, Dodds ASM, Sharp PJ, Chadwick A. (1981): J Endocrinol 91:88
6. Hall MR, Goldsmith AR. (1983): Gen Comp Endocrinol 49:270
7. Cavanaugh KP, Goldsmith AR, Holmes WN, Follett BK. (1983): Arch Environm Contam Toxicol 12:335
8. El Halawani ME, Burke WH, Dennison PT. (1980): Biol Reprod 23:118

424

9. Lea RW, Sharp PJ. (1982): Brit Poult Sci 23:451
10. Goldsmith AR, Burke S, Prosser JM. Gen Comp Endocrinol, in press
11. Patel MD. (1936): Physiol Zool 9:129
12. Goldsmith AR, Williams DM. 1980. J Endocrinol 86:371
13. Wentworth BC, Proudman JA, Opel H, Wineland MJ, Zimmerman MG, Lapp A. (1983): Biol Reprod 29:87
14. Burke WH, Dennison PT, Silsby JL, El Halawani ME. (1981): Adv Physiol Sci 33:109
15. Goldsmith AR. (1982): J Endocrinol 94:51
16. Dawson A, Goldsmith AR. (1982): Gen Comp Endocrinol 48:213
17. Silverin B, Goldsmith AR. Gen Comp Endocrinol, in press
18. Goldsmith AR, Edwards C, Koprucu M, Silver S. (1981): J Endocrinol 90:437
19. Cheng M-F, Burke WH. (1983): Horm Behav 17:54
20. Buntin JD. (1979): J Endocrinol 82:127
21. Opel H, Proudman JA. (1980): Poult Sci 59:2550
22. Donham RS, Dane CW, Farner DS. (1976): Gen Comp Endocrinol 29:152
23. Silver R, Goldsmith AR, Follett BK. (1980): Gen Comp Endocrinol 42:19
24. Ramsey SM, Goldsmith AR, Silver R. Gen Comp Endocrinol, in press
25. Goldsmith AR, Hall M. (1980): Gen Comp Endocrinol 42:449
26. Ebling FJP, Goldsmith AR, Follett BK. (1982): Gen Comp Endocrinol 48:485
27. El Halawani ME, Silsby JL, Fehrer SC, Behnke EJ. (1983): Gen Comp Endocrinol 52:67
28. Dawson A, Goldsmith AR. (1984): J Endocrinol 100:213
29. Dawson A, Goldsmith AR. (1983): J Endocrinol 97:253
30. Goldsmith AR, Nicholls TJ. (1984): Gen Comp Endocrinol 54:247
31. Dawson A, Goldsmith AR, Nicholls TJ. Physiol Zool, in press
32. Bex FJ, Bartke A. (1977): Endocrinology 100:1223
33. Bartke A, Klemcke HG, Amador A, Goldman BD, Siler-Khodr TM. (1983): J Reprod Fert 69:587
34. Goldsmith AR, Nicholls TJ. J Endocrinol, in press
35. Goldsmith AR, Nicholls TJ. (1984): J Endocrinol 101:RI
36. Goldsmith AR, Nicholls TJ. (1984): Gen Comp Endocrinol 54:256
37. Nicholls TJ, Goldsmith AR, Dawson A J Exp Zool, in press
38. Follett BK, Nicholls TJ. J Exp Zool, in press
39. Hamner WM. (1971). In: Menaker M (ed) Biochronometry. National Academy of Sciences, Washington DC, p 448
40. El Halawani ME, Burke WH, Dennison PT. (1980): Biol Reprod 23:815
41. Harvey S, Chadwick A, Border G, Scanes CG, Phillips JG. (1982). In: Scanes CG, Ottinger MA, Kenny AD, Balthazart J, Cronshaw J, Chester Jones I (eds) Aspects of Avian Endocrinology: Practical and Theoretical Implications. Texas Tech Press, Lubbock, p 41
42. Hall TR. (1982): J Endocrinol 92:303
43. Hall TR, Chadwick A. (1983): Gen Comp Endocrinol 49:135
44. Fehrer SC, Silsby JL, EL Halawani ME. (1983): Gen Comp Endocrinol 52:400
45. Assenmacher I. (1973): In: Farner DS, King JR (eds) Avian Biology. Academic Press, New York, vol 3:183
46. Jallageas M, Assenmacher I. (1979): Gen Comp Endocrinol 37:44
47. Thapliyal JP. Program of the 68th Session of the Indian Science Congress, Section of Zoology, Entomology and Fisheries, Varanasi, India, (1981): Presidential Address
48. Chaturvedi CM, Thapliyal JP. (1983): Gen Comp Endocrinol 52:279
49. Wieselthier A, van Tienhoven A. (1972): J Exp Zool 179:331
50. Woitkewitsch AA. (1940): Compt Rend (Doklady) Acad Sci URSS 27:741
51. Harvey S, Scanes CG, Chadwick A, Bolton NJ. (1978): Neuroendocrinology 26:249

52. Burke WH. (1983): Poult Sci 62:1394
53. Revault JP. (1976): Acta Endocrinologica 83:720
54. Walton JS, McNeilly JR, McNeilly AS, Cunningham FJ. (1977): J Endocrinol 75:127
55. Peters RR, Tucker HA. (1978): Endocrinology 103:229

Prolactin. Basic and clinical correlates
R.M. MacLeod, M.O. Thorner and U. Scapagnini (eds.),
Fidia Research Series, vol. I,
Liviana Press, Padova © 1985

Section VI
Comparative aspects of
prolactin production and function

PARTIAL CHARACTERIZATION OF TWO PROLACTINS FROM A CICHLID FISH

Jennifer L. Specker, *David S. King, Rodolfo J. Rivas, and Brett K. Young

Departments of Zoology and Genetics and Cancer Research Laboratory
University of California, Berkeley CA 94720

The identification of variant forms of both prolactin and growth hormone (GH) has opened up possible avenues for the explanation of the diverse activities ascribed to members of this family of hormones (1-3). Prolactin and GH variants are present in minor amounts relative to what have appeared to be the single dominant forms in various mammalian species (4,5). In the teleost fish that we study, *Oreochromis mossambicus*, a tilapia of the family Cichlidae, we have found two major forms of prolactin. We describe here some aspects of their chemistry and biology and conclude with a hypothesis about their possible physiological significance.

Methods for the purification of prolactin and GH from tilapia have been previously described (6,7) and the hormone preparations obtained from these methods have been characterized (8,9). In this earlier work, prolactin and GH were obtained by DEAE cellulose chromatography from a collection of lobes (rich in either prolactin or GH) which had been dissected from the tilapia pituitary and frozen. Given the possibility that stored and secreted forms of prolactin and GH may differ (10,11), the more recent efforts of our laboratory have been to obtain secreted prolactin and GH for the study of their physiological functions.

The regionalization of various cell types in the tilapia pituitary makes possible the organ culture of the rostral pars distalis (RPD) containing prolactin-secreting cells, or the proximal pars distalis (PPD) containing GH-secreting cells. This organizational simplicity has been utilized by Bern and colleagues in the study of prolactin and GH secretion from the tilapia pituitary: prolactin release can be induced by low osmotic pressure (12-14) and GH release can be stimulated by cortisol (15). We have incubated rostral and proximal lobes under the appropriate conditions for one to three weeks to obtain culture media rich in either prolactin or GH.

---

* Current address: Department of Zoology, University of Rhode Island, Kingston, RI 02881.

428

The purification of prolactin from hyposmotic medium by reversed-phase high performance liquid chromatography (rp-HPLC) has revealed the presence of a second form of prolactin. This second prolactin runs in its reduced state with an apparent molecular weight of 24 K_d, almost 4 K_d larger than the previously described prolactin from this species. The possibility that either prolactin is actually GH has been excluded by the simultaneous purification and characterization of tilapia GH (21 K_d).

The isoelectric points of the three proteins have been determined using ampholytes in a horizontal polyacrylamide gel (Fig. 1). Tilapia GH is similar to mammalian GHs, with pI 6.2. Unlike mammalian prolactins which are acidic, the 20 K_d prolactin is relatively neutral, with pI 7.5, and the 24 K_d prolactin is basic, with pI 8.5. It would appear that the uncharacteristically basic pI of the second prolactin precluded its earlier detection on basic Ornstein-Davis discontinuous gels, as this prolactin would be electrically neutral in the running gel and would not migrate toward the anode in this system (Fig. 2).

BIOLOGICAL PROPERTIES

Osmoregulation

The structural relatedness of the two proteins from the rostral lobe is indicated by their comparable physiological action in one type of bioassay. The classic bioassay

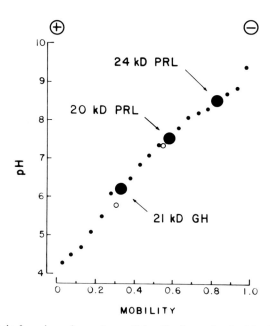

Figure 1. Isoelectric focusing of members of the tilapia prolactin-GH family using ampholytes (Bio-Lyte 3/10) in a horizontal polyacrylamide gel. Standard pI markers (open circles) are horse myoglobin (pI 7.35) and beta-lactoglobulin (pI 5.72).

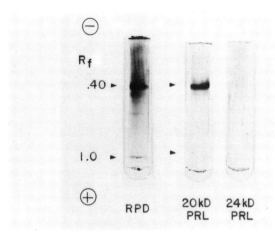

Figure 2. rp-HPLC-purified tilapia prolactins (10 ug of each) and one rostral pars distalis (RPD) from an adult male tilapia compared on basic discontinuous gels (Ornstein-Davis). The 24 K_d prolactin does not migrate in this system.

for prolactin activity in teleost fishes measures the ability of the preparation to prevent the loss of Na^+ that occurs when some species of hypophysectomized euryhaline fish are transferred from 1/3-strength seawater (isotonic to plasma) to fresh water (16,17). This so-called "Na^+-retaining bioassay" distinguishes mammalian prolactins from mammalian GHs (18,19) and has contributed to the concept of prolactin as the "freshwater-adapting hormone" of teleost fishes (20-22). A protocol that measures this feature of prolactin activity has been adapted using hypophysectomized juvenile tilapia (Specker and Nishioka, unpublished). In this test, the 20 K_d prolactin and the 24 K_d prolactin, but not tilapia GH, exhibited strong dose-dependent "Na^+-retaining" activity and were effective at doses as low as .01 pmol/g (about 20 ng/fish). Further, neither prolactins nor GH had any effect on plasma $[Ca^{2+}]$ or $[Mg^{2+}]$. Both proteins from the rostral lobe, then, can be defined as prolactins by their biological activity in the species from which they were extracted.

Growth

The ability of these three proteins to stimulate growth, as measured by an increase in distance from the nose to the fork in the tail (fork-length) as well as by an increase in weight, was measured using intact juvenile tilapia (average initial fork-length = 60 mm; average initial body weight = 3.3 g). Our first preparation (used in this bioassay) of 24 K_d prolactin contained some GH (< 20%) and the GH preparation was slightly contaminated with 24 K_d prolactin (< 5%). The fish were injected intraperitoneally

Table I. *Growth-promoting activity of mammalian and tilapia prolactins and GHs in intact juvenile tilapia*

| Treatment | n | Percent Increase (mean ± SE) | |
		Length	Weight
Control--not injected	8	4.8 ± 0.4	14.4 ± 1.8
Saline-injected	8	3.2 ± 0.6	8.4 ± 1.0
Ovine prolactin (30 IU/mg)	8	7.4 ± 1.0*	18.9 ± 2.8*
Bovine GH (0.92 IU/mg)	7	7.8 ± 1.8*	19.8 ± 5.5*
Tilapia GH	7	5.6 ± 1.0	22.1 ± 3.3*
Tilapia 20 K_d prolactin	15	5.7 ± 1.6	15.9 ± 1.9
Tilapia 24 K_d prolactin	7	7.3 ± 1.1*	21.8 ± 3.4*

* Significantly different from saline-injected control: ANOVA followed by Dunnett's test ($p < 0.05$).

every other day for 21 days with 1 ug of each of the hormones listed in Table 1. Both ovine prolactin and bovine GH increased weight and length gain in juvenile tilapia. Of the tilapia hormones, both the larger prolactin and GH increased weight gain, but only the 24 K_d prolactin stimulated an increase in length.

Enzyme-linked immunosorbent assay (ELISA)

The previous tilapia preparation (6), which appears to have been predominantly the 20 K_d prolactin from our analysis on rp-HPLC, was used to generate antibodies (9). The antisera from one rabbit (1:2000 dilution) was used in an enzyme-linked immunosorbent assay against each prolactin. This polyclonal antiserum bound both prolactins similarly (Fig. 3), suggesting that they share antigenic sites. However, the possibility that the hormone preparation used to generate the antiserum consisted of both prolactins cannot be excluded.

RATE OF RELEASE OF EACH PROLACTIN

Radiolabeled amino acid pulse-chase experiments using isolated pituitary lobes indicated that the release rates of the prolactins are similar. Briefly, after a one-hour pulse with [^{3}H]-leucine, the culture medium was sampled from incubations of 10 to 16 rostral lobes 0.5, 1, 4, 8, and 24 hours after the pulse. The medium was analyzed by rp-HPLC, and the column eluent was monitored by uv absorption (at 214 and 280 nm) and by a flow-through scintillation counter. The cumulative amount of each protein and the counts associated with it were virtually identical (Fig. 4) (Specker and King, unpublished), indicating that under the conditions tested, synthetic rates and release rates are similar.

ENZYME - LINKED IMMUNOSORBENT ASSAY

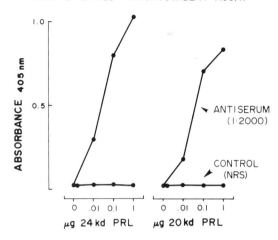

Figure 3. Enzyme-linked immunosorbent assay (ELISA) demonstrating that the antiserum generated against the 20 K_d prolactin also binds the 24 K_d prolactin. (NRS = normal rabbit serum.)

CUMULATIVE RELEASE — ONE PITUITARY

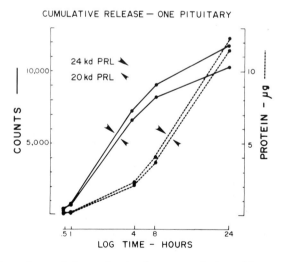

Figure 4. Cumulative release of the prolactins from one pituitary (the average of 16 cultured rostral lobes) taken from a freshwater-adapted tilapia, exposed to a 1 h pulse of [³H]-leucine, and cultured for 24 h in hypotonic medium.

REGULATION OF RELEASE

Factors regulating the release of prolactin and GH from organ-cultured lobes of the tilapia have been identified in part (13,14,23,24). The protocol for these studies has made use of the difference in mobility of tilapia prolactin and GH on basic Ornstein-Davis discontinuous gels (13,25). Briefly, the amount of hormone in the culture medium, as measured by densitometry, is compared to the amount of hormone remaining in the lobe, also measured by densitometry. We now know that the release of only the 20 K_d prolactin was measured in these studies, as the 24 K_d prolactin does not enter these basic gels. More recent experiments measured instead the optical density of both prolactins (stained with Coomassie blue) after electrophoresis on SDS-polyacrylamide gels. These experiments indicate that both somatostatin, a putative prolactin and GH inhibitory peptide in this species, and urotensin II, a somatostatin analog from the teleost caudal neurosecretory system (26), inhibit the release of both prolactins similarly (27). The issue of possible independent release of each prolactin remains of great importance to understanding the physiological significance of the two prolactins.

ORIGIN OF THE SECOND PROLACTIN

Our original aim was to determine whether the secreted form of prolactin differed from the stored form in this species (10). It has now become apparent that both prolactins that we have partially characterized are stored as well as released *in vitro*. Further, preliminary studies indicate that there are two major populations of mRNA in the rostral lobe whose protein products correspond with the 20 K_d prolactin and 24 K_d prolactin (Specker and Young, unpublished).

The total RNA from the rostral lobes was extracted and translated in a wheat germ cell-free system using [^{35}S]-methionine as a marker. As a control, the RNA from the proximal lobes was also translated. The proximal lobes are primarily "GH" cells but also contain some "prolactin" cells as a result of incomplete separation. The translation products were run in their reduced states on an SDS-polyacrylamide gel along with molecular weight markers and processed for fluorography. The fluorogram indicates that the rostral lobe has two predominant translation products in the correct size range to be the two prolactins (Fig. 5). The slightly larger molecular weights of the translation products may indicate the presence of signal sequences. The "GH lobe" contained, in addition to a small amount of products equal in size to those from the "prolactin lobe," a major and distinct product corresponding in apparent size to the tilapia GH prior to any post-translational modification (i.e. removal of the signal sequence). No further identification of the translation products has yet been attempted. However, it seems likely that each prolactin has its own mRNA, that is, that neither prolactin results from the post-translational modification of the other.

Clearly, the next question to be answered is whether the tilapia has two related genes, each encoding a protein with prolactin-like activity.

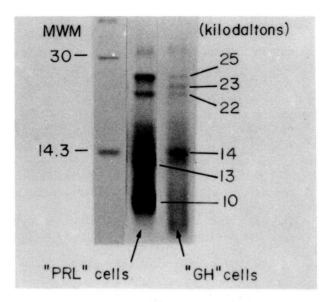

Figure 5. Fluorogram of the SDS-polyacrylamide gel of the translation products of the total RNA extracted from the rostral ("prolactin" cells) or proximal ("GH" cells) lobes of the tilapia pituitary.

WHY TWO PROLACTINS?

At the moment, this question has no clear answer. Our only evidence to date that the two prolactins may have discrete functions is that the 24 K_d prolactin succeeded, while the 20 K_d prolactin failed, to promote an increase in the length of juvenile tilapia. Although preliminary, these data are the first to indicate a growth-promoting role for prolactin in a juvenile teleost fish. Nicoll (28) has suggested that prolactin could well be considered the larval/fetal growth hormone for all vertebrate classes. One drawback with this interpretation of prolactin's functions among nonmammalian species has been that various mammalian prolactins previously used may be recognized not only as prolactins but also as GH (or even both) by distantly-related animals (28). Our study is important because we have used homologous prolactin to show effects on juvenile growth. Further, this somatotropic activity of tilapia 24 K_d prolactin is another example of an overlapping function of a member of the prolactin-GH-placental lactogen family (cf. 28,29).

The most intensively studied function of prolactin in teleost fishes has been its role in maintaining hydromineral balance (21,22). Both the 20 K_d prolactin and the 24 K_d prolactin were active in our "Na^+-retaining bioassay." However, there is also evidence that prolactin is a reproductive hormone in teleosts (1,30), possibly including tilapia (cf. 31). Tilapia are euryhaline and can reproduce in either seawater or fresh water. Secretion of prolactin as a reproductive hormone in seawater-adapted tilapia could have undesirable osmoregulatory consequences, since the smaller tilapia prolactin and mammalian prolactin are known to cause "Na$^+$- retention" in seawater-adapted tilapia (6,18). The presence of two prolactins (acting directly or acting indirectly via "synlactins"--32,33) may permit coordination of reproduction in environments of different salinities. Two prolactins and GH may also permit the growth of juvenile tilapia in different salinities. Tests of these hypotheses require a more through understanding of the physiology of the prolactin-GH family in tilapia. In addition to our previous proposal that the divergence of prolactin and GH about 400 million years ago (cf. 34) may have permitted the invasion of fresh water by primitive vertebrates (35), we now suggest that a second distinct prolactin may contribute to the coordination of osmoregulation, growth, and reproduction in this tilapia. The existence and roles of multiple forms of prolactin and/or GH in other fishes with different life histories invite investigation.

ACKNOWLEDGMENTS

We thank Professor Howard A. Bern for critically reading the manuscript and for support of all kinds, Professor Charles S. Nicoll for advice and encouragement, Richard S. Nishioka for advice and expertise, and Professor Harold Papkoff of the Hormone Research Laboratory, University of California, San Francisco, for comments and for supplying the antibodies. This work was supported by NIH Fellowhip AM 06596 to J.L.S., NSF Grant PCM 81-10111 to H.A. Bern, and NIH Grant CA 09041.

REFERENCES

1. Clarke WC, Bern HA. (1980): Horm Prot Pep 8:105
2. Nicoll CS. (1982): Perspect Biol Med 25:369
3. Bern HA. (1983): Amer Zool 23:663
4. Lewis UJ. (1984): Ann Rev Physiol 46:33
5. Sinha YN, Gilligan TA. (1984): Endocrinology 114:2046
6. Farmer SW, Papkoff H, Bewley TA, Hayashida T, Nishioka RS, Bern HA, Li CH. (1977): Gen Comp Endocrinol 31:60
7. Farmer SW, Papkoff H, Hayashida T, Bewley TA, Bern HA, Li CH. (1976): Gen Comp Endocrinol 30:91
8. Nagahama Y, Olivereau M, Farmer SW, Nishioka RS, Bern HA. (1981): Gen Comp Endocrinol 44:389
9. Nicoll CS, Farmer SW, Nishioka RS, Bern HA. (1981): Gen Comp Endocrinol 44:365
10. Bern HA. (1975): Amer Zool 15:937
11. Farmer SW, Bewley TA, Russell SM, Nicoll CS. (1976): Biochim Biophys Acta 437:562
12. Zambrano D, Clarke WC, Hajek A, Sage M, Bern HA. (1974): Acta Zool 55:202
13. Nagahama Y, Nishioka RS, Bern HA, Gunther RL. (1975): Gen Comp Endocrinol 25:166
14. Wigham T, Nishioka RS, Bern HA. (1977): Gen Comp Endocrinol 32:120
15. Nishioka RS, Grau EG, Bern HA. (1980): Amer Zool 20:859 (Abstract)
16. Ensor DM, Ball JN. (1969): Gen Comp Endocrinol 11:104
17. Dharmamba M. (1970): Gen Comp Endocrinol 14:256
18. Clarke WC. (1973): Gen Comp Endocrinol 21:498
19. Grau EG, Prunet P, Gross T, Nishioka RS, Bern HA. (1984): Gen Comp Endocrinol 53:78

20. Pickford GE, Phillips JG. (1959): Science 130:454
21. Hirano T. (1980): In: Cumming IA, Funder JW, Mendelsohn FAO (eds) Endocrinology 1980. Australian Acad Sci, Canberra, p 186
22. Loretz CA, Bern HA. (1982): Neuroendocrinology 35:292
23. Grau EG, Nishioka RS, Bern HA. (1981): Gen Comp Endocrinol 45:406
24. Grau EG, Nishioka RS, Bern HA. (1982): Endocrinology 110:910
25. Clarke WC. (1973): Can J Zool 51:687
26. Pearson D, Shively JE, Clark BR, Geschwind II, Barkley M, Nishioka RS, Bern HA. (1980): Proc Natl Acad Sci USA 77:5021
27. Rivas RJ, Nishioka RS, Specker JL, Bern HA. Program of the 4th International Congress on Prolactin, Charlottesville, VA (Abstract)
28. Nicoll CS. (1978): In: Robyn C, Harter M (eds) Progress in Prolactin Physiology and Pathology. Elsevier/North-Holland Biomedical Press, Amsterdam, p 175
29. Nicoll CS, Licht P. (1971): Gen Comp Endocrinol 17:490
30. de Vlaming VL. (1980): In: Barrington EJW (ed) Comparative Endocrinology. Academic Press, New York, vol 2:561
31. Edery M, Young G, Bern HA, Steiny S. Gen Comp Endocrinol, in press
32. Anderson TR, Rodriguez J, Pitts DS, Spencer EM, Nicoll CS. (1983): In: Spencer EM (ed) Insulin-like Growth Factors/Somatomedins. de Gruyter, Berlin/New York, p 71
33. Anderson TR, Pitts DS, Nicoll CS. (1984): Gen Comp Endocrinol 54:236
34. Martial JA, Cooke NE. (1980): In: MacLeod RM, Scapagnini U (eds) Central and Peripheral Regulation of Prolactin Function. New York, Raven Press, p 115
35. Specker JL, Ingleton PM, Bern HA. (1984): In: Mena F, Valverde CM (eds) Prolactin Secretion: A Multidisciplinary Approach. Academic Press, New York, p 17

Prolactin. Basic and clinical correlates
R.M. MacLeod, M.O. Thorner and U. Scapagnini (eds.),
Fidia Research Series, vol. I,
Liviana Press, Padova © 1985

Section VI
Comparative aspects of
prolactin production and function

LIGHT- AND ELECTRON-MICROSCOPIC IMMUNOCYTOCHEMICAL STUDIES ON PROLACTIN AND GROWTH HORMONE CELLS OF FISHES.

T. F. C. Batten, O. Skarphedinsson* and P. M. Ingleton

Department of Zoology, University of Sheffield, Western Bank, Sheffield S102TN, and *Fisheries Research Laboratory, M.A.F.F., Lowestoft NR33 OHT, UK

Immunocytochemical studies with antisera raised to teleostean and mammalian prolactin and growth hormone (GH) have been undertaken in an attempt to (a) identify the prolactin- and GH-secreting cells in various teleostean and non-teleostean fishes, (b) to determine the precise subcellular localization of these hormones, and (c) provide evidence of the immuno-relatedness of prolactin and GH in the different vertebrate groups. These studies might give further insight into the proposed evolutionary history of the two molecules (1,2).

Rabbit antisera were produced in our laboratory against the following hormones: chum salmon prolactin (sPRL), rainbow trout growth hormone (sGH), ovine prolactin (oPRL, Ferring), rat prolactin (rPRL, NIH), and rat growth hormone (rGH, NIH). The sPRL was a highly purified preparation kindly donated by Dr. H. Kawauchi (3), and the sGH was a partially purified secreted form of the hormone extracted from gels after electrophoresis of the medium from cultured pituitaries (4). All antisera were tested at dilutions of 1:200 to 1:10000, and used routinely at 1:1000. The unlabelled peroxidase-antiperoxidase (PAP) method of immunocytochemistry (5) was applied to 4 um sections of Bouin-Hollande Sublimate-fixed brain and pituitary. Spot sections from each series were stained with Herlant's tetrachrome for the tinctorial identification of the pituitary cell types.

Separate populations of prolactin and GH cells were identified in the trout, salmon parr and 17 other species of teleost from each taxonomic division (Table 1, Fig. 1). In species previously examined by histological, ultrastructural or immunocytochemical studies (4,6,7,8,9,10), cells corresponded well with the (presumptive) prolactin and GH cells of the rostral (RPD) and proximal pars distalis (PPD) respectively. The anti-sPRL antisera bound only to the acidophils forming the bulk of the RPD in all species. In contrast to the results of some other workers, our anti-oPRL gave no immunoreactivity and the anti-rPRL antisera gave only a slight, barely detectable staining of the same

438

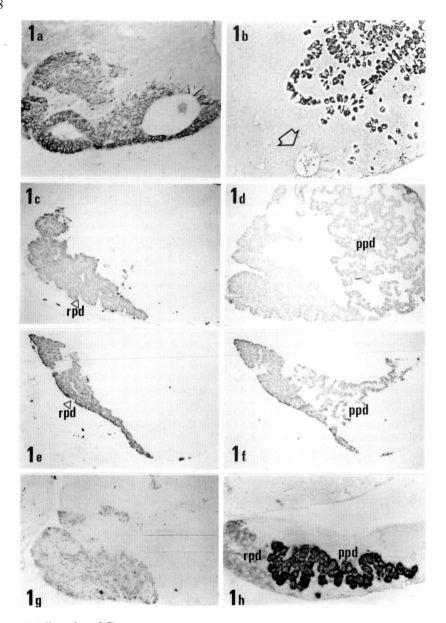

Figure 1: (all sections LS)

1a, 1b: Trout pituitary stained with anti-sPRL (a) and anti-sGH (b). Note the unstained RPD follicle, arrowed, in (b). x96.

1c, 1d: Near serial pike sections stained with anti-sPRL (a) and anti-sGH (b).
Note cross-reaction of anti-sGH with prolactin cells in (b). x90.

1e, 1f: Adjacent chromide sections with anti-sPRL (a) and anti-sGH (b).
Note cross-reaction as above. x96.

1g: Flounder, SW-adapted, showing poor staining of RPD with anti-sPRL. x96.

1h: Young molly, showing partial staining of prolactin cells with anti-sGH. x360.

cell population. In the salmonids and the eel, the prolactin-immunoreactive cells formed follicles (Fig. 1). The immunoreactivity of the cells was always much greater in
freshwater (FW) fishes, or FW-adapted euryhaline fishes, than in marine or high-salinity
adapted fishes (Table 1, Fig. 1). These results suggest that there is no species specificity
of the anti-PRL antisera among teleosts. This finding is surprising in view of the known
structural differences between chum salmon and tilapia prolactin molecules (3,11).

The anti-sGH antiserum stained the acidophilic cells of the PPD of all teleosts examined (Table 1, Fig. 1). In most species the immunoreactivity was intense, but in the
eel it was never very strong. The apparent lack of species specificity shown by this antibody suggests that, in the secreted form at least, GH might be very similar in all teleosts.
In some glands there was a cross-reaction of the anti-sGH associated with the prolactin
cells of the RPD (Fig. 1), which ranged from a very weak staining to immunoreactivity
of equal intensity to that shown by the PPD acidophils. When this cross-reaction occurred, it was unaffected by primary antiserum time, and it was not correlated with
phylogenetic status or environmental salinity. The reaction did show some correlation
with degree of sexual maturity, being much stronger in immature fishes. In the molly,
the prolactin cells of adult males or females did not bind the anti-sGH, whereas those
of 2 month old young showed considerable immunoreactivity (Fig. 1). This evidence
suggests that the prolactin cells of immature teleosts may store a protein which is more
antigenic to the anti-sGH than is the prolactin of mature individuals. This protein could
be a prohormone, isohormone or second protein with sequences common to the secreted
form of GH. It could also be the prolactin molecule itself, which, with maturity, becomes
less antigenically similar to sGH through loss of residues or through a conformational
change. Examination of pituitaries from immature fishes using anti-sGH preabsorbed
with sPRL might help clarify this hypothesis.

The subcellular localization of prolactin and GH on ultra-thin sections of
Karnovsky-fixed trout and molly pituitaries was examined using both the PAP method
and the immuno-gold method (12). Binding of the anti-sPRL to the prolactin cells of
the RPD and binding of the anti-sGH to the GH cells of the PPD occurred specifically
on the secretory granules, all of which gave a positive reaction (Figs. 3,4). Except for
occasional binding to lysosomes (associated with granule degradation), and some Golgi
saccules (condensing newly-formed granules), no other cellular compartment displayed
immunoreactivity. In accordance with the LM immunocytochemical observations anti-
sPRL was specific for the prolactin cells, whereas anti-sGH, in addition to a dense
staining of the GH cells, often gave a weak reaction with the prolactin cells. Both the
species of holostean fishes examined (*Lepisosteus* and *Amia*) had a large RPD composed almost entirely of acidophils arranged in follicles (cf.6,13). These cells were immunoreactive to anti-sPRL, but stained less intensely than those of teleosts (Fig. 2).
In contrast to the results of some previous studies (13), the RPD did not stain well with
antisera to mammalian prolactin: anti-oPRL was totally ineffective, and only slight staining was observed with anti-rPRL. The RPD cells were never seen to bind anti-sGH,
which in both species gave a weak reaction with numerous small acidophils scattered
throughout the PPD (Fig. 2). In *Calamoichthys*, a chondrostean fish, no immunoreactivity was observed with any of the antisera used, although acidophils, thought to secrete
prolactin (6,13), could be identified in the pars distalis. No immunoreactivity was noted

Table 1. *Reactivity of teleost prolactin and GH cells with antisera to sPRL and sGH*

Teleost Group	Species		Condition		Anti-sPRL	Anti-sGH
Salmonoidei (I)	Salmon	*Salmo salar* (1)	parr	FW	+ + + +	+ + + +
	Trout	*S. gairdneri* (6)	♀	FW	+ + + +	+ + + +
Esocoidei (I)	Pike	*Esox lucius* (2)	imm	FW	+ + + +	+ + + +
Cyprinoidei (II)	Carp	*Cyprinus carpio* (2)	nr	FW	+ + +	+ +
	Roach	*R. rutilus* (1)	nr	FW	+ + +	+ +
	Dace	*L. leuciscus* (1)	nr	FW	+ + +	+ +
	Chub	*L. cephalus* (1)	nr	FW	+ + +	+ +
	Minnow	*P. phoxinus* (1)	nr	FW	+ + +	+ +
Anguilloid.(III)	Eel	*A. anguilla* (5)	♀	FW	+ + + +	+
				SW	+ +	+
Cyprinodont.(V)	Killifish	*Fundulus kansae* (5)	♀	FW	+ + +	+ + + +
		F. heroclitus (5)		SW	+ +	+ + + +
	Molly	*Poecilia latipinna* (20)	♀ ♂imm.	FW	+ + + +	+ + + +
				SW	+ +	+ + + +
Percoidei (VII)	Sea bass	*Dicentrachus labrax* (1)	imm	SW	+ +	+ + + +
	Chromide	*Etroplus maculatus* (5)	imm	FW	+ + + +	+ + + +
	Tilapia	*T. grahami, T. alcalica*	♀ ♂	FW	+ + + +	+ + + +
		T. nigra, T. zillii (10)		SL	+ +	+ + + +
Pleuronect.(VII)	Flounder	*Platichthys flesus* (5)	imm	SW	+ +	+ + + +

No. of + indicates intensity of staining; nr, sex not recorded; imm, immature fish; FW, freshwater; SW, seawater; SL, 'soda lake' fish. No. of fish per group in brackets

in the pituitaries of elasmobranchs or hagfishes (Table 2). The lack of staining with antisera to the salmonid hormones may indicate that, with the exception of holosteans, the prolactin and GH molecules of lower fishes, are different from those of teleosts. These hormones have yet to be isolated from lower fishes and characterized, but there is immunological evidence in favor of their being more closely related to the tetrapod hormones than their teleostean counterparts (14). Results from immunocytochemical stainings must, however, be treated with caution. The anti-sPRL and anti-sGH may not be totally specific: a few short sequences, contained within unrelated peptides, might be sufficient for a positive reaction. This possibility is supported by the recent discovery of anti-sPRL and anti-sGH positive neurons in the central nervous system of an insect (Verhaert et al., unpublished observations). The poor immunoreactivity of the prolactin cells of fishes with antisera to rRPL and oPRL is surprising in view of the numerous earlier reports of their effectiveness (6,13), but this might be explained by the high specificity of antisera resulting from the low (usually 2) number of immunizing injections given.

The anti-sGH did not bind to any pituitary cells in the lungfish or tetrapod vertebrates, but the anti-sPRL gave positive results with lungfish, frog and newt (Table 2, Fig. 2). The immunoreactive cells corresponded to "type 1" acidophils (6), preferentially located towards the rostro-ventral part of the gland. Although prolactin cells could

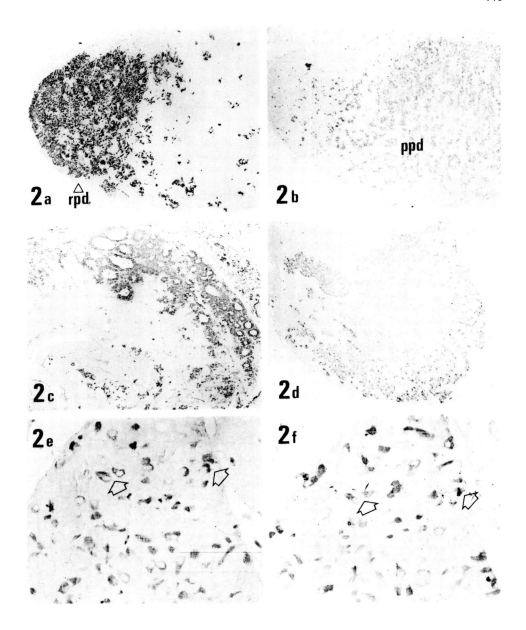

Figure 2: (all sections LS)

2a, 2b: *Lepisosteus* pituitary stained with anti-sPRL (a) and anti-sGH (b). x50.

2c: *Amia* pituitary showing anti-sPRL immunoreactive follicles. x50.

2d: Lungfish pituitary, stained with anti-sPRL. x50.

2e, 2f: Adjacent frog pituitary sections stained with anti-sPRL (a) and anti-rPRL (b). Arrows indicate same population of cells staining. x225.

442

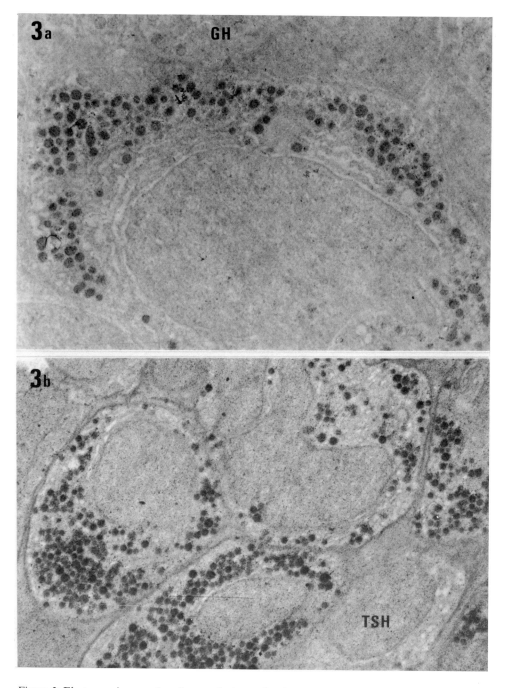

Figure 3: Electron micrographs of trout pituitary after immunocytochemical staining by the PAP method. (a) Prolactin cell stained by anti-sPRL, x10000, note the GH cell adjacent, which is unstained. (b) GH cell stained by anti-sGH, x7500, note the unstained TSH cell.

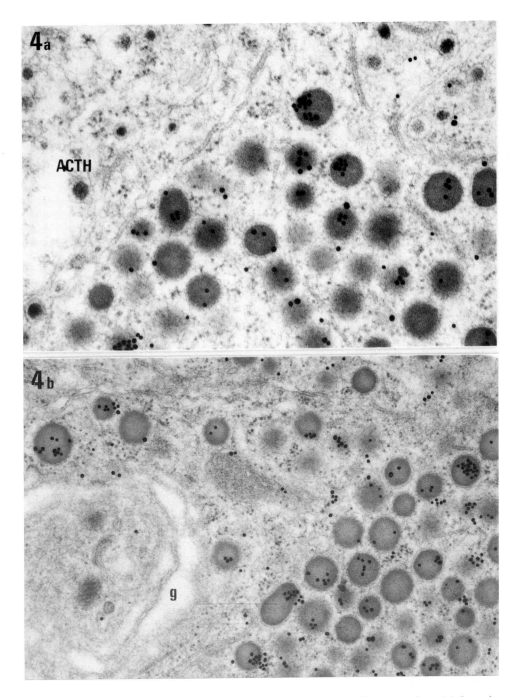

Figure 4: Immunogold EM immunocytochemical method on molly pituitary sections. (a) Granules of prolactin cell, stained by anti-sPRL, with no staining in adjacent ACTH cell, x45000. (b) Part of GH cell, stained by anti-sGH, note reaction on granules but not over golgi area, g. x30000.

Table 2. *Immunoreactivity of prolactin and GH cells in different vertebrate groups with antisera to sPRL, rPRL, oPRL, sGH, and rGH.*

Class	Species	Anti-sPRL	Anti-rPRL	Anti-oPRL	Anti-sGH	Anti-rGH
Cyclostomata	*Myxine* (2♀)	0	0	0	0	0
Elasmobranchi	*Scyliorhinus* (2♀)	0	0	0	0	—
	Raja (1nr)	0	—	—	0	—
Actinopterygii						
Chondrostei	*Calamoichthys* (4+)	0	0	0	0	0
Holostei	*Lepisosteus* (3+)	+	(+)	0	+	0
	Amei (4+)	+	(+)	0	+	0
Teleostei	See Table 1.	+ +-+ + + +	(+)	0	+-+ + + +	0
Crossopterygii	*Protopterus* (2♀)	+ + +	+	0	0	0
Amphibia						
Urodela	*Necturus* (3nr)	+ +	+ +	(+)	0	0
Anura	*Rana* (3nr)	+ +	+ + +	(+)	0	0
Reptilia						
Chelonia	*Chrysemys* (1 imm)	(+)	+ + +	—	0	—
Squamata	*Anolis* (1nr)	0	+ + +	+	0	—
Aves	*Gallus* (1♀)	0	0	—	0	—
	Taenopygia(1♀, 1♂)	0	0	0	—	—
Mammalia	*Rattus* (4♀)	0	+ + + +	+ +	0	+ + + +
	Felis (1♀)	0	+ + + +	+ + +	0	+ + +

No. of + signs indicates intensity of staining, 0 no staining, — not tested, (+) barely detectable, nr not recorded. No. of animals examined and sex in brackets.

be identified in the pituitaries of the reptiles and mammals with anti-mammalian prolactin antisera, they showed no immunoreactivity to anti-sPRL. The differences in immunoreaction of the pituitaries of teleosts and higher vertebrates to the various antiprolactin and anti-GH antisera were supported by absorption studies. Preabsorption of anti-sPRL (1:1000) with oPRL did not extinguish the immunoreactivity of teleost RPD, even at 100 uM concentration, whereas anti-rPRL (1:1000), tested on rat pituitary, was saturated by 1.0 uM oPRL. Similar results were obtained for preabsorption of anti-sGH and anti-rGH with rGH. Structural differences between the prolactin (and GH) molecules of the two vertebrate groups are probably responsible for the differences in antigenicity. This might involve a change in amino acid sequence in a critical part of the molecule, or simply a conformational change, perhaps resulting from a difference in disulphide bridging (3,11), which has hidden or exposed a particular antigenic sequence. The total lack of immunoreactivity of cells in bird pituitaries using antisera to teleost or rat prolactin and GH may be due to important differences in the molecules in this group. However, a more representative number of species must be examined before such conclusions can be drawn.

REFERENCES

1. Farmer SW. (1978): In: Gaillard PJ, Boer HH (eds) Comparative Endocrinology. Elsevier/North Holland, Amsterdam, p 413
2. Wallis M. (1981): J Mol Evol 17:10
3. Kawauchi H, Abe K-I, Takahashi A, Hirano T, Hasegawa S, Naito N, Nakai Y. (1983): Gen Comp Endocrinol 49:446
4. Ingleton PM, Stribley MF. (1977): Gen Comp Endocrinol 31:37
5. Sternberger LA, Hardy PH, Cuculis JJ, Meyer HG. (1970): J Histochem Cytochem 18:315
6. Holmes RL, Ball JN. (1974): The Pituitary Gland: A Comparative Account. Cambridge Univ Press, London
7. Follenius E, Doerr-Schott J, Dubois MP. (1978): Internat Rev Cytol 54:193
8. Nagahama Y, Olivereau M, Farmer SW, Nishioka RS, Bern HA. (1981): Gen Comp Endocrinol 44:389
9. Naito N, Takahashi A, Nakai Y, Kawauchi H, Hirano T. (1983): Gen Comp Endocrinol 50:282
10. Cook H, Cook AF, Peter RE, Wilson SW. (1983): Gen Comp Endocrinol 50:348
11. Farmer SW, Papkoff H, Bewley TA, Hayashida T, Nishioka RS, Bern HA. (1977): Gen Comp Endocrinol 31:60
12. Batten TFC, Hopkins CR. (1979): Histochemistry 60:317
13. Hansen GN. (1983): Acta Zool Suppl
14. Hayashida T, Papkoff H. (1984): In: Chan DKO, Lofts B (eds) Proc 9th Internat Symp Comp Endocrinol, Hong Kong Univ Press, Hong Kong (in press)

Prolactin. Basic and clinical correlates
R.M. MacLeod, M.O. Thorner and U. Scapagnini (eds.),
Fidia Research Series, vol. I,
Liviana Press, Padova © 1985

Section VI
Comparative aspects of
prolactin production and function

CONTROL BY HYPOTHALAMUS OF SYNTHESIS AND RELEASE OF PROLACTIN IN AN AVIAN SPECIES

A. Chadwick and K. O. Khoshaba

Department of Pure and Applied Zoology,
University of Leeds, Leeds LS 9JT UK

It is now well established that in birds the predominant hypothalamic influence is stimulatory even though there is some evidence for the existence of a prolactin inhibitory hormone which may be dopamine (1,2). A specific homologous radioimmunoassay for chicken prolactin has been used to determine plasma prolactin concentrations *in vivo* and pituitary homogenate and media concentrations after *in vitro* incubations (3,4). A stimulatory influence of serotonin on prolactin *in vivo* and *in vitro* has been demonstrated (5,6), which may exert some of its effect at the pituitary gland level. The ability of the mammalian pituitary gland to synthesize prolactin *in vitro* has been established using radiotracers (7) and several groups have used the technique to study prolactin cell physiology and in particular the role of monoamines and other neurotransmitters in controlling prolactin synthesis (8-10). Little work has been done on birds using this technique but radioactively labeled prolactin has been isolated from chicken pituitary glands by polyacrylamide gel electrophoresis following pituitary incubation with [^{14}C] leucine (11). The present study describes experiments performed to compare the total prolactin as determined by RIA in pituitary incubations with the prolactin synthesized de novo in these incubations.

Chickens were purchased as day olds and reared to different ages under 18 h light, 6 h darkness, with free access to food and water. Birds injected with pargyline received 75 mg/kg i.p. Estradiol was administered at a dose of 1 ug/kg in 10% ethanolic saline. Hypothalamic extract (12) was injected intravenously or added to incubation media at various concentrations. Pituitary incubations were performed using the method described by Hall et al. (1,2) except for the addition of L-(^{14}C) leucine to the incubation medium. In addition to determining prolactin by RIA (3,4) [^{14}C]- labeled prolactin was precipitated from aliquots of medium and pituitary homogenate using the same antiprolactin serum which was used in the RIA at the same dilution (1/3000). After 24 h the immune precipitate was centrifuged and solubilized in aqueous scintillator for counting in an auto-beta-counter. Results were expressed in ng/ml or ug/mg for total pro-

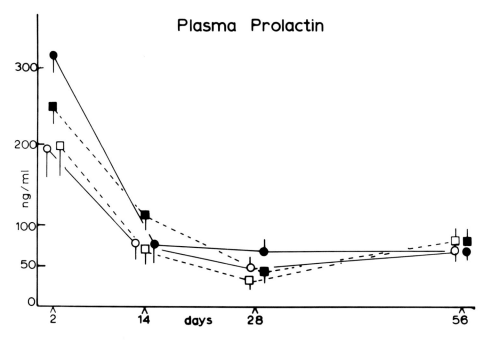

Figure 1. Plasma prolactin concentration (ng/ml) in male (○) and female (□) chickens of different ages. Open symbols: saline controls; closed symbols: injected pargyline i.p., 75 mg/kg, 2 h before death. Means ± SE (n = 10)

lactin or in cpm/mg pituitary for labeled prolactin. Pituitaries were collected from freshly killed broiler fowl from poultry packing stations as well as from experimentally treated birds. Figure 1 shows the circulating plasma prolactin concentration in male and female chicks at 2 days of age through to 8 weeks of age.

In both series one group was injected with pargyline while the other received control injections. Prolactin was higher in both sexes at 2 days than in older birds and the rather restricted pargyline treatment (2 h only) was effective in raising prolactin only in the 2 day old birds. Pituitary glands and mediobasal hypothalami from these birds were removed for *in vitro* incubation and the results are shown in Figures 2 and 3. It can be seen that there was a slight rise in total prolactin produced *in vitro* in the older birds, more marked in the females. Exposure to hypothalamic tissue produced a marked rise in prolactin in almost every group.

By contrast Figure 3 shows that de novo synthesized prolactin showed a progressive decline with increasing age. Further, unlike the results for total prolactin, the addition of hypothalamus produced an inhibitory effect on prolactin synthesis (females) or no effect at all (males). This finding was confirmed when pituitary glands from broiler fowl were incubated *in vitro*. Total prolactin was increased by up to 10X when pituitaries were incubated with hypothalamus, whereas the amount of newly synthesized prolactin either released into the medium or remaining in the pituitary was unchanged whether

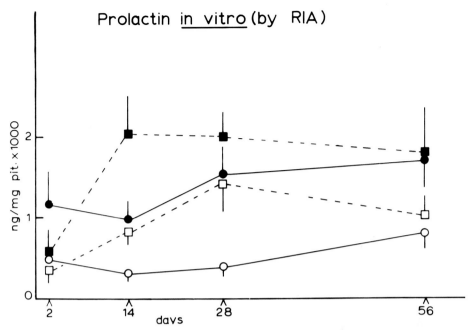

Figure 2. Total prolactin (ug/mg pit.wt.) (medium + pituitary) determined by RIA. 3 h *in vitro* incubation in Med. 199 + [¹⁴C] leucine. Birds of different ages as Fig. 1. ○: male; □:female; open symbols: pit. alone; closed symbols: pit. + medio-basal hypothalamus. Means ± SE (n = 10).

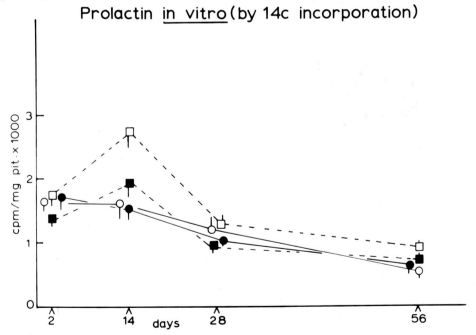

Figure 3. Newly synthesized prolactin (cpm/mg pit.) (medium + pituitary) determined by [¹⁴C] incorporation. 3 h incubation; symbols as Fig. 2; means ± SE (n = 10).

or not the hypothalamus was present. Chickens were treated in various ways known to cause changes in their circulating prolactin before investigating their pituitary prolactin secretory activity *in vitro*. Eight week old cockerels were treated with estradiol 17 beta (24 h), pargyline (2 h), or both. Circulating prolactin was elevated in experimentally treated birds as compared to saline injected controls, significantly so in the two pargyline treated groups. *In vitro*, hemipituitaries were incubated with or without hypothalami from the corresponding group. Hypothalamic stimulation of total prolactin was seen except in the case of the group receiving pargyline alone, where autonomous release was high. Once again the hypothalamus had no effect whatsoever on newly synthesized prolactin. Hypothalami from this experiment were also collected and pooled in the different groups prior to extraction. The extracts were administered i.v. to eight week old cockerels.

Figure 4 shows the rise in plasma prolactin concentration of these H.E. injected birds. H.E. prepared from the estrogen treated birds had the greatest stimulatory effect. After the final blood sample the birds were killed and their pituitaries and hypothalami removed for incubation *in vitro*.

Figure 5 shows the results for both total prolactin and newly synthesized prolactin. High autonomous release was still evident in two of the H.E. treated groups, even though circulating prolactin had returned to baseline values in every case. Hypothalamic stimulation of total prolactin was seen in every group. The total amount of newly synthesized prolactin differed slightly in the groups, being highest in the estradiol group. Once again the presence or absence of hypothalamic tissue made no significant difference to the total newly synthesized prolactin. Furthermore, in every case the amount of newly synthesized hormone remaining behind in the pituitary gland at the end of the incubation was only a small fraction of that released into the medium. These results have several implications with respect to the functioning of the prolactin-secreting cells of the avian pituitary gland. RIA has confirmed the stimulatory influence of the hypothalamus and hypothalamic factors *in vivo* and *in vitro*, which have been widely studied elsewhere (2,5). Despite this, it appears that in the same experiments the hypothalamus had no influence on the synthesis or the release of newly manufactured prolactin, as judged by [^{14}C] leucine incorporation. Prolactin synthesis has been shown by this method to occur *in vitro* by other workers (10) and the product accumulates in a time-related manner (unpublished observations). Synthesis appears to be enhanced in very young chicks despite the fact that RIA shows total prolactin release *in vitro* to be low. This observation might explain how the circulating prolactin concentration comes to be high at this age (Fig. 1) as has also been reported previously for late, unhatched embryos and one day old chicks (13). Little newly synthesized prolactin remains in the pituitary gland *in vitro* compared to that released into the medium (Fig. 5). This observation was made repeatedly and was seen consistently in the results reported here, suggesting that newly synthesized prolactin is discharged from the pituitary cell and leaves the pituitary gland rather than being retained in stored form. This result agrees with that of Piercy and Shin (14) for the rat, in which [^{3}H]-leucine-labeled prolactin was preferentially released from pituitary cells *in vitro* and not retained at all by the cells.

A second implication for pituitary cell functioning concerns the discrepancy between the relative amounts of total prolactin detected in the presence or absence of the hypothalamus as compared with the relative amounts of newly synthesized prolactin.

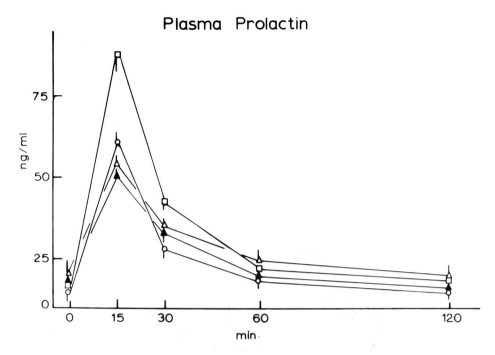

Figure 4. Plasma prolactin concentration (ng/ml) in 8 week old cockerels injected i.v. at time zero with H.E. from controls (▲), from estradiol injected cockerels (□), from pargyline injected cockerels (○), and from estradiol + pargyline injected cockerels (△). Estradiol 17 beta 1 ug/kg: 24 h paragyline: 75 mg/kg 2 h before death. Means ± SE (n = 10).

This discrepancy has been noted elsewhere (14). Since the total amount of hormone detected by RIA after incubation with hypothalamus is much greater than the amount apparently present at the start of the incubation one might expect synthesis to be proceeding apace under such circumstances. This is not borne out, however, by the synthesis results, which suggest little or no effect of hypothalamus on prolactin synthesis. This implies that the pituitary prolactin cells possess a considerable store of already synthesized prolactin which is not detected by RIA in pituitary homogenates and is not, of course, labeled with [14C]. It is well known that pituitary hormone secereting cells contain secretory granules, visible by classical staining techniques and at the fine structural level (15). It seems likely from the present results that the hormone present in these secretory vesicles and granules is in some non-immunoreactive form, awaiting the final stage of the secretory or discharge process during which it acquires its immunological and, presumably, its biological potency. Although this prolactin will also be precipitated by the procedure for determining newly synthesized hormone it will not be [14C] labeled and therefore will not be detected. Discharge of the secretory granules of the prolactin cells of the pituitary gland of the domestic fowl can be evinced by osmotic stress (15) which also brings about an elevation of circulating plasma prolactin (16).

452

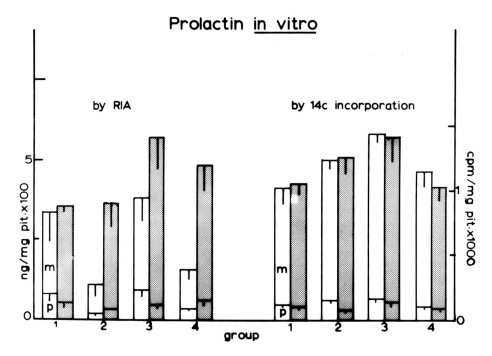

Figure 5. Total and newly synthesized prolactin after 3 h incubation of pituitaries from 8 week old cockerels seen in Fig. 4, removed at 120 min. Open columns: pituitary alone; shaded columns: pit. + hypothalamus; m: prolactin in medium; p : prolactin remaining in pituitary (for each histogram) 1: pits. from control group (▲); 2: from ○; *3: from* □; 4: from △ . Means ± SE (n = 5).

The effect of treatment with hypothalamic extract *in vivo* on circulating plasma prolactin suggests that perhaps this last stage in the secretory process for prolactin, at least in birds, is particularly under the influence of hypothalamic prolactin releasing factor or neurotransmitter agents.

REFERENCES

1. Hall TR, Chadwick A. (1979): Gen Comp Endocr 36:333
2. Chadwick A, Hall TR. (1983): In: Nistico G, Bolis L (eds) Progress in Non-Mammalian Brain Research III. CRC Press, p 79
3. Scanes CG, Chadwick A, Bolton NJ. (1976): Gen Comp Endocr 30:12
4. Lea RW, Sharp PJ, Chadwick A. (1982): Gen Comp Endocr 48:275
5. Harvey S, Chadwick A, Border G, Scanes CG, Phillips JG. (1982): In: Scanes CG, Ottinger MT, Kenney AG, Balthazart J, Cronshaw J, Chester-Jones I (eds) Aspects of Avian Endocrinology. Texas Tech. Press, Lubbock, p 41
6. Hall TR, Chadwick A, Harvey S. (1983): Comp Biochem Physiol 76C:151

7. MacLeod RM, Abad A. (1968): Endocrinology 83:799
8. MacLeod RM, Lehmeyer JE. (1974): Cancer Res 4:345
9. Lamberts SWJ, MacLeod RM. (1978): Endocrinology 103:1710
10. Slabaugh MB, Lieberman ME, Rutledge JJ, Gorski J. (1981): Endocrinology 109:1040
11. Hoshino S, Yamamoto K. (1977): Gen Comp Endocr 32:7
12. Follett BK. (1970): Gen Comp Endocr 15:165
13. Harvey S, Davison TF, Chadwick A. (1979): Gen Comp Endocr 39:270
14. Piercy M, Shin SH. (1981): Mol Cell Endocr 21:75
15. Tai SW, Chadwick A. (1976): IRCS Med Sci 4:209
16. Morley M, Scanes CG, Chadwick A. (1980): Comp Biochem Physiol 67A:695

Prolactin. Basic and clinical correlates
R.M. MacLeod, M.O. Thorner and U. Scapagnini (eds.),
Fidia Research Series, vol. I,
Liviana Press, Padova © 1985

Section VI
Comparative aspects of
prolactin production and function

EXTRACTABILITY OF RAT PITUITARY PROLACTIN: RAT AND BOVINE PROLACTINS ARE STORED DIFFERENTLY

Laurence S. Jacobs and Mary Y. Lorenson

University of Rochester School of Medicine and Dentistry
Rochester, NY 14642

A growing body of evidence indicates that the amount of prolactin detected by immunologic or biologic assay systems varies greatly in bovine pituitary homogenates, secretory granules, and granule subfractions depending on how these tissue preparations are handled and extracted (1-3). Addition of reduced glutathione (GSH) or other thiols increases detected prolactin (1,2), as does elevation of pH (2). In contrast, divalent cations, as well as cysteamine and certain of its aminothiol analogs, decrease detected prolactin (2,4-6).

A partial explanation for these effects is the fact that bovine prolactin is stored within secretory granules in an oligomeric disulfide-bonded form which possesses limited immunoreactivity (7). When GSH or other thiols reduce the intermolecular disulfides, immunoreactive monomeric hormone is released from the complex and made accessible to antibody (or cell surface receptor). The same thiols which increase prolactin detectability also augment prolactin release (1). Divalent cations interfere with hormone assayability, either by reacting directly with free hormonal thiols required for conversion, or by inhibiting enzymes which are involved in the process. These same divalent cations also inhibit prolactin release (8). Cysteamine (CySH) and its analogs exert inhibitory effects via a pH-dependent mechanism not fully understood, but which may serve to inhibit the conversion to monomer, thus maintaining prolactin in its poorly reactive storage form (4). Cysteamine exerts similar effects on tissue somatostatin (9-11). Again, inhibition of detectability parallels inhibition of hormone release or secretion.

The link between detectability and secretion may be effected via an osmotic mechanism, since the oligomeric hormonal forms ($n \geq 50$) of limited immunodetectability exert much less osmotic pressure than the monomers derived from them by thiol action. The marked increase in intragranular osmotic pressure which should occur with conversion to monomer may be one of the final events in the secretory process (7).

Though the selectivity of cysteamine effects on prolactin and somatostatin has not been explained (effects on GH, TSH, endorphins, and gonadotropins can be observed at high concentrations, but are minor compared to those seen with prolactin and somatostatin), a disulfide mechanism is now known to be involved (6). Local peculiarities or characteristics of specific disulfides may be important; for example, prolactin and somatostatin are the only hormones among those mentioned which have a cysteine residue precisely at the carboxyl terminus of the molecule.

These findings have suggested that the mechanisms of prolactin storage may have a design which helps to control secretory responses; if true, this would represent a newly recognized point of secretory regulation and a mechanism for cellular discrimination among secretagogues. Since so many investigators use rodents as experimental models, we decided to study rat pituitary homogenates and partially purified secretory granules to determine if the dramatic alterations in tissue prolactin values seen in bovine pituitaries also occur with similar treatments in rodent glands.

Homogenates of rat anterior pituitaries were made by the same methods and with the same buffers as we have used for bovine glands (1,2). General incubation protocols, assay methods, and statistical analyses have been described (1,2). Secretory granules were prepared by differential centrifugation from the 3500 rpm, 10 min homogenate supernatant; a 20 min, 12,000 rpm spin was followed by spins of equal length at 7700 and 5900 rpm, sequentially. The pellet top was gently rinsed between spins to minimize carry-over of mitochondria, and the final pellet was resuspended in buffer for immediate use, or in heavy sucrose (density > 1.2) for storage at -70 C. No density gradient step was used.

Elevated pH and GSH were tested first. Both treatments had markedly augmented bovine prolactin results, but had either inconsistent or quite small effects on rat pituitary prolactin (Tables 1 and 2). Of the 4 experiments with gland homogenates shown in Table 1, two showed a statistically significant change in prolactin with exposure to pH 10.5, and two did not, and the two differences were in opposite directions. The pooled homogenate data (n = 18) gave a pH 10.5 value which was 110.2 ± 4.5% of the pH 8.3 control. Two experiments with secretory granules showed an even smaller change, with an average increase of only 5%.

Addition of reduced glutathione at 5 mM usually had caused bovine prolactin increases of from 225 to 450%. However, under all conditions tested, with either homogenates or secretory granules, no rat prolactin increases were seen; rather, small but somewhat variable decreases were observed, ranging up to 28% in homogenates

Table 1. *Rat prolactin quantitation at alkaline pH*[a]

Tested Fraction		prolactin, % of pH 8.3 Control
Homogenate	1	111.5 ± 11.1
	2	112.0 ± 17.7
	3	86.3 ± 1.2*
	4	117.2 ± 4.2**
Granules	1	111.0 ± 1.9
	2	99.3 ± 5.8

[a] Exposure was at pH 10.5 for 60 min at 30 C or 180 min at room temperature. Both gave similar results, *P < 0.05, n = 3; **p < 0.01, n = 9.

and 22% in granules (Table 2). At 30 C (81.7 ± 2.4% of control) and 37 C (61.4 ± 3.9%), the decrease in rat prolactin was progressively larger than at room temperature (89.8 ± 6.6%) in the same experiment, compared to no added glutathione. The average

Table 2. *Rat prolactin quantitation with added glutathione* [a]

Tested Fraction		prolactin, % of Control
Homogenate	1	89.8 ± 6.6
	2	72.3 ± 4.3*
	3[b]	89.1 ± 5.3
	4[b]	98.1 ± 6.0
Granules	1	83.0 ± 0.6*
	2	77.9 ± 1.6*

[a] Exposure was at pH 8.3 and room temperature, to 5 mM GSH.
[b] 10 mM GSH was used in these 2 experiments.
* $p < .05$, n = 3.

GSH result, at room temperature, was 81.6 ± 5.5% for homogenates (n = 6) and 80.5 ± 4.4% for secretory granules.

When GSH and alkaline pH were combined, consistent increases in homogenate prolactin were seen in three separate experiments (118.9 ± 9.5%, 116.7 ± 5.8%, and 130.9 ± 6.8%); these included fresh and frozen homogenates, prepared from both young (150 gm) and old (> 450 gm) male rats. The combination of treat ments was without effect, however, in secretory granules; one experiment under each treatment condition was carried out, and the observed results were 100.5 ± 5.0% and 102.8 ± 4.0% of control.

Other concentrations of GSH were then tested, both at pH 8.3 and at pH 10.5, and in both freshly prepared and frozen pituitary homogenates. Though the pattern of response to GSH was similar with fresh and frozen samples, as shown in Figure 1, all the absolute prolactin values were higher if previously frozen homogenates were assayed, regardless of the pH or GSH concentration. The difference was about 30% under each set of conditions.

Table 3. *Effect of zinc on measured rat prolactin* [a]

Added Zinc, uM	Prolactin ug/ml	
	Homogenate	Granules
0	67.8 ± 1.1	107.0 ± 2.0
50	54.7 ± 4.0	74.0 ± 2.9
100	53.9 ± 1.6	72.8 ± 4.1
200	55.5 ± 1.0	
500		63.1 ± 3.7

[a] Exposure was for 180 min at room temperature. Maximum inhibition in homogenates, at 100 uM zinc, was 20.5%; in granules, at 500 uM, it was 41%.

458

The effects of time and temperature, without and with 5 mM GSH, are shown. in Figure 2. At room temperature, no additional prolactin was measured at 180 min as compared to 60 min, but at higher temperatures, modest increases occurred during the two additional hours of exposure; the bulk of the increase had occurred in the first hour. When 5 mM GSH was included, all the 180 min values were considerably below their temperature-specific controls, and were comparable to the zero time control value obtained at 4 C.

In the absence of any GSH or pH change, the effect of 180 min of incubation at room temperature was substantial: homogenate prolactin rose from 49.1 ± 1.7 to 90.5 ± 4.2 ug/ml, and granule prolactin from 35.9 ± 1.9 to 60.6 ± 6.4 ug/ml, 84% and 69% increases. This time-dependence was similar to that seen in bovine pituitary tissue, but smaller; at pH 10.5 with 10 mM GSH, changes in bovine prolactin exceeded 400%.

These data raised serious questions about the similarities and differences between bovine and rat tissue prolactin storage forms. We therefore decided to test other effectors which had presumably influenced measurable bovine prolactin via thiol:disulfide interchange reactions, including zinc and cysteamine. The effects of zinc are shown in

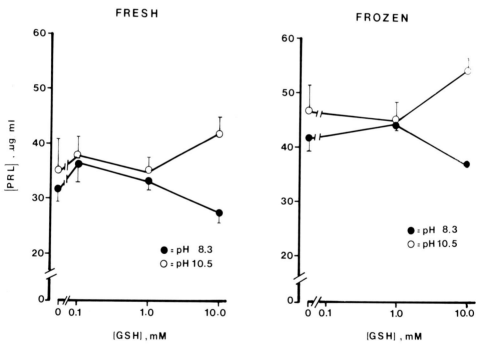

Figure 1. Influence of GSH at pH 8.3 or pH 10.5 on rat prolactin assayability in fresh and frozen pituitary extracts. Pituitary extracts, freshly prepared (left panel) or subjected to 3 freeze/thaw cycles at -70 C (right panel) were incubated with 0, 0.1, 1.0, or 10 mM GSH in 0.05 M Tris, HCl-0.18 M sucrose, pH 8.3 (●), or in buffer which had been adjusted to pH 10.5 with NaOH (○). EDTA (10 mM) was included in buffers containing GSH to prevent oxidation. After 3 h at room temperature, samples were diluted and immunoassayed. Data are presented as the mean ± SE (n = 3), and are taken from Ref. 12.

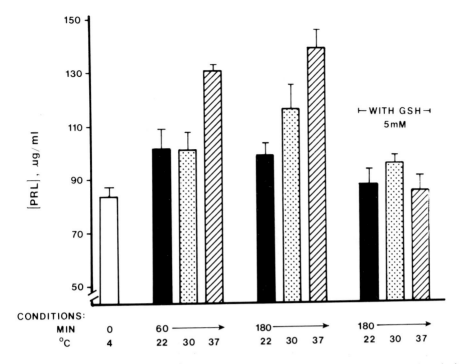

Figure 2. Influence of time, temperature, and 5 mM GSH on measurable rat prolactin. Pituitary homogenates were incubated in 0.05 M Tris-HCl - 0.18 M sucrose, pH 8.3 without or with 5 mM GSH/10 mM EDTA for 0, 60, or 180 min at 4C (□), 22 C (■), 30 C (▨), 37 C (▧) before dilution in RIA buffer. Data given are the mean ± SE for triplicate incubations, and are taken from Ref. 12.

Table 3. Though some inhibition was noted for both homogenates and granules, the magnitude of the effect was far less than that seen on bovine prolactin, and almost no dose-response relationship was seen up to 0.5 mM, a concentration that reduced bovine prolactin virtually to zero.

CySH and a variety of other thiols and thiol-active compounds were also tested. As shown in Table 4, in homogenates, homocysteine and mercaptoethanol inhibited prolactin more strongly than GSH; the effect of dithiothreitol was comparable to that of GSH. Consistent with the unexpected inhibitory effects of these thiols, the opposite of the stimulatory effects seen with bovine prolactin, agents which deplete GSH from tissue, diethyl maleate and diamide, caused brisk rises in prolactin to 135% and 147% of control. Results in secretory granules were not consistent; all tested compounds, including the thiols and the thiol-depletors, inhibited rat prolactin. Oxidized glutathione also inhibited.

The effect of CySH is shown in Table 5. With CySH, both the direction and magnitude of the change were comparable to the CySH effects seen previously on bovine

Table 4. *Influence of thiols and thiol-depleting agents on measured rat prolactin*

Addition	mM	Prolactin, % of no addition control	
		Homogenate	Granules
None		100.0 ± 3.5	100.0 ± 1.9
GSH	5	89.8 ± 6.6	77.9 ± 1.6
Homocysteine	5	66.3 ± 3.8	77.0 ± 1.5
Cysteine	5	107.0 ± 6.0	73.4 ± 4.4
Mercaptoethanol	1	67.6 ± 3.8	80.8 ± 3.0
Dithiothreitol	0.1	85.7 ± 8.8	55.8 ± 1.2
Diethyl maleate	10	135.0 ± 5.3	74.4 ± 8.2
Diamide	10	147.0 ± 8.6	60.2 ± 4.4

Exposure was for 180 min at room temperature. After dilution for assay, no compound was present at a concentration capable of interfering with the RIA.

prolactin (4). Thus, CySH was a potent inhibitor of rat prolactin detectability.

These results indicate a number of functional differences, and some similarities, between prolactin storage forms in rat and bovine pituitaries. Rat prolactin quantitation is inhibited, not enhanced, by exposure to glutathione and other simple thiols. Rat prolactin is essentially unaffected by pH 10.5 exposure, but bovine prolactin is increased. Whereas maximum values (439% of control) of bovine prolactin are measured following combined alkalinization and GSH exposure, that combination yielded only 15-30%

Table 5. *Cysteamine inhibition of rat prolactin detectability*

Cysteamine Dose, mM	Prolactin, ug/ml
0	67.8 ± 1.1
1	27.5 ± 2.2
5	18.9 ± 1.5
10	23.1 ± 2.5

This set of experiments was carried out at pH 7.2 and room temperature for 180 min. This pH had been shown to be optimal for demonstration of the CySH effect (4).

increases in rat prolactin in tissue homogenates, and no change at all in secretory granule prolactin. Time alone (180 min) yielded increases in rat prolactin which varied from 1.7-fold to 3.1-fold, whereas similar incubation for 180 min without GSH resulted in almost no change (11.8 ± 3.7% increase) in measured bovine prolactin (3). Zinc is a much more potent inhibitor of bovine than of rat prolactin, but the inhibitory potency of CySH is similar in both species.

We may conclude that maximal assayability of rat pituitary prolactin is not dependent on added thiols as for bovine prolactin; added thiols actually inhibit rat prolactin detectability. On the other hand, treatment time, even with plain buffer, exerts a powerful influence to increase rat prolactin; time alone, without thiols or alkaline pH, had almost no effect on bovine prolactin. The nature of the time-dependent process is unknown.

These differences are striking, and could be due to differences in granule membrane enzymes (or other membrane components), in non-hormonal intragranular constituents, or in the hormone storage forms themselves. Whatever the explanation, it must also account for the great similarity in cysteamine effects on both species of prolactin. We propose that rat tissue or granules may contain sufficient endogenous GSH to promote prolactin release; released bovine prolactin is insensitive to thiol augmentation, and may show decreases if intramolecular disulfide reduction alters conformation. If rat prolactin behaves similarly, this would help explain not only the prolactin results with added thiols, but also those with high pH and zinc, since GSH may bind zinc, and the high pH influence is probably in large part via disulfide interchange reactions. Additional study of how best to prepare tissue hormone for assay is likely to bring new insight to storage mechanisms, and thence to the regulation of secretion.

ACKNOWLEDGMENTS

This work was supported in part by research grants AM-21783 and AM-31326 from the NIADDK, and RR-00044 from the DRR, NIH.

REFERENCES

1. Lorenson MY, Jacobs LS. (1982): Endocrinology 110:1164
2. Lorenson MY, Robson DL, Jacobs LS. (1983): Endocrinology 112:1880
3. Lorenson MY. (1984), submitted
4. Lorenson MY. (1984): Endocrinology, in press
5. Jacobs LS, Lorenson MY. (1984): Endocrinology, in press
6. Lorenson MY, Jacobs LS. (1984): Endocrinology, in press
7. Lorenson MY, Lee Y-C, Miska SP, Jacobs LS. (1984): In: Mena F, Valverde CM (eds) Frontiers and Perspectives of Prolactin Secretion: A Multidisciplinary Approach. Academic Press, New York
8. Lorenson MY, Robson DL, Jacobs LS. (1983): J Biol Chem 258:8618
9. Szabo S, Reichlin S. (1981): Endocrinology 109:2255
10. Sagar SM, Landry D, Millard WJ, Badger TM, Arnold MA, Martin JB. (1982): J Neurosci 2:225
11. Palkovits M, Brownstein MJ, Eiden LE, Beinfeld MC, Russell J, Arimua A, Szabo S. (1982): Brain Res 240:178
12. Jacobs LS, Lorenson MY. (1984), submitted

Prolactin. Basic and clinical correlates
R.M. MacLeod, M.O. Thorner and U. Scapagnini (eds.),
Fidia Research Series, vol. I,
Liviana Press, Padova © 1985

Section VII
Physiological relevance of pituitary
and non-pituitary prolactins

REGULATION AND PHYSIOLOGICAL RELEVANCE
OF NONPITUITARY PROLACTIN

Daniel H. Riddick

Department of Obstetrics and Gynecology
University of Connecticut Health Center, Farmington, CT 06032

Shortly after the development of a specific radioimmunoassay for human prolactin, it was observed that amniotic fluid contained high concentrations of this molecule, up to 100-fold higher than in maternal serum (1). It was presumed that amniotic fluid prolactin originated from either the maternal or the fetal pituitary gland. In a series of experiments, radiolabeled prolactin was injected into both the maternal and fetal circulations of rhesus monkeys (whose amniotic fluid also contains high levels of prolactin) and the appearance of the radiolabeled prolactin in the amniotic fluid was monitored. During the two hours following injection, maternal and fetal serum levels of labeled prolactin fell precipitously while only very low levels of labeled prolactin could be detected in the amniotic fluid (2). Additionally, replacing amniotic fluid with physiologic saline was followed by a rapid reaccumulation of prolactin to prereplacement concentrations within 1-2 hours. Maternal circulating prolactin during gestation, and its response to ergocriptine, also differed markedly from amniotic fluid prolactin. Thus, maternal pituitary prolactin is produced in steadily increasing amounts throughout gestation, while amniotic fluid prolactin concentrations increase during the first half of gestation and subsequently fall during the last half of pregnancy (3,4,5). When maternal circulating prolactin concentrations during pregnancy are suppressed by ergocriptine, surgical removal, or radiation of the pituitary gland, amniotic fluid prolactin levels remain high and within the normal range (6,7,8).

With the maternal and fetal pituitary glands as unlikely sources of amniotic fluid prolactin, a further search for its source led to the examination of fetal membranes and maternal decidualized endometrium as possible local sources of prolactin production. Initially these investigations determined that prolactin was present in maternal endometrial decidua in high concentrations but not in amnion, chorion, or placenta. Additionally, incubation of these tissues *in vitro* demonstrated that decidua but not amnion, chorion, or placenta released prolactin into the incubation medium in amounts exceeding by many fold the amount of prolactin present initially in the tissue itself (9).

Following this initial report, two independent laboratories confirmed the de novo synthesis of human prolactin from amino acid precursors by decidualized endometrium of human pregnancy, by demonstrating the incorporation of tritated leucine into protein with immunologic and chromatographic properties indistinguishable from pituitary prolactin (10,11). Prolactin synthesis accounted for 3-5% of the total protein synthesis by decidua during *in vitro* incubations. The identity of this prolactin with pituitary prolactin was established subsequently by multiple biochemical and bioactivity criteria (12,13,14,15), and most recently by the demonstration that messenger RNA purified from human decidua hybridizes with a labeled DNA probe for human pituitary prolactin. No similar hybridization occurred with messenger RNA obtained from placenta or amnion (16). A nonpituitary source of prolactin, identical to pituitary prolactin, was thus firmly established.

SOURCES OF NONPITUITARY PROLACTIN

Nongestational endometrium

Prolactin is synthesized and released de novo by secretory endometrium in nonfertile cycles (17). Prolactin is not detectable in endometrium nor is it produced during *in vitro* incubation of endometrium until day 23 of an ideal menstrual cycle, at which time the first histologic evidence of decidualization of the endometrium occurs. Prolactin content of endometrial tissue and the capacity of endometrium *in vitro* to produce prolactin increase thereafter until the onset of menses (18). Furthermore, in luteal phase-deficient cycles where the histologic maturation of the endometrium is less than that expected by the subsequent onset of menses, prolactin production reflects the histologic maturity of the endometrium and thus the degree of decidualization rather than the cycle date (19).

Decidualized endometrium of pregnancy

If pregnancy occurs, prolactin production by decidualized endometrium continues in increasing amounts. The intrauterine presence of fetal or trophoblastic tissue, however, does not appear to alter the production of prolactin at least during early pregnancy (20). Thus, the *in vitro* production of prolactin by endometrium from early pregnancy is similar whether the implantation site is in the endometrial cavity or in the tubal mucosa, as long as the length of gestation is similar. The *in vitro* production of prolactin by decidua during pregnancy increases until midgestation and diminishes thereafter until term. A similar pattern in the concentration of amniotic fluid prolactin is observed. The close correlation between amniotic fluid prolactin concentration and the capacity of the decidua at different times during gestation to produce prolactin suggests that amniotic fluid prolactin is of decidual origin (21). That decidualized endometrium is the primary source of amniotic fluid prolactin is further substantiated by the demonstration that in excess of 40% of the total prolactin produced by decidual tissue itself is released and transported across the adherent amnion and chorion, while less than 3% of radiolabeled prolactin added to the medium on the decidual side of the fetal membranes crosses to the amniotic side during two hours of incubation (22). The "facilitated" transport of decidually produced prolactin requires an intact cellular contact between maternal decidua and fetal chorion (23). If this contact is disrupted, prolactin transport across the membranes fails to occur. The exact mechanism of transport from the decidual cells across the fetal membranes is unknown but may involve the microtubule system, since transport is inhibited in the presence of colchicine (24).

Immunofluorescent localization of prolactin has had varied results. Prolactin has been demonstrated with this technique in the amnion (25,26) and in the decidua and chorion, but other investigators could find no evidence of amniotic localization (27). Prolactin immunoreactivity has also been demonstrated in decidual cells by an immunoenzymatic method in early normal pregnancy, molar pregnancy, and tubal pregnancy (28). The discrepancy between *in vitro* production of prolactin by decidual tissue only and not by chorion, amnion, or placenta, and the above immunofluoresent findings, indicate either that the incubation conditions required for these tissues to produce prolactin have been inadequate to permit observation of the synthetic activity, the immunofluorescent studies are inconclusive, or the cells of the chorion and amnion through or past which prolactin must travel are intimately involved in the transport of prolactin but not in its synthesis.

Myometrium

Human myometrium produces a polypeptide identical to pituitary and endometrial prolactin by the criteria of immunoreactivity and gel chromatography (29). No prolactin is present initially in normal myometrium, but detectable amounts are produced during the first 24 to 48 hours of incubation. Prolactin has been reported present initially in tissue homogenates of uterine myomata (30). The exact cell of origin in the myometrium responsible for prolactin production is unknown at the present time. The presence of prolactin in myomatous tissue initially would suggest that the tissue has the capacity to produce prolactin *in vivo* as well as in tissue culture.

Connective tissue

Culture of rectus fascia has recently been observed to produce a polypeptide with immunoreactivity identical to that of pituitary and endometrial prolactin (unpublished observations). Its production is similar to that of myometrium in that there is no detectable prolactin initially in the tissue, but production begins at 24-48 hours of incubation and continues for at least six weeks during culture. The predominant cell type visible is the fibroblast, but the cell of origin is again unknown. Intestinal mucosa, skin, and liver produced no detectable prolactin *in vitro* during tissue culture.

CONTROL OF NONPITUITARY PROLACTIN PRODUCTION

Normal endometrium

Prolactin production during normal nonfertile cycles appears to be primarily under the control of progesterone. Prolactin production by endometrium has not been observed prior to one week after ovulation, at which time the first evidence of decidualization occurs around the spiral arterioles. When proliferative endometrium is cultured *in vitro* in the presence of progesterone, histologic decidualization of the tissue occurs. This transformation from proliferative to decidualized secretory endometrium does not occur in the absence of progesterone in the incubation medium (31). Furthermore, if estrogen is added to the culture medium in addition to progesterone, the production of prolactin by the tissue is inhibited. Although the endometrium in these experiments had already been exposed to estrogen *in vivo* during the first half of the menstrual cycle, stimulating receptors for progesterone, once such receptors have been induced, estrogen has an inhibitory effect on the secretion of prolactin *in vitro*.

Gestational decidual tissue

The requirement of progesterone for prolactin production by gestational decidua is less clear than for production by nonfertile endometrium. Progesterone has been shown to stimulate prolactin *in vitro* by gestational decidual tissue, an effect inhibited by estrogen (32). A similar study, however, has reported the reverse effects of progesterone and estrogen on the decidua of late pregnancy (33). These discrepant results are not reconcilable presently.

The regulatory effect of progesterone on prolactin production by the decidua of early pregnancy appears to be achieved by induction of the transcription of a stable message, since the effect, once initiated, does not require the continued presence of progesterone (34). This may explain the relatively small stimulatory effect reported for progesterone on prolactin production from term decidua. This tissue has already been exposed for long periods of time to extremely high levels of progesterone so that the effect may already be nearly maximal.

The known modulators of prolactin synthesis by pituitary cells (TRH, dopamine, ergocriptine) have no demonstrable effect on prolactin production by decidua *in vitro* (35). An adenylate cyclase system is present in the subcellular homogenates of human decidua, but dopaminergic binding does not occur (36). Furthermore, prolactin production *in vitro* is related directly to the calcium concentration in the medium (37) and inversely related to the arachidonic acid concentration (38).

As mentioned earlier, the replacement of amniotic fluid by physiologic saline is followed promptly by the re-establishment of prolactin concentrations comparable to those observed prior to saline replacement. There are several possible explanations for this observation. A large downhill concentration gradient may be present facilitating the diffusion of prolaction from regions of higher to lower concentrations. Disruption of decidual and fetal membrane cells by the saline environment may also occur, resulting in prolactin release from these tissues. Finally, prolactin synthesis and release by decidual cells *in vitro* could be under the control of an inhibitory substance which when diluted by saline exerts a diminished inhibition on prolactin synthesis and/or release, allowing it to be freely transported to the amniotic cavity. A substance inhibitory to gestational decidual prolactin production has been reported recently by independent investigators (39,40). This inhibitory substance is a polypeptide of approximately 12,000 Daltons which is not prolactin and which appears in the medium during incubation of decidua. Thus, it is possible that decidual prolactin *in vivo* is under an inhibitory control analogous to that of the pituitary gland.

A separate polypeptide of placental origin has been reported to stimulate the release of prolactin from term decidua. No measurable effect of this substance on the synthesis or release of other proteins by decidua was reported, nor was there any effect of the substance on prolactin release from dispersed rat pituitary cells (41).

Myometrium

The control of prolactin production *in vitro* by human myometrium differs in several respects from that of endometrium. Prolactin production by myometrium does not require the addition of hormones to the incubation medium but is observed after a 24-48 hour lag time in a simple DMEM medium. Furthermore, the addition of progesterone to the incubation medium significantly inhibits prolactin production whereas estrogen is markedly stimulatory (42). This is the reverse of what is seen in endometrium. In addition, the incubation medium from myometrial tissue culture contains a potent stimulator of myometrial prolactin production whereas the incubation medium from endometrium contains a potent inhibitor (43). A discrepancy in the effect of estrogen and progesterone on decidua and myometrium has also been reported for decidual and myometrial enzyme activity. Progesterone increases rat decidual enzyme activity whereas estrogen increases myometrial enzyme activity. Progesterone suppressed the stimulatory effects of estrogen on the myometrium (44).

Connective tissue

The production of prolactin by connective tissue is similar to that produced by myometrium in that no exogenous hormones are necessary for the production to occur. The effect of exogenous hormones on this production has not yet been studied. Both tissues undoubtedly have significant levels of prostaglandins released due to the tissue trauma, and this possibly may be the common factor in the stimulation of prolactin production by each. This is entirely speculatory, however.

PHYSIOLOGIC RELEVANCE OF NONPITUITARY PROLACTIN

A variety of functions have been suggested for extra-pituitary prolactin of uterine origin. Many of the functions appear unrelated, suggesting that they are not prolactin-dependent or that prolactin functions in a more basic physiologic fashion to facilitate a more specific action of other clinical mediators. Thus, nonpituitary prolactin may well act in a facilitory fashion, modulating cellular dynamics at the local tissue level.

Nongestational endometrial prolactin

Since prolactin becomes detectable at or near the time of implantation in the human being and is produced in increasing amounts thereafter, the likelihood of its involvement in the process of implantation and early expansion of the blastocyst is not unreasonable. Additionally, patients with luteal phase defects resulting in immature endometrial development also have diminished prolactin production from the endometrium, as mentioned previously. Such patients with luteal phase deficiency and a diminished prolactin production at the time of arrival of the blastocyst either fail to conceive or undergo repetitive early spontaneous abortions. Whether prolactin production is simply a biochemical marker of histologic maturity or is directly involved in the process of implantation remains speculative.

Another proposed function for endometrial prolactin is in the modulation of corpus luteal progesterone production. A direct effect of prolactin on luteal progesterone production and on the modulation of prostaglandin production by the ovary has been suggested. One mode of action may be in the depression of the production of intraluteal prostaglandins, postponing corpus luteal regression. That prostaglandins in the primate do not induce luteo-lysis does not exclude this possibility (45). Prolactin has been shown to function synergistically with chorionic gonadotropin in prolonging corpus luteal function in the human being when administered during the luteal phase of the cycle before luteal regression has begun (46). A luteotropin of decidual origin has recently been reported in the rodent (47). This decidual luteotropin can substitute completely for pituitary prolactin in maintaining corpus luteal function. Thus, in the absence of the uterus, ergocriptine suppresses pituitary prolactin and also corpus luteal progesterone production. If, however, decidual tissue is implanted following hysterectomy, the suppression of pituitary prolactin by ergocriptine does not diminish corpus luteal progesterone production. The mechanism of action appears to be control of luteal cell receptors for estradiol. Clearly, the interrelationship of corpus luteal progesterone production and endometrial maturity of development is critical for normal implantation and early growth of the blastocyst, as demonstrated by the reproductive failure experienced by patients with corpus luteal deficiency. Prolactin production by decidualized endometrium may be analogous to the decidual luteotropin in the rodent.

Decidual prolactin in gestation

The establishment of pregnancy during the early portions of gestation requires both a careful control of cell growth and proliferation and control of the immune response to avoid rejection of the trophoblast. That prolactin causes a dose-response proliferation of murine lymphoma cells has been used recently as a sensitive bioassay for prolactin (48).

Prolactin and growth hormone share similar binding to bioreceptors in keeping with a growth-promoting function. Additionally, prolactin stimulates the growth rate of newborn rodents, an effect inhibited by antiprolactin (49). Regulation of the immune response in early gestation is critical to the establishment of pregnancy. It has long been known that grafts of decidual tissue survive longer than those of other tissues, and the rejection of allografts in the uterine cavity is greatly retarded when the endometrium is decidualized (50). In addition trophoblastic transplants to nondecidualized tissues exhibit deep and rapid invasion of those tissues compared to the controlled and limited invasion in the decidualized endometrium (51). Prolactin may be involved in the development and functioning of the immune system in early gestation, similar to its role in the immune system in the mammary gland.

Of the many suggested biologic functions of decidual prolactin, its role in osmoregulation is by far the most widely studied. Prolactin is known to regulate sodium transport and, therefore, body fluid osmolality in a number of species of teleosts. The site of action may be the gill, the intestine, the kidney, or the urinary bladder depending upon the species. Analogous actions also occur in amphibians and aquatic avians.

Consequently, a similar role of prolactin in the regulation of electrolyte and water balance in amniotic fluid during primate and human gestation has been sought. Prolactin causes a diminished flux of water from the amniotic side of fetal membranes which is proportionate to the amount of prolactin present in the bathing media and is not reproducible by human placental lactogen or growth hormone. This effect is inhibited by antiprolactin in the bathing medium *in vitro* (52,53). Prolactin also has a direct effect on fetal water balance protecting against hemoconcentration in the fetal monkey when exposed to a hyperosmolar environment (54). The site of action in this process may be the intestinal tract, since it has been shown that prolactin modulates the transport of sodium and water by the mammalian intestine and gallbladder (55).

Receptors for prolactin have been described in human chorion with an affinity and capacity similar to those in the liver and mammary gland (56). Receptors for prolactin were not found in the decidua or umbilical cord. Indirect evidence for prolactin receptors in human amnion has also been presented (57). Of interest is the recent report of a prolactin receptor defect in the chorion laeve in patients with chronic idiopathic polyhydramnios and oligohydramnios (58). The binding of both prolactin and growth hormone to chorion laeve receptors increased as amniotic fluid volume decreased in normal patients. This pattern of binding was not present in patients with polyhydramnios. This is the first report of an abnormality in uterine prolactin production or action associated with a clinical disorder.

It is interesting to speculate that prolactin may be involved in calcium absorption by the fetal intestine. The fact that prolactin stimulates intestinal absorption of calcium in vitamin D deficient rats and the high concentrations of prolactin reaching the intestinal tract via fetal swallowing of amniotic fluid, make this possibility not unlikely (59). The mechanism for a positive calcium balance in the fetus might be provided in part by such a process.

That prolactin might influence surfactant production in type II pneumocytes of the fetal lung has been suggested, since receptors for prolactin are known to be present in the fetal lung and the concentrations of prolactin in the tracheobroncheal tree correlate with amniotic fluid concentrations and phosphatidylcholine (60). Prolactin has been reported to stimulate phosphatidylcholine production in human lung explants when present in addition to cortisol and insulin, but these findings have been difficult to reproduce. Also, abnormalities of fetal lung maturity have not correlated in general with amniotic fluid prolactin concentrations. This does not, however, rule out an abnormal response of the fetal lung to normal prolactin levels.

Myometrial prolactin

The rather unexpected finding that human myometrial tissue produces prolactin in culture has raised a number of interesting issues. First, the cell type of origin producing prolactin in the uterus may be diffusely present throughout the uterus rather than limited to the endometrial stromal cells themselves. Conversely, since the response of myometrium to estrogen and progesterone is the reverse of that observed in the endometrium, the possibility that there is present in the myometrium a stem cell for replacement of endometrial stromal cells is attractive. Transformation of smooth muscle cells into other stromal cellular forms has been described in the pulmonary trunk, the rat kidney, and human gastric mucosa (61,62,63). The myometrial-endometrial junction is irregular with interdigitation of smooth muscle and stromal cells. Furthermore, endometrial stromal sarcoma cells closely resemble smooth muscle cells. These observations suggest the presence of a mesenchymal stem cell existing in myometrium and possibly endometrium with the capacity to differentiate into a variety of cell types depending upon the location of the cell within the tissue and the local hormonal environment. It is also possible as has been previously suggested that the origin for this cell type is in the periphery, i.e. bone marrow, rather than within the uterus at all (64).

That myometrial prolactin may be involved in the control of labor has been suggested recently (65). Since prolactin is known to suppress prostaglandin production in ovarian tissue and prostaglandins are suppressed in myometrial tissue until shortly before or during active labor, this possible role for myometrial prolactin is exciting.

Fibroblasts

The finding of prolactin production *in vitro* by human fibroblasts obtained from the rectus fascia may represent either an anamoly of tissue culture or the fact that mesenchymal cells in general under the proper circumstances may produce physiologically important prolactin. The decidual reaction has been described as analogous in many respects to an inflammatory response. Prostaglandin production and inflammatory stimuli of all kinds may, in fact, transform quiescent fibroblasts into actively growing cells producing in the local environment factors responsible for the control and proliferation of those cells (66). The growth-regulating properties of prolactin have been suggested above. It is attractive to consider that prolactin production by connective tissue following tissue injury may be involved in the local control of cell proliferation necessary for the regeneration and healing of injured tissues. This is highly speculative but not unreasonable.

CONCLUSIONS

A number of hormones traditionally thought to be produced by a single endocrine organ have now been found present in a variety of different tissues of the body. The de novo synthesis and release of prolactin by the human uterus is the most widely studied of such hormones, but other hormones are similarly produced locally. For example, ACTH has been found in normal placenta, fetal lung, adrenal medulla, and in a number of locations in the brain. Such findings have resulted in a new and different concept of the origin and function of hormones. This does not negate classic concepts of endocrinology, but these findings do imply a much more complex control of cellular functions utilizing locally produced and locally acting chemical messengers for the specific and fine regulatory control of cellular functions. These changing concepts allow the action of a particular hormone such as prolactin to be limited to a given tissue in which it is produced without the need for exposure throughout the body when only one localized region requires it.

The uterus is an organ whose function is in a constant state of change during the normal cycle and gestation. The need for a rather slow but constant adjustment unrelated to the needs of the rest of the organism make local control not unexpected. The unique aspects of uterine function make it ideal for the study of local production of chemical messengers resulting in local control of cellular and tissue function. Furthermore, since many of the macromolecules produced by the uterus do not appear to enter the general circulation in significant quantities, the production and action of these hormones will be determined only by studying their production and action within the local tissue.

Although the uterus is an obvious example of a constantly changing organ, the need for careful local control of tissue regeneration and healing exists all the time in the organism, and this process is undoubtedly ultimately controlled at the local tissue level. The most fundamental understanding of endocrinology is that of communication via chemical messengers. Within this framework, the study of paracrine and autocrine functions in tissues will compose a large part of the exciting investigation in endocrinology over the next decade.

REFERENCES

1. Tyson JE, Hwang P, Friesen HG. (1972): Am J Obstet Gynecol 113:14
2. Josimovich J, Weiss G, Hutchinson D. (1974): Endocrinology 94:1364
3. Jaffe RB, Yuen BH, Keye WR, Midgley AR. (1973): Am J Obstet Gynecol 117:757
4. Rosenberg SM, Maslar IA, Riddick DH. (1980): Am J Obstet Gynecol 138:681
5. Chochinov RG, Ketupanya A, Maris IK. (1976): J Clin Endocrinol Metab 42:983
6. Bigazzi M, Ronga R, Lancranjan I, Ferraro S, Branconi F, Buzzoni P, Martorana G, Scarselli GF, Del Poso E. (1979): J Clin Endocrinol Metab 48:9
7. Quigley MM, Hammond CB, Handwerger S. (1976): Fertil Steril 27:1165
8. Riddick DH, Luciano AA, Kusmik WF, Maslar IA. (1979): Fertil Steril 31:35
9. Riddick DH, Kusmik W. (1977): Am J Obstet Gynecol 127:187
10. Golander A, Barrett J, Hurley T, Barrett J, Hizi A, Handwerger S. (1978): Science 202:311
11. Riddick DH, Luciano AA, Kusmik WF, Maslar IA. (1978): Life Sci 23:1913
12. Frame LT, Rogol AD, Riddick DH, Baczynski E. (1979): Fertil Steril 31:647

13. Golander A, Hurley T, Barrett J, Hizi A, Handwerger S. (1978): Science 202:311
14. Riddick DH, Luciano AA, Kusmik WF, Maslar IA. (1978): Life Sci 23:1913
15. Tomita K, McCoshen JA, Fernandez CS, Tyson JE. (1982): Am J Obstet Gynecol 42:420
16. Clements J, Whitefeld P, Cooke N, Healy DL, Matheson B, Shine J, Funder J. (1983): Endocrinology 112:1133
17. Maslar IA, Riddick DH. (1979): Am J Obstet Gynecol 135:751
18. Daly DC, Maslar IA, Rosenberg SM, Tohan N, Riddick DH. (1981): Am J Obstet Gynecol 140:587
19. Daly DC, Maslar IA, Rosenberg SM, Tohan N, Riddick DH. (1981): Am J Obstet Gynecol 140:587
20. Maslar IA, Kaplan BM, Luciano AA, Riddick DH. (1980): J Clin Endocrinol Metab 51:78
21. Rosenberg SM, Maslar IA, Riddick DH. (1980): Am J Obstet Gynecol 138:681
22. Riddick DH, Luciano AA, Kusmik WF, Masar IA. (1979): Fertil Steril 31:35
23. McCoshen JA, Tagger OY, Wodzicki A, Tyson JE. (1982): Am J Physiol 243:R552
24. Riddick DH, Maslar IA. (1981): J Clin Endocrinol Metab 52:220
25. Healy DL, Muller HK, Burger HG. (1977): Nature 265:642
26. McCoshen JA, Tomita K, Fernandez C, Tyson JE. (1982): J Clin Endocrinol Metab 55:166
27. Frame LT, Wiley L, Rogol AD. (1979): J Clin Endocrinol Metab 49:435
28. Meuris S, Soumenkoff G, Malengreau A, Robyn C. (1980): J Histochem Cytochem 28:1347
29. Walters CA, Daly DC, Chapitis J, Kuslis S, Prior JC, Kusmik W, Riddick DH. (1983): Am J Obstet Gynecol, in press
30. Daly DC, Maslar IA, Riddick DH. (1983): Society for Gynecologic Investigation (Abstract 218)
31. Daly DC, Maslar IA, Riddick DH. (1983): Am J Obstet Gynecol 145:672
32. Daly DC, Maslar IA, Riddick DH. (1983): Am J Obstet Gynecol 145:679
33. Rosenberg SM, Bhatnagar AS. (1983): Society for Gynecologic Investigation (Abstract 217)
34. Maslar IA, Roche J, LaFerla J. (1982): The Endocrine Society (Abstract 34)
35. Golander A, Barrett J, Hurley T, Barry S, Handwerger S. (1979): J Clin Endocrinol Metab 49:787
36. Rogol A. 1983, personal communication
37. Richards SR, Kim MH, Malarkey WB. (1982): J Clin Endocrinol Metab 54:820
38. Handwerger S, Barry S, Barrett J, Markoff E, Zeitler P, Cwikel P, Siegel M, (1981): Endocrinology 109:2016
39. Daly DC, Kuslis ST, Riddick DH. (1983): The Endocrine Society (Abstract #601) San Antonio, TX
40. Markoff E, Howell S, Barry S, Handwerger S. (1983): The Endocrine Society (Abstract #635) San Antonio, TX
41. Handwerger S, Barry S, Markoff E, Barrett J, Conn PM. (1983): Endocrinology 112:1370
42. Walters CA, Daly DC, Chapitis J, Kuslis S, Prior JC, Kusmik W, Riddick DH. (1983): Am J Obstet Gynecol 147:639
43. Walters CA, Kuslis S, Ying YK, Daly DC, Riddick DH. (1984): Society for Gynecologic Investigation (Abstract #241P) San Francisco, CA
44. Moulton BC. (1974): Biol of Reprod 10:526
45. Rothchild. (1981): Int Congress Series No 580, 10:51
46. Fried PH, Rakoff AE. (1952): J Clin Endocrinol Metab 12:321
47. Basury R, Jaffe RC, Gibori G. (1983): Biol Reprod 28:551
48. Tomita K, McCoshen JA, Friesen HG, Tyson JE. (1982): J Clin Endocrinol Metab 55:269
49. Sinha YN, Vanderlaan WP. (1982): Endocrinology 110:1871
50. Beer AE, Billingham RE. (1974): J Reprod Fertil (Suppl) 21:59
51. Kirby DRS, Cowell TP. (1968). In: Fleischmajer, Billingham (eds) Epithelial-Mesenchymal Interactions. Williams and Wilkins, Baltimore

52. Leontic EA, Tyson JE. (1977): Am J Physiol 232:R124
53. Leontic EA, Schrueffer JJ, Andreassen B, Pinto H, Tyson JE. (1979): Am J Obstet Gynecol 133:435
54. Josimovich J, Meriski K, Boccella L. (1977): Endocrinology 100:564
55. Mainoya JR, Bern HA, Regan JW. (1974): J Endocrinol 63:311
56. Herington AC, Graham J, Healy DL. (1980): J Clin Endocrinol Metab 51:1466
57. Leontic EA, Schrueffer JJ, Andreassen B, Pinto H, Tyson JE. (1979): Am J Obstet Gynecol 133:435
58. Healy DL, Herington AC, O'Herlihy C. (1983): J Clin Endocrinol Metab 56:520
59. Pahuja DN, DeLuca HF. (1981): Science 214:1038
60. Johnson JWC, Tyson JE, Wodzicki A, Friesen HG, Beck JC, London WT. (1982): Society for Gynecological Investigation Twenty-ninth Annual Meeting SGI Publishing, Dallas (Abstract #320)
61. Smith P, Health D, Padula F. (1978): Thorax 33:31
62. Cantin M, Araujo-Nascimento M, Benchimol S, Desormeaux Y. (1977): Am J Path 87:581
63. Boger A, Hort W. (1977): Virchows Archiv A Pathological Anatomy and Histology 372:287
64. Kearns M, Lala PK (1981): J Exp Med 155:1537
65. Healy DL, Hodgen GD. (1983): Obstetrical and Gynecological Survey 38:509
66. Finn CA. (1971): Adv Reprod Physiol 5:1

Prolactin. Basic and clinical correlates
R.M. MacLeod, M.O. Thorner and U. Scapagnini (eds.),
Fidia Research Series, vol. I,
Liviana Press, Padova © 1985

Section VII
Physiological relevance of pituitary
and non-pituitary prolactins

DECIDUAL LUTEOTROPIN: A PROLACTIN-LIKE HORMONE PRODUCED BY RAT DECIDUAL TISSUE

P.G. Jayatilak, L.A. Glaser, R. Basuray, P. A. Kelly[1] and G. Gibori

Department of Physiology and Biophysics, College of Medicine,
University of Illinois, Health Sciences Center, Chicago, Illinois 60612
[1]Laboratory of Molecular Endocrinology, McGill University,
Royal Victoria Hospital, Montreal, Quebec H3A 1A1 Canada

Several secretory products have been associated with the decidual tissue. Decidual cells secrete prostaglandins (1,2), relaxin (3,4), and in humans, prolactin (5-9). It was first hypothesized that the decidual tissue of the rat secretes a prolactin-like hormone by Gibori et al. (10). They found that inhibition of prolactin secretion in pseudopregnant rats causes a precipitous decline in luteal progesterone synthesis only in rats with decidual tissue. In the presence of decidual tissue, corpora lutea continue to secrete progesterone as if prolactin had not been removed from the circulation. Subsequently, it was found that the effect of the decidual tissue is exerted through a substance, decidual luteotropin, which reaches its sites of action by passage through the systemic circulation (11). Studies in pregnant rats have also revealed that the maternal part of the placenta, the decidua, produces a substance which sustains luteal cell function after prolactin withdrawal (12).

Recently, production of prolactin by decidualized human endometrium has been reported by several groups (5-9). Decidual prolactin has been found to be identical to its pituitary homologue (5,13). Antisera developed against human prolactin recognizes decidual prolactin (5,9,13), making quantitation of the hormone relatively easy. In the rat, decidual luteotropin does not cross-react with antisera to either rat or ovine prolactin (10). This has hampered the characterization of this hormone. With the use of highly luteinized ovaries as a source of prolactin receptors, we were able to identify, quantitate, and partially characterize rat decidual luteotropin.

Decidualization was induced by traumatization of the antimesometrial surface of both uterine horns on day 5 of pseudopregnancy with a hooked needle. On different days of pseudopregnancy, rats were sacrificed with an overdose of ether, the uterine horns were dissected out, kept on ice, and slit lengthwise. The decidual tissue was scraped off and weighed. Muscle was also obtained for use as a control tissue and similarly treated. Either decidual tissue or muscle was homogenized in a Polytron homogenizer with a short burst of 10 sec at 4 C in TEG buffer (50 mM Tris-HC1, 1 mM EDTA and 5% v/v glycerol, pH 7.4 containing 25 ug bacitracin, 10 ug pepstatin A and 174 ug phenylmethylsulfonyl fluoride per ml). The 25,000 x g supernatant of the homogenate was used for the determination of prolactin-like activity in a radioreceptor assay. For this assay, membranes of highly luteinized ovaries were used as a source of prolactin receptors. Prolactin bound to rat luteal membranes with high affinity (K_D = 46 pM) and specificity (Fig. 1). Ovine prolactin, bovine prolactin, and rat prolactin were all capable of displacing the [^{125}I]-ovine prolactin tracer from luteal prolactin receptors in a dose-related manner. Ovine LH and ovine FSH did not inhibit the binding of [^{125}I]-ovine prolactin to its receptor site. The inter- and intra-assay coefficients of variation were 8.9% and 5%, respectively. The sensitivity of this radioreceptor assay was 0.5 ng/tube. Graded dilutions of decidual tissue extracts yielded curves that were parallel to the ovine prolactin standard, indicating that decidual luteotropin and ovine prolactin compete for the same receptor sites on rat luteal membranes. Muscle extracts at similar dose levels did not displace prolactin binding. Utilizing this assay, the levels of decidual luteotropin were quantitated throughout pseudopregnancy.

The decidual tissue was isolated from rats on each day from days 6-15 of pseudopregnancy. Muscle was used as a tissue control. Tissue extracts were assayed in duplicate and in at least two aliquot sizes. The results of the time course experiments

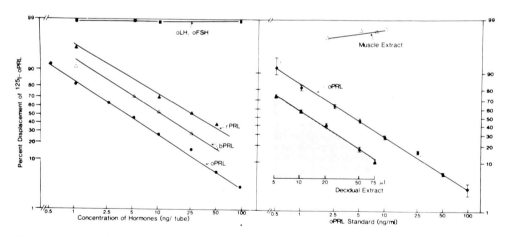

Figure 1. Competition of [^{125}I]-labeled ovine prolactin in the luteal radioreceptor assay with ovine, bovine, and rat prolactin and a serial dilution of decidual tissue extract. For the hormonal specificity of prolactin binding, luteal membranes were incubated with [^{125}I]-prolactin (100,000 cpm/ 100 ul) alone or with increasing concentrations (1-1000 ng) of ovine prolactin, bovine prolactin, rat prolactin, ovine LH, and ovine FSH. For the competition of ovine prolactin with decidual tissue extracts, 40 percent (w/v) homogenates of day 9 decidual tissue were prepared as outlined in the text and 5-200 ul were assayed in quadruplicate.

Table 1. *Decidual luteotropin (DLT) concentration throughout pseudopregnancy*

					Day of Pseudopregnancy				
	6	7	8	9	10	11	12	14	15
DLT (ng/gm)	57±11	87±13	317±72	472±88	248±54	214±36	141±22	45±3	48±1
	(10)	(15)	(14)	(22)	(17)	(17)	(12)	(5)	(5)

Decidual tissue was induced in day 5 pseudopregnant rats. The decidual tissue was obtained on the indicated days and the decidual extract from each rat was assayed in two aliquot sizes and in duplicate. The value shown represent the mean ± SE with the number of animals in parenthesis. They are expressed as ovine prolactin equivalents (NIAMDD ovine prolactin-16).

are shown in Table 1. Prolactin-like activity was detectable in decidual tissue as early as day 6, reached a maximum concentration on day 9, and declined thereafter. Muscle processed in a similar manner was found to be devoid of any prolactin-like activity. The time course was analyzed for significant differences between days by analysis of variance and found to be significant. ($p < 0.05$).

In the rat, decidual tissue proliferates vigorously for about 5 days following induction. Thereafter, the cells stop dividing and begin to regress. The decline in decidual luteotropin levels corresponds to the disappearance of the luteotropic effect of the decidua. From day 11, the decidual tissue of either pregnant or pseudopregnant rats loses its luteotropic activity and becomes unable to sustain luteal cell production of progesterone (12,14,15). In humans, the appearance of prolactin in the endometrium also coincides with the onset of decidualization at the time when implantation would occur.

To characterize decidual luteotropin, decidual tissue obtained from day 9 pseudopregnant rats was routinely used. A cytosolic fraction (9-10 ml) was obtained and applied to a column of Ultrogel AcA 54 (2.5 x 90 cm), eluted with TEG buffer, pH 7.4. The column was calibrated with a low molecular weight marker kit (Pharmacia) and elution fractions (10 ml) were analyzed by ovarian radioreceptor assay. As presented in Figure 2, the major component of decidual luteotropin had a V_e to V_o ratio of approximately 2.0, while a small shoulder eluted with a V_e to V_o ratio of 1.7. There was 60 to 80% recovery of the prolactin-like activity from the column fractions. Chromatography of the calibrated weight standards indicated that decidual luteotropin corresponds to a protein with a molecular weight of approximately 23,500 daltons.

To examine whether sulfhydryl compounds reduce decidual luteotropin, 100 ul dithiothreitol (DTT, 5 mM) solution in Tris buffer was incubated with 100 ul of day 9 decidual tissue cytosolic extract (40 percent v/v) for 60 min at 37 C. The control tubes were incubated with 100 ul of buffer only. Following incubation, the contents were dialyzed overnight in cold with 3 changes of buffer. The samples were subsequently assayed for prolactin-like activity. Incubation of decidual tissue extracts with DTT induced a 64% loss in activity (control 44.0 ± 2.8 vs DTT treatment, 17.1 ± 1 ng/g).

To examine the effect of DTT on the prolactin receptor, 100 ul of 5 mM DTT was incubated with 100 ug of ovarian membranes for 60 min at 37 C. Samples were washed twice; the pellet was then suspended and assayed for its ability to bind [125I]-

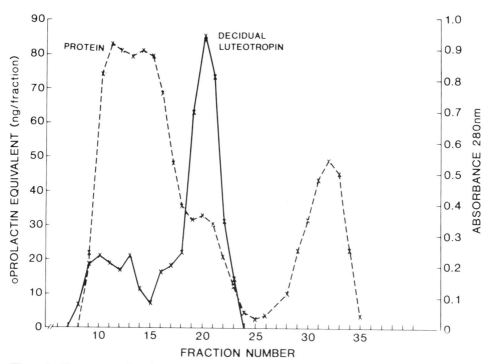

Figure 2. Chromatography of decidual tissue extract on a column (2.5 x 90 cm) of Ultrogel AcA54, equilibrated and eluted at 4 C with TEG buffer, pH 7.4. Elution fractions (10 ml) were analyzed by radioreceptor assay. The eluate was also assayed for protein content.

ovine prolactin. Pretreatment of receptors with DTT had no effect on their subsequent capacity to bind prolactin or decidual luteotropin (control, $17,727 \pm 909$ cpm vs DTT treatment, $18,636 \pm 909$). These findings suggest the presence of disulfide linkages in decidual luteotropin.

To determine whether decidual luteotropin is a protein, tissue was extracted in the absence of proteolytic inhibitors. Cytosolic extract (100 ug) was incubated with 100 ug of trypsin (15,000 units/mg protein) for 60 min at 37 C. The control tubes were incubated with Tris buffer. At the end of incubation, 200 ug trypsin inhibitor (10,000 units/mg protein) was added to all the tubes. The tubes were then assayed for the presence of prolactin-like activity. Digestion of decidual tissue extract with trypsin completely destroyed the hormone activity.

To investigate whether decidual tissue is a heat-stable protein, extracts were incubated for 16 h at 22 C, 1 h at 37 C, or boiled for 25 min. The tissue extract was then assayed for prolactin-like activity. The activity in the control tubes, kept at 4 C, was taken as 100%. As presented in Table 2, incubation of decidual extracts in moderate heat for long periods or at elevated temperatures for a short period resulted in a significant reduction in prolactin-like activity.

To examine whether decidual luteotropin is a glycoprotein, a cytosolic extract of decidual tissue obtained from day 9 pseudopregnant rats was applied to a column (10

Table 2. *Effect of temperature on decidual luteotropin activity*

Temperature (°C)	Time	Decidual Luteotropin Percent Activity Lost
20	16 h	33
37	1 h	16
100	0.25 h	100

The decidual tissue obtained from day 9 pseudopregnant rats was homogenized (30 percent w/v) in 25 mM Tris-HCl buffer (pH 7.4). A 25,000 x g supernatant fraction was incubated in triplicate at the indicated temperature and time. The extract incubated at 4 C was used as control. The control tube (73 ng of prolactin-like activity/gm of tissue) was taken as 100%.

ml syringe) packed with Concanavalin A Sepharose 4 B. The unadsorbed sample (non-glycosylated fraction) was washed with a starting buffer (0.1 M sodium acetate buffer, pH 6.1, containing 1 mM $MgCl_2$, $MnCl_2$, $CaCl_2$ and 1 M NaCl), collected and pooled. The adsorbed sample (glycosylated fraction) was eluted with 0.3 M alpha-D-methyl mannoside in the starting buffer. The eluates were pooled, dialyzed extensively, and then lyophilized, reconstituted and checked for the presence of prolactin-like activity by radioreceptor assay. All prolactin-like activity was found in the unadsorbed fraction. No activity was recovered in the glycosylated fraction. The results suggest that decidual luteotropin does not contain any carbohydrate moieties available to interact with the Concanavalin-A.

In summary, the characterization of decidual luteotropin indicates that it is a prolactin-like hormone because it competes with prolactin in a dose-dependent manner for the same receptor site on the luteal membrane. Decidual luteotropin appears to be a heat labile protein with disulfide bridge(s), and has a molecular weight of approximately 23,500. The time course of decidual luteotropic concentration closely corresponds to the luteotropic effect observed in pseudopregnant rats with decidualized uteri after the removal of pituitary prolactin (12,14,25). The results of the present investigation provide evidence that the rat can be used as an experimental animal model to further investigate the role of the prolactin-like hormone produced by the decidua.

ACKNOWLEDGMENTS

This work was supported by NIH grant HD12356 and NSF grant PCM 8112225.

REFERENCES

1. Anteby SO, Bauminger S, Zor U, Lindner HR. (1975): Prostaglandins 10:991
2. Sykes JA, Williams KI, Rogers AF. (1975): J Endocrinol 64:18 (Abstract)
3. Bigazzi M, Nardi E, Bruni P, Petrucci F. (1980): J Clin Endocrinol Metab 51:939
4. Bigazzi M, Nardi E, Petrucci F, Scarselli G. (1983): In: Bigazzi M, Greenwood FC, Casparri

G (eds) Biology of Relaxin and its Role in the Human. Excerpta Medica, International Congress Series No. 610, Amsterdam p 206

5. Golander A, Hurley T, Barrett J, Hizi A, Handwerger S. (1978): Science 202:311
6. Riddick DH, Luciano AA, Kusmik WF, Maslar IA. (1978): Life Sci 23:1913
7. Maslar IA, Kaplan BM, Luciano AA, Riddick DH. (1980): J Clin Endocrinol Metab 51:78
8. Kubota T, Kumasaka T, Yaoi Y, Suzuki A, Saito M. (1981): Acta Endocrinol 96:258
9. DeZiegler D, Gurpide E. (1982): J Clin Endocrinol Metab 55:511
10. Gibori G, Rothchild I, Pepe GJ, Morishige WK, Lam P. (1974): Endocrinology 95:1113
11. Castracane VD, Rothchild I. (1976): Biol Reprod 15:497
12. Basuray R, Gibori G. (1980): Biol Reprod 23:507
13. Tomita K, McCoshen JA, Friesen HG, Tyson JE. (1982): J Clin Endocrinol Metab 55:269
14. Gibori G, Basuray R, McReynolds B. (1981): Endocrinology 108:2060
15. McCoshen JA, Tagger OY, Wodzicki A, Tyson JE. (1982): Am J Physiol 243:R552

Prolactin. Basic and clinical correlates
R.M. MacLeod, M.O. Thorner and U. Scapagnini (eds.),
Fidia Research Series, vol. I,
Liviana Press, Padova © 1985

Section VII
Physiological relevance of pituitary
and non-pituitary prolactins

SUBCELLULAR LOCALIZATION OF DECIDUAL PROLACTIN BY DIFFERENTIAL AND DENSITY GRADIENT CENTRIFUGATION

S. Handwerger, S. Wilson, and P.M. Conn

Departments of Pediatrics, Physiology, and Pharmacology,
Duke University Medical Center, Durham, North Carolina

During pregnancy, decidual tissue synthesizes and releases a peptide which appears identical to pituitary prolactin by chemical, immunologic, and biologic criteria (1-3). However, despite the similarities, the mechanisms regulating the release of decidual and pituitary prolactins are different. Pituitary prolactin release is stimulated by cyclic AMP and calcium ionophores (4-6), neither of which stimulate release of decidual prolactin (7,8). Although both decidual and pituitary tissues contain estrogen receptors (9,10), estrogen stimulates the release of pituitary prolactin but has no effect on the release of decidual prolactin (8,11,12). Furthermore, while pituitary prolactin release is stimulated by thyrotropin-releasing hormone, vasoactive intestinal polypeptide, cholecystokinin, and prostaglandins, and is inhibited by dopamine and bromocriptine (for review, see 13), these hormones and drugs have no effect on decidual prolactin release (8,14). The secretion of decidual prolactin, unlike that of pituitary prolactin, is stimulated by a protein released by the placenta (15) and is inhibited by a protein (16) (other than prolactin) released by the decidua and by arachidonic acid (17).

Prolactin in the pituitary is stored in large secretory granules (18,19), but the intracellular localization of prolactin in decidual tissue is unknown. Since the difference in the mechanism of pituitary and decidual prolactin secretion might result, at least in part, from differences in the site of intracellular storage, we have compared the intracellular sites of the two hormones by differential and density gradient centrifugations. Human decidual tissue was obtained from women with normal pregnancies of 37-40 weeks gestation (3), and human pituitary tissue was obtained at autopsy within 2 hours of death. In the differential centrifugation studies, tissues were homogenized in 9 ml of 0.32 M sucrose per gram wet weight with 5 strokes of a glass-to-glass, motor-driven conical Duall tissue grinder (100-150 um clearance). The resulting homogenate was centrifuged at 800 x g for 10 minutes. The supernatant fluid was decanted and saved. The sedimented material was homogenized again in one-half the initial volume of 0.32 M sucrose and centrifuged at 800 x g for 10 minutes to produce a crude nuclear fraction. The supernatant fluid from both centrifugations was combined and centrifuged at 26,000 x g for 10 minutes to yield a crude mitochondrial fraction. The supernatant fluid was further centrifuged at 111,000 x g for 60 minutes to produce the microsomal fraction and the post-microsomal supernatant. In the density gradient centrifugation studies, the mitochondrial and microsomal fractions were fractioned using linear sucrose gradients of 0.32 M - 1.6 M sucrose or 0.5 M - 2.0 M sucrose. The gradients were centrifuged at 66,400 x g for 13.5 or 15.5 hours. Individual tubes were unloaded from the bottom using a peristaltic pump, and 20 or 21 fractions were collected from each. Identically prepared gradients overlaid with only 0.32 M sucrose were fractionated similarly and the sucrose concentration of each fraction determined by refraction using known standards. Human and rat prolactins were measured by homologous radioimmunoassays using kits supplied by the National Hormone and Pituitary Program, NIADDK, in which the human and rat prolactins did not cross react ($<0.001\%$).

Following differential centrifugation, 98% of prolactin in human pituitary tissue was detected in particulate fractions (Table II). The mitochondrial fraction contained 73.7% of the pituitary prolactin and the microsomal fraction contained 24.7%. Almost all of the thyrotropin-releasing (96%) hormone and LH (94%) in the pituitary was detected in the particulate fractions with most of the hormones in the mitochondrial fraction. In sharp contrast, $80.1 \pm 4.0\%$ of the prolactin in decidual tissue (mean $\pm$ SEM, n = 6) was present in the postmicrosomal supernatant with the remainder of the prolactin in the cytosol, equally divided between the mitochondrial and microsomal fractions (Table II).

Comparison of Table I and Table II shows that the decidual prolactin in the postmicrosomal supernatant did not result from rupture of secretory granules. When human decidual tissue and rat pituitary tissues were homogenized together prior to differential centrifugation, the subcellular distribution of decidual and pituitary prolactins in the combined homogenates were almost identical to that in the homogenates of the individual tissues.

Table I. *Differential centrifugation of rat pituitary and human decidual tissues.*

	Combined Homogenate		Rat Pituitary Homogenate
	pituitary prolactin	decidual prolactin	
mitochondrial fraction	58.3%	10.3%	61.0%
microsomal fraction	34.4%	9.5%	33.9%
post-microsomal supernatant	7.3%	80.2%	5.1%
prolactin centrifuged	1.7 ug	6.0 ug	1.5 ug
% recovery	79.9%	80.0%	89.0%

Human decidual tissue and rat pituitary tissue were homogenized together and then subjected to differential centrifugation. The percent of prolactin in each of the homogenate fractions is expressed as a percentage of the total prolactin in the non-nuclear fractions. Results of fractionation of combined homogenate are compared to those of rat pituitary homogenate processed in an identical manner.

Table II. *Differential centrifugation of human pituitary and decidual tissues*

	PITUITARY	DECIDUA (N=6) mean ± SE
mitochondrial fraction	73.3%	11.1 ± 2.3%
microsomal fraction	24.7%	10.8 ± 2.7%
post-microsomal supernatant	2.0%	80.1 ± 4.0%
prolactin centrifuged	193.2 ug	3.5 ± 1.0 ug
recovery	95.7%	85.1 ± 3.9%

The percent of prolactin in the pituitary and decidual homogenate fractions is expressed as the percent of prolactin in the non-nuclear fractions of the pituitary and decidua homogenates.

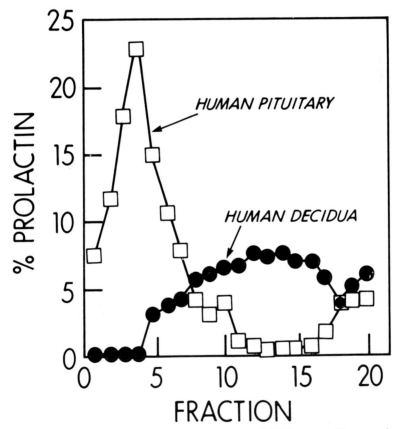

Figure 1. Density gradient centrifugation of the mitochondrial fraction of human pituitary and human decidual tissues through 0.5 - 2.0 M sucrose. The amount of prolactin in each of the fractions is expressed as a percentage of the total prolactin in the gradient tubes (pituitary 40.2 ug; decidua, 62 ng). An identical distribution of prolactin was obtained with the microsomal fractions of the tissues.

Following density gradient centrifugation of the microsomal and mitochondrial fractions of human pituitary homogenates, the prolactin, TSH, and LH sedimented as a sharp peak with a mean density of 1.22 g/cm³ (Fig. 1). These densities are similar to those previously reported for prolactin, thyrotropin-releasing hormone, LH, FSH, and growth hormone (for review, see 20). However, the prolactin in the microsomal and mitochondrial fractions of decidua was distributed over 90% of the gradient (Fig. 1). As in the differential centrifugation experiments, these marked differences between decidual and pituitary prolactin could not be attributed to the rupture of decidual granules. As shown in Figure 2, when human decidual and rat pituitary tissues were homogenized together prior to sucrose gradient centrifugation, the distribution of the two prolactins was still markedly different. The rat pituitary prolactin sedimented as

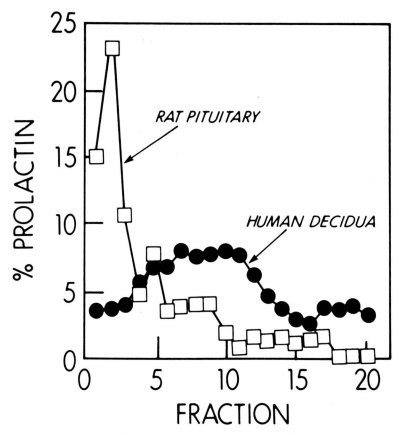

Figure 2. Density gradient centrifugation of the mitochondrial fraction of rat pituitary and human decidual tissues through 0.3 - 1.6 M sucrose. Rat pituitary and human decidual tissues were homogenized together prior to centrifugation. The prolactin in each fraction is expressed as a percentage of the total amount of prolactin (pituitary, 2.5 ug; decidua, 0.7 ug) in the gradient tubes. An identical distribution of prolactin was obtained with the microsomal fractions of the tissues.

a sharp peak, while human decidual prolactin in the particulate fractions was distributed over the entire gradient.

Although the biochemical studies reported here do not indicate the precise localization of prolactin in decidual tissue, they nevertheless clearly indicate that decidual tissue prolactin is not stored in secretory granules. The differences in the subcellular distribution of the two hormones may therefore explain, at least in part, the observed differences in the regulation of prolactin release from these tissues. The differences may also explain the observation that prolactin content of pituitary tissue on a weight basis, is 20-50 times greater than that of prolactin in decidual tissue (1,3).

ACKNOWLEDGMENTS

This research was supported by NIH grants HD06301, HD13220 and RCDA HDO337. Part of this work is in press elsewhere (21).

REFERENCES

1. Golander A, Hurley T, Barrett J, Hizi A, Handwerger S. (1978): Science 202:311
2. Riddick DH, Luciano AA, Kusmich WF, Maslar JA. (1978): Life Sci 23:1913
3. Golander A, Hurley T, Barrett J, Handwerger S. (1979): J Endocrinol 82:263
4. Bowers CY. (1971): Annals of New York Academy of Sciences 189:263
5. Tam WS, Dannies PS. (1980): J Biol Chem 255:6595
6. Stern JE, Conn PM. (1981): Am J Phys 240:504
7. Handwerger S, Golander A, Barrett J, Barry S, Conn PM. (1980): In: MacLeod RM, Scapagnini U (eds) Central and Peripheral Regulation of Prolactin Function. Raven Press, New York, p 311
8. Richards SR, Kim MH, Malarkey WB. (1982): J Clin Endocrinol Metab 54:820
9. Yudaev NA, Asribekova MK, Karpova SK, Murashko LE. (1981): Neurosci B Phy 11:443
10. Haug E, Naess A, Gautvik KM. (1978): Mol Cell Endocrinol 12:81
11. Tomika K, McCoshen JA, Fernandez CS, Tyson JE. (1982): Am J Obstet Gynecol 142:420
12. Markoff E, Zeitler P, Peleg S, Handwerger S. (1983): J Clin Endocrinol Metab 56:962
13. Fluckiger G, del Pozo E, von Werder K. (1982): In: Prolactin: Physiology, Pharmacology and Clinical Findings. Springer-Verlag, Berlin, p 24
14. Golander A, Barrett J, Hurley T, Barry S, Handwerger S. (1979): J Clin Endocrinol Metab 49:787
15. Handwerger S, Barry S, Markoff E, Barrett J, Conn PMC. (1983): Endocrinology 112:1370
16. Markoff E, Howell S, Handwerger S. (1983): J Clin Endocrinol Metab 57:1282
17. Handwerger S, Barry S, Barrett J, Markoff E, Zeitler P, Cwikel B, Siegel M. (1981): Endocrinology 109:2016
18. Racadot J, Vila-Porcile E, Peillon F, Oliver T. (1971): Ann Endocrinol (Paris) 32:298
19. Pasteels JL. (1972): In: Wolstenholme GEW, Knight J (eds) Livingstone, Edinburgh p 241
20. Hymer WC. (1975): In: Tixier-Vidal A, Farquhar MG Academic Press, New York p 137
21. Handwerger S, Wilson S, Conn PM. (1984): Mol Cell Endocrinol, in press

Prolactin. Basic and clinical correlates
R.M. MacLeod, M.O. Thorner and U. Scapagnini (eds.),
Fidia Research Series, vol. I,
Liviana Press, Padova © 1985

Section VII
Physiological relevance of pituitary
and non-pituitary prolactins

EVIDENCE FOR A GLYCOSYLATED PROLACTIN VARIANT IN HUMAN PITUITARY AND AMNIOTIC FLUID

S. Meuris, M. Svoboda, J. Christophe and C. Robyn

Human Reproduction Research Unit and Department of Biochemistry and
Nutrition, Faculty of Medicine, Université Libre de Bruxelles
Hôpital Saint-Pierre, B-1000, Brussels, Belgium

INTRODUCTION

Since the isolation of human pituitary lactogenic hormones and their availability for radioimmunoassays, evidence for a complex heterogeneity of these hormones has grown.

Two growth hormone (GH) molecules with different sizes coexist in the human pituitary. The major form (90%), and the first which has been isolated, possesses 191 amino acids. The minor form (10%) contains only 176 amino acids. This form is structurally identical to the major one except for a lack of 15 consecutive amino acid residues starting from position 32 in the primary structure (1). The minor form of GH or 20 K variant is biologically as active on growth as the major form but less immunoreactive. The radioimmunoassays available actually do not discriminate between the two forms.

Prolactin is heterogeneous when analyzed by gel filtration chromatography. In the pituitary as well as in serum from different species, three forms of the hormone exist. In man, besides the well characterized prolactin with a molecular weight (MW) of 23 K and 199 amino acids, two more forms with higher molecular weight are present: big prolactin (MW: 45 K) and big-big prolactin (MW > 100,000). Big prolactin probably is a dimeric form and big-big prolactin consists of more complex aggregates of prolactin molecules. The proportion of the three forms varies in physio-pathological conditions and seems to be influenced by endocrine factors (2-7). In addition, monomeric human prolactin also exists in three charge isomers (8).

Such molecular heterogeneity represents a severe handicap for the radioimmunoassay of these hormones. Indeed, the validity of a competitive assay depends on the antigenic similarity between the molecular forms present in the biological sample tested and the isolated molecule used as tracer. Since usual radioimmunoassay methods

488

cannot contribute to further elucidation of the physiological significance of the molecular heterogeneity of growth hormone and prolactin, it is essential to use procedures able to detect and possibly measure protein hormone variants in biological samples. To achieve this aim, we have developed a procedure, immunoperoxidase electrophoresis (IPE), as one approach fulfilling these requirements (9,10).

IMMUNOPEROXIDASE ELECTROPHORESIS

As reported by Meuris et al. (9,10), IPE combines the high separating power of sodium dodecyl sulfate polyacrylamide gel electrophoresis (SDS-PAGE) and the extreme sensitivity of the double bridge immunoperoxidase staining (Fig. 1). Here, we applied IPE to the analysis of the molecular heterogeneity of human lactogenic hormones. Crude homogenates of biological samples (tissue or biological fluid) can be directly analyzed by IPE without any preliminary purification steps (Fig. 1). After electrophoretic separation by SDS-PAGE, the proteins are transferred from the gel to the surface of a sheet of nitrocellulose filter membrane, by applying a transversal electric field (20V, 100 mA, 1 h) in an original apparatus designed for rapid electrofiltration (Biolyon, France). The proteins are fixed to the nitrocellulose filter membrane and the non-specific protein binding sites saturated with ovalbumin. The sheet of nitrocellulose

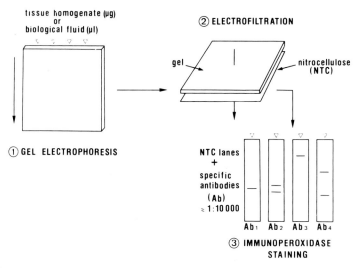

Figure 1. Schematic representation of immunoperoxidase electrophoresis (IPE) which includes a sodium dodecylsulfate polyacrylamide gel electrophoresis (SDS-PAGE) of the proteins contained in a tissue homogenate or in a biological fluid, an electrofiltration of the proteins on a nitrocellular membrane filter and a double bridge immunoperoxidase staining using specific antisera (Ab).

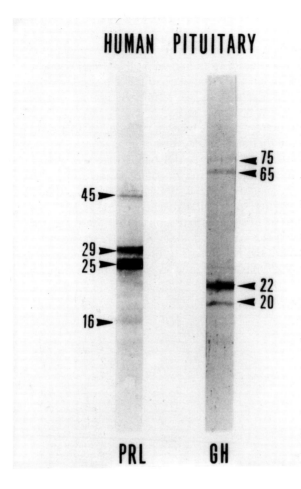

Figure 2. Immunoperoxidase electrophoresis (IPE) pattern of a human pituitary homogenate (left = 0.25 mg per lane; right = 0.025 mg per lane). The nitrocellulose strips were incubated with an anti-ovine prolactin serum and an anti-human growth hormone serum. Apparent molecular weights are indicated. Taken from Meuris *et al.* (9).

filter membrane is then stained by a double bridge immunoperoxidase technique using peroxidase-antiperoxidase complexes (10). Anti-prolactin and anti-GH sera are used at dilutions ranging from 1:10,000 to 1:100,000, dilutions similar to those used in radioimmunoassays (10).

The sensitivity of the staining procedure, i.e the smallest amount of antigen that can be distinguished from the background, is 0.01 fg, i.e. 100 molecules of lactogenic hormone per micron^2 (10).

HUMAN PROLACTINS

As shown in Figure 2, four prolactin-like immunoreactive bands are identified by IPE in total protein homogenates from human pituitary glands when using SDS-PAGE in the presence of 1% 2-mercaptoethanol (9,10). These bands, with 17 K, 25 K, 29 K, and 45 K apparent molecular weights, were similarly immunostained when using two anti-ovine and one anti-rat prolactin sera.

The IPE patterns were different when nitrocellulose strips obtained after SDS-PAGE of the same pituitary homogenates were immunostained with anti-human placental lactogen or GH sera (Fig. 2). Two major bands were then revealed corresponding to proteins with apparent molecular weights of 22 K and 20 K. The first band is GH itself (9,10). The second band is the 20 K GH variant (1,9,11). In addition, two slowly migrating forms with apparent molecular weights of 75 K and 65 K were also immunostained (Fig. 2). The most likely interpretation is that these last two forms are non-covalently bound aggregates of 22 K and/or 20 K GH molecules.

In order to compare the heterogeneity of human prolactin as seen by IPE in a homogenate of human pituitary gland and in a highly purified preparation, these two

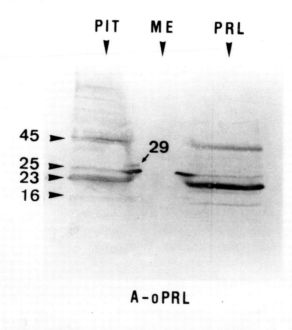

Figure 3. Effect of reduction on the immunoperoxidase electrophoresis pattern of a human pituitary homogenate (Pit) and a purified preparation of human pituitary prolactin PRL. Mercaptoethanol (ME) was allowed to diffuse in the polyacrylamide gel between the two lanes of protein samples prior to the electrophoresis. The nitrocellulose sheet was incubated with an anti-ovine prolactin serum (anti-oPRL). The 29 K form of prolactin is present only in the pituitary homogenate.

biological samples were submitted in parallel to protein reduction by 2-mercaptoethanol (ME) which was allowed to diffuse into the polyacrylamide gel prior to electrophoresis (Fig. 3).

The 45 K prolactin form disappears when completely reduced by ME and thus contains non-covalently bound prolactin molecules. When reduced, the 16 K and 23 K forms show somewhat higher molecular weights, 17 K and 25 K, respectively. The 29 K prolactin form appears after complete reduction in the homogenate of the human pituitary gland but not in the highly purified preparation of human pituitary prolactin. When unreduced, it migrates with an apparent molecular weight of 25 K similar to the reduced form of the known prolactin molecule (10,13). These changes in the migration rate of the molecular forms of prolactin as seen after reduction by ME are probably due to conformational changes resulting from the rupture of disulfide bridges. The 29 K prolactin form is found besides the 17 K and 25 K forms after adequate reduction in all human pituitary glands and represents 20-30% of the total prolactin immunoreactivity (10). The IPE pattern of prolactin variants obtained in total homogenates from prolactin-secreting adenomas is essentially similar to that obtained with homogenates of normal pituitary tissue (10,14). This suggests no basic alteration in the processing of the molecular forms of prolactin in these tumors.

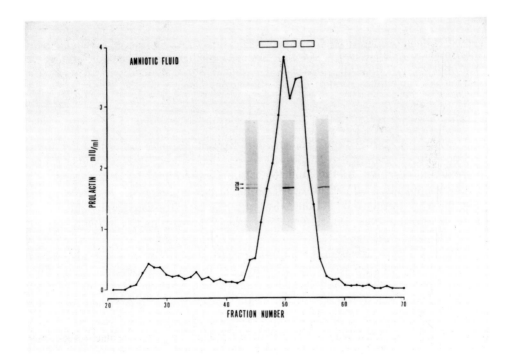

Figure 4. Profile of radioimmunoassayble prolactin obtained after gel filtration chromatography on Sephadex G 100 of human amniotic fluid. Three fractions of the main prolactin peak were analyzed by immunoperoxide electrophoresis (IPE). Taken from Meuris *et al.* (13).

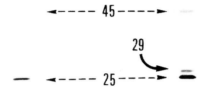

CONCANAVALIN-A   CONCANAVALIN-A
+
methyl-glucopyranose

Figure 5. Immunoperoxidase electrophoresis (IPE) pattern of a human pituitary homogenate passed through a concanavalin A sepharose column presaturated with methyl-glucopyranose (left) or not (right). Taken from Meuris *et al.* (13).

The 29 K prolactin is found not only in the pituitary gland but also in the human amniotic fluid, indicating that this form can be secreted and, thus, probably is not a pre-prolactin molecule (10,13). No 29 K prolactin was detected by IPE in the decidua (10). As demonstrated by IPE, the 29 K prolactin predominates in the ascending part of the main prolactin peak obtained by gel filtration chromatography of pituitary homogenates or amniotic fluids. The 25 K prolactin predominates in the descending part of the same peak (Fig. 4).

The 29 K human prolactin but not the 25 K form bound to concanavalin A when crude pituitary extracts or fractions of the main prolactin peaks obtained by gel filtration of these extracts were passed through a concanavalin A-sepharose column. As shown in Figure 5, this binding was suppressed when the concanavalin A-sepharose column was saturated with methyl glucopyranose (10,14).

The affinity of the 29 K prolactin for the lectin indicates that the 29 K prolactin is glycosylated while the 25 K form is not. The glycosylation of human prolactin is possible on theoretical grounds since this protein hormone contains an Asn-Leu-Ser sequence starting in position 31 of the primary structure (15). Thus, it can be anticipated that a sugar chain is attached to the Asn 31 of the human prolactin molecule. Recently,

Lewis et al. (16) reported the presence of a glycosylated form of prolactin in sheep pituitary.

Human prolactin and GH are heterogeneous with regard to their molecular sizes. The heterogeneity of GH molecules probably depends on a particular splicing of the primary transcript of the expressed GH gene. Glycosylation of prolactin represents a post-traductional event of the molecule. Factors influencing prolactin glycosylation and the physiological significance of the 29 K glycosylated prolactin are unknown. Because IPE is able to characterize the molecular heterogeneity of protein hormones in crude extracts or biological fluids, this procedure is adequate for protein processing studies and should be amenable to an immunoassay procedure.

ACKNOWLEDGMENTS

We thank Mrs. H. Preszow for her help in preparing the manuscript. We also thank Mrs. G. Bastin for her skillful assistance. This work was supported by grants 3.4501.81 and 3.4504.81 from the Fund for Medical Scientific Research (Belgium). S. Meuris received Senior Research Assistance from the National Fund for Scientific Research (Belgium)

REFERENCES

1. Lewis UJ, Bonewald LF, Lewis LJ. (1980): Biochem Biophys Res Commun 92:511
2. Guyda VS, Moon HK. (1975): J Clin Endocrinol Metab 41:953
3. Fang VS, Moon HK. (1975): J Clin Endocrinol Metab 41:1030
4. Gala RR, Van De Walle C. (1977): Life Sciences 21:99
5. Garnier PE, Aubert ML, Kaplan SL, Grumbach MM. (1978): J Clin Endocrinol Metab 47:1273
6. Benveniste R, Helman JD, Orth DN, McKenna TJ, Nicholson WE, Rabinowitz D. (1979): J Clin Endocrinol Metab 48:883
7. Sinha YN. (1980): Endocrinology 107:1959
8. Nyberg F, Roos P, Wide L. (1980): Biochim Biophys Acta 626:255
9. Meuris S, Svoboda M, Vilamala M, Christophe J, Robyn C. (1983): FEBS Lett 154:111
10. Meuris S. (1984): These d' agregation. Université Libre de Bruxelles
11. Singh RNP, Seavey BK, Lewis UJ. (1974): Endocrinol Res Commun 1:449
12. Meuris S, Svoboda M, Christophe J, Robyn C. (1984): Anal Biochem, in press
13. Meuris S, Svoboda M, Christophe J, Robyn C. (1984): FEBS Lett submitted
14. Meuris S, Svoboda M, Dewailly D, Lommel B, Fossati P, Christophe J, Robyn C. Proc 3rd European Workshop on Pituitary Adenomas (1983): p 18 (Abstract)
15. Pless DD, Lennarz WJ. (1977): Proc Natl Acad Sci USA 74:134
16. Lewis UJ, Singh RNP, Lewis LJ, Seavey BK, Sinha YN. (1984): Proc Natl Acad Sci USA 81:385

Prolactin. Basic and clinical correlates
R.M. MacLeod, M.O. Thorner and U. Scapagnini (eds.),
Fidia Research Series, vol. I,
Liviana Press, Padova © 1985

Section VII
Physiological relevance of pituitary
and non-pituitary prolactins

FURTHER STUDIES ON RAT PLACENTAL LACTOGENS

L. A. Glaser[1], I. Khan[1], G. J. Pepe[2], P. A. Kelly[3], and G. Gibori[1]

[1]Department of Physiology and Biophysics, University of Illinois College
of Medicine Health Sciences Center, Chicago, IL 60612
[2]Department of Physiology and Biophysics, Eastern Virginia Medical School
Norfolk, VA 23501
[3]Laboratory of Molecular Endocrinology, McGill University,
Royal Victoria Hospital, Montreal, Quebec, H3A 1A1, Canada

It is well established that at mid-pregnancy in the rat, the maintenance of luteal progesterone secretion shifts from the pituitary to the placenta and early studies provided evidence for the occurrence of a placental prolactin-like factor (1,2). With the use of bioassay techniques, both luteotropic and mammotropic activities were detected in the serum or placentas of mid-pregnant rats (3-8). The development of a radioreceptor assay using prolactin receptors from rabbit mammary gland (9) led to the quantification and measurement of rat placental lactogen (rPL), a prolactin-like hormone secreted during the second half of pregnancy (9-11).

Two peaks of prolactin-like material are detectable in the serum of pregnant rats by radioreceptor assay: one around days 11-14 and a second around days 17-21 of pregnancy (9). However, the luteotropic activity as determined by bioassay coincides only with the first peak of prolactin-like hormone in the serum (3-5). Previous reports have indicated that two lactogenic hormones, having different molecular weights and disappearance rates, circulate during pregnancy (10,12,13). The prolactin-like activity present in day 12 pregnant rat serum is comprised of 88% large molecular weight (LMW) and 12% small molecular weight (SMW) hormone (10). At late pregnancy, however, only the SMW hormone is present (10). As yet, it has not been determined whether the LMW hormone, the SMW hormone, or both hormones are necessary for maintenance of luteal steroidogenesis at mid-pregnancy.

Comparison of the levels of prolactin-like activity determined by bioassay and radioreceptor assay suggests that the mammary gland radioreceptor assay (MG-RRA) may not detect all of the luteotropic hormone present at mid-pregnancy. Therefore, a radioreceptor assay using particulate membranes from rat ovaries was developed (17). As shown in Figure 1, concentrations of LMW placental hormone present at mid-pregnancy were higher when measured by ovarian radioreceptor assay (O-RRA) than

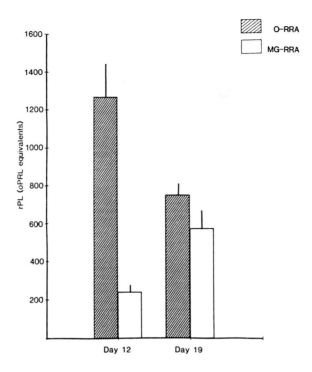

Figure 1. Measurement of peripheral rPL levels by ovarian and mammary gland radioreceptor assays. Peripheral serum was obtained by jugular venipuncture on days 12 and 19 of pregnancy. Values for rPL were determined by radioreceptor assay using particulate membranes from rat ovary (O-RRA) and rabbit mammary gland (MG-RRA). Values for day 12 were significantly different ($P < 0.01$).

by MG-RRA, but concentrations of the SMW placental hormone present on day 19 were found to be similar.

In order to determine the luteotropic potency of the two forms of rPL, an *in vivo* bioassay using day 6 pregnant rats was developed, with maintenance of pregnancy and progesterone secretion as the biological end-points. Day 12 pregnant rat serum was applied to a Sephadex G-100 column (2.5 x 65 cm) eluted with 0.1 M NH_4HCO_3, pH 8.3. The fractions comprising the peaks of SMW and LMW prolactin-like activity, as determined by O-RRA, were then combined to form two separate pools. The two partially purified hormone preparations were lyophilized and reconstituted in 0.9% NaCl.

On day 6 of pregnancy, rats were injected with 2-Br-ergocyptine (CB-154, 0.4 mg/0.25 ml 70% ethanol) to selectively inhibit pituitary prolactin surges. Prolactin withdrawal on day 6 of pregnancy was followed by diminished progesterone production and abortion (18). As presented in Figure 2, twice-daily injections of the amount of LMW rPL contained in 1 ml of day 12 pregnant rat serum reversed the effect of CB-154 and all animals remained pregnant. In contrast, administration of the SMW hormone alone did not maintain either pregnancy or progesterone levels. Administration of both molecular weight forms of rPL was also capable of maintaining luteal function. These results suggest that only the LMW prolactin-like hormone present in the circulation at midpregnancy has luteotropic properties.

The ability of a small amount of LMW placental hormone (2-3 ug ovine prolactin equivalents) to maintain corpus luteum function in pregnant rats indicates that it is an extremely potent hormone. One explanation for the tremendous luteotropic capacity of this substance is that it remains in the circulation for an extended period of time. Kelly et al. (10) reported the half-time disappearance rate of rPL to be 19.5 minutes on day 12 of pregnancy, about 2-3 times longer than the rate of ovine prolactin (6-8 minutes). However, even an extended half-life of 19.5 minutes is far too short to explain the potent and sustained luteotropic properties of the LMW hormone. Preliminary data from our laboratory indicated that placental prolactin-like activity is detectable in the peripheral serum for 3 days following the removal of the uterus on day 12 (19). This led to the speculation that the biological half-life of the LMW placental hormone

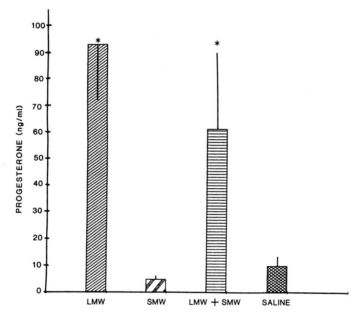

Figure 2. Effect of the large and small molecular weight placental prolactin-like hormones on progesterone production. The two molecular weight forms of placental lactogen were separated from 40 ml of day 12 pregnant rat serum by gel chromatography, lyophilized, and reconstituted in 40 ml saline, pH 7.4. All rats were treated with CB-154 (0.4 mg/rat) on day 6 of pregnancy. One ml of partially purified rPL, either large molecular weight (LMW), small molecular weight (SMW), or a combination of the two hormones (LMW + SMW) was injected s.c. twice on day 6 of pregnancy. Each bar represents the mean ± S.E. of values obtained from 3-4 rats 24 h after ECO administration. Values for the LMW and LMW + SMW groups were significantly different (P< 0.05) from the saline-treated group.

present on day 12 was much longer than previously reported. To investigate this hypothesis, we measured the rate of disappearance of both the LMW and SMW placental prolactin-like hormones. Pregnant rats were hysterectomized on days 12 and 19 of pregnancy and immediately thereafter serial blood samples were taken by jugular venipuncture from 0 to 48 hours. Prolactin-like activity in the serum was determined by O-RRA and the disappearance rates of rPL were calculated using an iterative computer program for non-linear regression (20). Results indicate that the disappearance rate of the placental luteotropin on day 12 is biphasic and comprised of two components: 31 min and 1063 min. The half-time disappearance rate of the lactogen found on day 19 of pregnancy, however, has only one component of 6 min. This is 5 times longer than the 1.2 minutes reported by Kelly et al. (10), yet it agrees closely with the disappearance rate of prolactin. The extremely slow disappearance rate of the LMW placental prolactin-like hormone on day 12 of pregnancy is remarkably consistent with the temporal data, suggesting its great luteotropic potency (14-16). Our results may provide a logical explanation for this occurrence.

Very little is presently known of the regulation of rPL secretion, yet it appears that the pituitary inhibits placental lactogen production. Levels of rPL in the serum increase after hypophysectomy on day 14 (21). We have recently obtained data suggesting that placental secretion of rPL increases after hypophysectomy (22). However, it remains possible that the pituitary also affects the clearance of these hormones and shortens their presence in the circulation. The disappearance rates of both forms of the hormone were determined on days 12 and 19 of pregnancy in rats hypophysectomized on day 12. The results of this experiment indicate that removal of the pituitary may prolong the disappearance rates of the placental prolactin-like hormones on both day 12 and day 19. The disappearance rates of the LMW hormone on day 12 were 41 min and 1443 min after hypophysectomy versus 31 min and 1063 min in intact rats. The disappearance rate of the SMW hormone was similarly prolonged from 6 to 10 min.

In summary, results of this investigation suggest that only the LMW placental prolactin-like hormone present at mid-pregnancy has luteotropic properties. Our data also indicate that the disappearance rate of the LMW hormone has only one short component. The slight but not significant decreases in the disappearance rates that occur after hypophysectomy on day 12 also suggest that the pituitary may increase the clearance of rPL in the circulation.

ACKNOWLEDGMENTS

This work was supported by NIH Grant 11119.

REFERENCES

1. Astwood EB, Greep RO. (1938): Proc Soc Biol Med 38:713
2. Ray EW, Averill SC, Lyons WR, Johnson RE. (1955): Endocrinology 56:359
3. Matthies DL. (1967): Anat Rec 159:55
4. Cohen RM, Gala RR. (1969): Proc Soc Exp Biol Med 132:683

5. Linkie DM, Niswender GD. (1973): Biol Reprod 8:48
6. Talamantes F. (1975): Gen Comp Endocrinol 27:115
7. Peters JM, Van Marle J. (1976): Acta Endocrinol 83:640
8. Malison JA, Swanson P, French LR. (1982): J Reprod Fert 64:25
9. Shiu RPC, Kelly PA, Friesen HG. (1973): Science 180:968
10. Kelly PA, Shiu RPC, Robertson MC, Friesen HG. (1975): Endocrinology 96:1187
11. Kelly PA, Tsushima T, Shiu RPC, Friesen HG. (1976): Endocrinology 99:765
12. Robertson MC, Friesen HG. (1981): Endocrinology 108:2388
13. Robertson MC, Gillespie B, Friesen HG. (1982): Endocrinology 111:1862
14. Gibori G, Antczak E, Rothchild I. (1977): Endocrinology 106:1584
15. Gibori G, Richards JS. (1978): Endocrinology 102:767
16. Gibori G, Richards JS, Keyes PL. (1979): Biol Reprod 21:419
17. Glaser LA, Kelly PA, Gibori G. (1984): Endocrinology, in press
18. Morishige WK, Rothchild I. (1974): Endocrinology 96:260
19. Khan MI, Glaser LA, Gibori G. Program of the 67th Annual Meeting of the Federation of American Societies for Experimental Biology, Chicago IL, (1983): p 316 (Abstract)
20. Jennrich R. In: Dixon WJ (ed) BMDP Statistical Software. University of California Press, Berkeley, p 290.
21. Daughaday WH, Trivedi B, Kapadia M. (1979): Endocrinology 105:210
22. Glaser LA, Sridaran R, Gibori G. Program of the 64th Annual Meeting of the Endocrine Society, San Francisco CA, (1982): p 307 (Abstract)

Prolactin. Basic and clinical correlates
R.M. MacLeod, M.O. Thorner and U. Scapagnini (eds.),
Fidia Research Series, vol. I,
Liviana Press, Padova © 1985

Section VII
Physiological relevance of pituitary
and non-pituitary prolactins

CHARACTERIZATION OF IMMUNOREACTIVE AND BIOACTIVE FORMS OF PROLACTIN IN THE RAT PITUITARY

Gul Mansur and W. C. Hymer

Department of Biochemistry, The Pennsylvania State University
University Park, PA 16802

The issue of prolactin heterogeneity in terms of molecular form and function has been carefully considered in the excellent review by Lewis (1). Structural heterogeneity can take many forms. It may reflect post-translational modification, e.g. molecular aggregation, interchain disulfide dimers, or proteolytically cleaved molecules; altered synthetic routes at the DNA level, as exemplified by the 20K GH variant; expression of multiple genes; or, finally, mRNA splicing variants. Several reports in the recent literature deal not only with the identification of such prolactin variants, but also with the issue of their relative biological (B) and immunologic (I) activities (2-5). In these studies variants are usually separated electrophoretically and their activities estimated by pigeon crop or mammary gland bioassays. Our approach has been to use polyacrylamide gel electrophoresis under native, denaturing, or denaturing + reducing conditions for separation; electrotransfer of proteins from gels to nitrocellulose paper according to the method of Towbin et al. (6); enzyme immunoassay (EIA) for identification of prolactin on the paper (hereafter referred to as EITB); electrophoretic elution of proteins from unstained gels, and, finally, assay of the dialyzed and lyophilized proteins by the NB2 lymphoma cell bioassay (7) and EIA (8).

When alkaline extracts of rat pituitary tissue were run on 15% native gels or 15% gels SDS in the presence or absence of mercaptoethanol, very different EITB patterns were obtained (Fig. 1). On native gels 8 discrete immunopositive bands were seen, 5 slowly migrating relative to the prominent band 6, and 2 fast moving. On SDS gels, aliquots of this same extract yielded numerous prolactin bands with apparent molecular weights in the ranges of 1) 97K-55K; 2) 31K; 3) 24K; and 4) 22K-17K species. Under reducing conditions the high molecular weight forms disappeared and new bands 15K, 13K, 10K, and 5K were apparently generated by this treatment. Further, the 24K monomer now migrated as 28K. These latter results parallel those of Mittra (3) who suggested on the basis of autoradiographic evidence that intact 24K molecules migrate slower due to unfolding of the molecule and cleaved 24K molecules migrate as 16K and

502

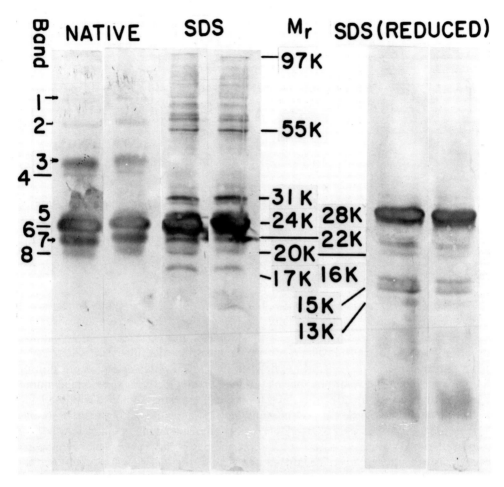

Figure 1. Enzyme-linked immunoelectrotransfer blot (EITB) of immunopositive prolactin bands after electrophoresis on 15% native gels (0.5 ug/lane); 15% SDS gels (1.0 ug/lane); and 15% SDS gels with 5% mercaptoethanol (1.5 ug/lane). Although not shown in the figure, prolactin forms migrating below 13K in the reducing conditions have apparent molecular weights of 10K and 5K.

8K species under reducing conditions. Sinha and Gilligan (5) have suggested that the frequency of these cleaved species may be small; the EITB patterns in Figure 1 tend to confirm this idea.

To determine the apparent molecular weights of prolactin contained within each of the 8 bands on native gels, molecules contained in each band region were recovered by electrophoretic elution and subsequently run on non-reducing SDS gels. Each band from the native gel is apparently composed of identical (approx. 13) prolactin species (Fig. 2). Proportions of these forms vary in the different native gel bands.

The biological and immunological activities of molecules recovered from each of 4 band regions (SDS gels) were different (Table 1). In each of 2 experiments, a majority of the bioactive hormone was associated with 17K-24K molecules. While approximately 80% of the immunoactivity was also recovered from this same region, considerable activity was associated with the 31K species.

How do these findings relate to those of others? Since different electrophoresis conditions, bioassays, and pituitary donors have been used (Table 2), comparison in more than a general way is difficult. In all 4 studies, the most bioactive molecules ap-

Table 1. *Biological and immunological activities of rat pituitary prolactin electrophoretically eluted from 15% SDS gels.*

	Bioactive prolactin		Immunoreactive prolactin	
	ng	% Recovered Hormone	ng	% Recovered Hormone
EXP #1				
97-55K	0.08	0.03	1.0	0.05
31K	0.03	0.01	473	21.4
24K	142	57.7	1173	51.4
22-17K	104	42.3	603	27.2
EXP #2				
97-55K	337	5.3	1023	0.8
31K	431	6.7	19804	15.0
24K	2677	41.8	58130	44.0
22-17K	2952	46.1	53026	40.2

In exp. 1, one pituitary equivalent was applied to a single gel. After electrophoresis, band areas from each of 10 lanes were cut from the unstained gel, pooled, and separated proteins electrophoresed into dialysis membranes (3.5K cutoff), dialyzed, lyophilized, and reconstituted in assay buffer. In exp. 2, 6 gels, each loaded with 1 pituitary equivalent, were similarly processed.

pear to be 17K-24K. Other bioactive forms in both Sinha's study and ours include some with high apparent molecular weight. There seems to be good agreement that the most immunoactive species is 24K.

The relatively high immunoactivity of the 31 K molecule is of interest. At the moment we are uncertain of its significance. Considering its size, we speculate that it may represent the biosynthetic precursor of the monomeric form.

While the function of these prolactin variants is still largely unknown, it is tempting to speculate on their possible significance to the organism. In Figure 3 we suggest 4 models; certainly there are more which could be offered.

504

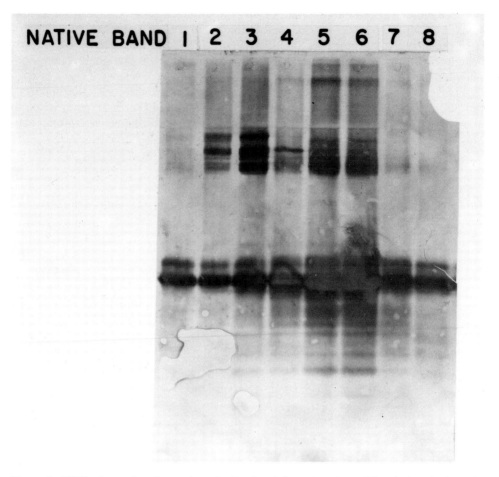

Figure 2. EITB of proteins electrophoretically eluted from 8 native gel bands (total of 5 gels) and subsequently electrophoresed on 15% SDS gels after dialysis and lyophilization. Each sample was reconstituted in 100 ul of SDS sample buffer and the entire sample was applied to the gel shown in this figure.

Model 1 is based on our findings in native gel systems. This model presumes that the 8 different prolactin bands in native gels are a reflection of prolactin "packets" in the extract. Each packet has the same makeup of prolactin molecules, but has different surface charge distributions. We do not know if these packets are the result of an extraction artifact, or exist in the cell as such. Model 2 presumes that 31K prolactin is contained within the cisternae of the endoplasmic reticulum. During processing, this form undergoes modification depending upon whether it is to be released immediately or stored. In the former case, the 31K molecule would be cleaved to bioactive forms ranging from 17K-24K at the cell surface. In the latter case, aggregates of 31K molecules

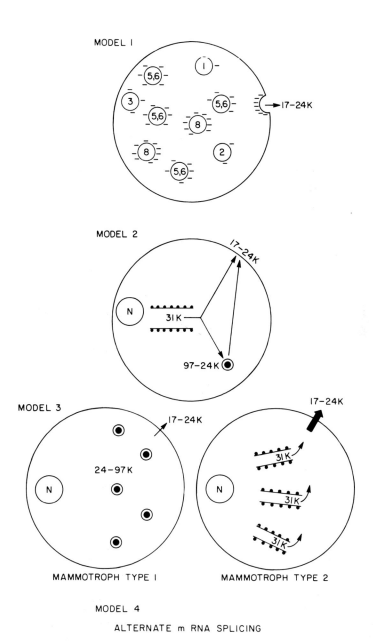

Figure 3. Models to help explain the functional significance in prolactin variants.

Table 2. *Comparison of characteristics among prolactin variants in four studies.*

	MITTRA (3)	SINHA (4)	ASAWARO-ENGCHAI (2)	THIS STUDY
Animal	Sprague-Dawley Rats	Rat (S/A Strain) & mice (SW strain) Sex not specified	Young or mature rats of Sprague-Dawley strain	F344 mature rats
Gel condition	15% SDC c̄ BME	15% Native	7.5% Native	15% SDS
Bioassay	Mouse mammary epithelial tissue (*in vivo*)	Pigeon-crop sac	Pigeon-crop sac	NB2 lymphoma cell
Immunoassay	RIA	RIA	RIA	EIA
Most Bioactive Species	16K	23K	1) Tissue = Area 4 2) Medium = Area 4	24K-17K
Other Bioactive Species	24K	31K > 20.5K > 62.5K	1) Area 2 > Area 3 2) Area 5 > Area 3	31K ≅ 97-55K
Most Immunoactive Species	24K	23K ≅ 20.5K	1) Area 4 2) Area 4	24K
Other Immunoactive Species	16K	31K > 62.5K	1) Area 2 > Area 3 2) Area 3 > Area 2 > Area 1 ≅ Area 5	22-17K > 31K > 97-55K

(perhaps with 24K, 22K forms?) would form during maturation of the secretion granule. Findings by the Jacobs group (9) suggest that hormone within the secretion granule is disulfide-linked. Further, its activity is greatly increased when exposed to thiols. Model 3 offers the intriguing possibility that heterogeneity of the mammotroph population is related to heterogeneity of prolactin molecules. Heterogeneity of cells in the mammotroph population is well known from cell separation studies (10). Recent evidence from our laboratory supports Model 3 (11). There is also a conceptually exciting "spin-off" to Model 3. Nicoll has pointed out that there are >85 different actions of prolactin in diverse biological systems (12,13). It is not known if prolactin variants are involved in these diverse activities. Is it possible that different subpopulations of mammotrophs produce/process hormone differently depending upon the ultimate prolactin target? If so, the pituitary is even more complex than we currently suspect it to be. In this specific regard, we have recently reported that there is diversity in biological activity of GH released from somatotroph subpopulations *in vitro* (14).

ACKNOWLEDGMENTS

The expert assistance of Kim Motter and Donna Bubeck in the prolactin assays is recognized, as is that of Theresa Peters in the typing of the manuscript. This work was supported by NIH Grant CA 23248.

REFERENCES

1. Lewis UJ. (1984): Ann Rev Physiol 46:33
2. Asawaroenchai H, Russell SM, Nicoll CS. (1978): Endocrinology 102:407
3. Mittra I. (1980): Biochem Biophys Res Commun 95:1750
4. Sinha YN, Gilligan TA. (1981): Endocrinology 108:1091
5. Sinha YN, Gilligan TA. (1981): Endocrinology 114:2046
6. Towbin H, Staehelin T, Gorgon J. (1979): Proc Natl Acad Sci 76:4350
7. Tanaka T, Shiu RPC, Gout PW, Beer CT. (1980): J Clin Endocrinol Metab 51:1058
8. Signorella AP, Hymer WC. (1984): Anal Bioch 136:372
9. Lorenson MY, Jacobs LS. (1982): Endocrinology 110:1164
10. Hymer WC, Hatfield JM. (1983): Methods In Enzymology 103:257
11. Hymer WC, Motter K, Hatfield JM, Mansur G. 7th International Congress of Endocrinology, Quebec City, (1984): (Abstract)
12. Nicoll CS. (1974): Handbook of Physiology, see 7: Endocrinology, Vol IV. part 2 ed 5. Am Physiol Soc, Washington, DC, p 253
13. Nicoll CS, Bern HA. (1972). In: Wolstenholme GEW, Knight J (eds) Lactogenic Hormones. Churchill Livingston, London, p 299
14. Grindeland RE, Hymer WC, Lundgren P, Edward C. American Physiological Society, San Diego, (1982): p 262 (Abstract).

Prolactin. Basic and clinical correlates
R.M. MacLeod, M.O. Thorner and U. Scapagnini (eds.),
Fidia Research Series, vol. I,
Liviana Press, Padova © 1985

IN VIVO RELEASE RATE OF NEUROTRANSMITTERS IN THE CONTROL OF PITUITARY PROLACTIN RELEASE

W. Wuttke, G. Flugge, H. Jarry, R. Wolf, M. Sprenger and A. Meyer-Fleitmann

Department of Reproductive Biology, German Primate Center
3400 Gottingen, FRG

In recent years no major breakthrough has been made in the understanding of hypothalamic mechanisms controlling anterior pituitary prolactin release. When talking about a prolactin inhibiting factor (PIF), dopamine is still the first candidate which fulfills most requirements for this function (1,2). The aminoacid neurotransmitter gamma aminobutyric acid (GABA) is also believed by some authors to have a PIF-like activity under physiological conditions (3-5). A peptidergic PIF still escapes our knowledge whereas a number of peptides are known to have stimulatory, i.e. prolactin releasing factor (PRF)-like activity. Vasoactive intestinal peptide (VIP), thyrotropin releasing hormone (TRH), angiotensin II, oxytocin, and vasopressin are clearly stimulatory to secretory mechanisms residing in the lactotrophs whereas a direct effect of endogenous opioid peptides is seen by some (7-9), but not by other (10) authors. This unsatisfactory situation prompted us to perform intrahypothalamic and intrapituitary perfusion studies utilizing the push-pull cannula technique. Intrapituitary perfusion allows measurement of catecholamines and a variety of neuropeptides which are drained from the median eminence through the portal vessels into the pituitary. Simultaneously the response of the lactotrophs to the stimulatory or inhibitory substances can be studied by measuring blood levels of prolactin. The results are presented by Duker *et al.* in this volume.

The perikarya of neurons producing the aforementioned PIFs and PRFs are primarily located in preoptic/anterior hypothalamic (MPO/AH) and in mediobasal hypothalamic (MBH) structures. Clusters of dopaminergic perikarya are located in the arcuate nucleus and are called the tuberoinfundibular dopaminergic (TIDA) neurons (11). While the perikarya of neuropeptide-producing neurons which are directly or indirectly involved in the regulation of anterior pituitary prolactin release are found in the MPO/AH and MBH, extrahypothalamic monoaminergic neurons located in the brainstem innervate these neuroendocrine structures in an apparently diffuse manner (12). There is some evidence that norepinephrine (NE) has an indirect stimulatory effect on pituitary prolactin release, thereby mediating steroid feedback signals during the course of the rat estrous cycle (13,14). It is of particular interest that MBH NE turnover correlates best with circulating prolactin levels under a variety of endocrine conditions such as proestrus, diestrus, ovariectomy, and ovariectomy plus estrogen treatment (14). There is also some evidence that an epinephrinergic (E) system also located in the upper brain stem participates in the regulation of anterior or pituitary hormone release (15). Possibly NE and/or E also have direct stimulatory effects at the lactotrophs (6).

Endogenous opioid peptides are stimulatory to pituitary prolactin release after systemic and intraventricular injection (16,17). Beta-endorphin injected intracerebroventricularly was shown to reduce TIDA turnover which may explain the effect of opioids as an indirect effect mediated via the dopamine system (17). On the other hand, we and others were able to stimulate prolactin release both *in vitro* and *in vivo* directly by opioid peptides from the lactotrophs provided they were under the inhibitory influence of dopamine (7-9).

As indicated earlier, GABA has a stimulatory effect on pituitary prolactin release which is clearly mediated within the central nervous system because the direct effect of GABA is inhibitory to the secretion of the lactotrophs. Pharmacological and biochemical evidence suggested the possibility that the neurotransmitter utilized by those estrogen receptive neurons, which mediate the negative and positive feedback action of estradiol on LH and prolactin secretion, are GABAergic (18-21).

Since this fragmentary knowledge stems primarily from pharmacological experiments or from experiments where neurotransmitter/neuropeptide concentrations or turnover rates were measured after appropriate endocrine manipulations, it appeared desirable to us to apply a method which allows a continuous record of hypothalamic catecholamine, GABA, and neuropeptide release rates and to compare these release rates with blood prolactin levels. Utilizing the push-pull cannula technique (22,23) which we (24) and others (25) adopted for neuroendocrine studies, we will now present some of our recent data.

RELEASE RATES OF DOPAMINE, NE, E, AND GABA IN THE MPO/AH AND IN THE MBH

Fractions of the artificial CSF used to perfuse this brain structure were collected continuously over 8 to 10 hours in 15 min fractions. The sensitivity of the radioenzymatic catecholamine assay allows additional measurement of GABA in the perfusate. All rats were stereotaxically implanted in the MPO/AH or in the MBH with the push-pull cannula at least one week prior to experimentation. They received a jugular vein catheter under light ether anesthesia for withdrawal of blood samples which were collected at the end of each 15 min fraction period. Blood prolactin levels were measured radioimmunologically. Animal models used were: a) intact male rats injected with the dopamine antagonistic drug sulpiride (100 ug intravenously per kg B.W.); b) female rats, ovariectomized at the time of implantation of the push-pull cannula 7 days before and 3 days prior to experimentation, pretreated with estradiolbenzoate (E2B, 25 ug for 3 days); and c) ovariectomized non-estrogen treated animals as controls.

COMBINED AUTORADIOGRAPHY AND IMMUNOCYTOCHEMISTRY

To demonstrate the existence of estrogen receptive neurons which might use GABA as neurotransmitter in the MBH, a combination of autoradiography of estradiol with immunocytochemistry with glutamic acid decarboxylase (GAD) antiserum (26) was used. Since GAD is the marker enzyme for GABA synthesis, demonstration of the brown peroxydase-antiperoxydase reaction product in estrogen concentrating neurons would be indicative of GABA formation within these neurons.

Push-pull cannula experiments in male rats

Figure 1 details blood LH and prolactin levels and the concentrations of catecholamines and GABA in the push-pull perfusate of the arcuate nucleus. Basal prolactin levels indicate that the animal was not stressed by the experimental conditions. The intravenous injection of sulpiride resulted in the expected prompt increase in blood prolactin levels. Interesting changes in catecholamine and GABA release rates as an obvious consequence of sulpiride treatment occurred: The release rates of all 3 catecholamines and of GABA were markedly increased in this animal. Such changes following intravenous injection of sulpiride were seen in a number of animals whereas a few others reacted only with increased hypothalamic dopamine and GABA release rates. The increased dopamine release following blockade of dopamine receptors can be interpreted to mean that the sulpiride inhibited autoreceptors at the TIDA neurons. In this case these neurons obviously have autoreceptors although others claim that TIDA neurons do not have such autoreceptors (27). The present results, however, are in agreement with findings of Gudelsky and Porter (28) who reported increased portal blood dopamine concentrations following treatment with haloperidol, another dopamine receptor blocking drug. The stimulatory effect of sulpiride on GABA and occasionally on NE and E release rates is obscure. Possibly the increased dopamine release inhibits the release of one or more other substances which is/are inhibitory to GABA and NE release. Thereby dopamine could indirectly disinhibit GABA and NE release.

Push-pull cannula experiments in female rats

In recent years we studied very extensively the release rates of catecholamines, aminoacid neurotransmitters, and a number of peptides into the MPO/AH. This structure is known to be involved in a number of neuroendocrine regulatory functions including the regulation of LH and prolactin secretion. While the majority of LHRH perikarya are located in this structure (29,30), little is known about the prolactin regulating neurons located here. Utilizing the pharmacological method to measure catecholamine turnover rates as well as the push-pull cannula technique to measure *in vivo* release rates in freely moving animals, it is now well established that preoptic norepinephrine and possibly epinephrine are stimulatory to the activity of LHRH neurons (31,32). Animals with high LH levels such as ovariectomized or proestrous or ovariec-

512

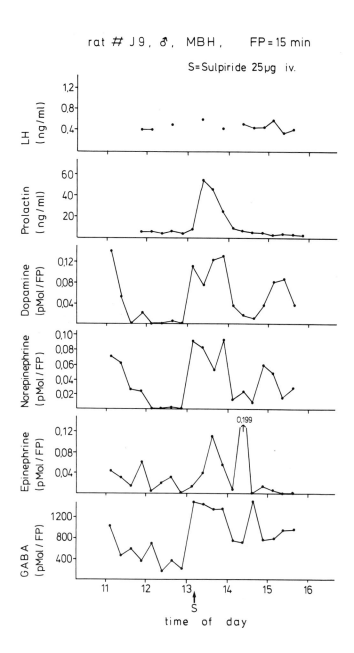

Figure 1. In vivo catecholamine and GABA release rates into the MBH of a male rat before and after injection of the dopamine receptor blocking drug sulpiride. Note increased catecholamine and GABA release following sulpiride and the increased blood prolactin levels.

rat # 135, ovx, E$_2$B, MPO, FP: 15min

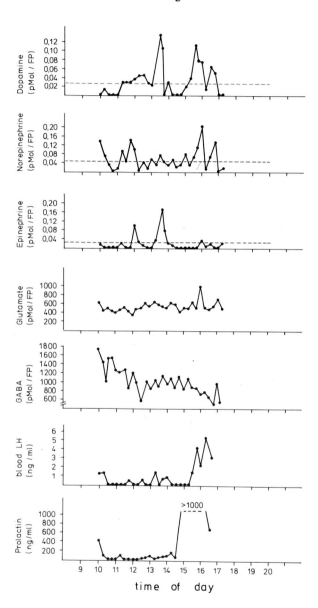

Figure 2. In vivo catecholamine and GABA release rates into the MPO of an ovariectomized, estrogen-primed rat. Note decreased GABA release at the time of expression of the positive feedback action of the estrogen on LH and prolactin levels.

tomized estrogen primed rats had high preoptic NE turnover (14,33,34) or release rates (35) whereas diestrous animals or animals under the negative feedback action of estrogens had low NE turnover and release rates. On the basis of NE turnover studies in other hypothalamic structures it is also well established that turnover changes may occur in one structure but not necessarily in others (19). Such changes in closely neighbored structures may even occur in opposite directions. Since the projection of noradrenergic axon terminals is very diffuse with little or no topographical orientation (12) we suggested that the specificity of such regional changes in turnover rates must be determined at the axon terminals and proposed that estrogen receptive neurons are involved in this mechanism. Presynaptic inhibition is a well-known phenomenon and often utilizes GABA as a presynaptically inhibitory neurotransmitter. On the basis of pharmacological and biochemical studies we were able to give some evidence for the validity of such a concept (19-21) but only recently, utilizing the push-pull cannula technique (35) and combined immunocytochemical and autoradiographic methods (36), were we able to give proof to our working hypothesis. Table 1 details mean catecholamine and GABA release rates into the medial preoptic/anterior hypothalamic area in ovariectomized animals with high and in diestrous rats with low LH levels. In both animal models prolactin levels are low. While no significant difference in dopamine release rates is observed, NE and E release rates in the ovariectomized rats are significantly higher than in diestrous animals whereas mean GABA release rates are significantly lower in OVX than in diestrous animals. Essentially the same can be seen in Figure 2 in which catecholamine and GABA release rates into the MPO/AH in an individual animal are shown. This animal was ovariectomized and treated with E2B for three days prior to experimentation. The animal had low LH and prolactin levels in the morning until the early afternoon and then prolactin levels rose abruptly followed by a steep increase in blood LH levels. The low hormone levels are due to the negative feedback action of estradiol and the high levels are the expression of the afternoon signal for the positive feedback action of the steriod (37). At the time of low hormone levels MPO/AH dopamine and NE release were low; they increased prior to and during the time of increasing prolactin and LH levels. With the exception of a few samples, E remained undetectable

Table 1. *Mean catecholamine (fmol/fraction), GABA (pmol/fraction) concentration in push-pull perfusate in the medial preoptic/anterior hypothalamic area and blood LH and prolactin levels of ovariectomized (OVX) and diestrous (D) rats*

Animal Models	DA	NE	E	GABA	LH	PRL
OVX	54 + 7	22 + 10	120 + 21	26 + 8	368 + 52	31 + 4
D	78 + 11	45 + 20*	27 + 5*	70 + 8	24 + 3	38 + 3

* $p < 0.01$ vs OVX

in this animal. In other, similarly treated rats, however, E was clearly detectable. The high morning and noon GABA release rates into the MPO/AH are in contrast to the decreasing GABA release rates at the time of the expression of the positive feedback signal in the afternoon. In a number of animals E release rates rose significantly at

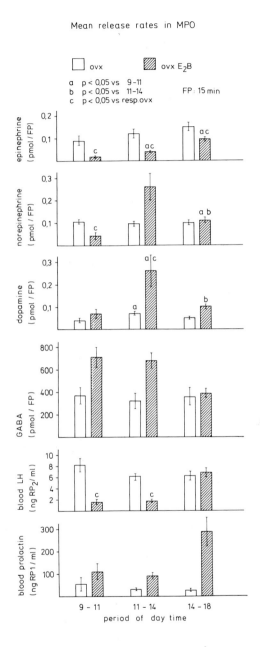

Figure 3. Mean catecholamine and GABA release rates into the MPO of OVX and OVX-estrogen-primed rats calculated for morning (9-11 hrs), noon (11-14 hrs) and afternoon (14-18 hrs). Note higher NE and E and lower GABA release at the time of increasing LH and prolactin levels in the estrogen primed animals. SEM are given on top of each bar.

the time of increasing pituitary prolactin and LH release. One observation made in the course of these experiments deserves further mention. In all animals in which estrogen resulted in a positive feedback action, spuriously high dopamine and/or NE release rates were observed during noon hours. This observation prompted us to calculate mean release rates in the morning (9.00 - 11.00 hrs), at noon (11.00 - 14.00 hrs) and in the afternoon (after 14.00 hrs). Figure 3 demonstrates that catecholamine release in ovariectomized animals is constant at the three daytime periods. Mean NE and E release is significantly higher than the release rates in ovariectomized estrogen-primed rats when they are under the negative feedback action of the steroid, i.e. in the morning. Significantly higher dopamine and NE release rates are observed during noon hours in the estrogen-primed animals and all three catecholamines are elevated in perfusates collected in the afternoon, i.e. at a time of the expression of the positive feedback action. Mean GABA release rates were high in animals with low LH levels and low in animals with high LH levels.

The high NE and dopamine release rates at noon may be causally related to the expression of the positive feedback action of estradiol later in the evening. They were observed only in animals which showed an afternoon surge of prolactin and LH. Possibly these secretory episodes of catecholamines in the MPO/AH reflect the biochemical signal of the so-called critical period at which time anesthetics can block the afternoon surge of prolactin and LH (42,43). This would also be in agreement with the observation that mechanisms regulatory to prolactin and LH surges reside in the MPO/AH (40,41,43).

To give final proof for the existence of a population of estrogen receptive neurons which utilize GABA as neurotransmitter we used the combined morphological method of autoradiography for estradiol and immunocytochemistry for glutamic acid decarboxylase (GAD) (26) and were indeed able to demonstrate that a large number of preoptic/anterior hypothalamic estrogen receptive neurons stain with a specific antibody against GAD (36).

Since the inverse release pattern of GABA and NE/E covariates best with blood LH levels under the different endocrine conditions, we conclude that these changes may be primarily involved in regulating the LHRH neurons, although prolactin regulatory mechanisms reside also in the MPO.

The question arises therefore whether mediobasal hypothalamic catecholamine or GABA release correlates better with blood prolactin levels. As indicated above, tuberoinfundibular dopamine neurons are strong candidates to be involved in inhibiting pituitary prolactin release (1,2) and MBH NE has been suggested to be stimulatory to hypothalamic mechanisms which in turn stimulate pituitary prolactin release (13,38). Furthermore, GABAergic mechanisms residing within the hypothalamus are also stimulatory to pituitary prolactin release (18,20,21,39). To test whether mediobasal hypothalamic catecholamine and GABA release rates correlate with blood prolactin levels, we recently utilized the push-pull cannula technique in the MBA also. Figures 4 and 5 detail 2 animals which were ovariectomized 7 days prior to experimentation and received injections of 25 ug of E2B for 3 days before the experiment. In one animal this estrogen priming resulted in dramatically increased prolactin and LH levels in the afternoon. In this animal GABA release rates into the MBH were relatively low at the beginning of the experiment. Just prior to the slowly increasing prolactin levels GABA release into the MBH increased more than 2-fold and remained at this high level during

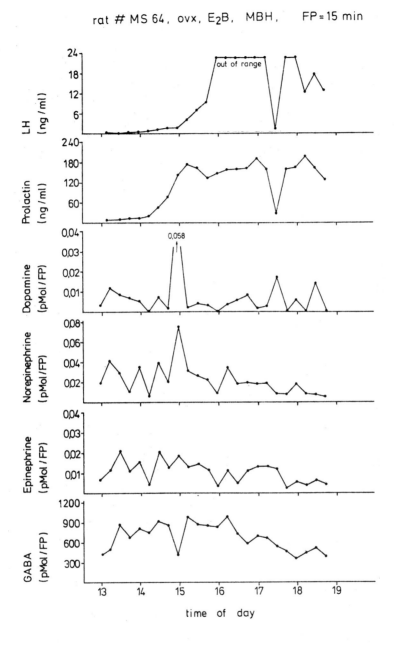

Figure 4. Catecholamine and GABA release in the MBH of an estrogen primed OVX rat. Note strong positive feedback effect of the estrogen on blood LH and prolactin levels in the afternoon. At the beginning of prolactin and LH surges catecholamine release is very high. GABA release remains higher during the time of high prolactin levels.

518

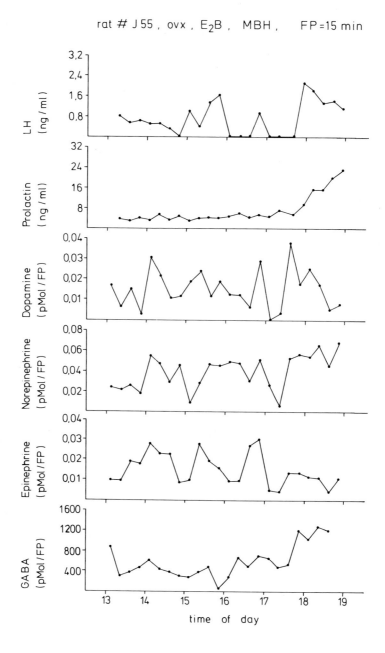

Figure 5. Catecholamine and GABA release in the MBH of an OVX estrogen primed rat which barely reacted to the estrogen. Few LH pulses correlate well with catecholamine pulses. The moderately increased blood prolactin levels are preceeded by increased hypothalamic GABA release.

the time of increased blood prolactin levels. GABA release rates slowly fell to those observed prior to increase of prolactin levels at a time when blood prolactin levels also decreased. Interestingly, spuriously high dopamine and NE release rates were observed in this animal just prior to the dramatic increase in blood LH levels. Such an apparent trigger signal was also observed in a number of other animals (see also Fig. 5). In Figure 5 estrogen injection resulted again in moderately increased blood prolactin levels during the afternoon hours which were again preceded by increased GABA release rates in the MBH.

This animal had extremely low LH levels and pulsatile episodic LH secretion occurred in the afternoon. Each of these pulses was accompanied by increased catecholamine release rates. Statistical evaluation of all data obtained in 12 such treated rats by means of correlation clearly indicated a significant correlation between hypothalamic GABA release rates and blood prolactin levels.

The latter observation prompted us also to test, by the combination of autoradiography and immunocytochemistry, whether estrogen receptive neurons might be GABAergic in the mediobasal hypothalamus. Figure 6 shows clearly that several estrogen retaining neurons stain with an antiserum against GAD. Hence, estrogen receptive GABAergic neurons exist also in the mediobasal hypothalamus.

Increased hypothalamic GABA release measured by the push-pull cannula technique correlates well with blood prolactin levels. Furthermore, our morphological studies

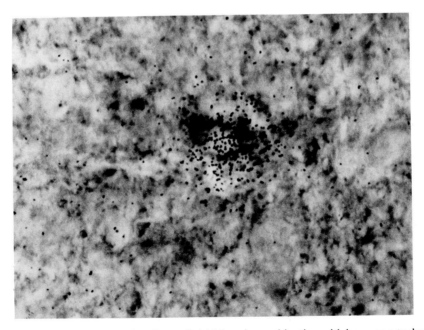

Figure 6. Autoradiogram of tritiated estradiol-17-beta in combination with immunocytochemical staining for glutamic acid decarboxylase. Black dots are indicative of radioactive estradiol. They accumulate over a GAD positive cell body located in the MBH of a female rat. GAD immunoreactivity is dark and surrounds the unstained nucleus of this cell. Numerous GAD immunoreactive patches can be found in the surroundings of this and/or other cells.

indicate that estrogen receptive neurons which use GABA as neurotransmitter exist in the hypothalamus. Possibly measurement of GABA release rates indicates their secretory activity. On the basis of these results it can be concluded that the well-known stimulatory effect of GABA on pituitary prolactin release is corroborated in this study. The mechanism of action of GABA remains unknown but it clearly does not involve inhibition of hypothalamic dopamine release since in none of the animals (including the male shown in the first part of this report) did intrahypothalamic dopamine release rates decrease at times of increasing prolactin levels. It is therefore safe to conclude that GABA, which is an inhibitory neurotransmitter, inhibits the release of either another non-dopaminergic PIF or of a substance which tonically inhibits the release of a prolactin-releasing factor. The role played by mediobasal hypothalamic catecholamines in regulating pituitary prolactin and LH release is not made clear by the present results. It appears that all 3 catecholamines may be released at high rates prior to expression of the positive feedback action of the injected estrogen. The most fascinating observation while utilizing the push-pull cannula technique was the missing correlation of hypothalamic dopamine release with blood prolactin levels. In fact, dopamine release may be episodically increased at the beginning of increased pituitary prolactin secretion. This is reminiscent of the observation published by Denef and Baes (42), who found that small amounts of dopamine applied in a pulsatile manner may be stimulatory to pituitary prolactin release. The observation of increased exposure of lactotrophs to dopamine at times of increased prolactin release is shared by our results obtained from intrapituitary perfusion (Duker, this volume). In these experiments, however, it also became clear that high dopamine concentration exerts the expected inhibitory action on prolactin secretion.

Research utilizing various techniques, including *in vivo* perfusion of circumscript brain areas with push-pull cannula, continues in our laboratory and will certainly allow a closer insight into the complex mechanisms which regulate the secretion of anterior pituitary hormones.

REFERENCES

1. MacLeod RM. (1976): In: Martini L, Ganong WF (eds) Frontiers in Neuroendocrinology. Raven Press, New York, p 169
2. Leong DA, Frawley LS, Neill JD. (1983): Ann Rev Physiol 45:109
3. Locatelli V, Cocchi D, Frigeria C, Betti R, Krogsgaard-Larsen P. Endocrinology 105:778
4. Libertun C, McCann SM. (1976): IRCS Med Sci 4:374
5. Enjalbert A, Ruberg M, Arancibia S, Priam M, Kordon C. (1979): Nature 280:595
6. McCann SM, Lumpkin MD, Mizunuma M, Khorram O, Ottlecz A, Samson WK. (1984): TINS:127
7. Enjalbert A, Ruberg M, Arancibia S, Fiore L, Priam M, Kordon C. (1979): Endocrinology 105:823
8. Voigt KH, Frank D, Duker E, Martin R, Wuttke W. (1984): Life Sci 33:507
9. Wuttke W, Duker E, Honma K, Demajo M, de-Lira SA, Lohse M, Mansky T. (1983): In: Calne et al. (eds) Lisuride and Other Dopamine Agonists. Raven Press, New York, p 175
10. Login IS, MacLeod RM. (1979): Europ J Pharmacol 60:253
11. Fuxe K, Hokfelt T. (1965): Acta Physiol Scand 66:243

12. Moore RY, Bloom FE. (1979): Ann Rev Neurosci 1:113
13. Carr LA, Conway PM, Voogt JL. (1973): Brain Res 133:305
14. Honma K, Wuttke W. (1980): Endocrinology 106:1848
15. Hokfelt T, Fuxe K, Goldstein J, Johansson O. (1974): Brain Res 66:235
16. Bruni JF, van Vugt D, Marshall S, Meites J. (1977): Life Sci 21:461
17. Lohse M, Wuttke W. (1981): Brain Res 229:389
18. Mansky T, Mestres-Ventura P, Wuttke W. (1982): Brain Res 231:353
19. Wuttke W, Mansky T, Stock KW, Sandmann R. (1981). In: Fuxe et al. (eds) Steroid Hormone Regulation of the Brain. Pergamon Press, Oxford, p 135
20. Lamberts R, Vijayan E, Graf M, Mansky T, Wuttke W. (1983): Exp Brain Res 52:356
21. Fuchs E, Mansky T, Stock KW, Vijayan E, Wuttke W. (1984): Neuroendocrinology 38:484
22. Gaddum JH. (1986): J Physiol 155:1
23. Myers RD. (1969): Physiol Behav 5:243
24. Ondo JG, Mansky T, Wuttke W. (1982): Exp Brain Res 46:69
25. Levine JE, Ramirez VD. (1982): Endocrinology 111:1439
26. Oertel W, Schmechel DE, Tappaz ML, Kopin IJ. (1981): Neuroscience 6:2689
27. Moore KE, Demarest KT. (1982), In: Martini L, Ganong WF (eds) Frontiers in Neuroendocrinology. Raven Press, New York p 161
28. Gudelsky GA, Porter JC. (1980): Endocrinology 106:526
29. Flerko B. (1980): Neuroendocrinology 30:56
30. Koskowski GP, Dees WL. (1984): J Histochem Cytochem 32:83
31. Sawyer CH, Clifton DK. (1980): Fed Proc 39:2889
32. Terry LC, Crowley WR, Lyoch C, Longserre C, Johnson MJ. (1982): Peptide 3:311
33. Wise PM, Rance N, Barraclough CA. (1981): Endocrinology 108:2186
34. Advis JP, McCann SM, Negro-Vilar A. (1980): Endocrinology 107:892
35. Wuttke W, Demling J, Fuchs E, Mansky T, Keck H, Lamberts R, Graf M. (1984). In: Naor et al. (eds) Hormonal Control of the Hypothalamo-Pituitary-Gonadal Axis, Plenum Press, New York, in press
36. Flugge G, Oertel W, Wuttke W. (1984): Nature, submitted
37. Freeman MC, Dupke KC, Croteau CM. (1976): Endocrinology 99:223
38. Fenske M, Wuttke W. (1976): Brain Res 104:63
39. Ondo JG, Pass KA. (1976): Endocrinology 98:1248
40. Kawakami M, Arita J. (1981): Exp Brain Res Suppl 3:274
41. Gunnet JW, Freeman ME. (1984): Neuroendocrinology 38:12
42. Everett JW, Sawyer CH. (1950): Endocrinology 47:198
43. Wuttke W, Meites J. (1972): Pflugers Arch Ges Physiol 337:71

Prolactin. Basic and clinical correlates
R.M. MacLeod, M.O. Thorner and U. Scapagnini (eds.),
Fidia Research Series, vol. I,
Liviana Press, Padova © 1985

PROLACTIN EFFECT ON *IN VIVO* STRIATAL DOPAMINERGIC ACTIVITY AS ESTIMATED WITH PUSH-PULL PERFUSION IN MALE RAT

J. C. Chen, A. D. Ramirez, and V. D. Ramirez

Department of Physiology and Biophysics, University of Illinois
Urbana, Illinois 61801

There is considerable evidence indicating that prolactin acts on the tuberoinfundibular dopaminergic neurons to modify synthesis and/or release of dopamine from these short-axon neurons (1-5). Whether prolactin modifies other CNS dopamine neurons is less clear, although an increasing number of experimental findings suggest that prolactin may also play an important role in controlling the activity of the nigrostriatal dopaminergic (NS-DA) system (6-8). Considerable knowledge has been gained in the past few years on the effect of prolactin on this long-axon neuronal system through studies examining the release rate of dopamine from *in vitro* striatal preparations (6,9), binding of dopamine agonists or antagonists to striatal membranes (10-13), and behavioral effects of prolactin, particularly grooming behavior (14-16). Therefore, it was of interest to investigate the possible role of prolactin on *in vivo* activity of the NS-DA system.

To this end, prolactin (rat or ovine in origin) was locally infused into the caudate nucleus (CN) of male rats bearing a push-pull cannula (PPC). These conscious unrestrained animals were then perfused *in vivo* and their biochemical and behavioral outputs were recorded. The perfusate from the CN was immediately injected into a high performance liquid chromatography with electrical detection (HPLC-EC) and the *in vivo* output of dopamine, 3-4 dihydroxyphenylacetic acid (DOPAC), 5-hydroxyindoleacetic acid (5-HIAA) and homovanillic acid (HVA) was subsequently measured as previously described (17).

To compare the *in vivo* output of the NS-DA system in animals acutely implanted with PPC versus chronically implanted animals, two groups of rats were studied. In the first group (n = 5), animals were anesthetized with Ketamine (9.1 mg/kg i.m.) and implanted with PPC. Approximately one hour following surgery, they were put back into their home cages and CN perfusion was initiated. Samples were collected at 20 minute intervals between 1200 and 1700 h and immediately analyzed for dopamine and

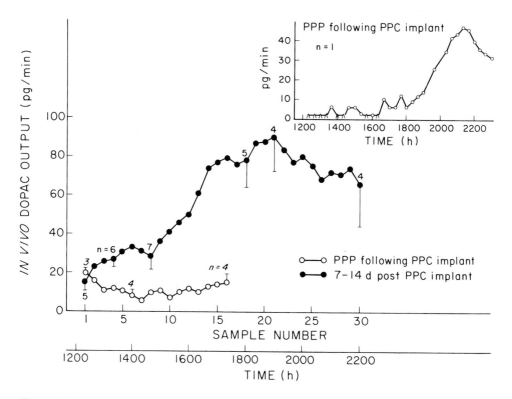

Figure 1. Comparison of the *in vivo* DOPAC output from the CN of acutely vs. chronically implanted male rats with PPC. The insert shows the DOPAC output profile from one acutely implanted animal. Numbers indicate corresponding sample size for each time period. In all cases the PPC reside in the effective perfusion area of the CN (see text and Fig. 6).

metabolites by HPLC-EC. The second group of rats (n = 7) were used 7-14 days after PPC implantation and were perfused between 1200 and 2200 h.

Figure 1 shows the output of DOPAC, an acidic and main metabolic product of dopamine, under these two conditions. In the chronic experiments, the data confirmed our previous findings (18) demonstrating a remarkable four-fold increase in DOPAC output between early afternoon hours (1200-1700 h) to plateau during the evening hours (1800-2200 h). This change in *in vivo* DOPAC output was a consistent finding across several animals although there were some variations in its magnitude and profile among individual rats. In the acute experiments, the results clearly indicate an absence of, or a rather prolonged delay in, the afternoon rise in DOPAC output from the CN which was also lower in magnitude than that from animals bearing chronic push-pull cannula. This indicates that the acute implantation procedure of PPC in the CN somehow impairs the function of the NS-DA system, emphasizing the importance of allowing a recovery period before push-pull perfusion (19). In the acute experiments, all animals were extremely lethargic and remained rather stationary in the corner of their cages for almost all of the push-pull perfusion session. In the chronic experiments, while the animals were being perfused, they went through their normal gamut of behaviors with bursts of activity including grooming, feeding, and exploratory behavior which interrupted resting and sleeping periods.

Therefore, the latter preparation was chosen to examine the effect of prolactin on the *in vivo* activity of the NS-DA system. One group of animals (n = 6) was infused for a 20 minute period with either rat prolactin or ovine prolactin (10 ng/ul NIAMDD-rPRL-RP-3; SIGMA; dissolved in modified Krebs-Ringer phosphate medium pH 7.4) at 1700 h or 1900 h. Following local perfusion of the CN with prolactin, at least three consecutive perfusates were collected and analyzed for neurochemical output. Figure 2 illustrates the effect of rat prolactin (approximately 0.1 uM) when it was perfused locally into the CN of rat No. 57 at 1900 h for a 20 minute period.

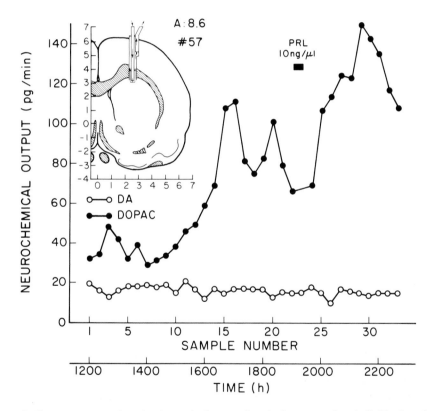

Figure 2. Spontaneous and prolactin-evoked neurochemical output of an individual rat bearing a PPC in the CN. Notice location of the tip of the cannula and the response to prolactin infused for *in* 20 min at 18 ul/min.

In this animal, after a spontaneous rise in DOPAC output which plateaued at approximately 1700-1800 h, prolactin evoked a two-fold increase in DOPAC output with

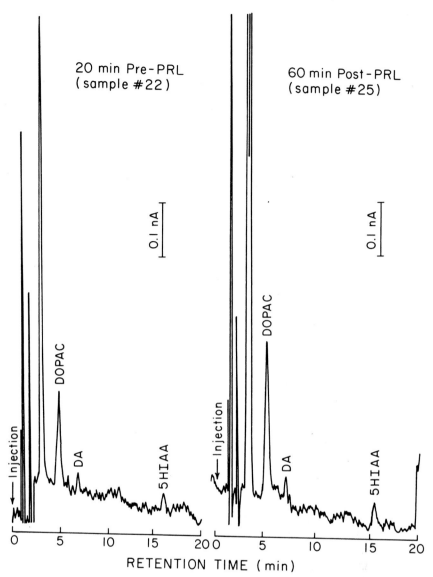

Figure 3. Chromatogram showing elution bands from perfusates from the CN of rat No. 57 of Fig. 2. Notice that after the solvent effect there is a large as yet unidentified peak that preceeds the elution band corresponding to DOPAC.

a maximal peak value of 150 picograms/min one hour after prolactin infusion and declined thereafter. Notice that dopamine output did not change either spontaneously or following prolactin infusion; there was a mean stable output of about 15 picograms/min during the entire PPP session.

Figure 3 shows the corresponding chromatogram of this experiment at 20 min before as compared with 60 min after prolactin infusion. The elution bands corresponding to dopamine and 5-hydroxyindoleacetic acid remained unchanged before, during or after prolactin infusion. The data also show that beside DOPAC, a major as yet unidentified and faster compound also markedly increased after prolactin infusion.

Figure 4 depicts the mean output of DOPAC, HVA, and dopamine before and after prolactin infusion in the six animals whose PPC were correctly placed in the effective site of the CN (see below).

In order to normalize the different infusion times of the hormone (either at 1700h or 1900h during the plateau phase of DOPAC output) the last time point of prolactin infusion was considered time zero. A significant elevation of DOPAC output was observed between 40 to 60 min after the termination of prolactin infusion without significant changes in either HVA or dopamine outputs. This effect of prolactin was not due to a high local concentration of proteins in the effective area of the CN since neither rat prolactin nor ovine prolactin (10 ng/ul, boiled at 100 C for 20 min), were effective in activating the striatal dopaminergic terminals of the CN. On the contrary, inactivated prolactin tended to inhibit DOPAC output with a significant minimum value of about 44 picograms/min at 60 min after prolactin infusion (Fig. 5).

In these same animals after a two hour recovery from this initial treatment, native prolactin infused in a similar manner and concentration (10 ng/ul for 20 min) caused a significant rise in DOPAC output at 20, 40, and 60 minutes after termination of prolactin infusion. Again, the increase in DOPAC output was specific to this neurotransmitter since neither 5-HIAA acid nor HVA outputs were affected by this treatment.

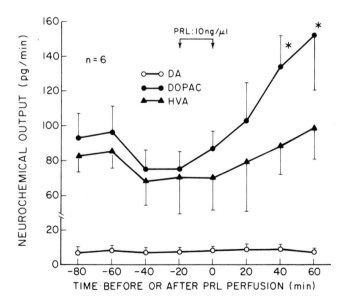

Figure 4. Stimulatory effect of native prolactin infused locally in the CN on DOPAC output. The stars indicate significant differences from values corresponding to 20 min before prolactin infusion (p < 0.05).

While the animals were perfused, their behaviors were recorded and scored one hour before and one hour after prolactin administration. Three types of reliably quantifiable behaviors were counted as discrete events: (1) Yawning (Y), (2) Stretch (STR), and (3) Stretch-Yawning Syndrome (SYS). In addition, the intensity of grooming (head, face, body, or genital) was scored by recording the duration of the behavior during the observational period as explained in Table 1.

An interesting topographic arrangement between the main position of the tip of the PPC in the CN and the rising phase of DOPAC output or the prolactin-evoked behavior was noticed after histological reconstruction of PPC placement in the CN of these animals. The spontaneous rising phase in DOPAC output was observed in 15 animals bearing PPC tips in the dorsal and anterior region of the CN (between A 8.6-9.4, DeGroots Rat Atlas). Individual positions of the tip of the PPC for these animals are shown in Figure 6, as well as a parasagittal view of the brain, depicting the extension of the "effective perfusion site" in the CN.

In seven rats with PPC in the CN, placed rostral or caudal to this region, no changes in DOPAC output were noticed during the PPP session. This functional topographic distribution of the *in vivo* activity of the CN clearly emphasizes the importance of topical innervation of the CN by dopaminergic terminals (20-23), and suggests that important functional difference may exist within discrete areas of the CN which ought to be considered in evaluating results implicating the effect of hormone or drugs on the function of the CN. As a case in point, only 9 of 13 rats with PPC in the effective perfusion area (i.e., showing the rising phase of DOPAC output) showed behavioral activation following prolactin infusion as shown in Table 1. The nine animals showed either yawning or SYS after prolactin administration while only one rat had one single yawn

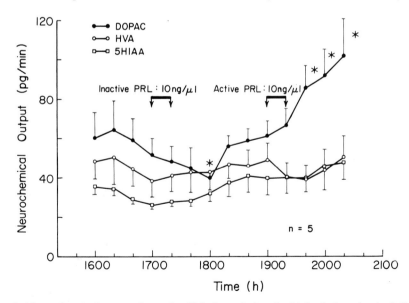

Figure 5. Neurochemical output from the CN of rats infused with boiled prolactin followed by native prolactin. Stars indicate significant differences from values corresponding to 20 min before treatment (p < 0.05).

Table 1. *Effect of prolactin locally perfused in the caudate nucleus (10 ng/ul/per minute for 20 min) on stretch (STR), stretch-yawning syndrome (SYS), yawning (Y), or grooming (GR) behavior of male rats bearing push-pull cannula. No effect (—), relative intensity of behavior (+), and frequency of events (Y, STR, SYS) are shown for each individual rat.*

			Number of individual Rat Perfused with Prolactin						
	76	136	168	173	175	178	181	195	196
Behavior				60 min pre-prolactin					
STR	—	—	—	—	—	—	—	—	—
SYS	—	—	—	—	—	—	—	—	—
Y	—	—	—	—	1	—	—	—	—
GR	—	—	—	+	—	+	+	+ +	—
Behavior				60 min post-prolactin					
STR	—	—	11	1	6	5	1	2	—
SYS	—	—	4	1	6	—	2	—	—
Y	5	3	—	—	1	1	3	2	2
GR	+ + +	+ + +	—	+ + +	+ + +	+ + +	+ + +	+ + +	+ + +

+ means a spontaneous short-burst of grooming during the 60 min observation period; + + means frequent bursts of grooming; + + + means 2 or more min of continuous grooming.

during the one hour pre-prolactin control period. This remarkable effect of prolactin was accompanied by intense, complex grooming behavior except in one animal. This confirms data reported previously by Drago et al. (14,15), although they believed that the effective brain site for the prolactin-evoked grooming behavior resided in the substantia nigra (SN) instead of the neostriatum. The fact that prolactin is capable of inducing yawning adds to the list of peptide hormones (24) known to stimulate this primitive behavior observed in different species of animals (25,26). One wonders about the physiological meaning of such clearcut behavioral effects induced by prolactin. Recently we have demonstrated that an extremely low dose of ovine prolactin (25 ng/100g bw) given subcutaneously into the neck of male rats is a powerful inducer of yawning after a latency of approximately 30-40 minutes. Higher doses appear to block this effect and the yawning is replaced by intense body and face grooming. (N. Laping and V. D. Ramirez, unpublished data). These results, and those of Drago et al. (14,15) indicate not only that prolactin is capable of modifying the activity of the NS-DA system, when the hormone is administered locally into a specific region of the brain, but also that this pituitary peptide can evoke NS-DA dependent behavior following systemic administration of prolactin. Therefore it appears that this hormone can cross the blood-brain barrier, as previously suggested by its measurement in the cerebrospinal fluid (27,28).

530

The present *in vivo* and previous *in vitro* data from our laboratory (9), indicate that prolactin can specifically alter NS-DA neurons through changes in either *in vitro* dopamine release or *in vivo* DOPAC output from corpus striatal dopaminergic terminals. Previously, it was demonstrated that levels of DOPAC in the striatum of rats tightly reflects the activity of the NS-DA system since electrical stimulation of the SN causes an increase in DOPAC levels whereas interruption of impulse flow through the NS-DA pathway causes decrease in DOPAC levels (29,30). Recently, voltametry recording from the CN of conscious male rats indicates that the major current signal feeding the voltameter is due to an increase in DOPAC and not dopamine release from this nucleus (31). Hence, in the male rat, the *in vivo* changes in DOPAC output appear to reflect the level of biological activity of the NS-DA system. In this context, it is interesting to recall that in freely moving male rats, a spontaneous rise in blood prolactin levels occurs during the afternoon hour of the photoperiod (32,33) which could be the

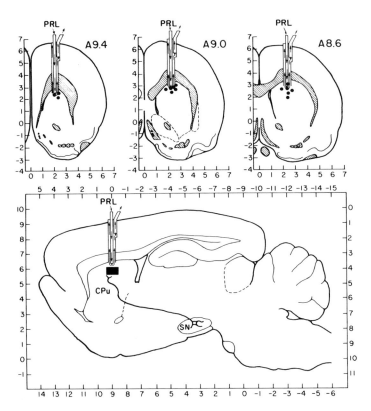

Figure 6. PPC position in the "effective area" of the CN (i.e. the area from which a spontaneous rise in DOPAC output can be detected) of 15 male rats perfused with prolactin. Of the 15 rats, two were not infused with prolactin and two animals received prolactin at times other than the plateau phase of DOPAC output (data not shown).

occurs during the afternoon hour of the photoperiod (32,33) which could be the physiological trigger of the spontaneous rise in DOPAC output observed under our experimental conditions in similar animal preparations. Additional studies in which injected anti-rat prolactin antibodies are used are required to prove such a hypothesis.

The behavioral components of the prolactin response induced either by local infusion into specific areas in the brain or through systemic injections of the hormone also reflect an activation of the nigrostriatal dopamine system. The functional complexity of this phenomenon is clearly evident from the present work, since not all of the animals that show changes in DOPAC output had a corresponding alteration in behavior or vice versa. We have not yet been able to identify a specific change in a chemical or chemicals from the CN with a corresponding specific component of the prolactin-evoked behaviors. It is known that dopamine neurons are somehow involved in inhibiting the activity of the yawning center (34,35), most likely through inhibition of cholinergic neurons (34,36). Therefore, it is feasible that prolactin may first activate the release of dopamine from CS dopaminergic terminals, with subsequent inhibition of the release of this neurotransmitter through the classic functional dopamine negative feedback loop, causing the disinhibition of the yawning center. This would explain the relatively late latency of the prolactin-evoked yawning behavior observed in these animals.

Finally, the present work indicates that our current methodology using PPC coupled to HPLC-EC is a suitable and useful experimental approach to examine correlates between in vivo output of neuroactive substances from specific brain areas and behavioral and physiological events which can only be investigated in conscious, freely behaving animals.

REFERENCES

1. Moore KE, Demarest KT. (1982): Frontiers in Neuroendocrinology 7:161
2. Porter JC, Gudelsky GA, Nansel DD, Pilotte NS, Foreman MM. (1980): Adv Sex Hormone Res 4:213
3. Gudelsky GA, Porter JC. (1980): Endocrinology 106:526
4. Demarest KT, Riegle GD, Moore KE. (1984): Neuroendocrinology 38:457
5. VanLoon GR, Shum A, George SR, Shin SH. (1982): Brain Res. Bull. 10:539
6. Perkins NA, Westfall TC. (1978): Neuroscience 3:59
7. Ramirez VD. (1983): In: Bhatnagar AS (ed) The Anterior Pituitary Gland. Raven Press, New York, p 97
8. DiPaolo T, Poyet P, Labrie F. (1982): Prog Neuro-Psychopharmacol Biol Psychiat 6:377
9. Chen YF, Ramirez VD. (1982): Endocrinology 111:1740
10. Hruska RE, Pitman KT, Silbergeld EK, Ludmer LM. (1981): Life Sci 30:547
11. Cronin MJ, Reches A, MacLeod RM, Login IS. (1983): Eur J Pharmacol 91:229
12. DiPaolo T, Poyet P, Labrie F. (1982): Life Sci 31:2921
13. Eva C, Glengio M, Ferretti C, Muccioli G, Portaleone P. (1982): Brain Res 251:388
14. Drago F, VanRee JM, Bohus B, Scapagnini U, DeWied D. (1984): Adv Biosc 6:377
15. Drago F, Bohus B, Gispen WH, Scapagnini U, DeWied D. (1983): Brain Res 263:277
16. Hutchison RE. (1978): In: Robyn C, Harter H (eds) Progress in Prolactin Physiology and Pathology. Elsevier/North Holland Biomedical Press, p 243
17. Chen JC, Rhee KK, Beaudyr DM, Ramirez VD. (1984): Neuroendocrinology 38:362
18. Ramirez VD. (1984): In: Bayon A, Drucker-Colin R (eds) In Vivo Release of Neuroactive

Substances in the Central Nervous System: Method, Findings and Perspectives. Academic Press, in press

19. Levine JE, Ramirez VD. (1980): Endocrinology 107:1782
20. Moore RY, Bloom FE. (1978): Ann Rev Neurosci 1:129
21. Strong R, Samorajsk T, Gottesfeld Z. (1982): J Neurochem 39:831
22. Tassin JP, Chermy A, Blanc G, Thierry AM, Glowinsky J. (1976): Brain Res 107:291
23. Veening JG, Cornelissen FM, Lieven PAJM. (1980): Neurosci 5:1253
24. Ferrari W, Gessa GL, Vargiut. (1963): Ann N.Y. Acad Sci 104:330
25. Rodriguez-Sierra JF, Terasawa E, Goldfoot DA, DeWied D. (1981): Horm Behav 15:77
26. Baldwin DM, Haun CK, Sawyer CH. (1974): Brain Res 80:291
27. Clemens JA, Sawyer BD. (1974): Exp Brain Res 21:399
28. Login IS, MacLeod RM. (1977): Brain Res 132:477
29. Roth RN, Murrin LC, Walters JR. (1976): Eur J Pharmacol 36:163
30. Elchiasak MA, Murrin LC, Roth RH, Maas JW. (1976): Psychopharmacol Commu 2 (5 and 6):411
31. Hefti F, Melamed E. (1981): Brain Res 225:333
32. Mattheij JAM, Swarts JJM. (1978): J Endocr 79:85
33. Hostetter MW, Piacsek BE. (1977): Biol Rep 16:495
34. Urba-Holmgren, Gonzalez RM, Holmgren B. (1977): Nature 267:261
35. Holmgren B, Urba-Holmgren R. (1980): Acta Neurobiol Exp 40:633
36. Yamada K, Furukawa T. (1980): Psychopharmacol 67:39

Prolactin. Basic and clinical correlates
R.M. MacLeod, M.O. Thorner and U. Scapagnini (eds.),
Fidia Research Series, vol. I,
Liviana Press, Padova © 1985

THE INTERRELATIONSHIP BETWEEN THE RAPID "TONIC" AND THE DELAYED "INDUCTION" COMPONENTS OF THE PROLACTIN-INDUCED ACTIVATION OF TUBEROINFUNDIBULAR DOPAMINE NEURONS

K. T. Demarest, G. D. Riegle and K. E. Moore

Departments of Pharmacology/Toxicology and Physiology
Michigan State University, East Lansing, MI 48824

Previous studies in our laboratories (1,2) have demonstrated that prolactin causes a delayed increase in the *in vivo* rate of dopamine synthesis and turnover in terminals of tuberoinfundibular neurons in the median eminence. Following systemic or intracerebroventricular administration of prolactin, or after pharmacologic manipulations (haloperidol, estradiol) which result in a prolonged increase in circulating prolactin concentration, an increase in the *in vivo* rate of dopamine synthesis and turnover is observed consistently after a delay of 12-16 h. This prolactin-induced increase in the activity of tuberoinfundibular dopamine neurons requires protein synthesis since it is blocked by cycloheximide pretreatment (3). Thus, it is thought that prolactin stimulates tuberoinfundibular dopamine neurons by either a direct action on these neurons or by altering the activity of afferent neuronal systems which project to the tuberoinfundibular dopamine neurons (Fig. 1).

Other investigators have demonstrated *in vitro* that prolactin can stimulate the synthesis and release of dopamine from tissue fragments of medial basal hypothalamus without any latent period (4-6). Attempts to demonstrate a rapid action of prolactin on dopamine synthesis and turnover in tuberoinfundibular neurons *in vivo* may have been hampered by the techniques employed to make these neurochemical determinations; that is, by estimating the rate of the alpha-methyltyrosine-induced decline of dopamine or the rate of DOPA accumulation after the decarboxylase inhibitor, 3-hydroxybenzylhydrazine (NSD 1015). By the nature of the pharmacologic manipulations associated with these *in vivo* estimates of dopamine synthesis and turnover, serum prolactin concentrations are elevated. Thus, "control" rates of dopamine synthesis and turnover in the median eminence represent values obtained in the presence of high circulating levels of prolactin, which probably activate any rapid prolactin action on tuberoinfundibular dopamine neurons. In the present studies the ability of the *in vivo*

534

administration of exogenous prolactin to stimulate tuberoinfundibular dopamine neurons was examined in rats which were pretreated with bromocriptine or were hypophysectomized to prevent prolactin-elevating effects of either alpha-methyltyrosine or NSD 1015. The results of the following studies will demonstrate that there are two components to the activation of tuberoinfundibular dopamine neurons by prolactin: a rapid 'tonic' component, which is responsive to acute changes in prolactin, and a delayed 'induction' component, which is activated by prolonged changes in prolactin concentrations. All of the following studies were performed in two-week ovariectomized rats. The activity of tuberoinfundibular dopamine neurons was estimated by measuring the rate of DOPA accumulation in the median eminence 30 min after the administration of NSD 1015 and is expressed as ng DOPA/mg protein (2).

Both bromocriptine pretreatment and hypophysectomy lower circulating levels of prolactin and decrease tuberoinfundibular dopamine neuronal activity, as measured by the rate of DOPA accumulation in the median eminence (6,7). Presumably, the abrupt decrease in circulating levels of prolactin reduces the activation of tuberoinfundibular neurons by this hormone. Thus, using these models it is possible to examine the acute actions of exogenously administered prolactin on tuberoinfundibular dopamine neurons. We studied the effect of intracerebroventricularly administered prolactin on the rate of DOPA accumulation in the median eminence of animals that were pretreated with bromocriptine, or its vehicle, 24 h prior to sacrifice (Fig. 2). As stated previously, bromocriptine decreased the rate of DOPA accumulation in the median eminence. In the vehicle-treated rats prolactin increased the rate of DOPA accumulation in the median eminence after 12 h but not 4 h, confirming previous reports (3,6). In the bromocriptine-treated rats prolactin increased DOPA accumulation back to 'control levels' after 4 h and caused a further increase above control levels by 12 h. Similar results were observed in hypophysectomized animals (data not shown). These results suggest

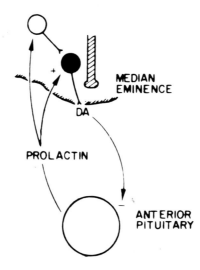

Figure 1. Schematic diagram of the stimulatory action of prolactin feedback on tuberoinfundibular dopaminergic neurons.

that there are two components to the action of prolactin on tuberoinfundibular neurons: a rapid 'tonic' component and a delayed 'induction' component.

Since previous studies demonstrated that the delayed action of prolactin on tuberoinfundibular dopamine neurons requires ongoing protein synthesis (3), the action of cycloheximide on the rapid and delayed actions of prolactin was examined in vehicle- and bromocriptine-pretreated rats (Fig. 3). Cycloheximide blocked the delayed (12 h) prolactin-induced increase in DOPA accumulation in the median eminence of both groups, but did not inhibit the rapid (4 h) action of prolactin in bromocriptine-treated rats. Thus, the delayed component appears to require the 'induction' of protein synthesis while the rapid 'tonic' component does not.

To examine the rapid 'tonic' component of prolactin feedback, the time course and dose-response of prolactin on tuberoinfundibular neurons were characterized. The effects of a continuous intravenous infusion of prolactin on the rate of DOPA accumulation in the median eminence of bromocriptine- pretreated rats were determined. The effect of endogenous prolactin secretion was thereby eliminated and it was possible to manipulate circulating levels of prolactin by altering the concentration of prolactin infused exogenously. Using this model, the continuous infusion of prolactin (at a rate of 1 ug/min) maintained serum prolactin concentrations at 500-700 ng/ml and increased DOPA accumulation in the median eminence within 2 h (Fig. 4). Varying the concentration of the prolactin infusion from 0.03-3 ug/min, yielded serum prolactin concentrations of 27 to 1106 ng/ml (Fig. 5). However, there was no clear dose-response relationship between the changes in trunk blood prolactin and the rate of DOPA ac-

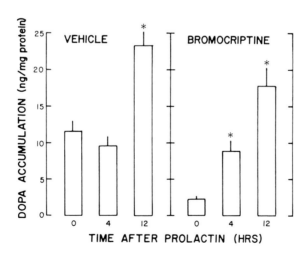

Figure 2. Time course for the effect of i.c.v. prolactin on the rate of DOPA accumulation in the median eminence of rats pretreated with bromocriptine. Rats were pretreated with bromocriptine (3 mg/kg, s.c.) or its vehicle 24 h prior to sacrifice followed by rat prolactin (10 ug/10 ul, i.c.v.) or its saline vehicle 4 or 12 h prior to sacrifice. Each column represents the mean and vertical line 1 S.E. of 8 determinations. *, values significantly different from the prolactin vehicle-treated (0 h) animals, p < 0.05.

cumulation in the median eminence after 4 h of continuous infusion; all doses of prolactin were equally effective. These results suggest that the rapid 'tonic' component of prolactin's action has a latency of approximately 2 h. Furthermore, prolactin does not induce a dose-related effect. Rather, sustained increases in serum prolactin concentrations appear to produce an all-or-none effect.

Additional studies were undertaken to examine the relationship between the rapid 'tonic' and the delayed 'induction' components of the prolactin mechanism. The 'induction' component was stimulated by pretreatment with haloperidol (2.5 mg/kg x 3 d) which elevates serum concentrations of prolactin. In previous studies this regimen both maintained a continuous increase in serum prolactin concentrations and resulted in maximal stimulation of DOPA accumulation in the median eminence. In the present studies, haloperidol pretreatment increased the rate of DOPA accumulation (Fig. 6). Administration of bromocriptine 4 hr prior to sacrifice decreased DOPA accumulation in the median eminence of vehicle-treated rats and blocked the haloperidol-induced increase. The ability of bromocriptine to decrease DOPA accumulation in vehicle- and haloperidol-treated rats appears to result from the decrease in circulating levels of prolactin since this action of bromocriptine is not observed in either vehicle-or haloperidol-treated rats which were administered ovine prolactin (10 mg/kg, ip) 4 h prior to sacrifice. These results demonstrate that the delayed 'induction' component increases the capaci-

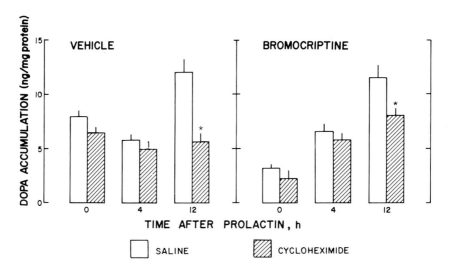

Figure 3. Effect of cycloheximide pretreatment on the prolactin-induced increase in the rate of DOPA accumulation in the median eminence of rats pretreated with bromocriptine. Rats were injected with bromocriptine (3 mg/kg, s.c.) or its vehicle 24 h prior to sacrifice. Cycloheximide (3 mg/kg, i.p.) or its vehicle was administered 1 h prior to the injection of rat prolactin (10 ug/10 ul, i.c.v.) or its saline vehicle at 12 or 4 h prior to sacrifice. Each column represents the mean and the verticle line 1 S.E. of 7-9 determinations. *, values from cycloheximide-treated animals (hatched columns) which are significantly different from their saline-treated controls (open columns), $p < 0.05$.

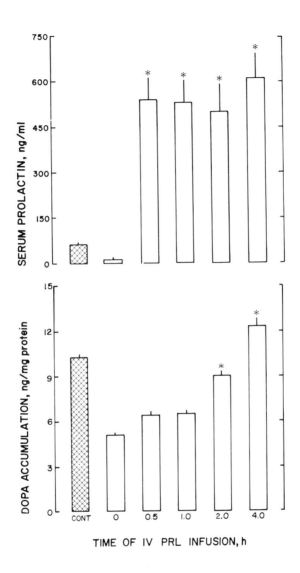

Figure 4. Time course for the effect of the continuous i.v. infusion of prolactin on serum prolactin concentrations and the rate of DOPA accumulation in the median eminence. Rats were implanted 3-5 days prior to experimentation with indwelling i.v. jugular cannulae. Bromocriptine (3 mg/kg, s.c.; open bars) or vehicle (CONT; hatched bars) was administered 4 h prior to sacrifice. All animals were continuously infused for 4 h with either saline or rat prolactin at a rate of 3.5 ul/min. Rat prolactin (NIAMDDK B-5; 1 ug/min) was administered 0, 0.5, 1, 2, and 4 h prior to sacrifice; the remaining time the rats received an infusion of saline. *, values from prolactin-infused animals which are significantly different from the bromocriptine-alone group (0 h), $p < 0.05$.

538

ty of tuberoinfundibular dopamine neurons to respond to prolactin. Nevertheless, this increased responsiveness can only be expressed via the rapid 'tonic' component and then only when circulating prolactin levels are elevated.

Using this haloperidol-bromocriptine model, studies were undertaken to examine the effect of activating the delayed 'induction' component of the prolactin feedback mechanism on the time course and dose-response for the action of prolactin to stimulate tuberoinfundibular neurons via the rapid 'tonic' component. The effect of continuous

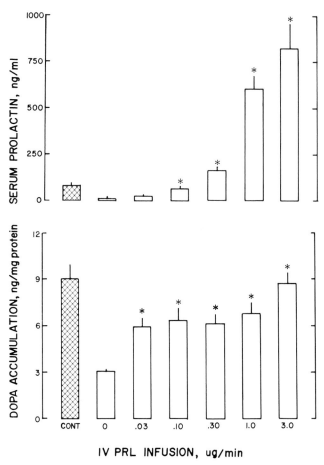

Figure 5. Dose-response for the effect of the continuous i.v. infusion of prolactin on serum pro-lactin concentrations and the rate of DOPA accumulation in the median eminence. Rats were implanted 3-5 days prior to experimentation with indwelling i.v. jugular cannulae. Bromocrip-tine (3 mg/kg, s.c.; open bars) or vehicle (CONT; hatched bars) was administered 4 h prior to sacrifice. All animals were continuously infused for 4 h with saline (CONT, 0 ug/min) or rat prolactin (NIAMDDK B-5; 0.03-3 ug/min) at a rate of 3.5 ul/min. *, values from prolactin-infused animals which are significantly different from the bromocriptine-alone group (0 ug/min), p < 0.05.

intravenous infusion of prolactin was studied in rats pretreated with haloperidol for several days (2.5 mg/kg x 3 d) followed by bromocriptine (10 mg/kg) 4 h prior to sacrifice. As reported earlier, haloperidol increased tuberoinfundibular dopamine neuronal activity, as evidenced by an increased rate of DOPA accumulation in the median eminence. This increase was attenuated by the bromocriptine treatment which decreased DOPA accumulation in both vehicle- and haloperidol-treated groups to similar low levels. A time course following the continuous infusion of prolactin (1 ug/min) demonstrated that DOPA accumulation in the median eminence of both vehicle- and haloperidol-treated rats was increased by 2 h (Fig. 7). The dose-response for continuous prolactin infusion revealed no clear-cut dose-related increase in either vehicle- or haloperidol-treated rats. Instead, all doses of prolactin increased the rate of DOPA accumulation in the median eminence, with a greater magnitude in the haloperidol-treated rats (Fig. 8). These results demonstrate that the increased responsiveness of tuberoinfundibular dopamine neurons to prolactin, as a consequence of activating the 'induction' component, is not characterized by a shortened onset of action or by an increase in the sensitivity of these neurons to the action of prolactin. Instead, an increased magnitude of response of these neurons to the actions of prolactin was observed.

The results of the present studies are depicted schematically in Figure 9. These results suggest that the 'tonic' component of the prolactin feedback mechanism increases tuberoinfundibular dopamine neuronal activity in response to short-term changes in

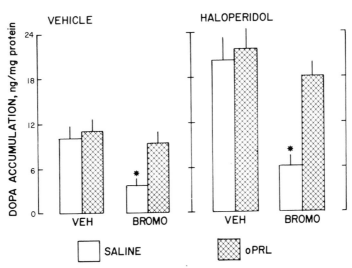

Figure 6. Effect of ovine prolactin and bromocriptine on the haloperidol-induced increase in the rate of DOPA accumulation in the median eminence. Rats were pretreated with 3 daily injections of haloperidol (2.5 mg/kg, s.c.) or its vehicle and were sacrificed 24 h after the last injection. Bromocriptine (10 mg/kg, i.p.) or its vehicle and ovine prolactin (NIAMDDK oPRL-16; 10 mg/kg, i.p) or its vehicle were administered 4 h prior to sacrifice. *, values significantly different from their appropriate vehicle-treated control groups, p < 0.05.

540

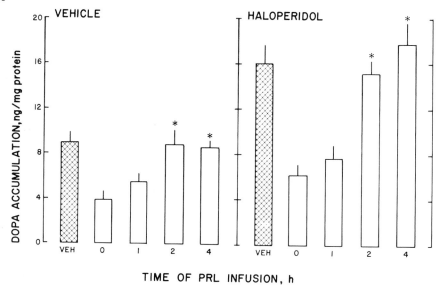

TIME OF PRL INFUSION, h

Figure 7. Effect of haloperidol pretreatment on the time course of stimulation of DOPA accumulation in the median eminence by continuous prolactin infusion. Rats, which were implanted 5 days prior to experimentation with indwelling i.v. jugular cannulae, received 3 daily injections of haloperidol (2.5 mg/kg, s.c.) or its vehicle and were sacrificed 24 h after the last injection. Bromocriptine (10 mg/kg, s.c.; open bars) or vehicle (VEH; hatched bars) was administered 4 h prior to sacrifice. All animals were continuously infused for 4 h with either saline or rat prolactin at a rate of 3.5 ul/min. Rat prolactin (NIAMDDK B-5; 1 ug/min) was administered 0,1,2, and 4 h prior to sacrifice; the remaining time the rats received an infusion of saline. * significantly (p < 0.05) different from bromocriptine-alone group (0 h)

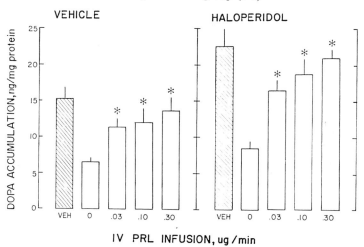

IV PRL INFUSION, ug/min

Figure 8. Effect of haloperidol pretreatment on the dose-response of stimulation of DOPA accumulation in the median eminence by continuous prolactin infusion. Experimental conditions were identical to those in Fig. 7. except that animals were continuously infused for 4 h with saline (VEH, 0 ug/min) or rat prolactin (NIAMDDK B-5; 0.03-3 ug/min) at a rate of 3.5 ul/min. * significantly (p < 0.05) different from bromocriptine-alone group (0 ug/min)

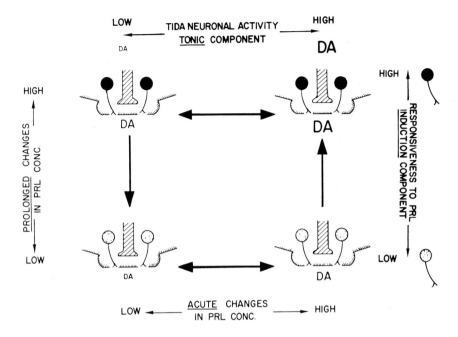

Figure 9. Schematic diagram depicting the interrelationship between rapid 'tonic' and delayed 'induction' components of the prolactin feedback mechanism. The greater size of dopamine represents increased activity of tuberoinfundibular dopaminergic neurons and the intensity of shading in the neuronal cell bodies represents increased capacity to respond to prolactin.

circulating prolactin concentrations and that the magnitude of response of tuberoinfundibular dopamine neurons to short-term increases in prolactin is determined by the preceding 'history' of the secretion of this hormone via the 'induction' component.

ACKNOWLEDGMENTS

These studies were supported by NIH grants AG02644 and NS09174, and by a Pharmaceutical Manufacturers Association Foundation Research Starter Grant and Career Development Award to K.T.D. The authors acknowledge Janet Keedy and Susan Stahl for technical assistance and Diane Hummel for manuscript preparation.

REFERENCES

1. Gudelsky, GA, Simpkins J, Mueller GP, Meites J, Moore KE. (1976): Neuroendocrinology 22:206
2. Demarest KT, Moore KE. (1980): Endocrinology 106:463

3. Johnston CA, Demarest KT, Moore KE. (1980): Brain Res 195:236
4. Perkins NA, Westfall TC. (1978): Neuroscience 3:59
5. Perkins NA, Westfall TC, Paul CV, MacLeod R, Rogol AD. (1979): Brain Res 160:431
6. Demarest KT, Moore KE. (1981): Neuroendocrinology 33:230
7. Demarest KT, Riegle GD, Moore KE. (1984): Neuroendocrinology 38:467

Prolactin. Basic and clinical correlates
R.M. MacLeod, M.O. Thorner and U. Scapagnini (eds.),
Fidia Research Series, vol. I,
Liviana Press, Padova © 1985

EFFECTS OF LONG-TERM TREATMENT WITH ESTRADIOL AND HALOPERIDOL ON SERUM CONCENTRATIONS OF PROLACTIN AND TUBEROINFUNDIBULAR DOPAMINERGIC NEURONAL ACTIVITY

K. E. Moore, G. D. Riegle, and K. T. Demarest

Departments of Pharmacology/Toxicology and Physiology,
Michigan State University, East Lansing, MI 48824

Short-term (3-5 days) treatment of rats with estrogens increases tuberoinfundibular (TIDA) neuronal activity, as revealed by an increased concentration of dopamine in hypophysial portal blood (1) and by increased rates of turnover and synthesis of dopamine in the terminals of these neurons in the median eminence (2,3). Since the latter effects are not seen in hypophysectomized rats it is believed that they result from the ability of estrogens to increase circulating concentrations of prolactin (2,4,5). Long-term (> two weeks) treatment with estrogens is reported to cause cytopathological changes in the arcuate nucleus (6) and to decrease the dopamine content in the median eminence (7).

The objective of the present study was to characterize the time course of the actions of, and the recovery from, the effects of estradiol on TIDA neurons and to determine the role of prolactin in these effects.

All experiments were performed in adult Long-Evans female rats that had been ovariectomized two weeks prior to the onset of treatments. Empty silastic capsules (SHAM) or identical capsules containing estradiol benzoate were implanted subcutaneously under ether anesthesia. Capsules were constructed (dimensions: 5 mm exposed length, I.D., 0.062 inch; O.D., 0.175 inch) (8) so that they maintained serum concentrations of 80-120 pg estradiol/ml serum for at least 18 days. By this time the anterior pituitaries were slightly hyperplastic but did not expand out of the sella turcica so as to compress the mediobasal hypothalamus. Blood was collected by orbital sinus puncture under light ether anesthesia and analyzed for prolactin by a double antibody radioimmunoassay according to directions and with reagents provided by NIADDK kits and reported on the basis of NIADDK-rat prolactin RP 1. The *in vivo* rate of dopamine synthesis was estimated by measuring the accumulation of DOPA in the terminals of TIDA neurons in the median eminence 30 min after the administration of NSD 1015 (100 mg/kg, ip), a decarboxylase inhibitor. Radioenzymatic assays were used to quantify dopamine and norepinephrine (NE) (9) and DOPA (2).

The time course for the effects of estradiol on serum prolactin concentrations, and on the rates of DOPA accumulation and dopamine and NE concentrations in the median eminence, is depicted in Figure 1. In the animals implanted with estradiol-containing capsules there was a progressive and sustained (for 18 days) increase in the serum concentrations of prolactin. Treatment with estradiol for 6 days increased the rate of dopamine synthesis in the median eminence. Since this relatively early effect of estradiol is not seen in hypophysectomized rats it is believed to result from the estradiol-induced increase in circulating prolactin concentrations (2). In animals treated with estradiol for an additional 6 days (sacrificed on day 12) the rate of DOPA accumulation in the median eminence was not significantly different from SHAM-controls, while in animals treated for 18 days with estradiol the rate of dopamine synthesis in the median eminence was actually less than control. Thus, although the serum prolactin concentrations remained elevated the TIDA neurons became unresponsive to the actions of this hormone. In contrast to the biphasic effect of long-term treatment with estradiol on the rate of dopamine synthesis, the concentration of dopamine in the median eminence declined progressively with time after implantation of the estradiol capsules. On the other hand, the NE concentration in this brain region did not change. The actions of estradiol were selective for TIDA neurons since there were no changes in the concentrations and rates of synthesis of dopamine in any other brain region studied (data not shown). That is, in animals treated for 1, 6, or 18 days with estradiol there were no changes in the

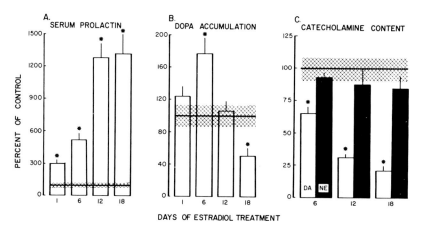

DAYS OF ESTRADIOL TREATMENT

Figure 1. Time course for the effects of estradiol on serum prolactin concentrations and the rates of DOPA accumulation and dopamine and norepinephrine concentrations in the median eminence.

Rats were implanted subcutaneously with empty (SHAM) or estradiol-containing capsules for 1, 6, 12, or 18 days prior to sacrifice. Horizontal lines and shaded areas represent means (set at 100%) ± 1 S.E. of values in SHAM controls; 100% represents: A, serum prolactin 26.1 ± 3.5 ng/ml; B, DOPA accumulation, 14.6 ± 1.9 ng/mg protein/30 min; C, dopamine (DA) and norepinephrine (NE) concentrations, 94.4 ± 7.9 and 31.2 ± 3.4 ng/mg protein, respectively. Each column represents the mean and vertical line 1 S.E. of 6-8 determinations made in estradiol-treated rats. *, values that are significantly different from the corresponding SHAM group (P<0.05).

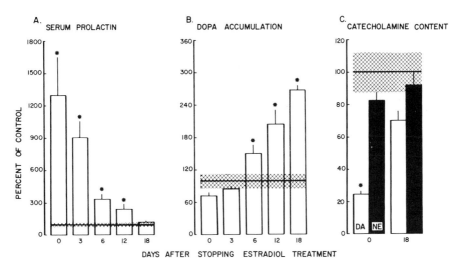

Figure 2. Serum prolactin concentrations, rates of DOPA accumulation and dopamine and norepinephrine concentrations in the median eminence at various times after the removal of estradiol-containing capsules.

Rats were implanted subcutaneously with empty (SHAM) or estradiol-containing capsules for 18 days. The capsules were removed and the animals were sacrificed on the same day (SHAM and Day 0) or 3, 6, 12, and 18 days later. Horizontal lines and shaded areas represent means (set at 100%) ± 1 S.E. of values in SHAM controls; 100% represents: A, serum prolactin 79.2 ± 11.6 ng/ml; B. DOPA accumulation 7.6 ± 0.9 ng/mg protein/30 min; C, dopamine (DA) and norepinephrine (NE) concentrations 145 ± 4.9 and 21.9 ng/mg protein, respectively. Each column represents the mean and vertical line 1 S.E. of determinations made in 8 rats implanted with the estradiol capsules. *, values that are significantly different from the corresponding SHAM group (p < 0.05).

dopamine concentrations or rates of DOPA accumulation in terminals of nigrostriatal (striatum), mesolimbic (nucleus accumbens, olfactory tubercle), or tuberohypophysial (posterior pituitary) dopamine neurons.

The next experiment was designed to determine if the effects of long-term treatment with estradiol on TIDA neurons were reversible. Empty (SHAM) or estradiol-containing capsules were implanted for 18 days and then removed. The serum concentrations of prolactin, the rate of DOPA accumulation in the median eminence, and the concentrations of dopamine and NE in the median eminence were determined on the day the capsules were removed (day 0) and on 3, 6, 12 and 18 days thereafter. The results are summarized in Figure 2. The serum concentrations of prolactin, which were markedly elevated after 18 days of estradiol treatment (day 0 in Figure 2), declined progressively once the capsules were removed, reaching control values within 18 days. The rate of DOPA accumulation in the median eminence, which was reduced in animals treated with estradiol for 18 days, promptly returned to control values (within 3 days)

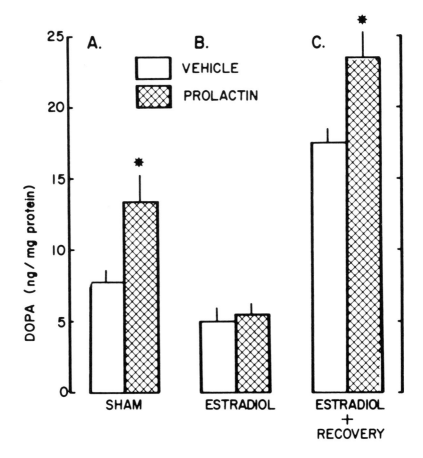

Figure 3. Effects of prolactin on the rate of DOPA accumulation in rats implanted with estradiol-containing capsules.

Rat prolactin (10 ug, hatched columns) or 0.9% saline vehicle (open columns) was injected icv 12 hr prior to sacrifice via previously implanted cannula guides in rats that were: A, implanted with empty capsules for 18 days (SHAM); B, implanted with estradiol-containing capsules for 18 days (ESTRADIOL); C, implanted with estradiol capsules for 18 days, with the capsules removed for 18 days prior to sacrifice (ESTRADIOL + RECOVERY). Each column represents the mean and vertical line 1 S.E. of 6-8 determinations. *, values that are significantly different from vehicle-injected controls.

after the capsules were removed, and then unexpectedly rebounded to values above control when examined 6-18 days after capsule removal.

The next question considered was, "If the estradiol activation of TIDA neurons is a result of the ability of this hormone to increase circulating prolactin levels, then why is the effect not sustained?" That is, estradiol maintained elevated serum prolactin concentrations for 18 days, while the TIDA neuronal activity, as estimated by the rate of DOPA accumulation in the median eminence, was increased for less than 12

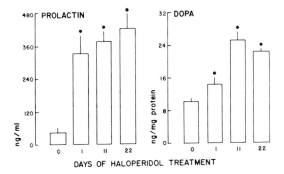

Figure 4. The effect of chronic haloperidol administration on the serum concentration of prolactin and the rate of DOPA accumulation in the median eminence.

Haloperidol (2.5 mg/kg, s.c.) or its 0.3% tartaric acid vehicle was administered daily for up to 22 days, and animals were killed 24 h after the 1st, 11th and 22nd injection. Each column represents the mean and the vertical line 1 S.E. of 7-8 determinations, *, values that are significantly different (p < 0.05) from vehicle-injected controls (0 days).

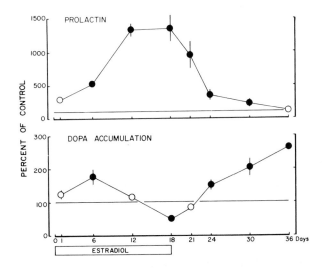

Figure 5. Composite time course for the effects of and recovery from chronic estradiol treatment. Horizontal lines represent values in animals implanted with empty capsules (SHAM). Circles represent means and vertical lines ± 1 S.E. of values in animals implanted with estradiol-containing capsules. Solid circles represent values in estradiol-treated animals that are significantly different (p < 0.05) from appropriate SHAM controls.

548

days. It was considered that estradiol may cause the TIDA neurons to become refractory to the actions of prolactin. To test for this possibility, rats that had been implanted previously with cerebroventricular cannulae were injected intracerebroventricularly (icv) with 10 ug of rat prolactin (B-3, courtesy of Dr. A. F. Parlow, NIADDK), or 10 ul of its saline vehicle, and the rate of dopamine synthesis in the median eminence determined 12 hours later. It has been shown previously that this treatment increases the rate of DOPA accumulation selectively in the median eminence (10). As depicted in Figure 3, 12 h after icv prolactin, the rate of DOPA accumulation was increased in the median eminence of SHAM control animals but not in that of rats that had been implanted with estradiol-containing capsules 18 days previously. Following removal of the estradiol capsules for 18 days, the TIDA neurons again became responsive to icv prolactin. These results suggest that the biphasic effects of estradiol on the rate of DOPA accumulation in the median eminence result from the fact that the TIDA neurons are first stimulated but then become refractory to the estrogen-induced increased circulating concentrations of prolactin.

Is the refractoriness of TIDA neurons in long-term estradiol-treated rats a consequence of the estradiol per se, or is it due to the continuously elevated concentrations of prolactin? To answer this question, dopamine synthesis in the median eminence was determined in animals in which prolactin was continuously elevated by daily treatment with haloperidol, a drug which increases prolactin secretion by virtue of its ability to block dopamine receptors in the anterior pituitary. The results of this study are summarized in Figure 4. Daily injections of haloperidol for up to 22 days caused a persistent increase in serum prolactin levels and a persistent increase in the rate of DOPA accumulation in the median eminence. Thus, continuously elevated serum concentrations of prolactin do not cause TIDA neurons to become refractory to the stimulatory actions of this hormone. Rather, the reduced responsiveness of TIDA neurons in rats treated chronically with estradiol appears to be the result of an action of estradiol per se.

SUMMARY

A composite picture of the time course of the effects of and recovery from chronic estradiol treatment is depicted in Figure 5. Long-term treatment of ovariectomized rats with estradiol causes a persistent increase in serum prolactin concentrations and a biphasic effect on TIDA neurons which is characterized by an initial increase followed by a decrease in activity. During the latter period TIDA neurons are unresponsive to the administration of prolactin. These effects are reversible once the estradiol-containing capsules are removed. That is, serum prolactin levels gradually fall to control values while TIDA neuronal activity increases progressively to a value above that seen in non-treated controls. The reason for the rebound increase is currently unknown, but at these later times TIDA neurons have regained their responsiveness to prolactin. Finally, the effects of long-term estradiol on TIDA neurons appear to be due to the action of the hormone per se and not to the continuously elevated circulating concentrations of prolactin.

ACKNOWLEDGMENTS

These studies were supported by NIH grants AG02644 and NS09174, and by a Pharmaceutical Manufacturers Association Foundation Research Starter Grant and Career Development Award to K.T.D. The authors acknowledge Mary K. Pryal, Janet Keedy, and Susan Stahl for technical assistance and Diane Hummel for manuscript preparation.

REFERENCES

1. Gudelsky GA, Nansel DD, Porter JC. (1981): Endocrinology 108:440
2. Demarest KT, Moore KE. (1980): Endocrinology 106:463
3. Fuxe K, Hokfelt T, Nilsson, O. (1969): Neuroendocrinology 5:107
4. Eikenburg DC, Ravitz AJ, Gudelsky GA, Moore KE. (1977): J Neural Transm 40:235
5. Wiesel FA, Fuxe K, Hokfelt T, Agnati LF. (1978): Brain Res 148:399
6. Casanueva F, Cocchi D, Locatelli V, Flauto C, Zambotti F, Bestetti G, Rossi GL, Muller E. (1982): Endocrinology 110:590
7. Dupont A, DiPaolo T, Gagne B, Barden N. (1981): Neurosci Lett 22:69
8. Freeman ME, Sterman JR. (1978): Endocrinology 102:1915
9. Umezu K, Moore KE. (1979): J Pharmacol Exp Ther 208:49
10. Demarest KT, Moore KE. (1981): Neuroendocrinology 33:230

Prolactin. Basic and clinical correlates
R.M. MacLeod, M.O. Thorner and U. Scapagnini (eds.),
Fidia Research Series, vol. I,
Liviana Press, Padova © 1985

POTENT STIMULATORY EFFECT OF LEUMORPHIN ON PROLACTIN SECRETION FROM THE PITUITARY IN RATS

Katsuyoshi Tojo, Yuzuru Kato, Hikaru Ohto, Akira Shimatsu, Norio Matsushita, Yasuhiro Kabayama, Tatsuhide Inoue, Noboru Yanaihara*, and Hiroo Imura

Second Medical Clinic, Department of Medicine, Kyoto University, Faculty of Medicine, Sakyo-ku, Kyoto 606, Japan and *Laboratory of Bioorganic Chemistry, Shizuoka College of Pharmacy, Shizuoka, Japan

Opioid peptides can be classified into three groups based on their precursor molecules (1). Beta-endorphin and alpha-endorphin represent the first group of peptides which are derived from preproopiomelanocortin (proACTH/beta-LPH). The second group of peptides include Met^5-enkephalin, Leu^5-enkephalin and some other related peptides which come from preproenkephalin A. Preproenkephalin B, the common precursor of the third group of peptides such as neo-endorphins and dynorphin, contains a leucine-enkephalin sequence with a C-terminal extension of 24 amino acids (2). This nonacosapeptide is named leumorphin (LM), in which the N-terminus of 13 amino acids is rimorphin (RM) (Fig. 1).

Recent studies have revealed that these opioid peptides are present in high concentrations in the hypothalamus and play an important role in regulating the pituitary function (3-5). However, the effect of LM on pituitary function remains to be elucidated. In the present study, we examined the effect of LM on prolactin secretion in the rat *in vivo* and *in vitro*. Wistar strain male rats were used throughout the experiments. In the first series of experiments, the animals were anesthetized with urethane (150 mg/100 g BW, ip) after overnight fasting. Test substances or control saline solution were injected into the lateral ventricle in a volume of 10 ul/rat or into the exposed jugular vein in a volume of 0.1 ml/100 g BW. Blood samples of 0.6 ml were withdrawn from the jugular vein immediately before and 10, 20, and 40 min after the injection (3). In the second series of experiments, animals were chronically implanted with intracerebroventricular and intraatrial catheters as previously described. Blood samples of 0.4 ml were withdrawn from the intraatrial catheters 20 min before, immediately before, and 10, 20, and 40 min after the injection of test substances iv or icv in conscious freely moving rats. The plasma was promptly separated and stored at -20 C until

552

```
Leu⁵-enkephalin : Tyr-Gly-Gly-Phe-Leu

α-neo-endorphin : Tyr-Gly-Gly-Phe-Leu-Arg-Lys-Tyr-Pro-Lys

β-neo-endorphin : Tyr-Gly-Gly-Phe-Leu-Arg-Lys-Tyr-Pro

dynorphin(1-17) : Tyr-Gly-Gly-Phe-Leu-Arg-Arg-Ile-Arg-Pro-Lys-Leu-Lys-
                  Tyr-Asp-Asn-Gln

      rimorphin : Tyr-Gly-Gly-Phe-Leu-Arg-Arg-Gln-Phe-Lys-Val-Val-Thr

     leumorphin : Tyr-Gly-Gly-Phe-Leu-Arg-Arg-Gln-Phe-Lys-Val-Val-Thr-
                  Arg-Ser-Gln-Glu-Asp-Pro-Asn-Ala-Tyr-Tyr-Glu-Glu-Leu-
                  Phe-Asp-Val
```

Figure 1. Amino acid sequences of leumorphin and related opioid peptides derived from preproenkephalin B.

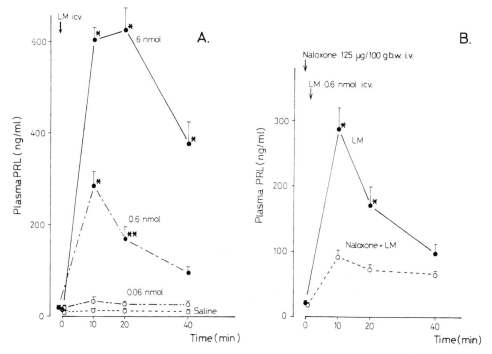

Figure 2. Effects of leumorphin (LM) and naloxone on plasma prolactin levels in urethane-anesthetized rats. A: LM was injected intraventricularly in a dose of 0.06, 0.6, or 6 nmol per rat. B: Naloxone was injected intravenously in a dose of 125 ug/100 g BW 3 min before the icv injection of LM (0.6 nmol/rat). All values are the mean ± SE of 5-8 animals in each group. Statistical significance is shown by asterisks (* $P < 0.01$ vs LM 0.6 or 0.06 nmol; ** $P < 0.05$ vs LM 0.06 nmol).

assayed. In the third series of experiments, prolactin release from rat anterior pituitary cells was examined *in vitro*, using a superfusion technique as previously described (7). Anterior pituitary cells were dispersed and placed on a small Sephadex G-25 column after incubation with medium F-10 for 48 hr at 37 C under 95% air-5% CO_2 atmosphere. The cell column was superfused by Krebs-Ringer bicarbonate buffer containing 10 mM glucose and 0.1% bovine serum albumin at a flow rate of 330 ul/min

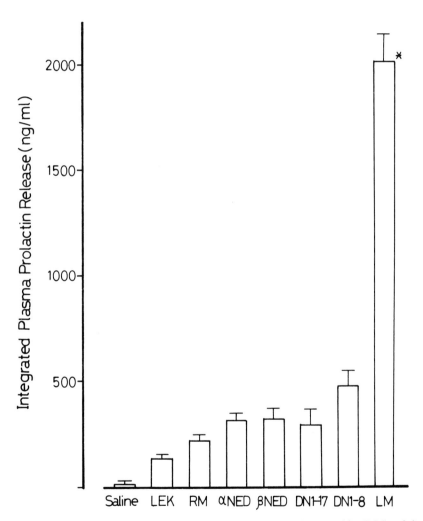

Figure 3. Effects of Leu^5-enkephalin (LEK), rimorphin (RM), leumorphin (LM), alpha-neo-endorphin (alpha-NED), beta-neo-endorphin (beta-NED), dynorphin 1-8 (DN 1-8) and dynorphin 1-17 (DN 1-17) on plasma prolactin levels in urethane-anesthetized rats. These peptides were injected intraventricularly in a dose of 6 nmol per rat. All values are the mean ± SE of integrated prolactin release in 6-8 animals. Statistical significance is shown by asterisks (* P < 0.01 vs others).

and the perfusate was collected every 5 min. Prolactin concentrations in the plasma and the perfusate were measured by specific radioimmunoassay using the kit supplied by the National Institute of Arthritis, Metabolism and Digestive Diseases (7). NIAMDD rat RP-1 was used as the standard. Duncan's new multiple range test was used for statistical evaluation.

Intraventricular injection of synthetic porcine LM in doses of 0.06, 0.6 and 6 nmol/rat caused a dose-related increase in plasma prolactin levels in urethane-anesthetized rats (mean ± SE peak prolactin: 33.5 ± 6.3, 286.5 ± 2.5 and 626.1 ± 44.1 ng/ml) (Fig. 2A). Plasma prolactin response to LM (0.6 nmol/rat icv) was blunted by naloxone (125 ug/100 g BW iv), a specific opiate antagonist, which was injected 3 min before the injection of LM (Fig. 2B). As shown in Figure 3, the stimulating effect of LM on prolactin release was the most potent and prolonged among the peptides derived from preproenkephalin B, when compared on a molar basis. In conscious rats, intraventricular injection of LM (0.6 and 3 nmol/rat) also raised plasma prolactin levels in a dose-related manner (mean ± SE peak prolactin: 39.9 ± 9.8 and 189.3 ± 23.9 ng/ml) (Fig. 4A), and the plasma prolactin response to LM (3 nmol/rat, icv) was blunted by the intravenous injection of naloxone (125 ug/100 g BW) (Fig. 4B). Intravenous injection of LM (10 ug/100 g BW) caused a significant increase in plasma prolactin

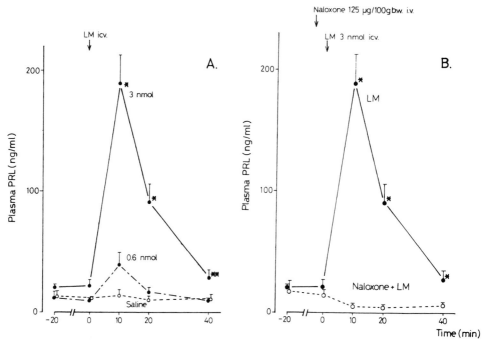

Figure 4. Effects of leumorphin (LM) and naloxone on plasma prolactin levels in conscious rats. A: LM was injected intraventricularly in a dose of 0.6 or 3 nmol per rat. B: Naloxone was injected intravenously in a dose of 125 ug/100 g BW 3 min before the icv injection of LM (3 nmol/rat). All values are the mean ± SE of 5-7 animals in each group. Statistical significance is shown by asterisks (* P < 0.01 vs LM 0.6 nmol; ** P < 0.05 vs LM 0.6 nmol).

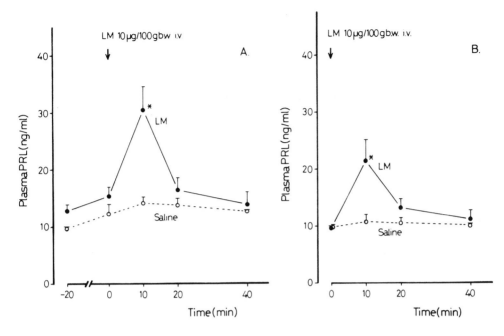

Figure 5. Effect of leumorphin (LM) on plasma prolactin (PRL) levels in conscious rats (A) and urethane-anesthetized rats (B). LM was injected intravenously in a dose of 10 ug/100 g BW per rat. All values are the mean ± SE of 5 animals in each group. Saline (100 ul/100 g BW) was injected in a control group. Statistical significance is shown by asterisks (* P < 0.05 vs control).

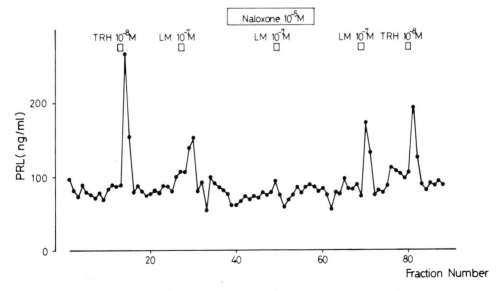

Figure 6. Effects of leumorphin (LM) (0.1 uM), TRH (0.01 uM) and naloxone (10 uM) on prolactin release from superfused rat anterior pituitary cells. LM and TRH were infused for 5 min and naloxone was infused for 30 min.

levels in conscious rats as well as anesthetized animals (mean ± SE peak prolactin: 30.5 ± 4.0 and 21.3 ± 1.7 ng/ml) (Figs. 5A and B). In *in vitro* studies, prolactin release from superfused anterior pituitary cells was stimulated by addition of LM (0.01, 0.1, and 1 uM) in a dose-related manner and prolactin release induced by LM (0.1 M) was blunted by naloxone (10 uM), which was concomitantly infused for 30 min (Fig. 6).

It is generally accepted that prolactin secretion is stimulated by opioid peptides such as enkephalins and endorphins (3-6). They have no direct effect on the pituitary and stimulate the secretion of prolactin possibly by acting in the hypothalamus to inhibit dopaminergic mechanisms (5,6,8). However, opioid receptors are known to exist not only in the hypothalamus but also in the pituitary (9). We have previously reported that alpha-neo-endorphin (alpha-NED), beta-neo-endorphin (beta-NED) and dynorphin (DN) stimulated prolactin secretion in the rat (7,10) and only alpha-NED showed a direct stimulatory action on prolactin release from the pituitary *in vitro*. In the present study, we have demonstrated that LM stimulates prolactin secretion by acting, at least in part, directly at the pituitary through an opiate receptor such as alpha-NED (7). LM is the most potent and long-acting stimulator of prolactin secretion on a molar basis among preproenkephalin beta-derived peptides examined. This potent stimulatory effect of LM on prolactin secretion cannot be explained only by its kappa-opioid receptor selectivity. LM is approximately equipotent with alpha-neo-endorphin and a little less potent than dynorphin in bioassays with guinea pig ileum and rabbit vas deferens (11,12). It is well established that the N-terminal tyrosine is necessary for the binding of opioid peptides to opioid receptors (13). It may be speculated that a C-terminal extension of amino acids of LM has a resistant action against deactivation of the peptide, or potentiates the binding activity of LM to the receptor. LM is a novel endogenous opioid peptide in the brain (14) and its physiological role must be further investigated.

ACKNOWLEDGMENTS

Supported in part by grants from the Ministry of Education and the Ministry of Health and Welfare, Japan.

REFERENCES

1. Imura H, Nakai Y, Nakao K, Oki S, Tanaka I, Jingama H, Yoshimasa T, Tsukada T, Suda M, Sakamoto M. (1983): J Endocrinol Invest 6:139
2. Kakidani H, Furutani Y, Takahashi H, Noda M, Morimoto Y, Hirose T, Asai M, Inayama S, Nakanishi S, Numa S. (1982): Nature 298:245
3. Kato Y, Iwasaki Y, Abe H, Ohgo S, Imura H. (1978): Proc Soc Exp Biol Med 158:431
4. Rivier C, Vale W, Ling N, Brown M, Guillemin R. (1977): Endocrinology 100:238
5. Meites J, Bruni JF, Van Vugt DA, Smith AF. (1979): Life Sci 24:1235
6. Kato Y, Hiroto S, Katakami H, Shimatsu A, Imura H. (1982): Proc Soc Exp Biol Med 169:95
7. Matsushita N, Kato Y, Shimatsu A, Katakami H, Fujino M, Matsuo H, Imura H. (1982): Biochem Biophys Res Commun 107:735
8. Matsushita N, Kato Y, Katakami H, Shimatsu A, Imura H. (1982): Endocrinol Jpn 29:277

9. Simantov R, Snyder SH. (1977): Brain Res 124:178
10. Kato Y, Matsushita N, Katakami H, Shimatsu A, Imura H. (1981): Eur J Pharmacol 73:353
11. Suda M, Nakao K, Yoshimasa T, Ikeda Y, Sakamoto M, Yanaihara N, Numa S, Imura H. (1983): Life Sci 32:2769
12. Yamamoto Y, Yanaihara C, Katsumaru Y, Mochizuki T, Tobe A, Egawa M, Imura H, Numa S, Yanaihara N. (1983): Regul Peptides 6:163
13. Judd AM, Hedge GA. (1983): Endocrinology 113:706
14. Nakao K, Suda M, Sakamoto M, Yoshimasa T, Morii N, Ikeda Y, Yanaihara C, Yanaihara N, Numa S, Imura H. (1983): Biochem Biophys Res Commun 117:695

Prolactin. Basic and clinical correlates
R.M. MacLeod, M.O. Thorner and U. Scapagnini (eds.),
Fidia Research Series, vol. I,
Liviana Press, Padova © 1985

TEMPORAL CHANGES OF PITUITARY DOPAMINE
AND BETA-ENDORPHIN CONCENTRATIONS
IN PUSH-PULL CANNULA EXPERIMENTS:
RESPONSE TO SUCKLING STIMULUS

Eva-Maria Duker, Wolfgang Wuttke,

Department of Reproductive Biology,
German Primate Center,
3400 Göttingen, FRG

The regulation of anterior pituitary prolactin release is incompletely understood. The lactotrophs contain receptors for dopamine, GABA, TRH, VIP, and estrogen and possibly for endogenous opioid peptides as well. At present, it is clear that dopamine or dopamine receptor agonists suppress prolactin release by a direct action on the pro-lactin cells (1). On the other hand, it has been proposed that concentrations of dopamine in the portal blood are far too low to cause a complete inhibition of prolactin release (2). Furthermore, dopamine at low concentrations (3), or when applied in a pulsatile manner, may even have stimulatory effects upon prolactin secretion (4).

It has also been proposed that GABA might serve as a prolactin inhibiting factor, and the existence of a GABA system similar to the tuberoinfundibular dopaminergic system has been postulated. Additionally, specific GABA receptors have been demonstrated in the pituitary. However, the concentrations of GABA needed to in-hibit the lactotrophs are much higher than those of dopamine. When given intraven-tricularly, GABA has a very strong stimulatory effect on pituitary prolactin release (5).

The question of whether endogenous opioid peptides, particularly beta-endorphin of hypothalamic or pituitary origin, may be involved in pituitary prolactin release is also a controversial issue. While some authors (6) could not find an effect of opioid peptides or morphine on dopamine-inhibited lactotrophs, others (7,8) including ourselves were able to stimulate pituitary prolactin release both *in vitro* and *in vivo* provided the lactotrophs were under the tonic inhibitory influence of dopamine.

In recent years, we have used the push-pull perfusion cannula technique for the study of neurotransmitter and neuropeptide release rates in various hypothalamic and limbic structures (9), and have adopted this method for the pituitary as well. All animals were implanted at least one week prior to experimentation. Figure 1 shows a schematic

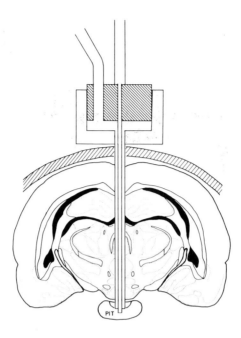

Figure 1. Implantation site of the push-pull cannula in the rat brain according to de Groot coordinates. Focal perfusion with artificial CSF at a flow rate of 25 ul/min was performed in the pituitary.

drawing of the size and location of the tip of the push-pull cannula in the anterior pituitary. A number of experimental models were studied with this technique. These experiments were carried out under the assumption that portal blood-borne catecholamines, GABA, and possibly peptides could be washed out of the pituitary, but still be able to exert their physiological effects and thereby modify blood prolactin levels. The sensitivity of radioenzymatic catecholamine and microenzymatic fluorometric GABA assays allows determination in fractions collected through the push-pull cannula over short periods of time (fraction period = FP = 15 min). Correlation of these putative prolactin regulating substances and blood prolactin levels may elucidate functional relationships.

The following experiments were performed in lactating rats. At the beginning of each experimental day, the experimenter had to manipulate and thereby stress the animals to connect them to the push-pull and blood collection tubing. As shown in Figure 2, this resulted in increased blood prolactin levels. Interestingly, under these conditions dopamine and GABA concentrations in the pituitary perfusates also were high at the time of high blood prolactin levels.

Since both putative PIFs are already high at the beginning of increased pituitary prolactin release, it is unlikely that the increase in the concentrations of the transmitters is due to the autoregulatory feedback action of prolactin. The results may in fact

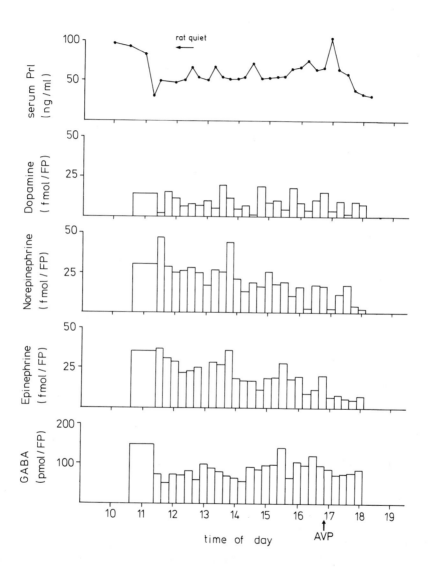

rat # E 143 ; pit ; day 9 lact. ;   FP = 15 min

AVP   0,1 µg iv.

Figure 2. Serum prolactin levels and catecholamine and GABA concentrations in the pituitary perfusates of a lactating rat. The experiment was conducted on day 9 after delivery.

562

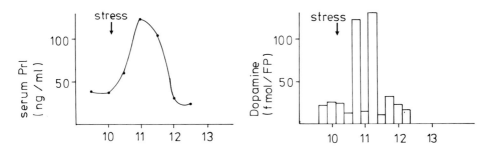

rat # E 46 ; ♀ ; day 5 lact.

Figure 3. Serum prolactin levels and dopamine concentrations in pituitary push-pull cannula perfusates of a rat on day 5 after delivery. At the beginning of the experiment the rat was stressed by the handling procedure.

indicate that stress is accompanied by pulsatile release of dopamine. This is shown in Figure 3, where low dopamine concentrations were measured between two fractions with high dopamine values. Blood prolactin levels in the stressed animal were also high. These results fit very well into a concept recently developed by Denef and collaborators (4), who showed that pulsatile application of low amounts of dopamine stimulates the secretory activity of the lactotrophs.

Similar results are shown in Figure 4, where stress also induced prolactin release, and dopamine measured in the intrapituitary perfusates also increased. Following the stress-induced period of high blood prolactin levels, they fell to basal values, at which time extremely high dopamine concentrations were measured in the perfusate. The dopamine release rates decreased abruptly at the time when the pups were returned to the mother, which resulted in a prompt increase in prolactin release. GABA concentrations in the perfusate did not fluctuate markedly. This experiment invites the following speculation: Moderately high, possibly pulsatile dopamine release from the tuberoinfundibular neurons may result in increased prolactin release, whereas constantly high dopamine release rates from the hypothalamus are suppressive to the secretory activity of the lactotrophs.

Figure 5 shows the concentrations of beta-endorphin in the push-pull perfusate of the pituitary in a lactating rat. Again this animal initially had high blood prolactin levels due to handling stress. At this time, beta-endorphin concentrations in the pituitary perfusates were also very high. They decreased in parallel with blood prolactin levels. When the rat was quiet and permitted the pups to suckle, blood prolactin levels increased again. This increase was also associated with slightly increased beta-endorphin concentrations measured in the pituitary perfusates. Although blood prolactin levels reached or even exceeded the height of prolactin observed under the initial stress conditions, beta-endorphin concentrations remained much lower than those observed under stress conditions. This experiment seems to indicate that the stress-induced increase in

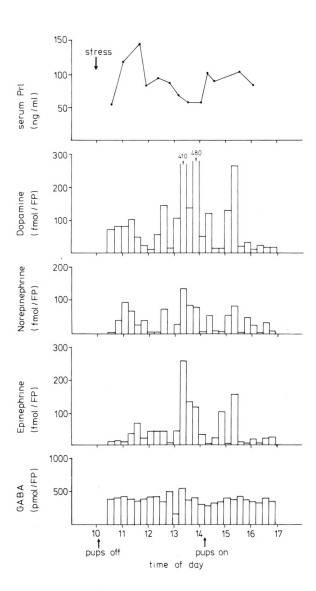

Figure 4. Serum prolactin concentrations and catecholamine and GABA concentrations in the push-pull cannula perfusates of a lactating rat on day 5 after delivery. The initial stress is due to handling of the rat.

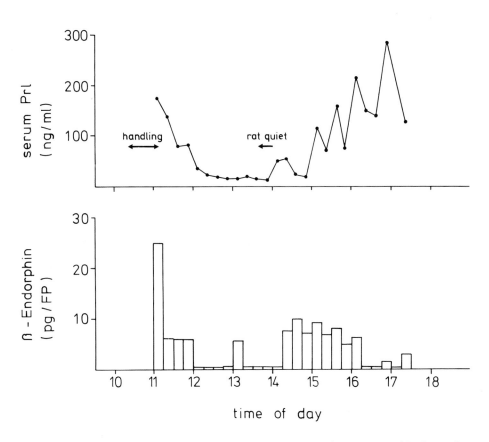

Figure 5. Serum prolactin levels and beta-endorphin concentrations measured in the perfusates. After the initial handling stress, the rat did not allow the pups to suckle which reflects in basal serum prolactin levels. When she started nursing again, blood prolactin levels increased.

beta-endorphin which is measured in pituitary perfusates is due to increased secretory activity of the pituitary proopiomelanocortin cell (i.e. the ACTH cell). On the other hand, the possibility that part of this beta-endorphin immuno-like reactivity is of hypothalamic origin cannot be excluded. It is known that suckling does not result in increased ACTH secretion (10). Therefore, the increase in beta-endorphin induced by the suckling stimulus may be indicative of increased beta-endorphin release from the pituitary pomc-cells.

In summary, we present evidence that the tuberoinfundibular dopaminergic neurons may be involved in the secretory activity of the lactotrophs in a manner much more dynamic than previously thought. Brisk release episodes of dopamine may result in stimulated activity of the lactotrophs whereas sustained and high release rates result in the well known inhibitory effect of dopamine on prolactin secretion. GABA does not seem to play a dominant role in the regulation of the lactotrophs, whereas pituitary as well as hypothalamic beta-endorphin levels may well participate in the regulation of the secretory activity of the lactotrophs.

REFERENCES

1. MacLeod RM. (1976): In: Martini L, Ganong WF (eds) Frontiers in Neuroendocrinology. Raven Press, New York, pp 169
2. De Greef WJ, Neill JD. (1979): Endocrinology 105:1093
3. Denef C, Manet D, Dewals R. (1980): Nature 285:245
4. Denef C, Baes M, Schramme C. (1984): Endocrinology 114:1371
5. Locatelli V, Cocchi D, Frigerio C, Betti R, Krogsgaard-Larsen P, Racagni G, Mueller EE. (1979): Endocrinology 105:778
6. Login IS, MacLeod RM. (1979): Eur J Pharmacol 60:253
7. Enjalbert A, Arancibia S, Priam M, Kordon C. (1979): Nature 280:595
8. Voigt KH, Frank D, Dueker EM, Martin R, Wuttke W. (1983): Life Sci 33:507
9. Ondo J, Mansky T, Wuttke W. (1982): Exp Brain Res 46:69
10. Riskind PN, Millard WJ, Martin JB. (1984): Endocrinology 114:1232

Prolactin. Basic and clinical correlates
R.M. MacLeod, M.O. Thorner and U. Scapagnini (eds.),
Fidia Research Series, vol. I,
Liviana Press, Padova © 1985

POSSIBLE INVOLVEMENT OF THE NUCLEUS ACCUMBENS IN SUCKLING INDUCED PROLACTIN RELEASE IN THE RAT

E. Fuchs, M. Baumert, R. A. Siegel, and W. Wuttke

German Primate Center, Department of Reproductive Biology
3400 Göttingen, FRG

It has become apparent in recent years that the neuroendocrine relationship between a lactating rat and her offspring is a dynamic rather than a static one (1,2). In the rat, prolactin releasing stimuli and maternal behavior are intimately correlated (2). Though suckling is the major stimulus controlling prolactin secretion in lactating rats, a number of other factors can also influence prolactin concentration in the circulation. Among these factors are the metabolic clearance rates of prolactin, the stage of lactation at which suckling is applied, and the length of the previous nonsuckling interval (1). Oxytocin-induced milk ejection reflexes occur only when the mother rats are suckled. They are then akinetic and appear to be dozing or sleeping and the EEG pattern during this time is synchronized (3). These studies strongly suggest that a "neural gate" which permits milk ejection is "open" during sleep.

Among all possible brain structures which may serve as a "neural gate" in the lactating behavior, the nucleus accumbens (NAC) seems to be of great importance. This nucleus is known to be involved in the regulation of extrapyramidal locomotor activity (for ref. see 4) and it appears that endocrine and behavioral tasks are integrated in this structure. For example, lesioning of the NAC in female rats disturbs both maternal behavior and lactation (5). Recent studies of dopamine (DA) turnover in the NAC have indicated that this area is also involved in the feedback regulation of prolactin in rats (6). This is in agreement with the finding that acute administration of prolactin to hypophysectomized male rats selectively accelerated DA turnover in the NAC (7). Taken together, these studies and those from our laboratory (8) suggest that prolactin may exert a direct influence on the NAC.

As shown by histochemical studies, the dense dopaminergic innervation of the NAC derives from the ventral tegmentum (see ref. 4). In addition, Hokfelt and collaborators (9) have shown that DA coexists with the octapeptide cholecystokinin (CCK) in a certain subpopulation of the mesolimbic neurons which arise in the A 10 region and innervate the NAC.

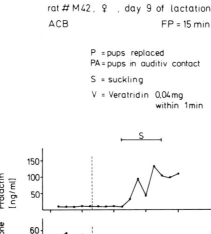

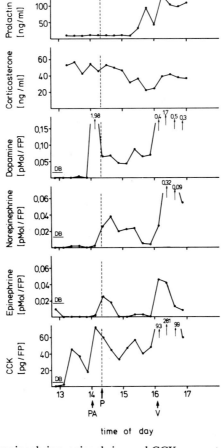

Figure 1. Dopamine, norepinephrine, epinephrine and CCK concentrations in 15 min perfusate fractions. (FP = fraction period) and prolactin and corticosterone plasma levels (samples withdrawn on the end of 15 min FP), DB: double blank The validity of the push-pull cannula technique is demonstrated by applying the depolarizing agent veratridine (V) at very low concentrations and a short exposure time to the perfusion medium. The marked stimulation of CCK and catecholamine release in response to veratridine indicates the neuronal origin of the peptide and the transmitters.

Biochemical studies provide evidence for the existence of intrinsic glutamate and gamma-aminobutyric acid (GABA) containing neurons as well as glutamatergic afferents in the NAC (for ref. see 4). The main glutamatergic excitatory projections to the NAC arise from the hippocampus. GABAergic fibres project from the NAC to the ventral globus pallidus, the substantia innominata, the substantia nigra, and the ventral tegmental area which is the site of origin of the mesolimbic dopaminergic neurons. At the present time the functional significance of the excitatory amino acid glutamate is not fully understood. However, *in vitro* studies suggest that glutamate as well as GABA both play a role in the regulation of motor activity by influencing dopaminergic mechanisms. The tonic inhibitory role of NAC GABA on the globus pallidus is interpreted as part of a functional link between limbic and motor system for the translation of motivation into action (10).

In view of these puzzling data it was tempting for us to utilize the push-pull cannula technique for focal perfusion of the NAC in the freely moving lactating rat in order to study the following questions: 1. Is there a temporal association between neurotransmitter/neuropeptide release and the time of replacement of pups to their mothers? 2. Is there a correlation between suckling-induced prolactin release and neurotransmitter/neuropeptide release rates under physiological conditions? 3. Is there any evidence that the co-storage of the neuroactive substances dopamine and CCK indicates co-release?

For the present experiments push-pull cannulae were implanted into the NAC (A:3,6; L:1,4; H:6,7) of pregnant rats according to the atlas of Pellegrino (11). Following spontaneous delivery mothers were implanted with a jugular vein catheter one day prior to the perfusion experiment. On the day of the experiment the litters were removed from the mothers for at least 6 hours. Push-pull perfusates and blood samples were collected for one hour in 15 min fractions prior to the replacement of the pups. During the next three hours behavior was recorded and perfusates and blood samples collected in 15 min fractions. In the perfusates catecholamines were determined radioenzymatically; GABA and glutamate were measured fluorometrically; CCK, plasma prolactin and corticosterone were determined using specific radioimmunoassays.

From many studies it is known that mother rats and their offspring have an ultrasonic communication system (1,2). In the experiment shown in Figure 1 pups were in auditory contact with their mother more than fifteen minutes before replacement to the cage. Under these conditions we observed an increase of DA and CCK release in the NAC. No changes in the prolactin concentration were apparent. Mothers showed motor activity and we could observe an activation of the adrenergic and noradrenergic system. A slight decrease in plasma corticosterone indicated a reduction in stress. More than one hour after replacement pups started suckling. At this time we recorded another increase of dopamine as well as CCK release. In several experiments the octapeptide CCK and catecholamines were measured in the same perfusates. As shown in Figures 1 and 2, dopamine and CCK profiles correlate very well. This suggests a co-release of these two neuroactive substances. At the time of maximal prolactin release, when the mothers were akinetic, we observed a pronounced release of GABA and glutamate. As a consequence of this akinesia may be induced, retained, or reinforced.

Looking at the activation of the dopamine/CCK system, the auditory communication between pups and mothers (Fig. 1) seems to be comparable to the situation when

570

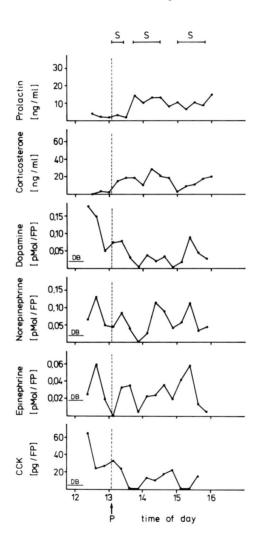

Figure 2. For details see Fig. 1.

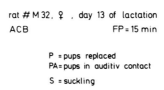

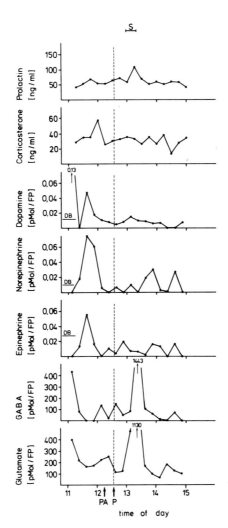

Figure 3. Dopamine, norepinephrine; epinephrine, GABA and glutamate concentrations in 15 min perfusate fractions. For further details see Fig. 1.

the young are replaced immediately to mothers without previous auditory contact (Fig. 2). In both cases no prolactin increase could be observed. Plasma prolactin levels seemed to vary independently from corticosterone titers, since we observed both an activation and an inhibition of the adrenocortical system as reactions to auditory contact or replacement of the pups. This specific activation in the CNS without changes in prolactin can be interpreted as a neuronal "stand-by position" induced by the presence of the litters alone.

When milk ejection reflexes occurred and pituitary prolactin release increased, the neuronal responses of the dopamine/CCK system were not different from the response seen when pups come in contact with the mother after separation. The more or less unspecific "stand-by position" had now changed to a very specific reaction induced by continuous suckling of the pups which increased the readiness of the mothers to open the "gate". A detailed analysis of all data revealed that the first suckling- induced plasma prolactin surge was always preceded by increased dopamine/CCK activity in the NAC. This result demonstrates the special "neural gate" function of the NAC. This "gating"-hypothesis states that dopaminergic input to the NAC from the ventral tegmental area modulates the ability of the limbic system input to communicate with GABAergic output to the globus pallidus (4). Release of GABA within the globus pallidus is assumed to inhibit motor responses (12). This dopaminergic activity within the NAC acts to open or close the "gate" between limbic system and motor system. Thus the NAC might serve to channel motivational input from the limbic system to the motor system, determining whether or not a particular motivated behavior takes place (4).

According to this we may speculate that the observed suckling- induced enhancement of dopamine/CCK NAC activity gives rise to the activity of GABAergic afferents to the globus pallidus, and there induces a reduction of motor activity. This may lead to akinesia and provoke in consequence a synchronization of the EEG pattern. Under this neuronal situation the mother is able to secrete oxytocin and prolactin and induce a contraction of the mammary glands and milk ejection.

At first view our neurochemical results are in contradiction to former publications where elevated endogenous prolactin levels induced higher dopamine-turnover in the NAC. These turnover studies were done in ovariectomized or male rats injected with prolactin (7, 13). Therefore, the physiological processes taking place in such animals are not comparable to processes in lactating rats.

From the methodological point of view our data demonstrate the validity and reliability of the push-pull cannula technique in studying the interactions among central nervous, endocrine, and behavioral processes under physiological conditions in freely moving animals. Our results may support an involvement of the mesolimbic dopaminergic system projecting to the NAC in the suckling- induced akinesia in the rat. The functional implication of the co-release of dopamine and CCK remains to be established.

ACKNOWLEDGMENTS

The excellent technical assistance of Mrs. J. Hagedorn and Mrs. M. Metten is gratefully acknowledged.

REFERENCES

1. Mence F, Pacheco P, Whitworth NS, Grosvenor CE. (1980): Frontiers Hor Res 6:217
2. Tindal JS. (1978): In: Larson B, Smith A (eds) Lactation, A Comprehensive Treatise. Vol. 4
3. Lincoln DW, Hentzen K, Hin T, van der Schoot P, Clarke G, Summerlee AJS. (1980): Exp Brain Res 38:151
4. Chronister RB, De France JF (eds) The Neurobiology of the Nucleus Accumbens, Haer Institute for Electrophysiological Research, Brunswick, Maine, (1981)
5. Smith MO, Holland RC. (1975): Physiol Psychol 3:331
6. Lofstrom A, Eneroth P, Gustafsson JA, Skett P. (1977): Endocrinology 101:1559
7. Fuxe K, Eneroth P, Gustafsson JA, Lofstrom A, Skett P. (1977): Brain Res 122:177
8. Hohn KG, Wuttke WO. (1978): Brain Res 156:241
9. Hokfett T, Skirboll L, Rehfeld JF, Goldstein M, Markley K, Dann O. (1980): Neuroscience 5:2053
10. Costa E. (1977): Adv Biochem Psychopharmacol 16:557
11. Pellegrino LJ, Pellegrino AS, Chusman AJ. (1979): A Stereotaxic Atlas of the Rat Brain, Plenum Press, New York
12. Roberts E. (1974): Adv Neurol 5:127
13. Fuxe K, Andersson K, Hokfelt T, Agnati LF. (1978): Prog Prolactin Physiol Pathol 95

Prolactin. Basic and clinical correlates
R.M. MacLeod, M.O. Thorner and U. Scapagnini (eds.),
Fidia Research Series, vol. I,
Liviana Press, Padova © 1985

6-METHYLTETRAHYDROPTERIN, A LIPOPHILIC COFACTOR FOR TYROSINE HYDROXYLASE, DECREASES SERUM PROLACTIN LEVELS AND INCREASES HYPOTHALAMIC DOPAMINE SYNTHESIS IN THE RAT

John F. Reinhard, Jr., Robert F. Butz, Gloria D. Jahnke, and Charles A. Nichol

Department of Medicinal Biochemistry, The Wellcome Research Laboratories, Research Triangle Park, NC 27709

One function of dopamine released from the A12 neurons of the arcuate nucleus is to tonically inhibit prolactin release from the pituitary (1). Dopamine biosynthesis depends upon the availability of tyrosine, oxygen, and a reduced pterin cofactor [6-(R)-L-erythro-5,6,7,8-tetrahydrobiopterin; BH_4] (Fig. 1). It has been demonstrated that BH_4 administration accelerates dopamine synthesis in striatum (2) and catecholamine synthesis in rat brainstem (3). While striatal dopamine synthesis and release is controlled through a variety of mechanisms (4), tuberoinfundibular dopamine synthesis appears to be regulated by the blood levels of prolactin (5), and these neurons do not appear to possess presynaptic autoreceptors (6). Thus, we reasoned that tuberoinfundibular dopamine synthesis and release might be responsive to alterations in the availability of exogenous tetrahydropterin cofactors which, in turn, should affect the levels of prolactin in blood. This hypothesis was tested by measuring rat serum prolactin levels following systemic administration of tetrahydropterin cofactors.

The present studies were undertaken with 6-methyltetrahydropterin since it is a good cofactor for tyrosine, tryptophan, and phenylalanine monooxygenases (7), and because it enters the brain more readily than the natural cofactor, BH_4 (8).

Male Wistar rats (175-250 g), obtained from the Charles River Breeding Laboratories (Wilmington, MA), were housed in wire mesh cages, permitted ad libitum access to food and water, and maintained on a 12-hour light-dark cycle for at least one week prior to use. To preclude diurnal variations in prolactin serum levels, experiments were conducted at approximately the same time each day (0900-1200 hours). Chromatographic standards and drugs were obtained from the Sigma Chemical Co. (St. Louis, MO), unless otherwise indicated. The 6-methyltetrahydropterin [6-(R,S-methyl)-5,6,7,8-tetrahydro-(3H)pteridinone; $6-MPH_4$] was synthesized by Dr. Eric

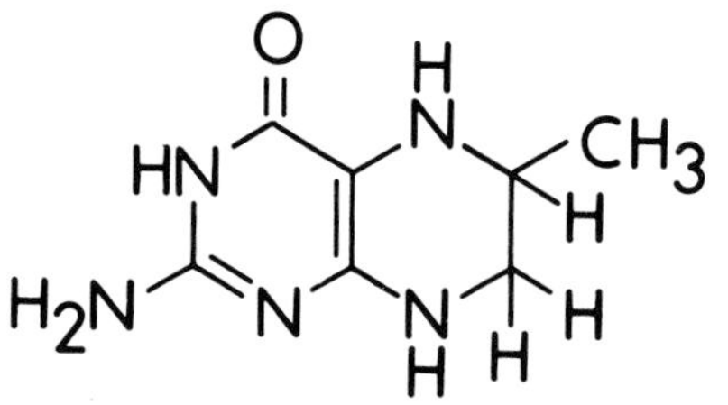

576

6-METHYLTETRAHYDROPTERIN

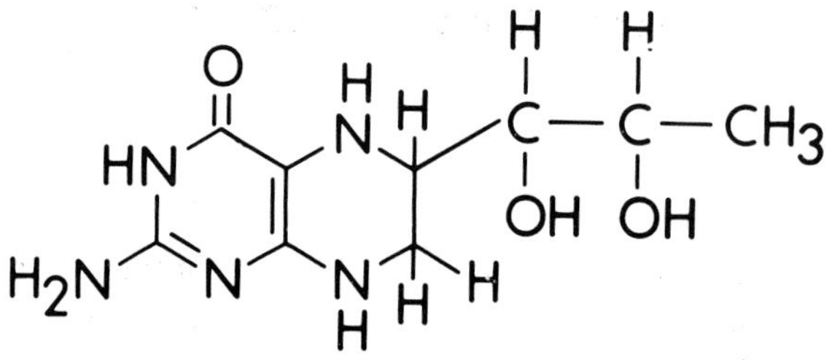

TETRAHYDROBIOPTERIN

Figure 1. Structures of 6-MPH$_4$ and the natural pterin cofactor, BH$_4$.

Bigham (Organic Chemistry Dept., The Wellcome Research Laboratories) and determined to be free of the 7-methyl isomer by NMR spectroscopy. Haloperidol was obtained from McNeil Laboratories (Spring House, PA).

Rat serum prolactin was measured by a double-antibody radioimmunoassay in a total volume of 0.5 ml (9). Reference prolactin (rPRL-RP-3) and antibody (PRL-S-8 and PRL-S-9) were obtained from NIADDK through the National Hormone and Pituitary Program (Baltimore, MD). The [125I]-rat prolactin was obtained from New England Nuclear (Boston, MA). The data are expressed as ng of prolactin (rPRL-RP-3 equivalents) per ml of serum. The interassay coefficient of variation was less than 10% while the amount of prolactin displacing 50% of the bound [125I]-prolactin was 1.38 ± 0.13 ng per tube.

Anterior hemipituitary incubations were performed as described (10), except that we measured release during a 2-hour interval. For experiments in which brain

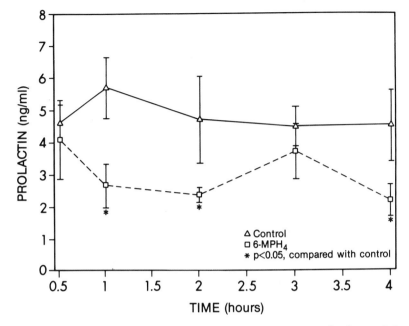

Figure 2. Time course effect of 6-MPH$_4$ on prolactin levels in serum. Animals were injected with 0.3 mmol/kg i.p., of the drugs or pH matched diluents (see Table 2 legend), and were killed at the times indicated following drug administration. The data are means ± S.E.M. of 5 animals per group. Asterisks denote significant differences from the time-matched control groups (p < 0.05), as assessed by t-tests.

catecholamine synthesis was measured (13), 3,4-dihydroxyphenylalanine (DOPA) was isolated on aluminum oxide columns and measured using liquid chromatography with electrochemical detection (11).

In initial experiments with 6-MPH$_4$, prolactin levels were measured at increasing intervals following a single dose of the pteridine. When compared with diluent-injected controls, 6-MPH$_4$ decreased prolactin at 1, 2, and 4 hours (Fig. 2); effects at longer times have not been determined.

We next examined the effect of increasing doses of 6-MPH$_4$ on prolactin levels. In these studies, the animals were killed 90 minutes after drug administration. The ED$_{50}$ for 6-MPH$_4$ was 0.33 ± 0.12 mmol/kg (Fig. 3).

To assess whether 6-MPH$_4$ reduced prolactin through a direct action upon the pituitary, we incubated anterior hemipituitaries with either 6-MPH$_4$, dopamine, or diluent (Table 1). For these studies, half of the pituitary was incubated with drug, the remainder with the diluent. While dopamine effectively suppressed prolactin release, no consistent effect was observed with 6-MPH$_4$ (1-10 uM).

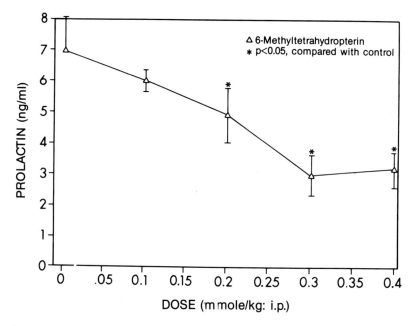

Figure 3. Dose-effect of 6-MPH$_4$ and BH$_4$ on rat prolactin levels in serum. Animals were injected with the tetrahydropterins, adjusted to pH 1.2 with 1 M HCl and added NaCl to reach isotonicity, or the diluent (see Table 2 legend), and were killed 90 minutes after drug administration. Asterisks denote significant differences from control groups as determined by two-way analysis of variance. The data are expressed as the means ± S.E.M. of 7-9 animals per group.

Table 1. *Effects of 6-methyltetrahydropterin and dopamine on in vitro release of prolactin from anterior hemipituitaries*

Additions	% of Control Prolactin Release
None	100%
6-MPH$_4$, 1 uM	83%
6-MPH$_4$, 3 uM	111%
6-MPH$_4$, 10 uM	90%
Dopamine, 3 uM	18%
Dopamine, 10 uM	23%

Anterior hemipituitaries were incubated, as described (10), for 2 hours with the compounds listed above. Data are the means of duplicate determinations which varied less than 16%. Control release averaged 108.83 ± 16.54 ng prolactin released per mg wet tissue weight per 2 hours.

Assuming that the pterin-induced reductions in prolactin were due to increased dopamine production and release, we administered 6-MPH$_4$ to animals which had also received an injection of the dopamine-receptor antagonist, haloperidol (0.27 umol/kg, i.p.). In these studies 6-MPH$_4$ (0.4 mmol/kg, i.p.), by itself, decreased serum levels of prolactin from 10.22 ± 3.95 ng/ml to 0.93 ± 0.49 ng/ml, while haloperidol increased the levels of prolactin to 26.73 ± 6.33 ng/ml. When haloperidol was co-administered with 6 MPH$_4$, the levels of prolactin were found to be 29.44 ± 9.87 ng/ml. Thus, haloperidol completely suppressed the decrease in prolactin produced by 6-MPH$_4$.

To test the possibility that 6-MPH$_4$ decreased serum prolactin by inhibiting monoamine oxidase, the tetrahydropterin was incubated *in vitro* with rat brain monoamine oxidase (12) and no significant inhibition of the deamination of either [^{3}H]-serotonin (6.9%) or [^{14}C]-phenylethylamine (8.0%) was observed when the enzyme was incubated with 0.1 mM 6-MPH$_4$ (H. White, personal communication).

Presuming that 6-MPH$_4$ reduced prolactin by acclerating the synthesis of dopamine within tuberoinfundibular neurons, we examined the effects of 6-MPH$_4$ on the accumulation of DOPA, both in hypothalamus and whole brain, following inhibition of L-aromatic amino acid decarboxylase with NSD-1015 (13). When 6-MPH$_4$ was injected 60 minutes before the NSD-1015, DOPA formation was accelerated by 36% in the hypothalamus, and only 15% in the remainder of the brain (Table 2).

Table 2. *The effect of 6 MPH$_4$ administration on the synthesis of catecholamines in hypothalamus and in the rest of brain*

Treatment	DOPA Accumulation (nmol/g x 30 min)	
	Hypothalamus	Rest of Brain
Diluent	1.33 ± 0.11 (8)	0.88 ± 0.05 (8)
6-MPH$_4$	1.81 ± 0.24 (7)*	1.01 ± 0.04 (8)*

Animals were first injected with 6-MPH$_4$ (0.3 mmol/kg, i.p.) or with its diluent (5.7 mM ascorbic acid, 0.12 M NaCl, adjusted to pH 1.24 with 1 N HCl), followed, 60 minutes later, by m-hydroxybenzylhydrazine (0.72 mmol/kg, i.p.), and were killed 30 minutes thereafter. Asterisks denote significant differences from the control means (p ≤ 0.05, as assessed by one-tailed t-tests). The numbers within parentheses are the number of animals per group.

It has been generally accepted that prolactin release from the pituitary is under tonic inhibitory control from dopamine, which is released into the hypophyseal blood vessels (1). These tuberoinfundibular dopamine neurons have cell bodies which lie in the basal hypothalamus (the A 12 group) and project to hypophyseal blood vessels in the median eminence (14). Since dopamine synthesis in vivo is limited by the levels of BH$_4$ (2), administration of an exogenous tetrahydropterin cofactor should accelerate dopamine synthesis and, in turn, decrease serum prolactin. Peripheral administration of 6-MPH$_4$, a tetrahydropterin cofactor for tyrosine hydroxylase, did produce a significant, sustained depletion of serum prolactin. The duration of the 6-MPH$_4$ effect may have its origin in the feedback control exerted upon tuberoinfundibular dopamine neurons. In the striatum, dopamine synthesis can be controlled by intraneuronal dopamine levels as well as by pre- and post-synaptic receptors (4). In contrast, the activity of tuberoinfundibular dopamine neurons is normally regulated by the levels of prolactin in blood (5). Moreover, these hypothalamic neurons do not appear to possess autoreceptors upon their terminals (6) which might limit the synthesis and release of dopamine.

Assuming that augmentation of dopamine synthesis is the mechanism by which tetrahydropterins lowered serum prolactin, then the effect should be dose-dependent and indeed this proved to the case since 6-MPH$_4$ decreased prolactin in the range of 0.1-0.4 mmol/kg.

One alternative explanation for the pterin-induced reductions in serum prolactin would be a direct effect of 6-MPH$_4$ on the pituitary. If this were so, incubation of anterior pituitaries with 6-MPH$_4$ should reduce prolactin release, but this did not happen. As expected, dopamine, incubated with anterior hemipituitaries, reduced prolactin release. If a metabolite of 6-MPH$_4$ were to act as a dopamine agonist, then turnover of dopamine in the CNS should decrease. However, since the dopamine metabolite, homovanillic acid, did not decrease in rat brain striatum 2 hours after drug administration (unpublished observations, J. Reinhard), we do not feel that 6-MPH$_4$ reduced prolactin by acting as a dopamine agonist. That the tetrahydropterin acted indirectly by promoting dopamine synthesis and release is suggested by the data with haloperidol. In these studies, the dopamine receptor antagonist reversed the decrease in prolactin produced by 6-MPH$_4$.

Demonstration that 6-MPH$_4$ actually increased dopamine synthesis was suggested by data which show that 6-MPH$_4$ augmented DOPA formation in intact hypothalami. Although whole hypothalamus contains dopamine and noradrenaline in addition to the tuberoinfundibular dopamine neurons, an acceleration of DOPA formation in this tissue is consistent with our hypothesis. The increase in DOPA formation in the remainder of the brain was only 15%. This lower response to the tetrahydropterin most probably reflects the recruitment of additional neuronal inhibitory mechanisms in response to the increased hydroxylation of tyrosine. However, specific nuclei within the "rest of brain" fraction may have been stimulated to a greater degree than the aggregate 15% response. One interpretation of these data is that the level of the reduced pterin cofactor, BH$_4$, in tuberoinfundibular dopamine neurons is inadequate for maximal levels of dopamine production. However, increases in dopamine production appear to be more readily sensed, and controlled, by some dopamine neurons than by others. The hormonally responsive tuberoinfundibular dopamine neurons would, according to this model, increase dopamine release which, in turn, would decrease prolactin release. The sensitivity of this system to the decreased levels of serum prolactin does not permit an instantaneous correction in the alteration of dopamine release and consequently the decrease in prolactin is prolonged.

An alternative mechanism of reduction in serum prolactin by 6-MPH$_4$ would involve an effect of the cofactor on adrenomedullary catecholamine synthesis. Increased levels of blood adrenaline and noradrenaline could theoretically stimulate pituitary dopamine receptors to reduce prolactin release. This is probably not the case since stressors which produce large elevations in blood catecholamines (15) also increase prolactin (16). Thus, the two phenomena appear to be unrelated.

One consequence of these studies is that tetrahydropterins might provide a selective means of depressing prolactin release in selected hyperprolactinemic states by promoting dopamine synthesis at sites where it is normally used, thus avoiding the likelihood of emesis.

REFERENCES

1. Weiner RI, Ganong WF. (1978): Physiol Rev 58:905
2. Kettler R, Bartholini G, Pletscher A. (1974): Nature 249:476
3. Reinhard JF Jr, Chao JY, Nichol CA. (1983): J Neurochem 41:S81
4. Nowycky MC, Roth RH. (1978): Prog Neuro-Psychopharm 2:139
5. Gudelsky GA, Simpkins J, Mueller G, Meites J, Moore KE. (1976): Neuroendocrinology 22:206
6. Demarest KE, Moore KE. (1979): J Neural Trans 46:263
7. Kaufman S. (1974): In: Wolstenholme GEW, Fitzsimons DW (eds) Aromatic Amino Acids in the Brain. Elsevier, New York, p 85
8. Kapatos G, Kaufman S. (1981): Science 212:955
9. Neill JD, Reichert LE Jr. (1971): Endocrinology 88:548
10. Meltzer HY, Simonovic M, Gudelsky GA. (1983): J Pharmacol Exp Therap 224:21
11. Reinhard JF Jr, Perry JA. (1984): J Liquid Chrom 7:1211
12. White HL, Glassman AT. (1977): J Neurochem 29:987
13. Carlsson A, Davis JN, Kehr W, Lindqvist M, Atack CV. (1972): Naunyn-Schmiedeberg's Arch Pharmacol 275:153
14. Bjorklund A, Moore RY, Nobin A, Stenvi U. (1973): Brain Res 51:171
15. Kvetnansky R, Sun CL, Lake CR, Thoa N, Torda T, Kopin I. (1978): Endocrinology 193:1868
16. Nicoll CS, Talwaker PK, Meites J. (1960): Am J Physiol 198:1103

Prolactin. Basic and clinical correlates
R.M. MacLeod, M.O. Thorner and U. Scapagnini (eds.),
Fidia Research Series, vol. I,
Liviana Press, Padova © 1985

Section IX
Experimental and clinical
effects of prolactin on behavior
and brain function

EXPERIMENTAL AND CLINICAL EFFECTS
OF PROLACTIN ON BEHAVIOR

Umberto Scapagnini, Filippo Drago, Giuseppe Continella, Francesco Spadaro, Giovanni Pennisi*, and Ida Gerendai**

Institute of Pharmacology and *Neurological Clinic, University of Catania
Medical School, Catania, Italy and **2nd Department of Anatomy, Semmelweis
University Medical School, Budapest, Hungary

The first indication that a humoral factor involved in lactation might cause behavioral effects came from the early studies of Lienhart (1), who described the induction of parental behavior in hens after the injection of serum from incubating animals of the same species. This factor may be prolactin since injections of this hormone induced laying hens to sit on eggs and to care for hatchlings (2). From these first observations considerable evidence has accumulated indicating that this hormone plays multiple roles in the behavioral expression of various animal species (3). In the last decade, evidence has been presented that prolactin can also influence human behavior. In fact, hyperprolactinemia is commonly associated with a loss of sexual performance both in men (4) and women (5).

The present chapter reviews the behavioral effects of prolactin induced by the exogenous administration of the hormone or by endogenously increased plasma prolactin levels that occur in rats bearing adenohypophysial homografts under the kidney capsule or those that underwent mastectomy and vagotomy. In addition, data are presented showing the possible involvement of prolactin in human sexual behavior and in opiate addiction.

BEHAVIORAL EFFECTS OF PROLACTIN IN LOW VERTEBRATES

The reports of Lienhart (1) on prolactin-induced parental behavior in hens have subsequently been described in a number of different birds (6,7). Prolactin has also been shown to induce parental behavior in cichlid fish (8) and may be involved in migration of fish (9), amphibians (10), and birds (11). The prolactin-induced migration in some birds is accompanied by increased nocturnal restlessness and food consumption

(11). In addition, prolactin can increase food consumption and promote feeding behavior in other species (12,13).

BEHAVIORAL EFFECTS OF PROLACTIN IN MAMMALS

Maternal behavior

Mammalian maternal behavior in several species consists of nest building and retrieval and caretaking of pups. The effects of prolactin on these parameters were first described by Riddle et al. (14), who observed that peripheral injections of the hormone induced maternal behavior in young male or virgin female rats when they were placed together with pups. Prolactin- induced maternal behavior has been established in a number of mammals, including rats, mice, and rabbits (15). However, the primary role of prolactin in inducing mammalian maternal behavior has recently been questioned (16).

The site of action of prolactin in inducing maternal behavior of rats may be the nucleus accumbens because its lesion results in reduction of post-partum behavior and impairment of lactational performance (17). Recently, Fuxe et al. (18) suggested that prolactin-induced maternal behavior in the rat involves the dopaminergic terminals in the nucleus accumbens, because its dopamine turnover was increased following injection of prolactin into hypophysectomized rats.

Feeding behavior

Mammals of other species also show stimulation of somatic growth and facilitation of feeding behavior after peripheral administration of prolactin (19).

Learning and memory

There is evidence for an effect of prolactin on learning processes. Banerjee (20) found that peripheral administration of prolactin slightly impairs the performance of conditioned avoidance responses in female rats. Furthermore, the hormone seems to abolish the emotional responses of these animals. In another study prolactin was reported to facilitate the acquisition of active avoidance behavior in male rats (21). Moreover, memory dysfunctions in men have been related to a low level of prolactin in the cerebrospinal fluid (22).

In a recent study, we presented evidence that prolactin-induced facilitation of active avoidance behavior in rats may involve central opioid transmission. In fact, the peripheral administration of the opiate receptor antagonist naltrexone reduced the behavioral effect induced by prolactin (22). It is worth mentioning that the involvement of central opioid transmission has also been postulated for other prolactin-induced behavior (Table 1).

Grooming behavior

One of the major behavioral changes following the induction of hyperprolactinemia in male rats is represented by increased grooming behavior (23). The intracerebroventricular (icv) administration of rat prolactin can also enhance grooming behavior in the rat (24). Since mastectomy or vagotomy seem to affect plasma prolactin levels, we have recently studied the effects of these surgical manipulations on grooming behavior of male rats (25). We found that hyperprolactinemia induced by right-side and bilateral mastectomy is accompanied by enhanced grooming activity of male rats, while left-side mastectomized animals with low levels of plasma prolactin display poor grooming activity (Table 2). Both left- and right-side vagotomy result in a significant increase in plasma prolactin levels. However, only left-side vagotomized rats exhibit increased levels of grooming behavior, while no difference exists between right-side vagotomized rats and control animals. These results suggest that changes in plasma prolactin levels induced by surgical manipulations can affect grooming activity in the rat. However, the hypothesis that the integrity of peripheral organs is important for the display of grooming behavior cannot be ruled out.

Table I. *Effects of opiate antagonists on active avoidance responses, responsiveness to electrical footshock (number of no responses) and grooming activity in hyperprolactinemic (HPRL) male rats.*

GROUPS	TREATMENT[a]	ACTIVE AVOIDANCE RESPONSES	RESPONS-IVENESS TO FOOTSHOCK	GROOMING SCORE
HPRL	Saline	13.2 ± 0.7^b	3.3 ± 0.7	72.3 ± 9.5
	Antagonist	$11.3 \pm 0.4*$	$1.3 \pm 0.5*$	$37.3 \pm 3.0*$
Control	Saline	9.3 ± 0.2	1.0 ± 0.3	10.4 ± 1.2
	Antagonist	9.8 ± 0.3	1.2 ± 0.3	8.9 ± 1.0

[a] Naloxone (1mg/kg) was used as antagonist for avoidance and grooming experiments and naltrexone (0.6 mg/kg) for footshock responsiveness. Each treatment group includes 6 animals.
[b] Values are mean $\pm$ SEM.
* Significantly different as compared to saline-treated group ($p < 0.05$, Student t test).

In a recent study on the time-course and element analysis of hyperprolactinemia-enhanced grooming behavior, it was found that this effect is time-dependent (23). In fact, it reaches the highest level 12 days after adenohypophysial homografts and declines to control levels on the 26th postoperative day. On the 10th and 12th day homografted animals exhibit relatively more genital grooming than the sham-operated rats, while the percent values of other elements of grooming behavior are slightly decreased.

The peripheral injection of the opiate receptor antagonist naloxone significantly reduces hyperprolactinemia-enhanced grooming behavior (Table 1). In addition to opioid activity, central dopamine activity has been implicated in prolactin-enhanced grooming. In fact, peripheral or intrastriatal injection of the dopamine antagonist haloperidol markedly suppresses prolactin-induced behavioral effect (26). Bilateral injections of prolactin in the striatum fail to induce grooming, whereas bilateral injections of the hor-

Table 2. *Effects of surgical manipulations on grooming behavior of male rats.*

Groups	(n)	PLASMA PRL (ng/ml)	Grooming Score
Sham-Mastectomy[a]	(10)	25.2 ± 1.5[b]	32.30 ± 3.0
Right-Side Mastectomy	(9)	62.1 ± 3.4*	56.87 ± 3.7*
Left-Side Mastectomy	(9)	8.1 ± 1.1*	20.12 ± 3.6
Bilateral Mastectomy	(10)	49.0 ± 2.9*	55.64 ± 2.6*
Sham-Vagotomy[a]	(6)	22.4 ± 3.6	27.11 ± 1.8
Right-Side Vagotomy	(6)	47.6 ± 3.3**	21.76 ± 1.3
Left-Side Vagotomy	(7)	41.0 ± 3.8**	46.89 ± 2.4**

[a] Animals with sham operation at the right and left side (in a 1:1 proportion) are pooled in this group.
[b] Values are mean ± SEM.
* Significantly different as compared to sham-mastectomy group ($p < 0.05$, Dunnett's test).
** Significantly different as compared to sham-vagotomy group ($p < 0.05$, Dunnett's test).

mone in the substantia nigra elicit the behavioral response. Thus, it is possible that the dopaminergic nigrostriatal system is involved in prolactin-enhanced grooming. In addition, a recent study demonstrated that the dopaminergic terminals in the nucleus accumbens also may play a role in prolactin-enhanced grooming (27). In fact, bilateral lesions in the nucleus accumbens induced by microinjections of of 6-hydroxydopamine suppress prolactin-enhanced grooming. The steady-state concentration of dopamine in the nucleus accumbens, measured by a radioenzymatic method, appeared to be increased in hyperprolactinemic male rats (Fig. 1). Other neurochemical effects of hyperprolactinemia include (28) a decrease in dopamine turnover in the substantia nigra, area tegmentalis ventralis, and gyrus cinguli, and an increase in the nucleus caudatus. Hyperprolactinemia also increases the noradrenaline turnover in the locus coeruleus, but decreases it in some terminal projections of the dorsal noradrenergic bundle, e.g. the gyrus dentatus and gyrus cinguli. Noradrenaline turnover in the substantia nigra appeared to be decreased in hyperprolactinemic animals. Prolactin decreases the turnover of acetylcholine in the striatum, and affects cholinergic transmission in the hippocampus and thalamus (29). Furthermore, hyperprolactinemia can influence the concentration of opioids (30) and increase the activity of glutamic acid decarboxylase activity in the striatum and substantia nigra (31).

Despite such a large number of neurochemical effects, it is difficult to correlate them with prolactin-induced excessive grooming or other behavioral changes.

ACTH can also enhance grooming behavior in the rat (32). In a recent study, the interaction between prolactin and ACTH in enhancing grooming behavior after icv administration has been investigated in intact and hyperprolactinemic rats (33). In intact rats, four hours after the icv injection of rat prolactin or ACTH, a subsequent administration of ACTH or rat prolactin induces the excessive grooming observed after the first injection. In hyperprolactinemic rats, which display excessive grooming 12 days after adenohypophysial homografting under the kidney capsule, icv injection of rat prolactin fails to enhance further the grooming activity while this behavior is substantially enhanced by icv injection of ACTH. Twenty-six days after surgery, the grooming activity of hyperprolactinemic rats was of the same magnitude as that of control animals.

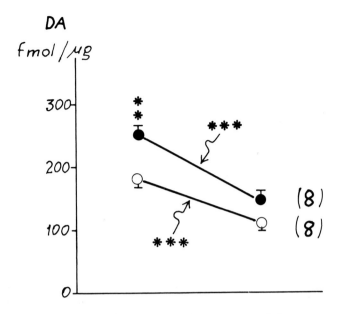

Figure 1. Steady-state concentration (left) and alpha-MPT-induced disappearance of dopamine in the nucleus accumbens of hyperprolactinemic (black circles) and control rats (white circles). Significant differences **vs controls (p<0.01) and ***vs steady-state concentration (p<0.001)

Icv injection of rat prolactin induced excessive grooming in control but not in hyperprolactinemic animals. In contrast, at this time icv injection of ACTH again induced excessive grooming in both hyperprolactinemic and control rats. These data suggest that although prolactin and ACTH may affect common neurotransmitter systems in the brain, the two hormones probably act on independent neural mechanisms in inducing excessive grooming in the rat.

Motor behavior

An altered sensitivity of striatal dopamine receptors has been postulated in hyperprolactinemic rats on the basis of nigro-striatal dopamine changes and prolactin-induced behavioral effects. In order to test this possibility, the behavioral responses induced by dopamine agonists or antagonists were studied in hyperprolactinemic rats. These animals seem to be more sensitive to amphetamine and apomorphine with respect to drug-induced stereotypies (34). Furthermore, hyperprolactinemia can significantly decrease haloperidol-induced catalepsy (35).

Sexual behavior

Although prolactin may physiologically stimulate gonadal function, chronic hyperprolactinemia fails to restore mating behavior in castrated male mice, and suppresses copulatory capacity in intact male rats and mice (37). Hyperprolactinemia is commonly associated with a loss of sexual capacity. However, a number of studies show that this effect is not common in all mammalian species (38).

The sexual impotence observed during treatment with neuroleptics has been associated with the neuroleptic-induced hyperprolactinemia. However, neuroleptics that hardly cross the blood-brain barrier fail to inhibit sexual behavior in male rats (38). Since it has been suggested that brain dopamine is involved in male sexual behavior (39), it is possible that blockade of brain dopamine receptors by neuroleptics that are able to cross the blood-brain barrier is responsible for the loss of sexual behavior observed during neuroleptic treatment.

In contrast to long-term hyperprolactinemic male rats, animals subjected to high levels of plasma prolactin for a short time display an enhancement of some parameters of copulatory behavior, i.e. a reduction in the mount and intromission latencies and an increase in mount and intromission frequencies (40). These findings suggest that the duration of hyperprolactinemia may be important for the change in sexual capacity of male animals.

Drug induced behavioral and adaptive responses

Prolactin also may play a role in drug-induced behavioral and adaptive responses of the rat. The inactivation of centrally present prolactin by specific antiserum administration results in an enhancement of acquisition of heroin self-administration behavior and in an inhibition of development of tolerance to the analgesic effect of morphine (41). It has been reported that hyperprolactinemia is accompanied by an inhibition of heroin self-administration in the rat (42). This effect is mimicked by icv injection of rat prolactin or peripheral administration of drugs that induce hyperprolactinemia, such as sulpiride or domperidone. Icv injection of anti-prolactin serum totally abolishes the effect of hyperprolactinemia on heroin self-administration behavior and facilitates it in normoprolactinemic rats. Furthermore, responsiveness to electrical foot-shock appears to be reduced in hyperprolactinemic rats (21) and this effect can be reversed by peripheral administration of naltrexone (Table 1). Morphine-induced analgesia can be potentiated in hyperprolactinemic rats (42).

BEHAVIORAL EFFECTS OF PROLACTIN IN HUMANS

Sexual behavior

The influence of prolactin on human sexual behavior has recently been reviewed (38). Sexual impotence has been described in men with chronic hyperprolactinemia due to hypophysial prolactin-secreting microadenomata (4). Accordingly, high levels of plasma prolactin have been found in men with loss of sexual capacity, but without signs of hypophysial hyperfunction caused by a tumor (43). Amenorrhea, infertility, and interference with gonadotrophic function have been reported in hyperprolactinemic women. A loss of sexual activity has been described in these subjects (44).

It is worth mentioning that all evidence showing an inhibitory action of prolactin on sexual capacity in man refers to chronic hyperprolactinemia. Thus, it is not known whether short-term hyperprolactinemia would also exert an inhibition of human sexual behavior. Furthermore, despite the large number of studies demonstrating an impairment of sexual capacity in hyperprolactinemic humans, the problem of decreased libido in these patients remains under debate.

A clinical study has shown that sexual impotence also can be present in men with low levels of plasma prolactin (45). In this study, the occurrence of ejaculatio precox was also described in hypoprolactinemic men.

Opiate addiction

On the basis of results obtained in hyperprolactinemic rats showing a resistance to heroin addiction (42), we have recently studied the effects of acute administration of a drug inducing hyperprolactinemia, domperidone, (1mg/kg iv) on acute opiate-withdrawal symptoms in heroin addicted patients. The subjects, addicted to heroin for 6-10 years, were observed for withdrawal signs and symptoms by a research nurse every 30 min, rating 21 items associated with withdrawal as present or absent. Furthermore, all patients completed a self-rating analogue scale to assess changes in nervousness, unpleasantness, energy, and irritability. The study revealed that domperidone-induced hyperprolactinemia can significantly reduce withdrawal signs in all addicted patients. Furthermore, treatment with domperidone reduced self-rating symptoms in addicted patients.

Because domperidone poorly crosses the blood-brain barrier, these findings suggest that reduction in withdrawal signs may depend on domperidone-induced hyperprolactinemia. These results may be of relevance for the treatment of acute opiate-withdrawal in humans.

Present data shows that prolactin possesses a complex behavioral profile in both animals and humans. Most of the behavioral effects of prolactin may be related directly or indirectly to an involvement of brain dopamine or opioids. However, the site of action, if unique, is not yet known. These findings prompt us to conclude that the brain and peripheral organs can be considered as target tissues for prolactin.

REFERENCES

1. Leinhart R. (1927): Compt Rend Soc Biol 97:1296
2. Riddle O, Bates RW, Lahr EL. (1935): Am J Physiol 3:352
3. Drago F. (1982): Prolactin and behavior, PhD Thesis, Univ Utrecht
4. Besser GM, Thorner MO. (1973): Pathol Biol 23:779
5. McNeilly AS. (1980): J Reprod Fertil 58:537
6. Nalbandov AV, Card LE. (1945): J Heredity 36:35
7. Crispens CG. Jr (1957): J Wildlife Management 21:462
8. Fiedler K, Bruss R, Christ H, Lotz-Zoller R. (1980): In: Brain and Pituitary Peptides, Ferring Symp. Karger, Basel, p 65
9. Lam TJ, Hoar WS. (1967): Can J Zool 45:509

10. Grant WC Jr, Grant JA. (1958): Biol Bull 114:1
11. Meier AH, Farner DS, King JR. (1965): Animal Behav 13:453
12. Licht P. (1967): Gen Comp Endocrinol 9:49
13. Zipser RD, Light P, Berm HA. (1969): Gen Comp Endocrinol 13:382
14. Riddle O, Lahr EL, Bates RW. (1934): Proc Soc Exp Biol Med 32:730
15. Zarrow MX, Gandelman R, Denenberg VH. (1971): Horm Behav 2:343
16. Baum MJ. (1978): Physiol Behav 20:87
17. Smith MO, Holland R. (1976): Physiol Psychol 4:361
18. Fuxe K, Eneroth P, Gustafsson J-A, Lofstrom A, Skett P. (1977): Brain Res 122:177
19. Bates RW, Milkovic S, Garrison MM. (1964): Endocrinology 74:714
20. Banerjee U. (1971): Neuroendocrinology 7:278
21. Drago F, Bohus B, Mattheij JAM. (1982): Physiol Behav 28:1
22. Drago F, Gispen WH, Bohus B. (1981). In: Takagi H, Simon EJ (eds) Advances in Endogenous and Exogenous Opioids. Kodansha, Tokyo, p 335
23. Drago F, Bohus B. (1981): Behav Neur Biol 33:117
24. Drago F, Canonico PL, Bitetti R, Scapagnini U. (1980): Europ J Pharmacol 65:457
25. Gerendai I, Drago F, Continella G, Scapagnini U. (1984): Physiol Behav 33:67
26. Drago F, Bohus B, Canonico PL, Scapagnini U. (1981): Pharmacol Biochem Behav 15:61
27. Drago F, Kovacs GL, Continella G, Scapagnini U. (1984): Biogenic Amines 1:75
28. Drago F, Kovacs GL, Continella G, Scapagnini U. (1984). In: Biggio G, Spano PF, Toffano G, Gessa GL (eds) Neuromodulation and Brain Function. Pergamon, Oxford, p 132
29. Wood PL, Cheney DL, Costa E. (1980): J Neurochem 34:1053
30. Panerai AE, Sawynok J, Labella FS, Friesen HG. (1980): Endocrinology 106:1804
31. Nicoletti F, Di Giorgio RM, Patti F, Rampello L, Condorelli DF, Amico-Roxas M, Canonico PL, Scapagnini U. (1981): Arch Int Pharmacodyn 249:153
32. Gispen WH, Wiegant VM, Greven HM, de Wied D. (1975): Life Sci 17:645
33. Drago F, Bohus B, Gispen WH, Scapagnini U, de Wied D. (1983): Brain Res 263:277
34. Drago F, van Ree JM, Bohus B, de Wied D. (1981): Europ J Pharmacol 72:249
35. Nicoletti F, Patti F, Ferrara N, Canonico PL, Giammona G, Condorelli DF, Scapagnini U. (1982): Brain Res 232:238
36. Hartmann G, Endroczi E, Lisak K. (1956): Acta Physiol Hung 30:53
37. Svare B, Bartke A, Doherty P, Mason I, Michael SD, Smith MS. (1979): Biol Reprod 21:529
38. Drago F. (1984): Neurosci Biobehav Rev, in press
39. Tagliamonte A, Fratta W, Del Fiacco M, Gessa GL. (1974): Pharmac Biochem Behav 2:257
40. Drago F, Pellegrini-Quarantotti B, Scapagnini U, Gessa GL. (1981): Physiol Behav 26:257
41. van Ree JM, de Wied D. (1977): Life Sci 21:315
42. Drago F, Scapagnini U. (1984): Brain Res, in press
43. Legros JJ, Chiodera P, Servalis J. (1980). In: de Wied D, van Keep PA (eds) Hormones and the Brain. MTP, Lancaster, p 205
44. Muller P, Musch K, Wolf AS. (1979). In: Zichella L, Pancheri P (eds) Psychoneuroendocrinology in Reproduction. Elsevier/North-Holland Biomedical Press, p 359
45. Deutsch S, Sherman L. (1979): Endocr Soc Meet abs 350

Prolactin. Basic and clinical correlates
R.M. MacLeod, M.O. Thorner and U. Scapagnini (eds.),
Fidia Research Series, vol. I,
Liviana Press, Padova © 1985

Section IX
Experimental and clinical
effects of prolactin on behavior
and brain function

PROLACTIN AND PITUITARY INVOLVEMENT IN MATERNAL BEHAVIOR IN THE RAT

Robert S. Bridges, Donna D. Loundes, Rosemarie DiBiase and Barbara A. Tate-Ostroff

Department of Anatomy, Laboratory of Human Reproduction and Reproductive Biology, Harvard Medical School, Boston, Massachusetts 02115, U.S.A.

At parturition, females show an immediate onset of caretaking behavior towards their young. In the rat, the behavioral responses exhibited by the parturient and lactating female are easily quantified. The responses displayed by a maternal lactating rat include retrieval of the young, crouching over the young, nest building, and defense of the young from intruders. Female rats that have never given birth do not exhibit these behavioral responses spontaneously although they can be induced to show many components of maternal behavior when placed in constant contact with foster young for an average period of 5-6 days (1,2). The underlying neural capacity to behave maternally toward young, therefore, is present in female rats from prepubertal life throughout adulthood (3). Events that transpire during pregnancy bring this underlying capacity to the surface, as evidenced by the immediate onset of maternal behavior present at parturition. Data from studies on rats indicate that changes in endocrine function during pregnancy play a major role in transforming the inexperienced female from a slow responder prior to birth to an immediate responder at the time of parturition.

The roles of specific hormones in the stimulation of maternal behavior have received considerable attention during the past ten to fifteen years. Most studies have examined the roles of estradiol (E_2), progesterone (P), prolactin, and more recently, oxytocin (4-12). While well defined roles for E_2 and P have been elucidated, the involvement of prolactin in the induction of maternal behavior in mammals remains uncertain. A role for prolactin in the stimulation of maternal behavior in the rat has lacked strong experimental support. (10,12-16).

An early report of an action of prolactin on maternal behavior in the rat was that of Riddle and colleagues (17). They reported an enhancement of maternal behavior in intact nulliparous female rats after repeated prolactin injections and a number of days of contact with foster young. Attempts to replicate the finding of Riddle et al. have been unsuccessful (13,14). More recently, researchers have measured the effects of drugs that interfere with prolactin release on maternal behavior in rats after hysterectomy and ovariectomy during the latter stages of gestation, a procedure that results in a rapid onset of maternal behavior towards foster young (18). Treatment of rats with either CB-154 (15) or apomorphine (16) failed to disrupt the onset of maternal behavior induced by the combination of hysterectomy and ovariectomy on day 16 of gestation and estradiol benzoate administration. In another study, ectopic pituitary transplants given to ovariectomized, nulliparous rats failed to stimulate maternal responsiveness (12).

During the past few years we have developed a model for the study of the hormonal regulation of maternal behavior in the rat (7,19). This model employs the administration of known amounts of steroids using hormone-filled Silastic capsules. Using this mode of hormone delivery, we found that maternal behavior was facilitated in ovariectomized, nulliparous rats that were administered physiological levels of estradiol and progesterone in specified combinations. In the present set of experiments, we have used one of these hormone regimens to reexamine the role of the pituitary gland and prolactin in the induction of maternal behavior in hypophysectomized rats.

In our initial experiment, the effects of sequential exposure to progesterone and estradiol on the rate of induction of maternal behaviors were measured in hypophysectomized and nonhypophysectomized female rats. Hypophysectomized and nonhypophysectomized nulliparous female rats (Crl:CD(SD)BR) weighing 201-225 grams were obtained from Charles River Breeding Laboratories, Inc., Wilmington, Massachusetts. Upon their arrival in our laboratory, all rats were individually housed in translucent polypropylene cages (20 x 45 x 25 cm) in light- (lights on 0500-1900 h) and temperature- (21-24 C) controlled rooms. Food (Purina rat chow) and water were available ad libitum throughout all studies. Two to three days after arrival in our laboratory, half of the hypophysectomized (hypox) rats were ovariectomized and given 3 x 30 mm P-filled Silastic capsules (Dow Corning, 602-305) s.c. (19). The remaining hypox females were ovariectomized and implanted with blank Silastic capsules. The day of ovariectomy and P or blank implantation was designated treatment day 1. Nonhypophysectomized (nonhypox) females were ovariectomized 2-3 weeks after their arrival in our laboratory. One week after ovariectomy half of the nonhypox females were given 3 x 30 mm P-filled Silastic capsules, while the remaining nonhypox rats were given blank capsules. Again, the day of P or blank capsule implantation was designated treatment day 1. On day 11 of treatment, P and blank capsules were removed from all hypox and nonhypox rats. At the same time, 2-mm E_2-filled capsules were implanted into the P-treated groups. Animals previously exposed to blank capsules were given another blank capsule on day 11. Behavioral testing began on day 12 between 0930 and 1100 h, approximately 22-24 hr after P removal and E_2 insertion. Latencies to exhibit maternal behaviors in a home cage text were measured following the standard procedure employed in our laboratory (19). Behavioral responses exhibited towards three 3-8 day old foster young were recorded daily during 1-hr test sessions. All animals were tested for 11 consecutive days or until they exhibited full maternal behavior (retrieval of all 3 pups and grouping them in the nest) for two consecutive days, whichever first occurred. At the end of testing on test day 11, all rats were sacrificed. Blood was collected for subsequent prolactin determinations, and at autopsy the sella turcica was examined for the presence of pituitary fragments and paired adrenal weights were recorded. Rats with detectable serum prolactin levels, pituitary fragments, or elevated adrenal

Table 1. *Effect of hypophysectomy on steroid-induced maternal behavior in ovariectomized, nulliparous rats.*

Treatment groups	Behavioral Responses			
	Carry Young	Group Young in Nest	Crouch Over Young	Full Maternal Behavior
Hypophysectomized				
Steroid-Treated (11)	7.5 ± 1.3	8.1 ± 1.3	8.7 ± 1.2	8.1 ± 1.3
Controls (10)	5.3 ± 1.5	7.9 ± 1.2	8.3 ± 1.1	7.9 ± 1.2
Nonhypophysectomized				
Steroid-Treated (11)	1.9 ± 0.3*	2.0 ± 0.3*	2.5 ± 0.4*	2.0 ± 0.3*
Controls (12)	8.3 ± 0.7	8.7 ± 0.6	8.6 ± 0.9	9.0 ± 0.7

Steroid-treated females were exposed to P from days 1-11 and E_2 from day 11 to the completion of testing. Controls were exposed to blank implants. Behavioral testing began on treatment day 12 and continued through day 22. The scores represent the mean latency in days ± SEM for animals to exhibit the behavioral responses. *$P <0.01$ when compared with nonhypophysectomized controls. The numbers in parentheses are the Ns for the groups.

weights were dropped from the study prior to statistical analyses.

The effects of hypophysectomy on steroid-induced maternal behavior are shown in Table 1. Whereas P and E_2 treatment facilitated maternal behavior in animals with intact pituitary glands, hypophysectomized rats failed to respond to the identical hormone regimen. Rats with intact pituitary glands responded maternally towards foster young with an average latency of about 2 days compared to a latency of 8-9 days in nonhypox control females. Hypophysectomized rats that were either exposed to steroids or no steroids required 5-8 days before they behaved maternally towards young (see Table 1). These findings demonstrate that the presence of the pituitary gland is required for this steroid-facilitated maternal behavior.

Data from a second study provides additional support for a role of the anterior pituitary gland in the regulation of maternal behavior (20). At the most recent meeting of the American Association of Anatomists, we reported that placement of the anterior lobe of the pituitary gland under the kidney capsule of hypophysectomized, steroid-treated female rats stimulated a rapid onset of maternal behavior (20). In this study two groups of ovariectomized, hypophysectomized, nulliparous rats were implanted s.c. with P-filled Silastic capsules on treatment day 1. At this time, females in one group had the anterior lobes of two pituitary glands grafted under their kidney capsules. On day 11, P implants were removed and each female was given an estradiol capsule. When females were tested for maternal behavior, rats bearing ectopic pituitary grafts responded rapidly (50% responded within 30 minutes) and significantly faster than sham-grafted controls (p < 0.01). The latency to display complete maternal behavior for the graft recipients was about 2 days, while the latency for the controls was 8 days. In addition, blood levels of prolactin as measured by radioimmunoassy were elevated in graft recipients and highest in those recipients that responded maternally with the shortest

594

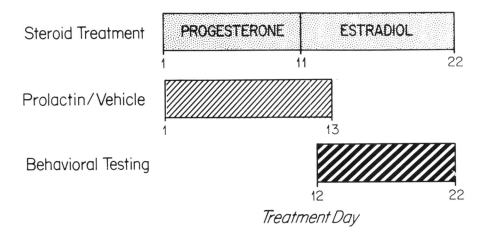

Figure 1. Experimental protocol used in the study on the effects of prolactin on maternal behavior. Rats were hypophysectomized 2-3 days prior to treatment day 1. See text for additional details.

latencies. A significant positive correlation was found between the rapidity of onset of maternal behavior in these animals and circulating prolactin levels ($p < 0.05$). These findings indicated that the anterior pituitary gland participates in the steroid-induced stimulation of maternal behavior in inexperienced female rats, and suggested to us that one behaviorally active pituitary agent may be prolactin.

In the third experiment, therefore, the possible involvement of prolactin in the induction of maternal behavior has been examined. The experimental approach employed was similar to that used in the previous studies except that hypophysectomized animals were treated with prolactin or vehicle in combination with P and E_2. The experimental protocol is shown in Figure 1. Hypophysectomized rats were ovariectomized and implanted with 3 x 30 mm P-filled Silastic capsules on treatment day 1. Half of the females were injected twice daily from days 1-13 with ovine prolactin (NIADDK oPRL-16) at a dose of 500 ug/injection. Controls were injected with the polyvinylpyrrolidone-saline vehicle (21,22) twice daily. On day 11, the P implants were removed and each rat was implanted with a 2 mm E_2-filled Silastic capsule. Behavioral testing began on day 12, 22-24 hr after P removal/E_2 insertion and 1 hr after the morning prolactin/vehicle injection. Testing continued for 11 days through treatment day 22. After testing on day 22, all rats were sacrificed, a blood sample collected, the sella turcica examined for the presence of pituitary fragments, and paired adrenal weights recorded. As in earlier studies, data on adrenal weights in combination with the inspection of the sella turcica and the measurement of serum prolactin by radiommunoassay provided a basis for the establishment of complete hypophysectomy. Rats with elevated adrenal weights, detectable serum prolactin, or pituitary fragments were dropped from the study prior to analysis of the behavioral data.

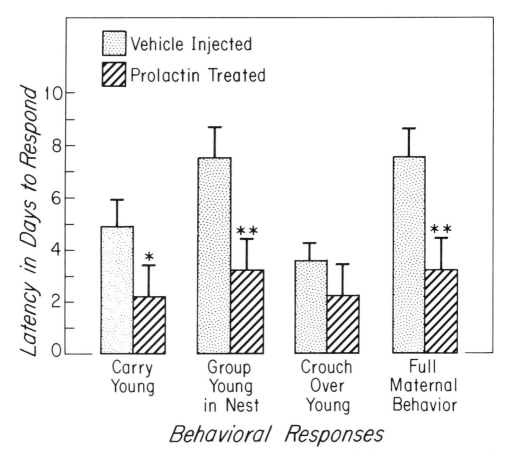

Figure 2. Effects of prolactin treatment on maternal behavior in hypophysectomized, gonadec-tomized, steroid-treated female rats. *P < 0.05 when compared with controls (Mann-Whitney U Test). **P < 0.01 when compared with controls (t-test & Mann Whitney U test).

The effects of prolactin treatment on maternal behavior are shown in Figure 2. Prolactin stimulated a rapid onset of maternal responsiveness in hypophysectomized, ovariectomized, steroid-treated, nulliparous rats. The latencies to carry a rat pup, group young in the nest, and show full maternal behavior were significantly shorter in prolactin-injected females than in control rats (p < 0.05 to <0.01). Prolactin treatment did not affect crouching latencies; both prolactin and vehicle-injected animals exhibited relatively short crouching latencies.

As shown in Table 2, the comparable body and adrenal weights found in this experiment indicate that prolactin's behavioral actions most likely did not result from its effects on the general health of the animal. Both groups lost similar amounts of weight during the course of the experiment, the loss primarily being associated with the chronic exposure to estradiol from days 11-22.

Table 2. *Body and adrenal weights in steroid-treated, hypophysectomized, ovariec-tomized, nulliparous rats after prolactin or vehicle administration.*

Treatment	Body Weights (g)				Adrenal Weights (mg)
	Day 1	Day 22	Δ Days 1-11	Δ Days 1-22	Day 22
Prolactin	184 ± 2	165 ± 4	-2.2 ± 2.4	-19.3 ± 4.6	21.5 ± 1.4
Vehicle	187 ± 2	158 ± 4	-6.9 ± 1.8	-28.7 ± 3.4	22.9 ± 0.8

Changes in body weights are represented by Δ

These results are the first to demonstrate an effect of prolactin on maternal behavior in hypophysectomized rats and suggest to us that during gestation, prolactin helps to prime the female to respond maternally towards her young at parturition. It would appear that the elevated titers of prolactin in the circulation during the first half of gestation (23,24) in combination with the prepartum increase in prolactin secretion (25,26) in the rat help stimulate the onset of maternal behavior in this species. Presently, it is not known whether prolonged exposure to prolactin throughout gestation or acute exposure to prolactin prepartum is sufficient to stimulate maternal behavior. If indeed prolonged exposure to prolactin is required for the full expression of maternal behavior at parturition, one would expect that removal of the pituitary gland during pregnancy would interfere with the establishment of maternal behavior at parturition.

In a final experiment, we have examined this possibility by measuring maternal behavior in rats hypophysectomized after mid-pregnancy. Sixteen rats were hypophysectomized on day 14 of gestation. Day 1 of pregnancy was designated the day sperm was found in the vaginal lavage. Gravid females were checked hourly for the onset of delivery beginning the morning of day 22 of gestation. The time of delivery onset was noted and animals were observed continuously throughout parturition. All females gave birth to live young on day 22 or 23 of gestation. One hour after birth of the last young, litters were removed and the number of live and dead young recorded. At this time, six young were placed throughout the homecage and the mother's behavioral responses to the young recorded during a 1-hr test. Incidences and latencies to retrieve pups, group the young in the nest, and crouch over young were noted. The following day at 1000 h, 18-27 hr postpartum, this test was repeated. On day 4 or 5 postpartum (day 27 post-sperm positive), trunk blood was collected from all females. Implantation sites were counted, the sella turcica examined for pituitary fragments, and adrenal weights recorded. Sera were subsequently assayed for prolactin content. Two animals were not included in the data analysis because they were found to have elevated serum prolactin concentrations 4-5 days postpartum.

The behavioral responses of the hypophysectomized females are shown in Figure 3. Eighty-three percent (83%) of the females hypophysectomized on day 14 of gestation exhibited complete maternal behavior between 1-2 hr postpartum. All females were completely maternal the following day, a finding similar to that previously reported

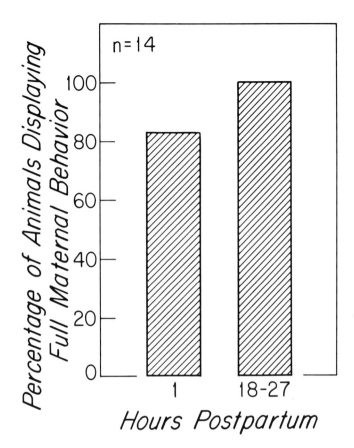

Figure 3. Maternal behavior postpartum in primiparous rats hypophysectomized on day 14 of gestation. Full maternal behavior was defined as retrieval of the 6 test young, grouping them in the nest, and crouching over the pups within the 1-hr test period. The 18-27 hr postpartum test session was conducted between 0900 and 1100 h the day after parturition.

(27). The percentage of live births/implantation sites was 87.2% ± 2.7%, and the average number of live births for the hypophysectomized animals was 9.1 ± 0.7 pups. These findings indicate that hypophysectomy did not adversely suppress fetal survival. The mean paired adrenal weight at autopsy for these hypophysectomized mothers was 27.7 mg ± 1.0 mg.

The findings of this final study raise an interesting possibility, namely, that in the absence of pituitary prolactin secretion the conceptus, through its hormonal secretions, may communicate with the mother, priming her to respond to her young at the birth. Given prolactin's behavioral action in the previous experiment, it is tempting to speculate that a prolactin-like substance secreted by the conceptus, possibly a placental lactogen, could help stimulate maternal behavior at the time of parturition. A system through which the fetal-placental unit could communicate with the mother is an attractive possibility. When we place these findings in the perspective of the endocrine events of pregnancy, our results indicate that prolactin and/or prolactin-like substances act during pregnancy in combination with the steroids, E_2 and P, to stimulate the spontaneous onset of maternal care shown by new mothers. The sites and mechanisms of action of prolactin in the regulation of maternal behavior remain to be elucidated.

When one tries to account for the discrepancies in the literature pertaining to the effects of prolactin on maternal behavior, one is led to hypothesize that prolactin (and perhaps prolactin-like molecules) affects maternal behavior over a prolonged period during gestation, rather than just acutely during the prepartum period. Furthermore, the action of prolactin appears to be dependent upon the presence of sufficient gonadal steroids, i.e., estradiol and progesterone, during this prolonged priming period. If one applies these hypotheses to preexisting data, it is possible to account for the majority of negative and positive findings in the literature. Specifically, acute disruption of prolactin secretion with drugs after surgical termination of pregnancy (15,16) might not be expected to disrupt the onset of maternal behavior, since these treated females had been exposed to high titers of prolactin and placental lactogen for 16 days prior to surgery and behavioral testing. Likewise, administration of prolactin (13,14) or ectopic pituitary transplants (12) to female rats in the absence of the gonads or necessary steroidal priming would also not be expected to stimulate the rapid onset of maternal care in inexperienced females. Finally, when one examines Riddle et al.'s data (17), one is struck by the fact that Riddle and his colleagues used intact females given prolactin for 1-2 weeks before any effects were noted. By today's behavioral standards, Riddle's work could only be considered suggestive. Yet, our data support the conclusion reached by Riddle (17), namely, that prolactin can stimulate maternal behavior in rats.

In summary, we have demonstrated that a steroid treatment which stimulates maternal behavior in ovariectomized rats with intact pituitary glands fails to facilitate maternal behavior in hypophysectomized, ovariectomized rats. Second, we reiterate our previously reported finding that a rapid onset of maternal behavior is found in hypophysectomized, ovariectomized, steroid-treated rats bearing ectopic anterior pituitary lobe grafts. Third, we have demonstrated that exogenous prolactin administration to steroid-treated, hypophysectomized, ovariectomized rats stimulates maternal behavior, whereas treatment with the prolactin vehicle fails to enhance maternal care. Finally, we report that in pregnant rats, hypophysectomy does not disrupt the establishment of maternal behavior. These results indicate that the pituitary gland, through its secretion of prolactin, and possibly the conceptus through its hormonal secretions, normally help stimulate the establishment of maternal behavior in the newly parturient female.

ACKNOWLEDGMENTS

We would like to thank Dr. Paul Doherty, Mr. Frank Menniti, and Mr. Paul Ronsheim for their excellent scientific and technical assistance in conducting these studies and Mr. Steve Borack for his photographic skills. This research was aided by Basil O'Connor Starter Grant No. 5-311 from the March of Dimes Birth Defects Foundation, NSF Grant BNS 80-14670, and NIH Grant HD 16856 awarded to RSB, a grant from the Andrew W. Mellon Foundation awarded to Harvard Medical School, Laboratory of Human Reproduction and Reproductive Biology, and NIH Center for Population Research Grant 1P30-HD06645 awarded to the Laboratory of Human Reproduction and Reproductive Biology.

REFERENCES

1. Rosenblatt JS. (1967): Science 156:1512
2. Cosnier J, Couturier C. (1966): C R Soc Biol 160:789
3. Bridges RS. (1974): Physiol Behav 5:219
4. Moltz H, Lubin M, Leon M, Numan M. (1970): Physiol Behav 5:1373
5. Zarrow MX, Gandelman R, Denenberg VH. (1971): Horm Behav 2:343
6 Siegel HI, Rosenblatt JS. (1975): Physiol Behav 14:465
7. Bridges RS, Russell DW. (1981): J Endocrinol 90:31
8. Pedersen CA, Prange AJ Jr. (1979): Proc Natl Acad Sci USA 76:6661
9. Pedersen CA, Ascher JA, Monroe YL, Prange AJ. (1982): Science 216:648
10. Bridges RS, Goldman BD, Bryant LP. (1974): Horm Behav 5:219
11. Numan M, Leon M, Moltz H. (1972): Horm Behav 3:29
12. Baum MJ. (1978): Physiol Behav 20:87
13. Lott DF, Fuchs SS. (1962): J Comp Physiol Psychol 65:1111
14. Beach FA, Wilson JR. (1963): Psychol Rep 13:231
15. Numan M, Rosenblatt JS, Komisaruk BR (1977): J Comp Physiol Psychol 91:146
16. Rodriguez-Sierra JF, Rosenblatt JS. (1977): Horm Behav 9:1
17. Riddle O, Lahr EL, Bates RW. (1935): Proc Soc Exp Biol Med 32:730
18. Rosenblatt JS, Siegel HI. (1975): J Comp Physiol Psychol 89:685
19. Bridges RS. (1984): Endocrinology 114:930
20. Bridges RS, DiBiase R, Doherty PC. (1984): Anat Rec 208:23A
21. Morishige WK, Rothchild I. (1974): Endocrinology 95:260
22. Richards JS, Williams JJ. (1976): Endocrinology 99:1571
23. Butcher RL, Fugo NW, Collins WE. (1972): Endocrinology 90:1125
24. Smith MS, Neill JD. (1976): Endocrinology 98:696
25. Amenomori Y, Chen CL, Meites J. (1970): Endocrinology 86:506
26. Linkie DM, Niswender GD. (1972): Endocrinology 90:632
27. Obias MD. (1957): J Comp Physiol Psychol 50:120

Prolactin. Basic and clinical correlates
R.M. MacLeod, M.O. Thorner and U. Scapagnini (eds.),
Fidia Research Series, vol. I,
Liviana Press, Padova © 1985

Section IX
Experimental and clinical
effects of prolactin on behavior
and brain function

PSYCHOLOGICAL DISTRESS IN HYPERPROLACTINEMIC WOMEN

Maire T. Buckman

Department of Medicine, VAMC and University of New Mexico,
Albuquerque, New Mexico 87131

A few uncontrolled studies published in the mid to late 1970's suggested that unphysiologic hyperprolactinemia in women might be associated with psychological distress. These studies were followed in the early 1980's with reports that hyperprolactinemia may represent an independent risk factor for anxiety and depression in hyperprolactinemic amenorrheic women (1), and, in a preliminary study by our group, that restoration of euprolactinemia with bromocriptine treatment resulted in amelioration of distress (2).

In order to further explore the possible relationship between psychological distress and elevated serum prolactin concentrations, we undertook a study to examine whether hyperprolactinemic women suffered distress similar to, more than, or less than that suffered by control subjects, family practice patients, and non-psychotic psychiatric out-patients (3) (Study 1). In a separate study we further examined the effect of bromocriptine administration to lower serum prolactin concentrations on psychological parameters in a 12 week placebo controlled double blind study of 8 hyperprolactinemic subjects (4) (Study 2). The latter study, submitted for publication as a short communication (4), will be presented here in greater detail.

METHODS

Study 1 and 2. Fourteen hyperprolactinemic women participated by informed consent in the studies. Serum prolactin concentrations on four or more separate days were greater than 30 ng/ml in each patient with a range from 31 to 1,253 ng/ml (normal less than 24 ng/ml). All demonstrated a blunted or absent prolactin response to phenothiazine, perphenazine administration indicating autonomous prolactin regulation consistent with the presence of pituitary adenomas (5). All patients had been referred to the endocrine clinic because of galactorrhea, menstrual dysfunction and/or infertility. Some patients had been diagnosed before referral as suffering from hyperprolactinemia and in others the diagnosis was made during evaluation. No patient was referred because of psychiatric symptoms and none had neuro-opthalmologic signs or symptoms. Goldman perimetry was normal in all patients. CT scans were non-diagnostic or consistent with pituitary adenomas. Three patients had undergone incomplete trans-sphenoidal adenomectomies several years prior to inclusion in the study. Anterior and posterior pituitary function had been assessed by standard dynamic testing techniques in each patient and in 4 abnormalities were uncovered: partial hypopituitarism in 3 and primary hypothyroidism in one. All patients received appropriate hormone replacement therapy and had been on a stable treatment program for at least 6 mos. prior to inclusion in the study. The identical treatment regimen was maintained in all patients during the 12 week double blind study. None of the patients had other systemic illnesses and none were on drugs known to affect prolactin secretion.

Study 1. Hyperprolactinemic patients were compared with 25 consecutive non-psychotic women admitted for outpatient psychiatric care who were anxious, depressed, or both by DSM-III criteria, with 29 consecutively admitted women attending the family practice clinic with a variety of representative illnesses, and with 26 randomly selected women employees of a factory and an office complex in the same city.

Study 2. Seven women successfully completed this study. In addition, one hyper-prolactinemic man was included in the study. Patients were admitted consecutively and at the time the study was initiated, no sex bias was introduced.

STUDY DESIGN

Study 1. Self-rating scales were administered to individuals in the 4 groups.

Study 2. A double blind simple crossover trial of bromocriptine and placebo with random allocation to treatments was performed. Each treatment block lasted 6 weeks. Bromocriptine mesylate treatment was started with 1.25 mg with food qd and increased over 5 days to 2.5 mg bid. In order to avoid observer bias and to maintain the double blind design, the prescribing physician did not know what the prolactin levels were during the study. Prolactin levels were determined before treatment and at weeks 1, 6, 7 and 12 so that there were 2 estimations of prolactin during each treatment phase.

PSYCHOLOGICAL ASSESSMENTS

To eliminate the possibility of observer bias, validated self-rating scales were administered instead of observer rating scales. Detailed description of these tests and discussion of their validation is presented elsewhere (3,4).

Study 1. Two distress scales were selected for this study: the Symptom Rating Test (SRT) and the Symptom Questionnaire (SQ). The SRT consists of 4 self-rating scales that are state measures of anxiety, depression, somatic symptoms, and feelings of inadequacy. The SQ has evolved from the SRT and it is also a state measure consisting of less well known series of questions based on the original list of symptoms in the SRT, which the subjects answer "yes" or "no." It contains 4 scales based on factor analyses: anxiety, depression, hostility, and somatic symptoms. Each scale is subdivided into a symptom subscale and a corresponding well-being subscale (six items each) -- "relaxed," "contented," "friendly," and "somatic well-being." The scores on the well-being subscales serve as checks of consistency for the results obtained with the symptom subscales.

Study 2. During this study, several self-rating scales were administered at each visit at the clinic and twice at home: the standard Beck Depression Inventory (BDI), the SRT, the SQ, a relative 5-point global self-rating scale of distress and an absolute 5-point self-rating scale of libido (with cues from 1 = "very satisfactory" to 5 = "totally absent"). The various scales used for this study differ in self-rating methods and have somewhat different psychometric properties; several scales were administered in order to check the consistency of the results.

PROLACTIN ASSAY

Serum prolactin was measured by a homologous double antibody radioimmunoassay system as previously described (5).

STATISTICAL ANALYSES

Study 1. Analysis of covariance with age as covariate was compared with age-adjusted means. The analyses were repeated using Dunnett's test. The results obtained using the 2 analytical methods were similar and only the results obtained with Dunnett's test are reported here.

Study 2. The data were analyzed by the standard analysis of variance for crossover design.

RESULTS

Study 1

Hyperprolactinemic women were significantly more hostile, depressed and anxious than family practice patients or nonpatient employees on the SRT and the SQ (Table 1). On the other hand, the scores were similar for hyperprolactinemic and psychiatric outpatients indicating a significant level of distress among hyperprolactinemic women.

The SRT inadequacy scale scores showed similar results: hyperprolactinemic women were similar to psychiatric patients and both felt significantly less adequate than either family practice patients or nonpatient employees.

Study 2

Bromocriptine treatment was associated with a decrease in serum prolactin concentrations in all patients. Following 6 weeks of treatment prolactin was normal (less than 24 ng/ml) in 6 subjects and substantially decreased in 2 (from 144 and 94 on placebo to 33 and 24 ng/ml, respectively, on bromocriptine). At the end of each 6 wk study period mean ± SD serum prolactin was 70 ± 49 on placebo and 17 ± 10 ng/ml on bromocriptine ($p < .001$).

Table 1. *Symptom Questionnaire Scores of Hyperprolactinemic Women and Female Nonpsychotic Psychiatric Patients, Family Practice Patients, and Nonpatient Employees[a]*

Scale or Subscale	Group Scores[b]								Differences Between Hyperprolactinemic Women and Other Groups (Q)[c]		
	Hyperprolactinemic Women (N=14)		Psychiatric Patients (N=25)		Family Practice Patients (N=29)		Nonpatient Employees (N=26)		Psychiatric Patients	Family Practice Patients	Nonpatient Employees
	Mean	SD	Mean	SD	Mena	SD	Mean	SD			
Hostility scale	13.1	4.6	9.8	7.2	5.2	4.7	5.2	4.4	1.96	4.70[d]	4.64[d]
Hostility symptoms	10.6	4.1	7.9	6.4	4.6	4.4	4.8	3.8	1.85	4.10[d]	3.91[d]
"Friendly"	2.5	2.0	1.8	1.8	0.7	1.4	0.4	1.0	1.28	3.61[d]	4.01[d]
Depression scale	12.2	4.6	14.3	7.2	5.3	4.8	3.2	3.4	1.18	4.06[d]	5.15[d]
Depressive symptoms	9.9	3.7	11.0	5.4	4.0	3.8	2.5	2.6	0.82	4.52[d]	5.53[d]
"Contented"	2.3	2.0	3.2	2.2	1.3	1.7	0.7	1.1	1.61	1.71	2.63[e]
Anxiety scale	12.8	3.8	14.8	7.8	7.1	5.4	4.6	4.2	1.15	3.01[d]	4.30[d]
Anxiety symptoms	8.8	3.4	11.4	5.9	5.8	4.9	3.1	3.1	1.67	2.01[e]	3.71[d]
"Relaxed"	4.0	1.9	3.5	2.2	1.3	1.8	1.5	1.6	0.64	4.13[d]	3.87[d]
Somatic scale	10.1	4.8	11.1	7.4	10.4	6.7	5.6	4.4	0.80	0.47	1.98
Somatic symptoms	6.2	3.3	7.5	5.6	7.0	5.3	3.5	3.3	1.11	0.83	1.52
"Somatic well-being"	3.9	2.09	3.6	2.0	3.4	1.9	2.1	1.6	0.23	0.52	2.63[e]

[a] The mean (±SD) ages of the respective groups are 27.5±3.6 years, 30.0±8.4 years, 35.0±13.7 years, and 35.2±13.2 years.
[b] A higher score indicates more distress or more psychopathology on all scales and subscales.
[c] Dunnett's test with 90 degrees of freedom (two-tailed).
[d] $p < .01$.
[e] $p < .05$.
(Reproduced from Ref. 3 with permission)

The scores on self-rating tests were high before treatment and while on placebo and decreased significantly on bromocriptine (Table 2).

No changes were observed on the somatic scales or the somatic well-being scale.

On most measures there was a progressive and substantial decrease in distress with the passage of time while being treated with bromocriptine whereas there were only small and inconsistent changes with placebo. The changes in depression scores were representative of the changes observed on the 2 drug regimens (Fig. 1). On all 3 depression scales (SRT, SQ, and BDI), bromocriptine treatment resulted in a progressive improvement in scores over the 6 week study period and on 2 scales these changes were statistically significant (SRT and SQ). The improvement in scores was parallel to the fall in serum prolactin concentration. In contrast, no consistent trend in depression scores or serum prolactin was observed during the placebo treatment period.

The changes in spontaneously reported physical symptoms and signs of hyperprolactinemia, such as cessation of galactorrhea (occult in most) or return of menstruation, were not conspicuously different during the 2 treatment periods. The difference in self-rating scores of those patients who had drug first and placebo second did not differ from those who had the treatments in reverse order. When the scores of the only male patient were excluded and the analyses repeated, the results remained essentially the same.

Table 2. *Serum prolactin and self-rating scores of distress and well-being at the end of each treatment period in hyperprolactinemic patients ($N = 8$) in a crossover study of bromocriptine and placebo for six weeks each. Higher Score indicates more distress or more psychopathology on all scales and subscales. NS = Not Significant.*

	Bromocriptine Mean ± SD		Placebo Mean ± SD		F (1,6)	p value
Beck Depression Inventory	3.8	4.1	14.8	13.1	4.92	NS
Symptom Rating Test						
Anxiety	2.0	1.9	4.3	3.7	2.37	NS
Depression	2.5	2.7	6.3	4.5	7.48	(<.05)
Inadequacy	2.1	2.2	5.9	3.6	7.17	(<.05)
Symptom Questionnaire Subscales						
Anxiety	2.0	3.0	5.8	4.4	6.67	(<.05)
Relaxed	1.0	4.4	2.9	3.3	6.89	(<.05)
Depression	2.3	3.2	6.8	3.8	17.12	(<.01)
Contented	0.6	4.9	1.9	4.4	3.53	NS
Hostility	4.0	4.7	8.3	4.5	9.67	(<.05)
Friendly	0.3	5.5	2.0	3.8	7.5	(<.05)
Global Scale	1.9	1.1	3.8	1.0	9.36	(<.05)
Self Rating of Libido	1.4	.5	2.8	1.7	7.14	(<.05)

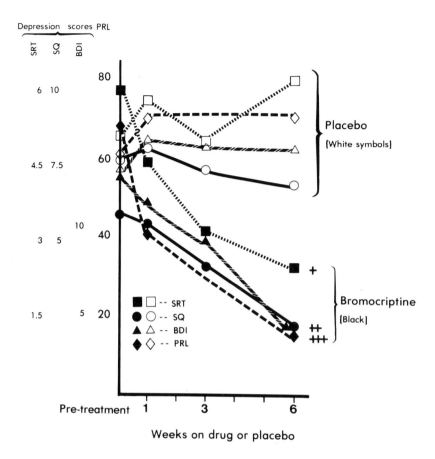

Figure 1. Changes in depression scores of the Symptom Rating Test (SRT), Symptom Question-naire (SQ), the Beck Depression Inventory (BDI) and prolactin (PRL) levels during a crossover study of bromocriptine and placebo for 6 weeks each. The pre-treatment scores are the means at the beginning of the treatment block (that is, the scores before the study if the treatment was first, or at the point of crossover if the treatment was second). + p <.05, + + p <.01 (SQ), + + + p <.001

DISCUSSION

In the current study, hyperprolactinemic women suffered significant anxiety, depression, hostility, and feelings of inadequacy compared to controls. This distress did not seem to be related to illness alone since other patients seeking medical care at a family practice clinic did not exhibit a similar pattern of psychopathology.

Bromocriptine treatment for 6 weeks resulted in significant reduction of most of the distress parameters with improvement in general well-being and in libido. Differences between the psychological effects of bromocriptine and placebo were striking even though only 8 patients completed the study. It is rare to detect statistically significant effects of psychotropic agents in placebo controlled studies with samples of this size (6). Thus, bromocriptine treatment exerted a powerful effect on relieving distress in hyperprolactinemic subjects.

The role of abnormal prolactin secretion in the pathogenesis of the psychological distress of hyperprolactinemia is unclear. Three possibilities warrant consideration. First, hyperprolactinemia per se may evoke anxiety, depression, hostility, and feelings of inadequacy and may impair libido by a direct central nervous system effect. It has been suggested that the diminished libido and impaired sexual function in hyperprolactinemic men is a direct result of abnormal prolactin activity in the central nervous system (7). This hypothesis derives from observations that achievement of euprolactinemia correlates better with restoration of libido and sexual function than serum testosterone levels (7,8). Bromocriptine enhances central nervous system dopaminergic tone and may increase sexual behavior by this mechanism (9) rather than via its prolactin lowering effect. The observation that bromocriptine is ineffective in men with impotence and normal endocrine function (10) has been used to argue against an intrinsic dopamine mechanism; however, since brain dopaminergic tone may be normal in euprolactinemic impotence and diminished in hyperprolactinemic impotence (11), this observation does not mitigate against a role for bromocriptine enhanced dopaminergic tone in the improved libido and sexual function in hyperprolactinemic men. To definitively delineate the possible direct effect of prolactin on the neuroendocrinology of mood disorders, non-pharmacologic intervention to restore normoprolactinemia must be pursued. Unfortunately, this may be a formidable task. Since the advent of effective dopamine agonist therapy, surgery for prolactin secreting pituitary adenomas is much less common than it once was. Furthermore, a control group of matched patients with non-hormone producing adenomas of similar size requiring surgical intervention may be difficult, if not outright impossible, to find. Development of a multi-center study to examine this issue would be a minimum requirement for this type of investigation.

In contrast to a possible direct effect of prolactin on modulating mood, hyperprolactinemia may induce distress indirectly via alterations in other gonadal (i.e. decrease in estrogen and progesterone) and adrenal (i.e. increase in DHEA and DHEA-S) hormones. Decreased estrogen secretion has been implicated in the mood disorders of postmenopausal women. However, when Fava et al (1) compared psychological test scores in normo- and hyperprolactinemic amenorrheic women (both groups have estrogen deficiency), they found the hyperprolactinemic women to be significantly more distressed than the euprolactinemic ones. This study suggests that hyperprolactinemia induced distress in excess of that attributable to suppressed hypothalamic-pituitary- ovarian-uterine cyclic function. The possible role of other prolactin-induced hormonal changes in the dysphoria of hyperprolactinemia has not been explored.

Finally, hyperprolactinemic distress may evolve from brain dopamine depletion resulting in concomitant but unrelated manifestations of hyperprolactinemia and distress. It has been suggested that prolactin secreting pituitary tumors may arise as a consequence of inadequate dopaminergic tone or sensitivity (11). Likewise, dopamine depletion may play a role in some depressive disorders (12). Thus, both hyperprolactinemia and depression may be independently derived from a dopamine depletion syndrome and both would be expected to respond to dopamine agonist treatment. In fact, bromocriptine treatment has been found to have antidepressant effects. Theohar et al

(13) performed a double-blind multicenter trial comparing bromocriptine with standard doses of imipramine and found that bromocriptine was generally as effective as imipramine in ameliorating depression. Doses of bromocriptine utilized in these studies ranged from 10 to 60 mg qd, which is substantially more than the 5 mg qd utilized in the present study. Whether 5 mg qd would also be effective in depressed patients is unknown, and warrants further investigation.

The current study suggests a high level of psychological distress in hyperprolactinemic patients. Bromocriptine administration lowered serum prolactin concentrations and also significantly improved symptoms of depression, anxiety, hostility, and inadequacy and increased libido and global well-being. Thus, psychological distress can be added to the symptom complex of hyperprolactinemia. Since the level of hyperprolactinemic dysphoria may be severe, i.e. similar to that observed in psychiatric out-patients, psychological distress should be considered an independent indication for drug treatment of hyperprolactinemic patients.

ACKNOWLEDGMENTS

I gratefully acknowledge the participation of my colleagues in these studies: Drs. Robert Kellner, Giovanni Fava, John Mattox, and Dorothy Pathak; the assistance of the Clinical Research Center nursing staff in performing some of the studies; and Sandoz, Inc. for generously providing bromocriptine and the matched placebo.

These studies were supported by a grant from the Veterans Administration (Merit Review) and by NIH-DRR-GCRC RR00997

REFERENCES

1. Fava GA, Fava M, Kellner R, Serafini E, Mastrogiacomo. (1981): Psychother Psychosom 36:122
2. Buckman MT, Kellner R. (1982): No. 174 Program and Abstracts of the 64th Annual Meeting of the Endocrine Society (Abstract)
3. Kellner R, Buckman MT, Fava GA, Pathak D. (1984): Am J Psychiatry 141:759
4. Buckman MT, Kellner R. (1984): Am J Psychiatry, in press
5. Buckman MT, Peake GT. (1978): Horm Metab Res 10:400
6. Kellner R, Sheffield BF, Simpson GM. (1978): Prog Neuropsychopharmacol 2:197
7. Franks S, Jacob HS, Martin N, Nabarro JDN. (1978): Clin Endocrinol 8:277
8. Carter JN, Tyson JE, Tolis G, Van Vliet S, Friesen HG. (1978): N Engl J Med 299:847
9. Tolis G. (1980). In: Krieger DT, Hughes JC (eds) Prolactin: Physiology and Pathology in Neuroendocrinology. Sinauer Publishers, Sunderland, Mass, p 321
10. Ambrosi B, Rossella B, Travaglini P, Weber G, Peccoz PB, Rondend M. Elli R, Faglia G. (1977): Clin Endocrinol 7:417
11. Marin C, Martin MD, Schriock ED, Jaffe B. (1983): Western J Med 139:663
12. Bertilsson L, Asberg M, Lantto O, Scalito GP, Traskman L, Tybring G. (1982): Psych Rev 6:77
13. Theohar C, Fisher-Cornellsen K, Akesson HO, Ansari J, Gerlach J, Harper P, Ohman R, Ose E, Stegink AJ. (1981): Curr Ther Res 30:830

Prolactin. Basic and clinical correlates
R.M. MacLeod, M.O. Thorner and U. Scapagnini (eds.),
Fidia Research Series, vol. I,
Liviana Press, Padova © 1985

Section IX
Experimental and clinical
effects of prolactin on behavior
and brain function

EFFECTS OF ENDOGENOUS HYPERPROLACTINEMIA ON ADAPTIVE RESPONSES TO STRESS

Filippo Drago, Shimon Amir*, Giuseppe Continella, M. Concetta Alloro, and Umberto Scapagnini

Institute of Pharmacology, University of Catania Medical School, Catania, Italy, and *The Weizmann Institute of Science, Isotope Laboratory, Rehovot, Israel

The application of stressor stimuli activates complex mechanisms which lead to the adaptation of the body to environmental changes. Adaptation is accomplished mainly through neuroendocrine, behavioral, and autonomic responses. A sufficiency of evidence indicates that prolactin secretion from the adenohypophysis responds to different types of stressor stimuli. Swingle et al. (1) first described the occurrence of pseudopregnancy in female rats subjected to different kinds of stress. Later, it was found that stress promotes milk secretion, suggesting the possible involvement of prolactin (2). In 1965, Grosvenor described in detail the stress-induced depletion of prolactin from the adenohypophysis (3).

In parallel with the development of psychoneuroendocrine research concerned with the effect of stress on prolactin secretion, the brain as a target organ for this hormone received more and more attention. Animal experiments and further human observations led to the notion that prolactin influences behavioral adaptation to environmental changes (4). In addition, evidence has been presented recently that prolactin may also affect stress-induced autonomic responses, e.g. changes in the motility of gastric musculature and gastric acid secretion, and in thermoregulation (5).

The present paper, dealing with the role of prolactin in adaptive responses to stress, shows that this hormone may exert multiple effects under stress conditions. In fact, prolactin seems to affect neuroendocrine, behavioral, and autonomic responses to stress. These findings suggest that stress-induced hyperprolactinemia is not a mere consequence of stress activation, but may play a role in the physiological mechanisms leading to restoration of body homeostasis.

610

INFLUENCE OF PROLACTIN ON ACTH-CORTICOSTERONE SYSTEM

The influence of prolactin on ACTH-corticosterone responses to stress has been studied in rats bearing adenohypophyseal homografts under the kidney capsule. Under these conditions, adenohypophyseal homografts secrete high amounts of prolactin and little, if any, of the other pituitary hormones (6). Fourteen days after surgery, it has been found, basal plasma corticosterone levels in hyperprolactinemic rats are higher than those of intact or sham-operated animals (7). This increase in plasma corticosterone levels appears to be accompanied by hypertrophy of the adrenal glands, observed in post-mortem examination of hyperprolactinemic rats. The question rose as to whether the increased secretory activity of adrenal glands in hyperprolactinemic rats is due to a direct effect of prolactin or to an activation of adenohypophyseal ACTH. In order to answer this question, we have measured plasma corticosterone levels in hypophysectomized rats made hyperprolactinemic by adenohypophyseal homografts under the kidney capsule. Table 1 shows that these animals exhibit high basal levels of plasma corticosterone in spite of hypophysectomy. These findings suggest that higher plasma corticosterone levels in hyperprolactinemic rats depend on a direct action of prolactin on adrenal glands.

When a physical stress is applied, hyperprolactinemic rats show a suppression of the three-fold increase in plasma corticosterone levels observed in sham-operated animals given the same type of stress stimulus (Table 2).

Table 1. *Influence of hyperprolactinemia on plasma corticosterone levels in rats under basal conditions.*

GROUPS	(n)	PLASMA CORTICOSTERONE LEVELS (ug/100 ml)
Intact	(12)	25.2 ± 2.6
Sham-Operated	(12)	20.1 ± 2.7
Hyperprolactinemic	(10)	44.2 ± 3.8*
Hyperprolactinemic + Hypophysectomized	(10)	40.6 ± 4.2*

Values are mean ± SEM
* Significant difference vs intact group (p < 0.05, Dunnett's test)

A number of authors have described a protective effect of hyperprolactinemia against stressor stimuli. Thoman et al. (8) have found that hyperprolactinemic lactating rats exhibit a marked resistance to stress-induced changes in body temperature and a diminished secretory activity of adrenal glands under stress conditions. Further, the differences between lactating and non-lactating animals are accentuated as lactation increases, and disappear following weaning of the young animals. The same authors (9) have also demonstrated that lactating rats show a marked suppression of plasma corticosterone levels after application of different types of stressor stimuli. Other authors have confirmed these findings (10,11).

Table 2. *Influence of hyperprolactinemia on plasma corticosterone levels in rats subjected to physical stress.*

GROUPS	(n)	PLASMA CORTICOSTERONE LEVELS (ug/100 ml)
Sham-Operated Controls	(12)	67.3 ± 5.7
Hyperprolactinemic	(10)	41.3 ± 2.8*

Values are mean ± SEM
* Significant difference vs controls (p < 0.05, Student's t-test)

An increase in the secretory activity of adrenal glands in hyperprolactinemic rats has been reported above. This effect has been found by others (12,13). Thus, it is possible that the increase in plasma corticosterone levels due to hyperprolactinemia causes, in turn, a reduction in ACTH secretion from the adenohypophysis (7). This can account for the suppression of the ACTH-corticosterone system under stress conditions. To verify this hypothesis, we have measured plasma ACTH levels in hyperprolactinemic and sham-operated control rats either under stress conditions or after intraperitoneal injection of vasopressin. It was found that hyperprolactinemic rats show a decrease in basal plasma ACTH levels as compared to controls and no increase after either application of physical stress or injection of vasopressin.

These results suggest that high levels of plasma prolactin can modify the response of the ACTH-corticosterone system to stress. This effect can be considered as a protection against stress-induced changes mediated by the ACTH-corticosterone system.

INFLUENCE OF PROLACTIN ON STRESS-INDUCED BEHAVIORAL CHANGE

The organism's adaptation to the dynamically changing environment requires a chain of behavioral responses in order to preserve homeostasis (14). Hormones of pituitary origin, which are secreted in response to stress, exert central effects resulting in modification of adaptive behavior like avoidance, approach, or even aggressive and sexual responses. A number of experiments have been performed on the influence of prolactin on stress-induced behavioral changes and adaptation. It was found that hyperprolactinemic rats exhibit a facilitated acquisition of active avoidance behavior (15), a reduced responsiveness to footshock (15), and an enhanced approach performance in sexual behavior (16). Another behavioral change occurring in rodents in conflict or stress situations is in grooming (17). It has been reported that hyperprolactinemia or intracerebroventricular injection of prolactin causes an enhancement of grooming behavior in the rat (6,18). Most of these prolactin-induced behavioral changes seem to involve opioid transmission in the brain. In fact, peripheral administration of opiate receptor antagonists, such as naloxone or naltrexone, inhibits prolactin-induced facilitation of active avoidance behavior, reduction in responsiveness to footshock, and enhancement of grooming (19).

It is worth mentioning that other pituitary hormones, secreted in response to stress, share the behavioral profile of prolactin. In fact, hormones such as ACTH, MSH, vasopressin, and beta-endorphin may facilitate avoidance behavior, exert analgesic effects, and enhance grooming (20-22).

INFLUENCE OF PROLACTIN ON STRESS-INDUCED GASTRIC ULCERS

In light of the possible protective action of prolactin against stress-induced autonomic changes, a series of experiments has been performed on the influence of this hormone on the development of gastric ulcers induced by cold-plus-restraint stress in the rat. Hyperprolactinemia, as induced by pituitary homografts under the kidney capsule, appears to inhibit the development of gastric ulcers in this model (Table 3). Furthermore, when hyperprolactinemic rats are treated with indomethacin, an inhibitor of

Table 3. *Influence of hyperprolactinemia on development of gastric mucosal lesions after cold-plus-restraint stress in rats*

GROUPS	(n)	NO LESIONS	PETECHIAE	ULCERS
Normoprolactinemic	(8)	12.8	12.8	75.0
Hyperprolactinemic	(9)	77.7*	11.1	11.1*
Hyperprolactinemic + Indomethacin	(6)	16.6	16.6	66.6
Normoprolactinemic Non-Stressed	(8)	100.0		

Values are expressed as % of rats exhibiting mucosal lesions
* Significant difference vs controls ($P < 0.05$, Fischer's test)

prostaglandin synthesis, prior to stress application, the cytoprotective effect of prolactin is completely abolished. This finding suggests that the cytoprotective effect of prolactin on stress-induced gastric ulcers requires an intact prostaglandin synthesis pathway.

The possible mechanism of the cytoprotective effect of prolactin on stress-induced gastric ulcers is not known. In fact, Pillai et al. (23) have recently described a contractile effect of prolactin on guinea pig isolated ileum. Also, the administration of high doses of prolactin seems to increase intestinal transit in mice (24). A marked hyperplasia of ileum mucosa has been found in hyperprolactinemic lactating rats (25). Recently, prolactin-like immunoreactivity has been detected in human intestinal mucosa (26). These findings support the hypothesis of a direct action of prolactin on the gut. However, a possible mediation of brain mechanisms cannot be ruled out.

INFLUENCE OF PROLACTIN ON STRESS-INDUCED HYPERTHERMIA

The effect of hyperprolactinemia on core temperature has recently been investigated in rats before and after the application of restraint stress (5). Hyperprolactinemia is accompanied by a significant decrease in core temperature of freely moving rats, as observed for four days after pituitary homografts. Hyperprolactinemia-induced hypothermia can be totally reversed by intraperitoneal injection of naloxone. In normoprolactinemic rats, intraperitoneal administration of naloxone causes a small but significant decrease in core temperature and an attenuated rise in temperature following the application of restraint stress. After application of restraint stress, core temperature of hyperprolactinemic rats rose to the level of non-stressed normoprolactinemic rats (Table 4). However, hyperprolactinemic rats injected intraperitoneally with naloxone showed no increase in core temperature after restraint stress application. These findings suggest that prolactin may exert a protective effect against stress-induced hyperthermia and this effect seems to involve brain opioid neurotransmission.

Different types of stressor stimuli can induce a rise in body temperature (27). However, it is of great interest that most of the pituitary hormones secreted in response to stress cause hypothermia when administered exogenously. This is true for ACTH and MSH (28), vasopressin (29), and beta-endorphin (30). As reported above, the same hormones exert similar effects on adaptive responses to stress. Thus, prolactin shows a profile of action on stress-induced behavioral and autonomic changes which is similar to that of other pituitary hormones.

Table 4. *Influence of hyperprolactinemia on core temperature of rats before and after the application of restraint stress, and the effect of peripheral administration of naloxone (1 mg/kg, intraperitoneally)*

Groups	(n)	Basal conditions	20 min after injection of saline of naloxone	Restraint stress
NPRL + Saline	(10)	37.1 ± 0.3	37.1 ± 0.4	38.3 ± 0.3
NPRL + Naloxone	(10)	37.1 ± 0.3	$36.5 \pm 0.3^*$	$37.3 \pm 0.2^*$
HPRL + Saline	(10)	$35.8 \pm 0.2^*$	$35.6 \pm 0.4^*$	$36.9 \pm 0.3^*$
HPRL + Naloxone	(10)	$35.8 \pm 0.2^*$	37.1 ± 0.3	37.0 ± 0.2

Values are mean ± SEM expressed in mmHg
In parentheses the number of animals per each group
NPRL = Normoprolactinemic; HPRL = Hyperprolactinemic
* Significant difference vs NPRL ± saline ($p < 0.05$, Dunnett's test)

In conclusion, adaptation to environmental changes requires a chain of neuroendocrine, behavioral, autonomic, and metabolic responses in order to preserve organism homeostasis. The organization of this repertoire of adaptive responses is ensured by integrative central nervous mechanisms. However, hormonal systems also represent a special integrative role in adaptive processes. It is well known that stimuli which provoke changes in emotionality leading to fear, anxiety, or disappointment are among the most potent of all stimuli affecting the release of prolactin from the adenohypophysis (2,3). However, abundant evidence is available suggesting not only that the release of this hormone is a concomitant of emotional behavior, but also that the brain may serve as a target organ of prolactin (4).

It is difficult to define the functional meaning of the protective effect of prolactin on stress-induced neuroendocrine, behavioral, and autonomic changes. It is worth mentioning that physiological hyperprolactinemia occurs immediately before and after parturition. During these phases, a protection against stress-induced modifications could be of relevance for the defense of the fetus or the offspring.

614

ACKNOWLEDGMENTS

Part of the experiments described in this chapter were funded by a grant from the Consiglio Nazionale delle Ricerche (Rome, Italy) awarded to Filippo Drago for work at the Weizmann Institute of Science in Rehovot (Israel). The Authors wish to thank Mr. S. Maugeri (Institute of Pharmacology, University of Catania Medical School) for his precious help in preparing the manuscript.

REFERENCES

1. Swingle WW, Seay P, Perlmutt J, Collins EJ, Barlow G Jr, Fedor EJ. (1951): Am J Physiol 167:586
2. Nicoll CS, Talwalker PK, Meites J. (1960): Am J Physiol 198:1103
3. Grosvenor CE. (1965): Endocrinology 77:1037
4. Drago F. (1982): Prolactin and Behavior, PhD Thesis, Univ Utrecht
5. Drago F, Amir S. (1984): Brain Res Bull 12:36
6. Drago F, Bohus B. (1981): Behav Neur Biol 33:117
7. Drago F, Scapagnini U. (1984). In: Kvetnansky R, Axelrod J (eds) Stress: The Role of Catecholamines and Other Neurotransmitters. Gordon and Breach, New York, in press
8. Thoman EB, Wetzel A, Levine S. (1970): Commun Behav Biol 2:165
9. Thoman EB, Conner RL, Levine S. (1970): J Comp Physiol Psychol 70:364
10. Kamoun A. (1970): J Physiol (Paris) 62:5
11. Endroczi E, Nyakas CS. (1974): Endocrinologie 63:1
12. Voogt JL, Sar M, Meites J. (1969): Am J Physiol 216:655
13. Doherty PC, Smith MS, Bartke A. (1980): Endocr Soc Meet abs 704
14. Bohus B. (1975). In: Gispen WH, van Wimersma Greidanus TJB, Bohus B, de Wied D (eds). Progress in Brain Research vol 42. Elsevier, Amsterdam, p 275
15. Drago F, Bohus B, Mattheij JAM. (1982): Physiol Behav 28:1
16. Drago F, Pellegrini-Quarantotti B, Scapagnini U, Gessa GL. (1981): Physiol Behav 26:277
17. Gispen WH, Isaacson RL. (1981): Pharmac Ther 12:209
18. Drago F, Canonico PL, Bitetti R, Scapagnini U. (1980): Europ J Pharmacol 65:457
19. Drago F, Gispen WH, Bohus B. (1981). In: Takagi H, Simon EJ (eds). Advances in Endogenous and Exogenous Opioids. Kodansha, Tokyo, p 335
20. de Wied D. (1969). In: Ganong WF, Martini L (eds). Frontiers in Neuroendocrinology. Oxford University, NY, p 97
21. Olson RD, Kastin AJ, Kastin GA, Coy DH. (1982). In: Shah NS, Donald AG (eds). Endorphins and Opiate Antagonists in Psychiatric Research. Plenum, NY, p 61
22. de Wied D, Bohus B, van Wimersma Greidanus TJB. (1974). In: Integrative Hypothalamic Activity, Progress in Brain Research vol 41. Elsevier, Amsterdam, p 417
23. Pillai NP, Ramaswamy S, Gopalakrishnan V, Ghosh MN. (1981): Europ J Pharmacol 72:11
24. Gopalakrishan V, Ramaswamy S, Pillai PN, Ghosh MN. (1981): Europ J Pharmacol 74:369
25. Muller E, Dowling RH. (1981): Gut 22:558
26. Stevens FM, Shaw C. (1982): Br Med J 284:1014
27. Stewart J, Eikelboom R. (1979): Life Sci 25:1165
28. Glyn JR, Lipton JM. (1981): Peptides 2:117
29. Crine AF, Bredart S, Legros JJ. (1981): Horm Behav 15:226
30. Martin GE, Bacino CB. (1979): Europ J Pharmacol 59:227

Prolactin. Basic and clinical correlates
R.M. MacLeod, M.O. Thorner and U. Scapagnini (eds.),
Fidia Research Series, vol. I,
Liviana Press, Padova © 1985

Section IX
Experimental and clinical
effects of prolactin on behavior
and brain function

EFFECT OF CHRONIC HYPERPROLACTINEMIA ON TUBEROINFUNDIBULAR DOPAMINERGIC NEURONS: HISTOFLUORESCENCE IN MALE RATS

Carol Phelps and Andrzej Bartke

Department of Anatomy, University of Rochester School of Medicine, Rochester, N.Y., and Department of Obstetrics and Gynecology, University of Texas Health Science Center, San Antonio, Texas

With the recent advent of sensitive hormone-assay and radiologic techniques, clinical diagnosis of pituitary adenomas as prolactin-secreting has increased, to the extent that 40% of adenohypophysial tumors are estimated to be "prolactinomas" (1), including the majority of those previously thought to be functionless (2). The etiology of prolactinomas remains largely unknown, but a defect in hypothalamic prolactin-inhibitory dopaminergic function is implied, particularly by the response of human prolactinomas to dopamine-agonist drugs (2). Thus, naturally occurring and experimentally induced hyperprolactinemia in laboratory rats have been developed as model systems. Hyperprolactinemia and spontaneous prolactinoma are commonly associated with aging in rats (3); this phenomenon has been linked with findings of decreased hypothalamic dopamine concentrations (4), turnover (5), and portal blood content (3). Prolactinomas induced by chronic estrogen treatment, particularly with diethylstilbestrol (DES), show morphological and functional similarities to human tumors (6,7,8) and diminished hypothalamic dopamine function has ben found after tumor induction (6). It has been proposed that these deficits are indicative of dopamine neuronal death in hyperprolactinemic states either associated with aging or experimentally induced (9,10). This is an especially significant question in light of recent studies which indicated intact hypothalamic dopamine secretory responses in aged rats (11).

Similarly, recent biochemical assessment of tuberoinfundibular dopamine neuron function in rats rendered hyperprolactinemic by DES treatment (12) indicated that high circulating prolactin stimulated dopamine synthesis in media basal hypothalamus and median eminence (ME), provided that DES treatment had been withdrawn, while dopamine content in those areas was depressed. In animals subjected to continuous DES, dopamine levels were also decreased and dopamine synthesis was comparable to controls. The findings emphasize that measurement of dopamine levels is not adequate for assessing ME-afferent neuron function. More importantly, tuberoinfundibular dopamine neurons appear to remain viable during DES treatment and prolonged hyperprolactinemia. The studies further indicated that 8 weeks' treatment with DES induces a permanent prolactinoma; pituitary hypertrophy and peripheral prolactin levels of 1 ug/ml persisted for 4 months after DES withdrawal.

Based on the question of hypothalamic dopamine neuronal toxicity by hyperprolactinemia, and especially on the latter biochemical findings, studies were initiated to pro-

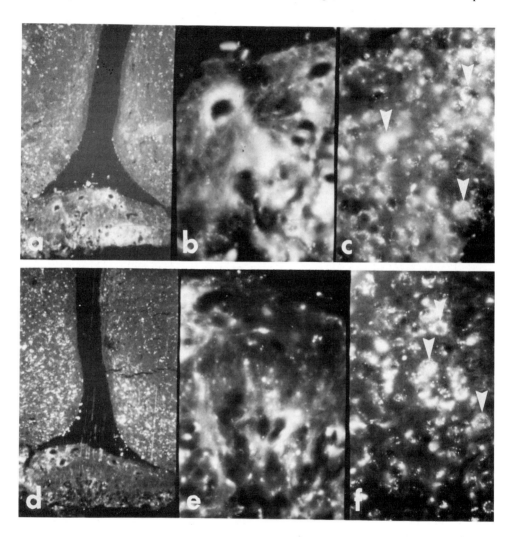

Figure 1. Tuberoinfundibular histofluorescence, Falck-Hillarp method, in aged (32 mo) male rats. A-C, in an animal whose anterior pituitary was histologically normal. D-F, in a rat bearing a large (150 mg) hemorrhagic spontaneous adenohypophysial tumor. A,D / arcuate nucleus - median eminence, 49X; B,E / central median eminence, 197X; C,F - A12 dopamine perikarya (arrows), 197X.

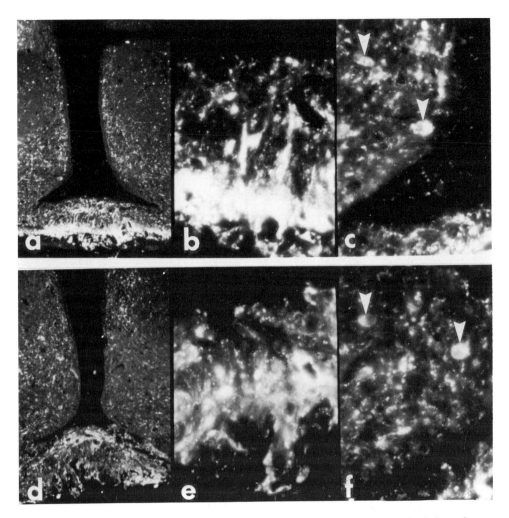

Figure 2. Tuberoinfundibular fluorescence, aluminum-formalin (ALFA) method, in male rats treated 8 wks with a DES (8 mg) implant, and sacrificed 10 months after DES withdrawal (at 18 m.o.) A-C, in a control animal bearing an empty implant. D-F, in a DES-treated rat: bright contact zone and A12 perikaryal fluorescence are visible. A,D = arcuate nucleus - median eminence, 49X; B,E = central median eminence, 197X; C,F = A12 dopamine perikarya (arrows), 197X.

vide morphologic correlates of tuberoinfundibular dopamine neuronal function in aged rats and in rats treated with DES, either continuously or for 8 weeks, and sacrificed several months following DES withdrawal. Specifically, the experiments were directed to determine 1) whether tuberoinfundibular neuron cell number is indeed reduced in either naturally-occurring or induced hyperprolactinemic states, 2) whether histofluorescence is qualitatively different in continuously DES-treated rats versus rats subjected to DES treatment followed by withdrawal, and 3) whether tuberoinfundibular histofluorescence differences exist between spontaneous and induced hyperprolactinemia.

Histofluorescence induction in brain and subsequent fluorescence microscopy were used to assess hypothalamic perikaryal dopamine and terminal dopamine in the external contact (perivascular) zone of the median eminence. The basic method employed involved rapid extirpation and freezing of brains, followed by freeze-drying and paraformaldehyde treatment, as originally described by Falck et al. (Falck-Hillarp method, 13). Some tissue was treated by the fluorescence-enhancing aluminum-formaldehyde ("ALFA", 14) or rapid aqueous formalin-glutaraldehyde ("FAGLU", 15) method. Neither the ALFA nor the FAGLU method is appropriate for quantitation in comparative studies, because each animal is individually perfused and brain tissue treated for fluorescence. Following fluorescence induction, ALFA- or Falck-Hillarp-treated brains were paraffin embedded, serially sectioned coronally at 8-10 um, and examined microscopically; FAGLU-prepared brains were examined as 30 um coronal vibratome sections. The dopamine neurons which terminate in the ME external or contact zone have perikarya located in catecholaminergic regions A12 (arcuate nucleus) and possibly A14 (periventricular region, rostral to A12), according to the classification by Bjorklund and colleagues (16), but not confined to classical nuclei. The groups are continuous, but are often, and here, arbitrarily divided at the rostral extent of the ME.

The pituitary prolactin cell population was examined immunocytochemically (ICC) in rats from each group (aged, DES continuous treatment, and DES followed by withdrawal). The type of ICC was influenced by fixation, chosen a priori in each case for histofluorescence. FAGLU perfusion/fixation is inadequate for subsequent prolactin ICC; ALFA-perfused pituitaries were embedded, sectioned, and stained for prolactin ICC by the peroxidase- antiperoxidase (PAP)-DAB method (17). Pituitaries from rats designated for Falck-Hillarp fluorescence were either embedded and processed as above, or enzymatically dissociated, maintained in culture for 4 days, and subsequently processed for prolactin ICC (8). The prolactin cell population in young (6 m.o.) F344 male rats, as quantitated by the latter method, is large, numbering approximately 32% (19).

AGED RATS

Basal hypothalamic histofluorescence and gross pituitary morphology, were examined in a total of 55 Fischer 344 male rats, ages 20-32 months. As previously reported for aged males (18), dopamine fluorescence in the external ME was depressed, compared with that in young rats, as shown in Figure 1A-C. Bright perikarya were, however, observed through the extent of A12 and A14. Serum prolactin levels were elevated (60.0 $\pm$ 20.5 ng/ml, n = 3) in 32 m.o. rats with "normal" pituitaries; prolactin cell numbers were comparable to those found in younger F344 males accounted for (see Table I).

Pituitaries in which a focal or large tumor was observed were processed and examined histologically; the extent of examination was based on the fixation used to prepare brain tissue. The incidence of such spontaneous tumors was: a total of 6 focal (but grossly visible, at least 0.5 mm) tumors were discovered - 1 in a 20 m.o. rat, 1 in a 27 m.o. rat, and 4 in 30 m.o. animals; 3 large (pituitaries weighing 100 mg) tumors

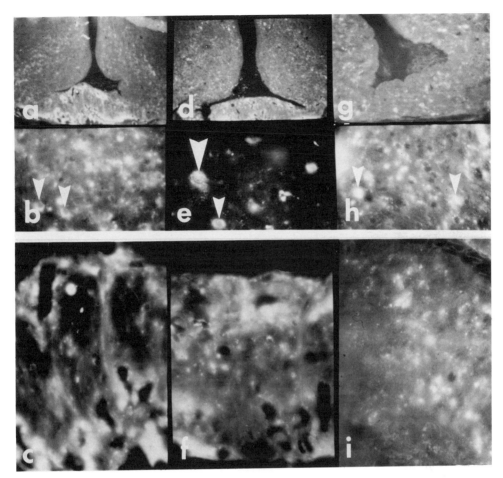

Figure 3. Tuberoinfundibular histofluorescence, Falck-Hillarp method, in young adult (6 months old) male rats subjected to continuous DES treatment, via subcutaneous capsule implant (8 mg DES). A-C, in a control animal, bearing an empty capsule. D-F, in a rat treated 50 days with DES: terminal fluorescence, in external ME, is visibly reduced. G-I, in an animal treated continuously for 70 days with DES: ME fluorescence is nearly absent, but fluorescent perikarya are identifiable (H). A,D = arcuate nucleus and median eminence, 38X; G = ventral arcuate n. and m.e., 96X; B,E,H = A12 dopamine cell bodies (arrows), 153X; C,F,I = central median eminence, 197X.

were found - 1 each in 20, 27, and 32 month old rats. No qualitative difference in A12/A14 or ME fluorescence was notable in rats with focal tumors. These small tumors were characterized histologically by increased vascularization, pale cytoplasmic staining, dark pyknotic nuclei, and nearly absent prolactin immunoreactivity.

Among rats with large spontaneous tumors, ME fluorescence was qualitatively suppressed (see Fig. 1, D-F) but brightly fluorescent and morphologically normal perikarya were extant throughout the A14/A12 region. Because such tumors were randomly and infrequently encountered, they were processed individually and no attempt at A12/A14 cell body quantitation was made. Prolactin cell ICC showed 49% of one pituitary (shown in 1 D-F) to be prolactin-positive (see Table I); cellular content of prolactin was reduced in this animal, which is different from tumors induced by DES (8,12).

DES-INDUCED HYPERPROLACTINEMIA

First examined were 8 rats treated for 8 wks. with DES, followed by DES capsule removal and a potential recovery period of 10 months. Brains from 2 control and 2 DES-treated rats were prepared by the rapid FAGLU method; 4 such animals were prepared by the ALFA method, for enhanced histofluorescence. Anterior pituitaries were homogeneously enlarged; other animals from the same DES-treatment group had plasma prolactin levels of 1.5 ± 0.2 ug/ml (12). Prolactin ICC in ALFA-perfused, DES-treated pituitaries showed increased vascularity, adenomatous changes, and intense homogeneous prolactin immunoreactivity. Brain histofluorescence in a DES-treated and in a control rat are compared in Figure 2.

Median eminence contact zone fluorescence was bright in both animals of Figure 2, but terminal varicosity density in this region was slightly decreased in the DES-treated brains, i.e., approximately 3+ compared with 4-5+ in the untreated rat, according to the fluorescence rating introduced by Fuxe (20). Such a decrease was most notable in rostral median eminence. Bright A12 and A14 perikarya were observed in all animals (see Figure 2C,F); neither distortion nor abnormalities in these cells was noted. Counts on selected comparable coronal A12 regions revealed no significant differences between control and DES-treated brains; numbers of A12 perikarya on one side of the midline third ventricle in single sections ranged from 5 to 18 in control, and from 3 to 14 in DES-treated brains; 50 to 75% of cells were visibly nucleated. Numbers of A12 perikarya have been reported to increase with age, beginning at 12 months (19). No attempt was made at total quantitation or statistical comparison, because brains were individually perfused and treated to induce fluorescence.

Even though chronic hyperprolactinemia was induced by 8 weeks DES and pituitaries appeared tumorous, recovery by tuberoinfundibular neurons after 10 months DES withdrawal was suspected. Therefore, a group of rats subjected to chronic DES implantation was prepared and examined. Eight rats (4 with empty silastic capsule implants) were divided into groups sacrificed 50 and 70 days after DES implantation. Brains were prepared for histofluorescence by rapid freezing after decapitation (Falck-Hillarp method) so that they could be simultaneously freeze-dried and reliably compared and so that anterior pituitaries could be enzymatically dissociated, maintained *in vitro*, and processed for prolactin ICC, in order to quantitate each prolactin cell population, as well as A14 and A12 populations. The results of prolactin cell quantitation for this group are shown in Table I, compared with cell counts obtained in preparations from aged rats. DES-induced prolactin cell hyperplasia was progressive with time of DES treatment.

Histofluorescence was examined and fluorescent perikarya were counted, in areas A12 and A14 in 10u serial coronal sections. Fluorescence photo-micrographs comparing a control brain with brains treated 50 and 70 days with DES, are shown in Figure 3.

Table I. *Prolactin Cell Populations in Aged and/or Tumorous Fischer 344 Male Rat Pituitaries*

Animals	Serum PRL (ng/ml)	PRL release *in vitro* (ng/1000 cells/day)	% PRL cells
"Normal" AP: 6 months old	—	—	32.9 ± 4.6 (n = 4)
27-32 months old	60.0 ± 20.5 (n = 5)	8.9 ± 1.6	34.6 ± 2.7 (n = 7)
AP Tumors spontaneous 32 months old	294 (n = 1)	5.8	48.9 ± 6.7 (n = 1)
DES-induced 6 months old			
50d DES	—	—	36.6 ± 2.9
70d DES	—	—	80.0 ± 4.1

Prolactin levels in serum, cell cultures and immunochemical preparations were determined for individual animals. DES treatment: continuous silastic capsule implants, with 8 mg DES.

Dopamine histofluorescence of A12 and A14 neurons, in perikarya and in terminal varicosities in the median eminence, of control animals was typical of that previously reported for young F344 male rats (19). Perikaryal fluorescence was dull, but cell bodies were identifiable as small, typically round profiles, and were numerous; 8-10 such perikarya can be seen in a single 40X field in Figure 3B. Dopamine fluorescence in the external median eminence (3A,C) was extremely intense, consisting of dense patterns of varicosities adjacent to capillaries and probable tanycytes. In rats treated 50 days with DES (Fig. 3D-F) ME fluorescence intensity was decreased, notably in terminal densities in the contact zone (Fig. 3F). Perikaryal number was comparable to controls in 50-day treated rats, but the fluorescence intensity in cell bodies was quite intense, and cell bodies in A12 and A14 often appeared enlarged (see 3E). As in untreated animals, the perikarya were round, the majority nucleated, and cytoplasmic fluorescence had a reticular appearance, which is typical for freeze-dried tissue. In animals subjected to 70 days continuous DES (Fig. 3G-I), tuberoinfundibular fluorescence was dramatically decreased. Terminal fluorescence in ME was nearly absent, and the ME itself was thinner (note that the photomicrograph 3G is at higher magnification than are 3A or 3D); this phenomenon was probably effected, at least in part, by the physical size of the pituitary (116 and 154 mg), with suprasellar extension, in one case (shown in fig. 3G-I), which displaced the ME. Yellow to orange fluorescence, indicative of lipofuscin deposits, was greater in 70 d treated tuberoinfundibular regions, in fluorescent and non-fluorescent perikarya; this appearance was similar to that seen in very old rats (19). Cell bodies (A12) were fewer in one treated brain than in control rats, duller in intensity than in 50d-treated rats, but, when observed, were round and often nucleated profiles.

Cell counts for A14 and A12 in continuously DES-treated rats are compared with their untreated controls in Table II. Raw counts were corrected for periodicity of sampling (X10, because counts were made in every 10 um serial section), but were not corrected for error due to cells missed or recounted based on average diameter. Such a correction requires camera lucida tracings of each cell profile, and the rapid fading of the dull A12/A14 dopamine fluorescence during microscopic examination introduces secondary error via such drawing. Cell diameters for A12 and A14 perikarya have been calculated in this way (21); A12 perikarya were 13.5 ± 0.4 um, and A14 dopamine cells were 13.1 ± 2.2 um for young male F344 rats; diameters were slightly but not

Table II. *Perikaryal Counts of Tuberoinfundibular Dopamine Neurons in DES-treated F344 Male Rats*

Animal	DES	Ap wt (mg)	A14		A12	
			Nucleated	Total	Nucleated	Total
C1	—	17.4	210	570	970	2240
C2	—	11.2	190	440	1320	1950
T1	50d	63.1	200	400	1080	2100
T2	50d	66.3	200	490	940	1850
C3	—	9.0	220	450	1010	2240
C4	—	11.7	210	440	1080	1810
T3	70d	115.8	100	290	210	630
T4	70d	154.1	240	380	1810	2060

DES treatment was performed by subcutaneous implantation of a silastic capsule containing 8 mg DES. Control rats were implanted with empty capsules and were sacrificed with age matched treated rats as indicated by animal numbers. Brains were processed together for histofluorescence induction. The pituitary of rat T3 extended dorsally and anteriorly from the sella turcica, displacing the ME.

significantly larger in aged rats. The correction factor for cell size in that study was 0.714 for A12 perikarya and is valid for studies in which section thickness is trivial compared with cell size (22); that was not the case in the present examination. It is suspected that cell diameters, as shown by histofluorescence, differed among control and DES-treated rats. These considerations taken together, the effect of DES treatment and the resultant hyperprolactinemia on A12/A14 cell numbers is proportionally indicated by raw counts. Numbers of fluorescent perikarya were lower in DES-treated brains; the effect was marked with longer treatment time.

Histofluorescence examination of prolactin-inhibitory hypothalamic dopamine neurons, in combination with biochemical studies, reveals that the major effect of hyperprolactinemia is on ME content of dopamine. Spontaneous hyperprolactinemia, as occurs in aged rats, is compatible with normal dopamine neuron function (11), as reflected in A12/A14 cellular appearance and ME terminal fluorescence. Prolactin cell hyperplasia in very large spontaneous tumors in aged rats results in significant elevation of peripheral prolactin, but only has slight effect on hypothalamic dopamine fluorescence.

The effect of DES-induced hyperprolactinemia must be separately considered. Chronic DES treatment had profound effect on TIDA neurons as well as on the pituitary lactotroph population. A marked increase occurred between 50 and 70 days' DES treatment, with regard to effect on TIDA neurons as well as on pituitary response. At 50 days DES the histofluorescence effect was reflective of dopamine neuron stimulation, and increased dopamine turnover resulting in intense perikaryal fluorescence and decreased ME dopamine terminal density. After 70 days continuous DES, ME fluorescence was virtually absent and perikaryal dopamine intensity was at control or lower levels.

The decrease in perikaryal numbers in DES continuously-treated rats may well indicate a reduced threshold for obvious fluorescence. No indications of cell death were observed.

After DES treatment followed by withdrawal, dopamine fluorescence appeared to rebound to normal levels, although, significantly, prolactin levels remained high.

Neurons of the arcuate (A12) area have been shown to concentrate estrogens, by combined histofluorescence and autoradiographic examination (23). Dopamine levels in ME increase (24) and dopamine turnover is low after castration (25); steroids subsequently increase dopamine turnover (25). These previous reports imply a direct effect of DES on hypothalamic dopamine neurons. That implication is supported by the present report. Impressive rebound/recovery was exhibited by dopamine neurons after DES withdrawal.

Thus, hyperprolactinemia itself, as examined by histofluorescence and biochemical measurements, appears to exert no permanently toxic effect on hypothalamic dopamine nueurons. There appears to be a prolactin suppressive effect on ME content/fluorescence, which may simply indicate increase dopamine turnover.

The studies indicate that differences in dopamine neuron effect exist among models exhibiting spontaneous states of hyperprolactinemia induced by continuous DES, and induced by DES treatment followed by withdrawal. Continuous DES treatment appears to exert a direct effect, indicating that spontaneous prolactinoma, or prolactinoma effected by DES treatment and withdrawal, are preferred models for the clinical problem of prolactinoma etiology with regard to hypothalamic inhibition.

ACKNOWLEDGMENTS

The authors are indebted to Ms. Barbara Planchard, Ms. Mary Pat Hogan and Ms. Janice White for technical preparation and analysis. The contribution in use of histofluorescence-preparatory and microscopic equipment in the laboratory of J. R. Sladek, Jr., is greatly appreciated. The studies were financially supported by PHS Grants HD 18243 (CP)and HD12671 (AB).

REFERENCES

1. Faglia G, Giovanelli MA, MacLeod RM (eds) (1980): Proc Serono Symp, vol 29, Academic Press, London
2. Thorner MO, Perryman RL, Rogol AD, Conway BP, MacLeod RM, Login IS, Morris JL. (1980): J Clin Endocrinol Metab 53:480
3. Gudelsky GA, Nansel DD, Porter JC. (1981): Brain Res 204:446
4. Riegle GD, Miller AE. (1978). In: Schneider (ed) The aging reproductive system, Raven Press, NY, p 159
5. Demarest KT, Riegle GD, Moore KE. (1980): Neuroendocrinology 31:222
6. Casanueva F, Cocchi D, Locatelli V, Flauto C, Zambotti F, Bestetti G, Rossi GL, Muller E. (1982): Endocrinology 110:590

7. Wiklund J, Gorski J. (1982): Endocrinology 111:1140
8. Phelps C, Hymer WC. (1983): Neuroendocrinology 37:23
9. Porter JC, Nansel DD, Gudelsky GA, Reymond MJ, Pilotte NS, Foreman MM. (1980): Peptides 1:135
10. Sarkar DK, Gottschall PE, Meites J. (1982): Science 218:684
11. Novelli A, Cocchi D, Calderini G, Toffano G, Muller EE. (1983): Gerontology 29:362
12. Morgan WW, Steger RW, Smith MS, Bartke A, Sweeney CA. (1984): Neuroendocrinology (in press)
13. Falck B, Hillarp HA, Theime G, Torp A. (1962): J Histochem Cytochem 10:348
14. Ajelis V, Bjorklund A, Falck B, Lindvall F, Loren, Walles B. (1979): Histochemistry 65:1
15. Furness JB, Heath JW, Costa M. (1978): Histochemistry 57:285
16. Bjorklund A, Moore RY, Nobin A, Stenevi U. (1973): Brain Res 51;71
17. Sternberger LA. (1979): Immunocytochemistry 2nd ed, Wiley, NY
18. Phelps C. (1984): Endocrinology 115 (suppl):(abs)
19. Hoffman G, Sladek JR Jr. (1980): Aging 1(1):27
20. Fuxe K. (1965): Z Zellforsch 65:573
21. Selemon L. (1982): Ph.D. Dissertation, Center for Brain Research, University of Rochester
22. Konigsmark BW, Kalyanaraman VP, Corey P, Murphy EA. (1969): Johns Hopk Med J 125:146
23. Grant LD, Stumpf WE. (1974): In Stumpf, WE and Grant LD (eds) Anatomical Neuroendocrinology, Karger, Basel, p 445
24. Advis JP, McCann SM, Negro-Vilar A. (1980): Endocrinology 107:892
25. Fuxe K, Hokfelt T. (1969): Neuroendocrinology 5:107

Prolactin. Basic and clinical correlates
R.M. MacLeod, M.O. Thorner and U. Scapagnini (eds.),
Fidia Research Series, vol. I,
Liviana Press, Padova © 1985

Section IX
Experimental and clinical
effects of prolactin on behavior
and brain function

EFFECTS OF HYPERPROLACTINEMIA ON DOPAMINE UPTAKE INTO STRIATAL SYNAPTOSOMES *IN VITRO*

K. A. Gregerson and M. Selmanoff

Department of Physiology, University of Maryland, School of Medicine,
Baltimore, MD 21201

There is a growing body of evidence that prolactin can modulate the function of dopaminergic terminals in the corpus striatum. Prolactin has been shown to increase the electrically-induced release of preloaded, tritium-labeled dopamine from superfused striatal slices (1) and the spontaneous efflux of endogenous dopamine from male, but not female, striatal fragments *in vitro* (2). In addition, prolactin-induced grooming behavior has been demonstrated in male rats. This effect is blocked by injection of the dopamine receptor blocker haloperidol directly into the neostriatum (3). Relevant to this are reports that hyperprolactinemia increases the density of dopamine receptors in the caudate nucleus (4,5). We have previously reported an effect of prolactin on dopamine transport in the caudate nucleus in the form of increased steady-state uptake of dopamine into striatal synaptosomes following *in vivo* prolactin administration (6).

Although the manifestations of an action of prolactin on striatal dopamine transport are evident, the molecular mechanisms involved are unknown. In the present report, the effect of prolactin on dopamine uptake by isolated presynaptic striatal nerve terminals (synaptosomes) has been examined with particular attention focused on the unidirectional, carrier-mediated influx of dopamine. The use of synaptosomes allows measurement of the kinetics of unidirectional neurotransmitter transport in controlled media on a time scale approaching physiologically relevant parameters (7).

In these studies, adult male Sprague-Dawley rats were administered ovine prolactin (4 mg/kg, sc, every 8 h) for 48 hours. Controls received a similar regimen of the vehicle which was 0.01 M sodium bicarbonate buffer. Animals were decapitated between one and two hours after the last injection when serum concentrations of ovine prolactin were approaching peak levels (1000-2000 ng/ml; see ref. 8). Caudate nuclei were immediately removed and pooled according to treatment prior to preparation of synaptosomes for uptake experiments.

Synaptosomes were prepared from the pooled caudate nuclei according to a modification (9) of the method of Hajos (10). The P_2 pellet was resuspended in a physiological saline solution at concentrations of approximately 30 ug protein per ml as determined by the method of Bradford (11). All experiments were carried out at 30 C. Dopamine uptake was performed in a reaction volume of 0.25 ml containing (final concentrations) 75 mM NaCl, 70 mM N-methyl-D-glucamine, 5 mM KCl, 1 mM CaCl$_2$, 2 mM MgCl$_2$, 10 mM Tris Hepes (pH 7.4), 10 mM glucose, 0.25 mM ascorbic acid, 0.1 mM pargyline, 0.1% bovine serum albumin, plus 0.02 - 1.0 uM dopamine (specific activity approx. 2000 cpm/pmol). For assay of dopamine uptake in the absence of sodium, NaCl was replaced with N-methyl-D-glucamine to maintain a constant ionic stength. Uptake was initiated by addition of 10 ul of synaptosomes to the incubation solution and was terminated by the addition of 3 ml of ice-cold incubation solution followed immediately by rapid filtration over a glass fiber filter. The filter was then washed with three successive 3 ml aliquots of the ice-cold solution. Uptake of dopamine was determined from the counts retained on the filters.

Studies measuring the steady-state incorporation of dopamine into the synaptosomes were undertaken to determine if the effect of ovine prolactin was specifically associated

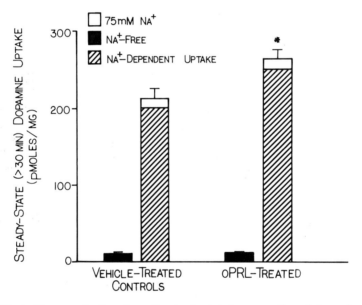

Figure 1. Effect of hyperprolactinemia on the steady-state incorporation of dopamine into striatal synaptosomes. Synaptosomes were prepared from caudate nuclei of male rats treated for 48 hours with either ovine prolactin or vehicle (see text for details) and were suspended in incubation solutions (30 C) containing 75 mM Na (open bars) or 0 Na (shaded bars; Na replaced by N-methyl-D-glucamine). The concentration of dopamine was 0.1 uM. Uptake was terminated after 30 min by rapid filtration on glass fiber filters. Na-dependent uptake (lined bars) was calculated as the difference between total and Na-independent intake. The data have been corrected for the amount of radioactivity retained on the filters in the absence of synaptosomes. The error bars represent S.E.M. of 12 determinations.
* These values (both total uptake in the presence of 75 mM Na and the Na-dependent component) differ at $p < 0.001$ from corresponding values of vehicle-treated controls.

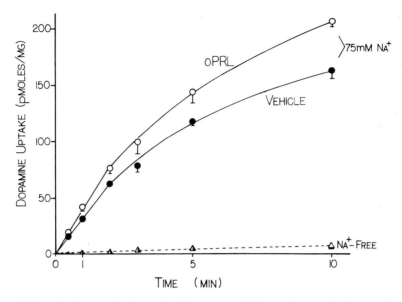

Figure 2. Effect of ovine prolactin on the time course of dopamine uptake into striatal synaptosomes. Uptake into synaptosomes prepared from ovine prolactin- (○, △) and vehicle-treated (●, ▲) rats was determined as described in the text and legend to Fig. 1. Concentration of dopamine in the incubation solutions was 0.1 uM. Concentration of Na was 75mM (○,●) or 0 (△ , ▲). Error bars represent S.E.M. of five determinations from one of three similar experiments and are shown when larger than the dimensions of the symbols.

with a sodium-dependent component of uptake, since sodium (Na) is a requirement for the carrier-mediated process of catecholamine transport (12,13). Figure 1 illustrates dopamine incorporation into striatal synaptosomes after a 30-minute incubation at 30 C. Most (>95%) of the uptake at 0.1 uM dopamine concentration was Na-dependent. Ovine prolactin treatment significantly increased total synaptosomal dopamine content with a mean increase over control values of approximately 20%. However, no difference in dopamine uptake between treatment groups was observed in the absence of added external Na. Thus, this effect of prolactin is specific to the Na-dependent component of steady-state dopamine accumulation (Fig. 1), which suggests that prolactin somehow modulates the activity of the dopamine carrier.

In order to characterize the kinetics of the carrier-mediated dopamine transport, we studied the time course of Na-dependent and Na-independent dopamine uptake. Dopamine accumulation into rat striatal synaptosomes was linear with time for at least two minutes and subsequently decreased, reaching a plateau between 10 and 20 minutes (Fig. 2; data after 10 min not shown). In the absence of sodium, dopamine uptake was also time-dependent but represented only 2-3% of the initial rate in the presence of sodium. Treatment with ovine prolactin increased the uptake of dopamine in the presence of Na at all times measured, consistent with the steady-state uptake measurements. It is noteworthy that the ovine prolactin-induced increase (approx. 20%) was the same at all times, including the initial uptake period and final plateau values. Ovine prolactin exposure had no effect on the Na-independent component of dopamine uptake. It appears that hyperprolactinemia can enhance the rate and steady-state accumulation of dopamine in the presence of sodium.

The effect of prolactin on the Na-dependent uptake of dopamine could be mediated either by a direct effect on the carrier (i.e., a change in the density and/or affinity of the carrier) or indirectly via a change in the driving force for the Na-coupled carrier. In order to test the first possibility, we studied the dependence of the initial uptake (measured at one minute of accumulation) on the dopamine concentration. In the presence of Na, the initial rate of dopamine uptake was saturable with increasing dopamine concentration (Fig. 3) while in the absence of Na, dopamine uptake was linearly related to the dopamine concentration. Again, ovine prolactin treatment affected only the Na-dependent component of dopamine uptake and the degree of stimulation was constant throughout the range of dopamine concentrations tested.

A double reciprocal plot of the data presented in Figure 3 is shown in Figure 4. This analysis of the Na-dependent component of dopamine uptake indicated an increased maximum velocity of uptake (Vmax) following ovine prolactin treatment (Fig. 4). The estimated Vmax values were 76.5 pmol/min/mg in the ovine prolactin group as compared to 63.8 pmol/min/mg in controls. However, no change in the apparent affinity of the transport process for dopamine was seen (K_M = 0.14 uM for controls and 0.13 uM for ovine prolactin-treated animals). In four similar experiments, K_M values for both controls and treated synaptosomes ranged from 0.13 to 0.17 uM, similar to other published estimates of dopamine uptake affinities in striatum (12-14). Although the maximum dopamine uptake varied substantially between experiments (from 41.5 to 83.3 pmol/min/mg for controls and 52.1 to 94.8 pmol/min/mg for ovine prolactin-treated preparations), within experiments the ovine prolactin-induced increase was always significant and ranged from 14 to 24% over controls.

In this report, two mechanisms for the accumulation of dopamine by striatal presynaptic nerve terminals have been demonstrated: 1) a minor Na-independent pathway that comprises less than 5% of total dopamine uptake under physiological conditions and 2) a Na-dependent pathway which probably represents the carrier system that catalyzes the reaccumulation of dopamine subsequent to the presynaptic action potential. Precedent exists for such a mechanism in amine transport in that co-transport with Na has been reported for synaptosomal uptake of gamma-aminobutyric acid (GABA) (15) and norepinephrine (16) and has been suggested for dopamine (17). It is thought that this process derives its ability to transport the neurotransmitter against its concentration gradient by utilizing the free energy stored in the sodium electro-chemical gradient. Therefore, this process should be affected by the transmembrane Na concentration gradient and/or electrical potential. The initial rate of dopamine uptake into synaptosomes has, in fact, been shown to increase as a graded function of external Na concentration (17). It also has been demonstrated that conditions that depolarize synaptosomes either at constant external potassium concentrations (i.e., with veratridine, which opens voltage-gated Na channels; see ref. 13) or by increasing external potassium concentrations (B.K. Krueger, personal communication), inhibit dopamine uptake. Thus, under physiological conditions, the major pathway for dopamine uptake appears to be a sodium-dopamine cotransporter.

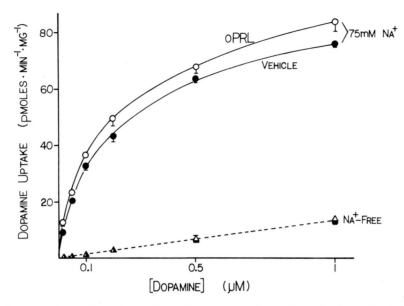

Figure 3. Dependence of uptake on dopamine concentration: effect of ovine prolactin. Uptake into synaptosomes prepared from ovine prolactin- (○,○) or vehicle-treated (●, ▲) rats was measured for one minute in the presence of 75 mM Na (○,●) or in the absence of Na (Δ, ▲). Error bars represent S.E.M. of five determinations from one of four similar experiments and are shown when larger than the dimension of the symbols.

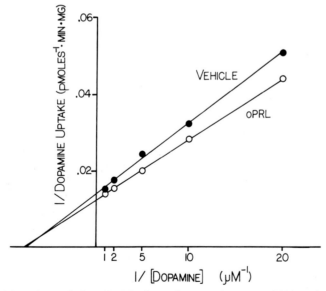

Figure 4. Double reciprocal plot of 1/Na-dependent uptake versus 1/dopamine concentration. Data are replotted from Fig. 3. Synaptosomes were prepared from ovine prolactin-treated rats (○) or vehicle-treated controls (●). The lines drawn are least-squares fits to the data points.

The present data demonstrate that when male rats are exposed to elevated levels of prolactin *in vivo*, nerve terminals subsequently isolated from the corpus striatum exhibit enhanced dopamine uptake activity. This effect is confined to the Na-dependent component of dopamine influx, suggesting an action of prolactin on the carrier-mediated transport of dopamine in the striatum. Alteration of the activity of the sodium-coupled dopamine uptake could potentially be expressed through several mechanisms: either direct (changes in the carrier itself) or indirect (changes in the driving force on the carrier). Lineweaver-Burk analysis of the data indicated no change in the apparent affinity of the carrier for the dopamine after ovine prolactin treatment, but the maximal rate of uptake (Vmax) was increased over controls. Since conditions of the external media (substrate concentrations, pH and temperature) were maintained constant between the two groups of synaptosomes, an increase in Vmax in the absence of altered affinity might suggest an increased density of uptake sites. However, as seen in Figures 1 and 2, striatal synaptosomes prepared from ovine prolactin-treated rats developed a greater steady-state accumulation of dopamine than did control preparations. If one assumes that the proportion of total protein comprised by intact, functional synaptosomes remained the same between the preparations (i.e., the treatment did not alter the relative yield or internal volume of synaptosomes) then the increased steady-state accumulation must reflect a greater dopamine concentrating ability in the ovine prolactin-exposed synaptosomes. An increased transmembrane dopamine concentration ratio ($[dopamine]_i/[dopamine]_o$) would require a greater driving force for dopamine uptake and could not be accounted for by only an increased carrier density. Prolactin would affect striatal dopamine uptake by inducing a change in the transmembrane Na electro-chemical gradient, thereby changing the driving force for dopamine uptake. This would be consistent with both a change in Vmax and a change in steady-state accumulation. Alternatively, a shift in the dynamic equilibrium existing between the cytoplasmic and vesicular pools of intraneuronal dopamine could lead to greater steady-state accumulation of dopamine without a change in the actual transmembrane dopamine concentration gradient. Thus, enhanced synaptic vesicle pumping or an increased number of vesicles per nerve terminal also would be consistent with our present data. The present results do not allow us to eliminate all of the above possibilities. However, the use of the synaptosome preparation should prove to be a powerful tool in examining each of them in turn and thereby elucidating the molecular mechanisms involved.

In summary, the maximal rate of uptake of dopamine is greater following prolactin treatment (Figs. 3 and 4), as is the steady-state accumulation (Fig. 1). In the absence of altered carrier affinity, an increase in carrier density could account for the former observation but would not be sufficient for the latter. The enhanced capacity for dopamine accumulation in terminals from hyperprolactinemic rats could result from increased binding of intrasynaptosomal dopamine within storage granules or from increased transmembrane driving force on dopamine uptake coupled with the sodium electro-chemical gradient.

It would be premature to suggest that these observed alterations in dopamine uptake are direct actions of prolactin in the caudate nucleus. Although others have demonstrated a direct effect of prolactin on the release of dopamine from isolated striatal fragments (1,2), we have not determined that in our model the ovine prolactin itself reaches this area of the brain. The effects seen may be secondary to an action of prolactin on the steroid output of the testis or adrenal gland or both. Nevertheless, the evidence is that hyperprolactinemia can, either directly or indirectly, produce alterations in dopamine transport into nigrostriatal terminals. Furthermore, these alterations, produced *in vivo*, are such that significant increases in the uptake of dopamine can still be measured following isolation of the striatal nerve terminals *in vitro*. There is ample precedent for modulatory effects of prolactin on behavior in mammals (18). The corpus striatum, a basal ganglia structure involved in the processing of motor, sensory, and motivational sensations (19), is a possible site of action for these effects. Future studies may elucidate the specific role of prolactin in the modulation and integration of synaptic transfer of dopamine in the corpus striatum.

ACKNOWLEDGMENTS

The authors would like to express their appreciation to Drs. Dieter K. Bartschat and John M. Hamlyn for critical review of this manuscript. Ovine prolactin was generously provided by Dr. Albert Parlow through the NIADDK Rat Pituitary Hormone Distribution Program. This work was supported by NIH Grant NS-14611 and RCDA NS-00731 awarded to M.S. and NRSA HD-06481 awarded to K.A.G.

REFERENCES

1. Perkins NA, Westfall TC. (1978): Neuroscience 3:59
2. Chen Y-F, Ramirez VD. (1982): Endocrinology 111:1740
3. Drago F, Bohus B, Canonico PL, Scapagnini U. (1981): Pharmacol Biochem Behav 15:61
4. Hruska RE, Pitman KT, Silbergeld EK, Ludmer LM. (1982): Life Sciences 30:547
5. Di Paolo T, Poyet P, Labrie F. (1982): Life Sciences 31:2921
6. Gregerson KA, Selmanoff M. (1983): Soc Neurosci Abst 9:319
7. Drapeau P, Blaustein MP. (1983): J Neuroscience 3:703
8. Selmanoff M, Gregerson KA. (1983): Proc Soc Exp Biol Med 175:398
9. Krueger BK, Ratzlaff RW, Stricharz GR, Blaustein MP. (1979): J Membr Biol 50:287
10. Hajos F. (1975): Brain Research 93:485
11. Bradford MM. (1976): Analyt Biochem 72:248
12. Harris JE, Baldessarini RJ. (1973): Life Sciences 13:303
13. Holz RW, Coyle JT. (1974): Molec Pharmacol 10:746
14. Annunziato L, Leblanc P, Kordon C, Weiner RI. (1980): Neuroendocrinology 31:316
15. Blaustein MP, King AC. (1976): J Membr Biol 30:153
16. Sammet S, Graefe K-H. (1979): Naunyn-Schmiedeberg's Arch Pharmacol 309:99
17. Bruinvels J. (1975): Nature 257:606
18. Nicoll CS. (1974): Handbook of Physiology, Section 7; Endocrinology Vol IV, Greep RD, Astwood EB (eds). Washington, DC: American Physiological Society, pp 253-267
19. Marsden CD. (1980): Trends in Neuroscience 3:284

Prolactin. Basic and clinical correlates
R.M. MacLeod, M.O. Thorner and U. Scapagnini (eds.),
Fidia Research Series, vol. I,
Liviana Press, Padova © 1985

Section IX
Experimental and clinical
effects of prolactin on behavior
and brain function

HYPERPROLACTINEMIA AND THE OPIOID HYPOTHALAMIC SYSTEMS

D. Cocchi, F. Petraglia*, I. Ganzetti, M. Parenti, A. R. Genazzani*, and E. E. Muller

Department of Pharmacology, School of Medicine, University of Milan, 20129 Milano and*Department of Clinical Obstetrics and Gynecology, University of Modena, 41100 Modena, Italy

It is known that hyperprolactinemia induces alterations in the hypothalamic opioid system; long-lasting hyperprolactinemia, either physiological (lactating rats) or experimentally-induced (rats with a transplanted prolactin-secreting tumor), provokes decrease of beta-endorphin (beta-EP) and met-enkephalin (ME) concentrations in the hypothalamus (1). In view of the inhibitory role exerted by opioids on luteinizing hormone (LH) release (2), hyperproduction of opioid peptides may contribute to the reduction of LH secretion present in hyperprolactinemic subjects (3). Supporting this proposition is the finding that in ovariectomized rats, injections of naloxone completely reversed the inhibitory effect of hyperprolactinemia on the progesterone mediated LH surge (4).

It has been observed recently by our group that rats with experimentally- induced hyperprolactinemia have an altered endocrine responsiveness to opiate agonists and antagonists (5). In that study we showed that female rats treated for three days with ovine prolactin (250 ug/rat twice daily) exhibited a higher LH increase after naloxone than control rats. On the contrary, administration of FK 33-824, a potent analog of met-enkephalin, evoked a much lower increase of prolactin levels in ovine prolactin-treated rats than in controls. Similarly, FK 33-824 did not elicit any prolactin rise in rats rendered hyperprolactinemic by transplantation of two ectopic pituitaries under the kidney capsule (5).

With the aim of correlating functional and biochemical aspects of opioid function, in the present study we have determined, in these two animal models of experimentially-induced hyperprolactinemia, hypothalamic concentrations of beta-endorphin-like immunoreactivity (beta-EP-LI) and of met-enkephalin (ME), according to previously described methods (6,7). As shown in Figure 1, female rats treated for three days with ovine prolactin exhibited significantly lower hypothalamic concentrations of beta-EP-LI than saline- treated controls (P < 0.01, Fig. 1, lower part).

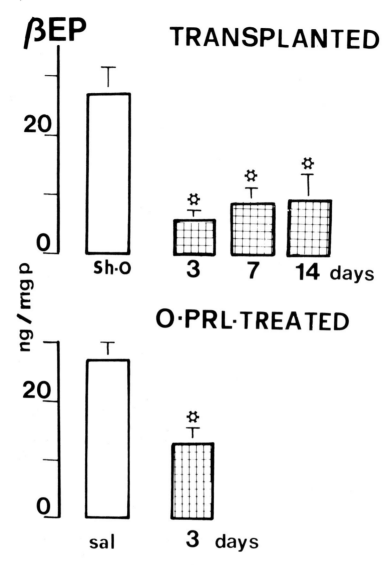

Figure 1. Beta-endorphin-LI (β-EP) concentrations in the hypothalamus of female rats bearing two additional ectopic pituitaries under the kidney capsule (transplanted rats, upper part) or treated with ovine prolactin (250/ug twice daily for 3 days, lower part). Transplanted rats were killed 3, 7, and 14 days after surgery. Each column represents the mean ± SEM of 5-7 determinations. Open columns represent sham operated (Sh-o) or saline treated (sal) animals. *p at least <0.05 vs control group

A similar pattern was present in female hyperprolactinemic rats 3, 7, and 14 days after transplantation of two additional anterior pituitaries under the kidney capsule (P < 0.05, Fig. 1, upper part). In both experimental models, no differences were detected in the hypothalamic levels of ME in comparison to control rats. Determination of the absolute concentrations of a given peptide is by no means predictive of the function of a given neuronal system. In our specific case, since hyperprolactinemic rats had a higher LH response to the opiate receptor antagonist naloxone and an impaired prolactin response to the opioid agonist FK 33-824, the decrease in hypothalamic beta-EP-LI we observed may be taken to indicate the presence of an enhanced opiatergic tone in the hypothalamus.

Many studies have reported diminished concentrations of beta-EP-LI and ME (8,9) in the hypothalamus of aged male rats, although the functional significance of this alteration has never been explored. To clarify this point we next decided to evaluate in aged rats the prolactin responsiveness to the same opioid agonist and antagonist used in the above previously reported studies.

We studied aged female rats since reportedly, in contrast with males (10), they are hyperprolactinemic (11). In all, 28 aged female rats (Charles River, 20-22 months) were used, of which 14 bore a prolactin-secreting adenoma, identified by both inspection of the pituitary at autopsy and detection of very high baseline prolactin levels. All the experiments were performed in the morning, disregarding the day of the estrous cycle in young rats and the disruption of the cycle in the old ones (most of which were in

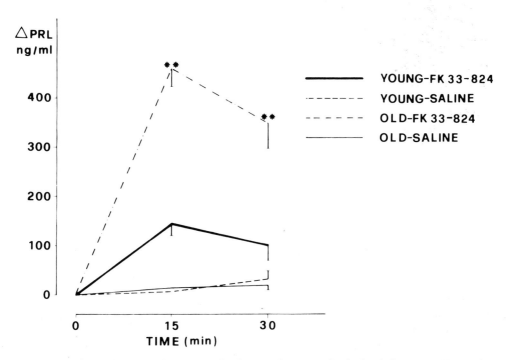

Figure 2. Effect of FK 33-824 (0.5 mg/kg ip) on plasma prolactin levels in young (6 months) and old (20-22 months) female rats. Due to the difference in basal prolactin levels between the two age groups, results are expressed as differences (Δ) between prolactin values at each time interval and baseline. **P<0.01 vs young + FK 33-824

persistent estrous). In a first experiment young and old rats received an acute injection of FK 33-824 (0.5 mg/kg ip) and were sampled 15 and 30 minutes later by the retroorbital plexus. Basal prolactin levels were 113.0 ± 28.8 ng/ml in aged and 7.9 ± 1.6 ng/ml in young female rats ($p < 0.01$).

As shown in Figure 2 the prolactin increase after FK 33-824 was significantly higher in old than in young rats ($p < 0.01$ at 15 and 30 minutes).

The differing responsiveness to the opioid could not be accounted for by the different weight and, hence, different drug dose administered to old vs young animals (mean weight old rats 402 ± 11.6 g, mean weight young rats, 265 ± 27 g). In fact, when we administered the same absolute dose of FK 33-824 (0.15 mg/rat), to young and old rats, once again a greater prolactin response was present in old animals (the difference in prolactin being 710 ± 133 ng/ml in old rats and 494 ± 155 ng/ml in young rats; data not reported).

Administration of naloxone (5 mg/kg sc) instead evoked a consistent rise of plasma LH levels in young rats (the difference being $\pm 51 \pm 15.7$ ng/ml) but failed to alter basal LH levels in aged rats. Basal LH levels were similar in the two groups (51.8 ± 22 ng/ml in young and 50.1 ± 2.3 ng/ml in old rats, data not shown).

In contrast to the results obtained in aged male rats, in females, beta-EP-LI levels in the hypothalamus do not decrease with advancing age (Table 1). These data were obtained from a small sample of animals (5 per group), and therefore need corroboration; nevertheless a sex difference is envisaged in the process of aging of hypothalamic opioid systems. Results similar to ours have been reported by Forman et al. (12) in constant estrous old female rats.

Furthermore, it seems that the opioid neurons in the hypothalamus of aged female rats are insensitive to the feedback action of high prolactin levels which, in young rats, produces a decrease of beta-EP-LI (1, and Fig. 1).

Table 1. *Hypothalamic concentrations of beta-endorphin like-immunoreactivity (beta-EP-LI) and met-enkephalin (ME) in old and young female rats.*

Age	beta-EP-LI (ug/g)	ME (ug/g)
6 months	3.68 ± 0.95[a]	0.98 ± 0.02
24 months	4.98 ± 0.79	0.99 ± 0.05

[a] Each number is the mean $\pm$ SEM of 5 determinations.
Animals were killed by microwave irradiation. After decapitation, brains were rapidly removed and the medial basal hypothalamus separated by taking optic chiasm as the cephalic limit, the anterior commissure as an horizontal reference, and the line between the posterior hypothalamus and the mamillary bodies as the caudal limits.

Based on the presence of unchanged beta-EP-LI levels in the hypothalamus of aged female rats, the cause of the enhanced prolactin responsiveness to FK 33-824 (see above) may be related to an alteration of the function of some neurotransmitters located "downstream" from opioid receptors.

Reportedly, opioid peptide-induced stimulation of prolactin release is mediated by an inhibition of tuberoinfundibular dopaminergic (TIDA) function (13) and/or by activation of hypothalamic serotoninergic neurons (14,15). Aging in rats is associated with an impairment of the TIDA system. Gudelsky et al. (16) found that the concentrations of dopamine in pituitary stalk plasma of aged male rats is less than half that in young male rats. Similar results have been reported in old female rats (17). The possibility might be suggested that in aged animals the impairment of the TIDA system allows the higher prolactin responsiveness to opioids. However, this hypothesis seems unlikely, for young female rats bearing an estrogen-induced prolactin-secreting tumor in which, as in old rats, an impaired TIDA function is present, exhibited complete unresponsiveness to the prolactin-releasing effect of FK 33-824 (18).

Let us consider now the biochemical state of the other neural system which mediates the prolactin response to opioids, namely the serotoninergic system. Based on the rate of accumulation of serotonin (5-HT) which follows blockade of monoamine oxidase, an increased serotonin metabolism has been postulated in aged male rats (19). Were such an alteration present also in aged female rats, this would be an event relevant to the prolactin hyperresponsiveness following administration of the opioid agonist. We have determined the concentrations of serotonin and of its main metabolite, 5-hydroxyindoleacetic acid (5-HIAA), in the hypothalamus of these rats. As it appears from Table 2, 5-HT and 5-HIAA concentrations in aged and young female rats are similar, suggesting that in old female rats the function of serotoninergic system is preserved, but not enhanced.

However, administration of 5-hydroxytryptophan, the immediate 5-HT precursor, induced a significantly higher prolactin release in old than in young rats (Fig. 3)

Table 2. *Hypothalamic concentrations of serotonin (5-HT) and 5-hydroxy-indoleacetic acid (5-HIAA) in old and young female rats.*

Age	5-HT (ug/g)	5-HIAA (ug/g)
6 months	1.48 ± 0.06[a]	1.00 ± 0.05
24 months	1.41 ± 0.02	0.93 ± 0.02

[a] Each number is the mean ± SEM of 5 determinations.
Animals were killed by decapitation, brains were rapidly removed and the medial basal hypothalamus separated according to the procedure described in Table 1. 5-HTP and 5-HIAA were assayed by HPLC, with electrochemical detection according to the method of Lackovic et al. (20).

($p < 0.05$ at 15 minutes). This finding would indicate that the hypothesis previously put forward is correct. In fact, despite the normal neuronal content of 5-HT and 5-HIAA, aged female rats would be characterized, as males, by hyperactivity of the hypothalamic serotoninergic system.

An alternative hypothesis to explain prolactin hyperresponsiveness to both FK 33-824 and 5-HTP would be that of an increased activity of the neuronal system manufacturing the still unknown prolactin-releasing factor (PRF) associated with or induced in aged female rats by the decreased activity of the TIDA system. Experimental evidence suggests in fact that PRF and not dopamine mediates the effect of 5-HT on prolactin release (21).

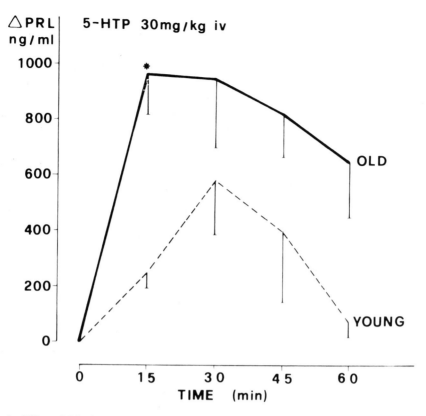

Figure 3. Effect of 5-hydroxytryptophan (5-HTP 30 mg/kg iv) on plasma prolactin levels in young (6 months) and old (22 months) female rats. Blood samples were obtained through a catheter permanently inserted in the jugular vein. Data are expressed as differences between prolactin values at each time interval and baseline. *P<0.05 vs young rats.

Considering now the LH response to naloxone, it appears that a catecholaminergic neuronal circuit is the main mediator of such response. Prior blockade of alpha adrenergic receptors or suppression of hypothalamic noradrenaline (NE) and adrenaline (E) levels rendered naloxone, administered intracranially or systemically, ineffective in stimulating LH release in steroid-primed ovariectomized rats (22,23). In addition, blockade of opiate receptors with naloxone promptly activated LH-RH release, concomitantly with NE and E release from preoptic area and medial basal hypothalamus *in vitro* (24).

The ineffectiveness of naloxone to stimulate LH release in aged female rats, a result similar to that already reported in old male rats (25), may be related to the defective NE function in aged animals (26). It has to be recalled, however, that the impaired LH response to naloxone might also be due to a defect in LH-releasing hormone (LH-RH) synthesis, (27) and/or lower pituitary responsiveness to LH-RH (28).

In all, these results allow us to draw the following conclusions:
a) Hyperprolactinemia exerts a feedback action on the hypothalamic beta-EP system,

probably enhancing its function (higher LH response to naloxone, impaired prolactin response to FK 33-824).

b) Aged female rats, despite a very high basal prolactin secretion, show normal levels of beta-EP-LI and ME in the hypothalamus and an opposite pattern of hormonal responsiveness (higher prolactin response to FK 33-824 and defective LH rise after naloxone) with respect to the experimental models of hyperprolactinemia.

c) Both endocrine responses seem to be unrelated to primary alterations in the hypothalamic opioid system, but rather would reflect alterations in other neuronal systems located "downstream" the opioid receptors.

d) Assessment of hypothalamic opioid concentrations is per se meaningless to predict the functional state (in terms of endocrine responses) of the opioid systems. The compartmentalization of the opioid systems that control different neuroendocrine functions and different neurotransmitters subserving their action are more crucial in this context.

ACKNOWLEDGMENTS

This work was supported by a special research program, "Mechanisms of Aging", C.N.R. Rome. Miss Maria Lupo provided skillful secretarial assistance.

REFERENCES

1. Panerai AE, Sawynok J, La Bella FS, Friesen HG. (1980): Endocrinology 106:1804
2. McCann SM. (1982). In: EE Muller and RM MacLeod (eds) Neuroendocrine Perspectives. Elsevier Biomedical Press, Amsterdam vol 1:1
3. Grossman A, Moult PJA, McIntyre H, Evans J, Silverstone T, Besser GM (1982): Clinical Endocrinol 17:379
4. Carter DA, Cooper IS, Inkster SE, Whitehead SA. (1984): J Endocr 101:57
5. Penalva A, Novelli A, Parenti M, Locatelli V, Muller EE, Cocchi D. (1984): Brain Res, in press
6. Petraglia F, Penalva A, Locatelli V, Cocchi D, Panerai AE, Genazzani AR, Muller EE. (1982): Endocrinology 111:1224
7. Yang HYT, Hong JS, Costa E. (1977): Neuropharmacology 16:303
8. Forman LJ, Sonntag WE, Van Vugt DA, Meites J. Neurobiol of Aging 2:281
9. Missale C, Govoni S, Croce L, Bosio A, Spano PF, Trabucchi M. (1983): J Neurochem 40:20
10. Novelli A, Cocchi D, Calderini G, Toffano G, Muller EE. (1983): Gerontology 29:362
11. Cocchi D, Novelli A, Petraglia F, Calderini G, Muller EE. (1984); In: Biggio G, Spano PF, Toffano G, Gessa GL (eds) Neuromodulation and Brain Function. Pergamon Press, Oxford
12. Forman LJ, Sonntag WE, Hylka VW, Meites J. (1983): Life Sci 33:993
13. Gudelsky GA, Porter JC. (1979): Life Sci 25:1697
14. Spampinato S, Locatelli V, Cocchi D, Vicentini L, Bajusz S, Ferri S, Muller EE. (1979): Endocrinology 105:163
15. Koenig JA, Mayfield MA, McCann SM, Krulich L. (1979): Life Sci 25:853
16. Gudelsky GA, Nansel DD, Porter JC. (1981): Brain Res 204:446
17. Reymond MJ, Porter JC. (1981): Brain Res Bull 7:69
18. Casanueva F, Cocchi D, Locatelli V, Flauto C, Zambotti F, Bestetti G, Rossi GL, Muller EE. (1982): Endocrinology 110:590

19. Simpkins JW, Mueller GP, Huang HH, Meites J. (1977): Endocrinology 100:1672
20. Lackovic Z, Parenti M, Neff NH. (1981): Europ J Pharmacol 69:347
21. Martin JB, Reichlin S, Brown GM. (1977): Clinical Neuroendocrinology. FA Davis Company, Philadelphia, p 134
22. Kalra SP (1981): Endocrinology 109:1805
23. Kalra SP, Simpkins JW. (1981): Endocrinology 109:776
24. Leadem et al. (unpublished) in Kalra SP, Kalra PS. (1984): Neuroendocrinology 38:418
25. Steger RW, Sonntag WE, Van Vugt DA, Forman LJ, Meites J. (1980): Life Sci 27:747
26. Simpkins JW, Mueller GP, Huang HH, Meites J. (1977): Endocrinology 100:1672
27. Wise PM, Ratner A. (1980): Neuroendocrinology 30:15
28. Wise PM, Ratner A, Peake GTI, J Reprod Fert 47:363

Prolactin. Basic and clinical correlates
R.M. MacLeod, M.O. Thorner and U. Scapagnini (eds.),
Fidia Research Series, vol. I,
Liviana Press, Padova © 1985

THE ROLE OF VASCULAR CHANGES IN THE ETIOLOGY OF PROLACTIN SECRETING ANTERIOR PITUITARY TUMORS

Richard I. Weiner, Kathleen A. Elias, and Florianne Monnet

Department of Obstetrics, Gynecology, and Reproductive Sciences,
University of California San Francisco, School of Medicine,
San Francisco, California 94143

The etiology of prolactin secreting tumors is unclear. One obvious hypothesis is that hyperprolactinemia and lactotroph hyperplasia are a consequence of escape from inhibitory regulation by the hypothalamus. Prolactin secretion is tonically suppressed by the hypothalamic hormone dopamine, and blockade of the action of dopamine results in hyperprolactinemia. That dopamine is also involved in the control of cell division of lactotrophs is suggested by several observations. Short term blockade of dopamine receptors with an antagonist results in increased mitotic activity and DNA content of the anterior pituitary (1,2). Destruction of the tuberoinfundibular neurons which produce dopamine leads to an increase in the density of lactotrophs (3). Finally, GH_3 cells, a rapidly dividing cell line derived from a prolactin producing tumor, are unresponsive to the action of dopamine due to the absence of dopamine receptors (4,5).

Three possible mechanisms by which lactotrophs could excape dopamine inhibition are: (1) destruction of the tuberoinfundibular neurons; (2) resistance of lactotrophs to the action of dopamine; and (3) vascularization of a region of the anterior pituitary by an artery carrying systemic blood containing a subphysiologically active concentration of dopamine. This chapter will focus on the recent findings of our study of the role of vascular changes in the etiology of estrogen-induced tumors in rats.

Several studies have demonstrated that in many mammalian species the blood supply of the anterior pituitary gland is exclusively via the hypophyseal portal vascular system (6). The hypophyseal portal system is a true portal system starting and ending in a capillary plexus (Fig. 1). Blood is carried to the primary portal capillaries via the superior, middle, and inferior hypophyseal arteries (6). The primary capillary plexus is drained via the long and short portal vessels to a secondary capillary plexus in the anterior pituitary. Blood from the primary capillary plexus contains high levels of dopamine released from nerve terminals in close apposition to these capillaries. If a region of the anterior pituitary was to receive a direct arterial blood supply, the concentration of

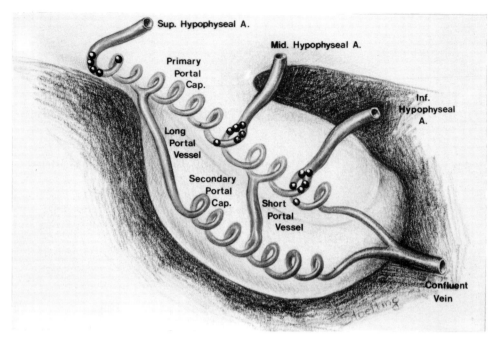

Figure 1. A diagrammatic representation of microspheres lodged in the primary portal capillaries of the hypophyseal portal vascular system. This drawing is based on the work of Page et al. (6). (from Monnet et al. [9])

dopamine in this region would be decreased by dilution with systemic blood. The concentration of dopamine in systemic blood during pregnancy is approximately 10-30 times lower than in portal blood (7).

We chose two models in rats to study the role of vascular changes in lactotroph proliferation: hyperplasia induced by mechanical destruction of the tuberoinfundibular neurons and tumors induced by estrogen. Testing a vascular hypothesis necessitated the development of a rapid technique to identify the presence of a direct arterial blood supply. Microspheres (15 um diameter polystyrene spheres), when injected into the left ventricle of the heart, are trapped in the first capillary which they reach since they are too large to traverse the capillary lumen. Therefore, they should not reach the secondary capillary plexus in the anterior pituitary, but should reach the neural lobe (Fig. 1). Confirming the earlier work by Goldman and Sapirstein (8), we demonstrated in Sprague-Dawley (S-D) rats that 15 um microspheres were unable to reach the anterior pituitary; however, numerous spheres reached the neural lobe (Fig. 2). In control animals injected first with microspheres and then perfused with Microfil, a vascular cast material, no microspheres were observed in the anterior pituitary gland but microspheres were trapped in small arterial branches of the primary capillary plexus supplying the median eminence (Fig. 3). If microspheres are observed in the anterior pituitary following some treatment the only way they could reach the gland would be via an artery directly supplying the gland (Fig. 4).

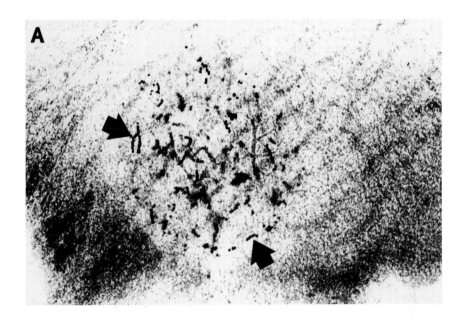

Figure 2. (A) Photomicrograph of a transilluminated cleared pituitary gland of a control rat. Microspheres (15 um) were observed within the neural lobe (arrows) in large numbers. No microspheres can be observed in the surrounding anterior pituitary gland. (B) Photomicrograph of the pituitary gland of a rat with a MBH lesion. The distribution of microspheres within the neural lobe (arrows) was identical to controls. (from Monnet et al. [9])

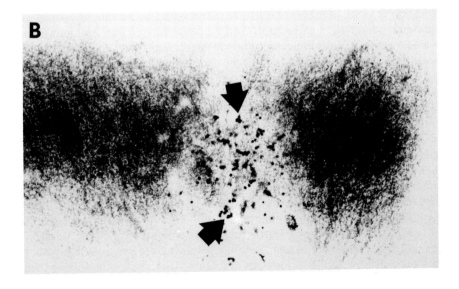

DESTRUCTION OF TUBEROINFUNDIBULAR NEURONS

It has been hypothesized that regional changes in the blood supply of the anterior pituitary could result from blockade of a portion of the portal blood supply, e.g. a thrombis in a long portal vessel. We have previously demonstrated that destruction of the medial basal hypothalamus (MBH) with a modified Halasz knife results in hyperprolactinemia and apparent hyperplasia of the lactotrophs of the anterior pituitary (3). This procedure not only destroys the tuberoinfundibular neurons, but results in extensive destruction of the primary portal capillaries in the median eminence and long portal vessels (Fig. 5). Therefore, we studied whether these lesions resulted in vascular changes in the anterior pituitary associated with the increased density of lactotrophs (9).

One month following lesions in female ovariectomized S-D rats no microspheres were observed in the anterior pituitary. However, a large number of microspheres still reached the neural lobe (Fig. 2b). From these findings it was clear that the inferior hypophyseal artery was spared by the lesion leaving a direct arterial blood supply to the neural lobe. The inferior hypophyseal artery supplying the neural lobe is a branch of a pontine artery and is below the plane of section of the lesions (Fig.4).

In the lesioned animals, the anterior pituitary received its entire blood supply from the neural lobe via the short portal vessels. This explains the observation that prolactin levels rise within minutes after the lesion, a finding inconsistent with a gland disconnected from its blood supply. Furthermore, it explains why there is little necrosis of the gland as shown by the weight of the gland and histological evaluation (3).

That the anterior pituitary gland can be supplied directly by an artery following total interruption of its blood supply was demonstrated by studies in which anterior pituitaries were transplanted under the kidney capsule. Small numbers of microspheres reached glands (30.8 ± 6.3, $n = 6$) transplanted under the kidney capsule. Observations from vascular cast experiments suggested that the capillary plexus in the gland was reconnected with small arteries from the capsule.

These findings speak to the considerable potential of the hypophyseal portal vascular complex to respond to a massive insult. It has been estimated that normally 30 percent of the blood supply of the anterior pituitary is via the short portal vessels (11), whereas following the lesion almost all of its supply is from this source. That partial destruction of the plexus results in arterial revascularization of a region of the anterior pituitary seems very unlikely from these experiments.

One question which arises from these findings is: Why doesn't long term destruction of the tuberoinfundibular neurons lead to formation of large prolactin secreting tumors? If removal of dopamine inhibition is all that is necessary, why aren't tumors formed? Indeed, there appears to be increased hyperplasia of lactotrophs following the lesion. A three-fold increase in lactotroph density was observed by morphometric analysis of immunostained sections (3). One possible explanation for the lack of further growth could be related to additional effects of the lesions. Numerous other endocrine systems of potential importance in controlling cell growth, e.g. the adrenal and thyroid glands were also affected by the lesions. Furthermore, the animals were ovariectomized at the time of lesioning, removing ovarian steroids. Clearly estrogens play a pivotal role in the control of cell division in lactotrophs as discussed in detail in the following section.

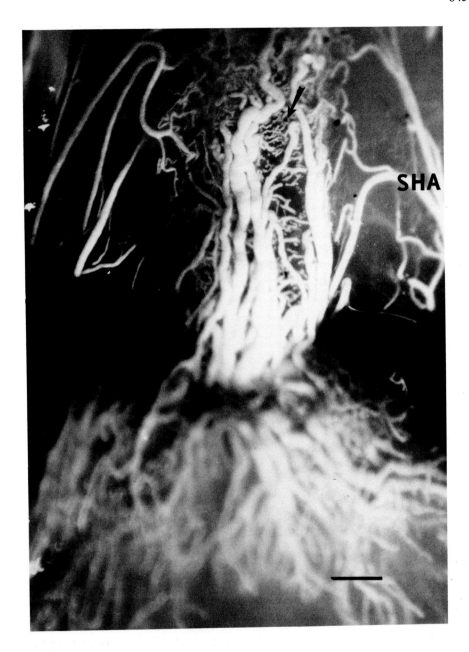

Figure 3. A photomicrograph (150x) of the ventral view of a control Sprague-Dawley rat brain. Animals were injected sequentially with microspheres followed by Microfil cast material. Microspheres (arrows) can be seen trapped in the median eminence in the vicinity of the small terminal branches of the superior hypophyseal artery (SHA). No microspheres can be seen in the anterior pituitary. Bar indicates 100 um. (from Elias and Weiner [10])

ESTROGEN INDUCED ANTERIOR PITUITARY TUMORS

The second model we examined for vascular changes in the anterior pituitary was estrogen induced tumors. We used two strains of rat, the Fischer 344 (F344) from Harlan Laboratories, which is extremely sensitive to the tumorigenic action of estrogen on the anterior pituitary, and the S-D from Simonsen Laboratories which is relatively insensitive (1)). Animals were ovariectomized and implanted with empty or 17 beta-estradiol (E_2)-filled Silastic capsules 1 cm long. Ten, 26, or 63 days post-implantation the animals were anesthetized and 2 million microspheres injected into the left ventricle of the heart. The pituitary weight, serum prolactin levels, and number of microspheres reaching the gland were determined. Prolactin levels were measured using the NIADDK radioimmunoassay.

The F344 rats showed a dramatic 6-fold increase in pituitary weight with chronic E_2 treatment (Fig. 6). Serum prolactin levels were also greatly increased. In contrast, the pituitary weight only doubled in S-D rats while serum prolactin levels were dramatically increased (Fig. 7). This dissociation between the effect of estrogen on growth of the anterior pituitary and prolactin synthesis was previously reported by Wiklund et al. (12).

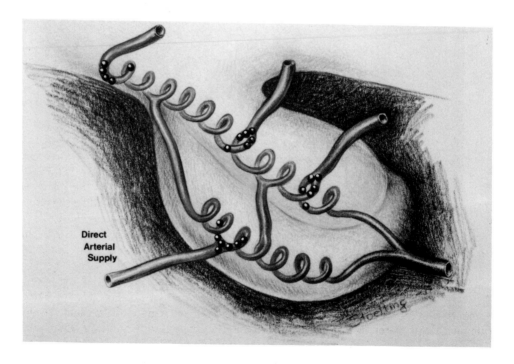

Figure 4. A diagrammatic representation of the hypophyseal portal blood supply of the rat. An aberrant artery is shown directly supplying the anterior pituitary. Microspheres are shown trapped both in the primary portal capillaries, as would normally occur, and also in the region of the anterior pituitary supplied by the aberrant vessel. (from Elias and Weiner [10])

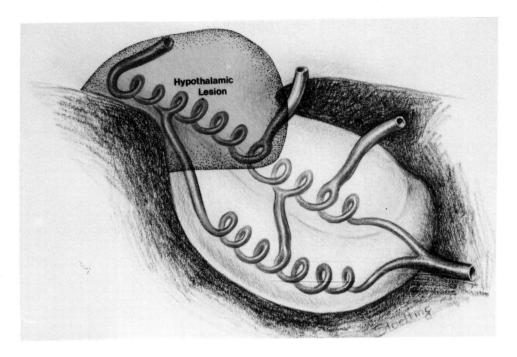

Figure 5. A diagrammatic representation of the region destroyed by the MBH lesion (shaded area). The inferior hypophyseal artery is spared by this lesion. (from Monnet et al [9])

Associated with the discrepancy in the sensitivity of the two strains to the tumorigenic action of E_2 was a dramatic difference in the numher of microspheres reaching the anterior pituitary. After 26 days of E_2 treatment the anterior pituitary of F344 rats contained 935 ± 307 microspheres while that of the S-D rats contained 165 ± 88 microspheres. While relatively few microspheres were observed in all S-D controls, 2 out of 13 F344 controls contained over 100 microspheres. This finding suggested that the vascular changes observed in these 2 animals could represent early stages in tumor development caused by endogenous estrogens. No change was observed in the number of microspheres trapped in the posterior pituitary following E_2 treatment.

As previously mentioned, S-D controls sequentially injected with microspheres and Microfil cast material had no arteries entering the gland (Fig. 3). After 63 days of E_2 the enlarged anterior pituitaries of F344 rats contained extensive areas of necrosis. Large numbers of microspheres were observed in the non-infarcted regions of the gland. Vessels filled with cast material could be observed entering the anterior pituitary which contained microspheres in the vicinity of their terminal branches (Fig. 8). Arteries were observed entering the gland from the dura. The bilateral dural vessels in this photomicrograph originated from the basilar artery. In other instances (not shown) dural vessels were demonstrated to be branches of the internal carotid and posterior communicating arteries. In anterior pituitaries which were sectioned, microspheres could be observed throughout the gland.

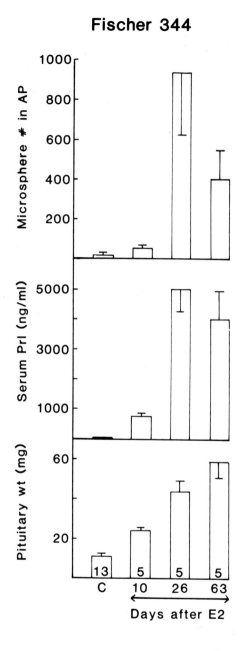

Figure 6. Anterior pituitary weight, serum prolactin levels, and number of microspheres in the anterior pituitary of ovariectomized Fischer 344 rats implanted with blank or E_2-filled Silastic capsules for various times. (from Elias and Weiner [10])

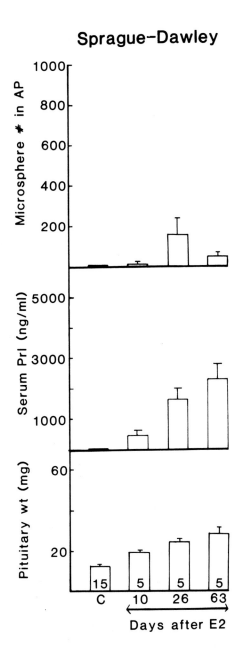

Figure 7. Anterior pituitary weight, serum prolactin levels, and number of microspheres in the anterior pituitary of ovariectomized Sprague-Dawley rats implanted with blank or E$_2$-filled Silastic capsules for various times. (from Elias and Weiner [10])

We have utilized the term tumor to describe the E_2 induced enlargement observed in these experiments. It is important to realize that the changes we observed in anterior pituitary morphology represent a diffuse hyperplasia of lactotrophs (13). Longer term estrogen treatment has been reported to result in the development of neoplastic prolactin secreting adenomas, i.e. regionalized areas of the gland comprised predominantly of one rapidly dividing cell type which is no longer under physiological regulation (14).

Our studies demonstrate the formation of new arteries (arteriogenesis) that directly enter the anterior pituitaries of rats with E_2 induced prolactin secreting tumors. The degree of arteriogenesis of the anterior pituitary closely paralleled the sensitivity of the two strains to the tumorigenic action of E_2. Although this correlation doesn't establish a cause and effect relationship it is consistent with our initial hypothesis that regions of the anterior pituitary receiving systemic blood could escape from dopaminergic regulation.

Clearly estrogen has multiple sites of action in stimulating tumor formation. Estrogen stimulates mitotic activity in the anterior pituitary (2) either by a direct action on the lactotrophs or via autocrine, paracrine, or endocrine interactions. Damage to the tuberoinfundibular dopamine neurons has been demonstrated by a decrease in dopamine fluorescence in aged female rats with spontaneous prolactin secreting tumors as well as in young females given E_2 (16). In rats with chronic hyperprolactinemia induced by E_2, dopamine concentrations in the median eminence are significantly reduced while norepinephrine and serotonin are unchanged (17). This reduction in hypothalamic dopamine may be due to the hyperprolactinemia that develops, although other studies (18) implicate a direct action of E_2 on the brain. Therefore, arteriogenesis in concert with those other mechanisms may result in tumorigenesis.

The mechanisms involved in arteriogenesis are unknown. One obvious hypothesis would be to analogize the process to angiogenesis (formation of capillary sprouts with eventual development of a microcirculatory network; 19). The growth of numerous solid tumors has been shown to be dependent on angiogenesis (20). Possibly E_2 stimulates the production of a factor which stimulates the growth and reorganization of endothelial cells of arteries supplying the dura or inhibits production of an inhibitory factor. The idea of the existence of an inhibitory factor is appealing since the occurrence of arteriogenesis in the anterior pituitary would disrupt normal hypothalamic regulation. An additional hypothesis is that the growth of the gland within the bony casing of the brain would result in compression of the gland against the dura, stimulating growth of dural arteries into the gland. This appears unlikely since anterior pituitaries transplanted under the kidney capsule of animals treated with E_2 undergo arteriogenesis.

E_2 induced cell division of lactotrophs can be blocked by the administration of the potent dopamine agonist bromocriptine (CB-154) (2). Therefore, we wondered if arteriogenesis of the anterior pituitary would also be blocked in these animals. Ovariectomized F344 rats were implanted subcutaneously with empty or E_2-filled Silastic capsules. Half the animals in both groups were also implanted with a 5 mg pellet of CB-154. Animals were anesthetized 21 days later and injected with 1 million 15 um microspheres. Pituitary weight, serum prolactin levels, and the number of microspheres reaching the anterior pituitary were determined.

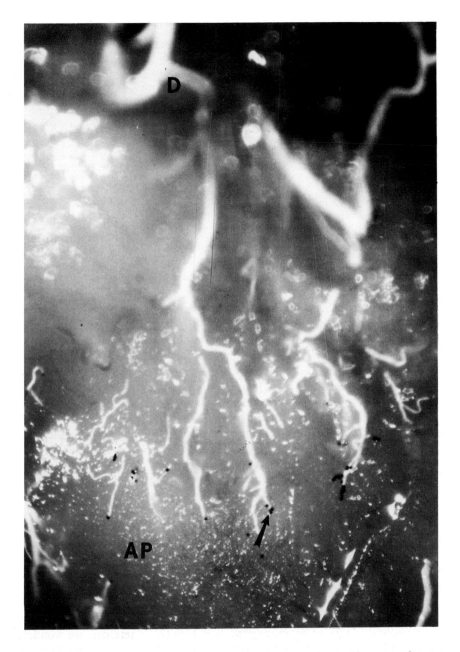

Figure 8. A photomicrograph of the ventral surface of a female Fischer 344 rat treated with estradiol for 55 days (118x). The dura (D) has been reflected. Arteries filled with cast material can be seen coursing from the dura to the anterior pituitary (AP). Microspheres (arrows) can be observed in the AP in the region of the fine branches of the arteries. In subsequent dissections the arteries supplying the dura were shown to be branches of the basilar artery. The dark appearance of extensive regions of the AP is the result of infarctions (from Elias and Weiner [10]).

E$_2$ treatment resulted in large increases in pituitary weight, serum prolactin levels, and the number of microspheres found in the anterior pituitary (Table 1). These

Table 1. *Inhibition of E$_2$ Induced Tumors by Bromocriptine (from Elias and Weiner (21))*

Groups	Control	E$_2$	CB-154	E$_2$ + CB-154
Anterior pituitary weight (mg)	12.2 ± 0.7	54.4 ± 4.5	9.6 ± 0.6	18.5 ± 0.8
Serum prolactin (ng/ml)	25.2 ± 10	4345 ± 989	12.7 ± 3	476.4 ± 89
Number microspheres	8.5 ± 1	1214 ± 250	8.6 ± 2	59 ± 13

effects were dramatically reversed by simultaneous administration of E$_2$ and CB-154. The inhibition of arteriogenesis as demonstrated by the large decrease in the number of microspheres reaching the gland was relatively proportional to the inhibition of growth of the anterior pituitary. Again we have not established the primacy of arteriogenic response in tumor formation, but these data in conjunction with the previous study clearly establish an important role for arteriogenesis in tumor growth.

A vascular hypothesis is particularly attractive in explaining the etiology of prolactin secreting adenomas in the human. It can explain the focal nature of the adenomas (22) and their excape from dopamine inhibition (23). Rather than suggesting that arteriogenesis occurs in response to estrogenic stimulation we feel that a direct arterial blood supply to a region of the anterior pituitary may be a fairly common anomaly in people. We base this speculation on postmortem observations that 22.5% of all pituitaries contained adenomas (24). Tumor frequency was independent of age or sex and the vast majority of immunostainable tumors were prolactin producing (25). The possibility exists that these large numbers of small non-functional tumors are associated with a direct arterial blood supply to a region of the anterior pituitary. Further stimulation of these focal areas of hyperplasia by tumor promoting agents (e.g. estrogens) could then lead to development of functional tumors.

ACKNOWLEDGMENTS

This work was supported by NIH Grant HD09835 and the Mellon Foundation

REFERENCES

1. Jacobi JM, Lloyd HM. (1981): Neuroendocrinology 33:97
2. Lloyd HM, Meares JD, Jacobi J. (1975): Nature 255:497
3. Cronin MJ, Cheung CY, Weiner RI, Goldsmith PC. (1982): Neuroendocrinology 34:140
4. Faure N, Cronin MJ, Martial J, Weiner RI. (1980): Endocrinology 107:1022
5. Cronin MJ, Faure N, Martial J, Weiner RI. (1980): Endocrinology 106:718
6. Bergland RM, Page RB. (1978): Endocrinology 102:1325
7. Ben-Jonathan N, Oliver C, Weiner H, Mical R, Porter J. (1977): Endocrinology 100:452
8. Goldman H, Sapirstein LA. (1962): Endocrinology 71:857

9. Monnet F, Elias KA, Fagin K, Neill A, Goldsmith P, Weiner RI. (1984): Neuroendocrinology 39:251
10. Elias K, Weiner RI. (1984): Proc Natl Acad Sci USA 81:4549
11. Porter J, Hines M, Smith K, Repass R, Smith A. (1967): Endocrinology 80:583
12. Wiklund J, Wertz N, Gorski J. (1981): Endocrinology 109:1700
13. Lloyd RV. (1983): Am J Pathol 113:198
14. Holtzman S, Stone JP, Shellabarger (1979): Cancer Res 39:779
15. Daniel P, Prichard M. (1975): Acta Endocrinologia (Suppl 201) 80:1
16. Sakar DK, Gottschall PE, Meites J. (1982): Science 218:684
17. Smythe GA, Brandstaten JF. (1980): Aust J Biol Sci 33:329
18. Eikenburg DC, Ravitz AJ, Gudelsky GA, Moore KE. (1977): J Neurol Transm 40:235
19. Clifton KH, Meyer RK (1956): Anat Rec 125:65
20. Folkman J Cotran R. (1976): Int Rev Exp Pathol 16:207
21. Elias K, Weiner RI. (1985): Endocrinology (submitted)
22. Jaffe RB. (1981): In: Jaffe RB (ed) Prolactin. Elsevier, New York, p 180
23. Barbarino A, DeMarinis L, Menini E, Anile C. (1978): J Clin Endocrinol Metab 47:1148
24. Costello RT. (1936): Am J Pathol 12:205
25. Burrow GN, Wortzman G, Rewcastle NB, Holgate RC, Kovacs K. (1981): N Engl J Med 304:156

Prolactin. Basic and clinical correlates
R.M. MacLeod, M.O. Thorner and U. Scapagnini (eds.),
Fidia Research Series, vol. I,
Liviana Press, Padova © 1985

INHIBITION OF DIETHYLSTILBESTROL-INDUCED PITUITARY TUMOR DEVELOPMENT IN BLIND-ANOSMIC FEMALE FISHER-344 RATS

Christopher A. Leadem

Department of Anatomy, College of Medicine, University of Arizona, Tucson, AZ 85724

The pineal gland of rodents has long been known to produce profound changes in the neuroendocrine-reproductive axis (1). Blinding or the placement of hamsters in short photoperiods results in a regression of the reproductive organs within three months that is preventable by the prior removal of the pineal gland. Similar effects can be elicited in rats if, in addition to blinding, prepubertal animals are rendered anosmic by olfactory bulbectomy (2). This procedure apparently sensitizes the rat to the anti-gonadotrophic effects of an activated pineal gland in that anosmia alone has little or no effect on gonadal function in rats. Pinealectomy largely prevents the effects of blinding and olfactory bulbectomy in rats. All of these effects of blinding or short photoperiods can be mimicked by the daily afternoon administration of the pineal hormone melatonin both in hamsters (3) and anosmic rats (4).

Paralleling these changes in reproductive physiology in blind-anosmic (BA) rats are alterations in pituitary function. Prolactin synthesis, storage, and release are all reduced in BA rats (5,6); furthermore, this effect is not a consequence of gonadal regression (7). The ultrastructural morphology of gonadal cells correlates well with these functional alterations (8). Blinding and anosmia result in a marked decrease in cell size from that seen in intact rats. There are scant arrays of rough endoplasmic reticulum, small Golgi complexes with few immature secretory granules, few mature secretory granules, and rare exocytosis patterns. Combined blinding and induced anosmia not only cause a potent hypotrophy of individual mammotrophs but also produce profound changes in the entire population of these cells. It is well documented that the anterior pituitary of BA rats weighs approximately 50% of that in control animals (2,9). We reported that this weight reduction is accompanied by a 30% decrease in the total DNA content of the gland (5-7), thus indicating a considerable reduction in pituitary cell number. Furthermore, light microscopic immunocytochemistry of mammotrophs revealed that the number of these cells is decreased in BA rats in proportion to the decrease in anterior pituitary size (8); this apparently accounts for the majority of the reduction in anterior pituitary cell number. Pinealectomy significantly prevents all of these effects. We concluded, therefore, that the pineal causes both hypotrophy and hypoplasia of mammotrophs.

The hypoplastic effect of the pineal on prolactin cells apparently occurs primarily around the time of puberty. In a study of the temporal development of the inhibitory influences of the pineal on mammotrophs (10) it was found that one week after blinding and olfactory bulbectomy, when rats were 31 days old (just prior to puberty), there were no significant alterations of mammotroph activity, pituitary weight, or pituitary cell number from that seen in control animals. At four weeks after treatment, when the animals were 52 days old (post-pubertal), there were the expected (11) pubertal increases in pituitary weight and pituitary cell number, and in prolactin synthesis, storage, and release in intact animals. Significantly, combined blinding and induced anosmia severely retarded the development of all of these parameters. Once again, the effects were largely preventable by pinealectomy. The pineal, therefore, can by some mechanism inhibit the normal development of mammotrophs that occurs at puberty. This inhibition includes an almost complete abolition of the mammotroph hyperplasia expected at this time.

Since the pineal of blind-anosmic rats apparently inhibits the normal proliferation of prolactin cells that occurs at puberty, it was of interest to determine whether this prolactin-inhibitory effect could affect the abnormal proliferation of mammotrophs in experimentally-induced prolactinomas. To test this possibility we chose to use the diethylstilbestrol (DES)-treated Fisher 344 (F344) rat. This model was originally described by Dunning et al. (12) who found that female F344 rats developed pituitary adenomas that were 40 times the size of normal pituitaries within seven weeks of treatment, whereas the other rat strains tested required much longer time periods (23-42 weeks) for more modest tumor growth (6-10 times normal). With this finding many subsequent studies have been performed to further characterize these tumors. The tumors have been found to be composed primarily of degranulated prolactin cells (13,14) and to contain high levels of prolactin (13). The tumor tissue exhibits a sizable increase in protein synthesis with a marked augmentation in prolactin production (15). Additionally, serum prolactin levels are increased 100-fold in these animals (14). In a recent study, Wiklund et al. (16) have followed the temporal development of DES-induced pituitary tumors in Fisher 344 rats. Pituitary weight and DNA content exhibited significant increases as little as two weeks after initiation of treatment and continued increasing exponentially for eight weeks. Prolactin synthesis, on the other hand, was significantly increased over control animals at the earliest time point tested (1 week). An increase in pituitary DNA synthesis parallels the time course for prolactin synthesis in these animals (17). Furthermore, Phelps and Hymer (18) have shown that there is a marked hyperplasia and hypertrophy of immuncytochemically-stained mammotrophs in these tumors.

The DES-treated F344 rat appears to be one of the better experimental models currently available for the study of prolactinoma control. As with the findings in humans, dopamine agonists have been shown to affect pituitary tumors in estrogen-treated rats. Bromocriptine has been observed to interfere with the stimulatory actions of short-term estrogen treatment on pituitary DNA synthesis and prolactin secretion and to increase pituitary concentrations of prolactin in these rats (19,20). Furthermore, Kalberman et al. (21), using the DES-treated Fisher 344 rat, found that after six days of treatment with bromocriptine, pituitary tumor weight, serum prolactin levels, and pituitary DNA synthesis were all reduced in comparison to vehicle-treated controls. These data appear to be at odds with those studies which have delineated a potent antidopaminergic effect of estrogens on prolactin cells (22,23). These differences could be due to the fact that the antidopaminergic action of estrogens may be an acute effect of these steroids that dissipates during chronic treatment, or to the fact that the chronically-treated prolactin cells still retain enough sensitivity to dopamine to respond to the potent and long-lasting agonistic effects of bromocriptine. Interestingly, Casanueva et al. (24) have found that rats chronically treated with estrogens failed to demonstrate either a stimulation of pro-lactin release in response to dopamine antagonist administration or an inhibition of prolactin secretion after injection of nomifensine, an activator of central dopaminergic activity. Moreover, these authors found progressive reductions of hypothalamic dopamine concentrations in these animals as well as pathological changes in the ar-cuate nucleus. These data indicate that, as has been expected in humans with prolac-tinomas (25), there may be a central defect in dopaminergic neurons that contributes to the induction and growth of prolactinomas.

To investigate the influence of combined blinding and anosmia on prolactinoma development in the present study, adult female Fisher 344 rats (120-130 g, Charles River Laboratories) were either blinded and olfactory bulbectomized, or sham-olfactory bulbectomized. Blinding and olfactory bulbectomy were performed as previously describ-ed (5). Sham bulbectomy was similar to olfactory bulbectomy in all regards with the exception of aspiration of the bulb tissue. Animals were allowed to recover for two weeks in a 14:10 light:dark photoperiod. At this time animals were assigned to one of the following groups: sham-operated animals that received empty implants (Sham), sham-operated animals that received 5 mg DES implants (Sham-DES), and blind-anosmic rats that received 5 mg DES implants (BA-DES). The implants were made from Silastic tubing as described by Wiklund et al. (16) and implanted subcutaneously in the in-terscapular region. All animals were sacrificed eight weeks after the initiation of DES-treatment, body and reproductive organ weights were recorded, and trunk blood was collected for subsequent prolactin radioimmunoassay. The anterior pituitary of each animal was weighed and one half of the gland incubated *in vitro* to determine the rate of prolactin synthesis. The *in vitro* incubations were performed by placing each hemipituitary in 0.5 ml of minimum essentials medium containing 10 uCi [^{3}H]-leucine that had been gassed previously for one hour with 95% O_2: 5% CO_2. The hemipituitaries were then incubated for five hours at 37 C in a Dubnoff metabolic shaker with constant shaking and gassed with 95% O_2: 5% CO_2. At the end of the incuba-tions the media were saved and the hemipituitaries weighed and then sonicated in 0.5 ml phosphate-buffered saline. Serum, media, and pituitary homogenates were radioim-munoassayed for immunoreactive prolactin using a kit supplied by the National Pituitary Program. Newly synthesized prolactin was assayed by polyacrylamide gel electrophoresis followed by scintillation counting of the prolactin bands (5). Pituitary content of DNA, RNA and protein were determined by colorimetric assay (26). All data were analyzed by one-way analysis of variance followed by the Newman-Keuls multiple range test.

As expected, chronic treatment with DES resulted in profound changes in the pituitaries of female F344 rats. After eight weeks of exposure to DES, anterior pituitary

Table 1. *The effects of blinding and anosmia (BA) on diethylstilbestrol (DES)-induced alterations in body, ovarian and uterine weights as well as anterior pituitary DNA, RNA, and protein content*

Treatment	n	Body Wt(g)	Ovarian Wt(mg)	Uterine Wt(mg)	DNA (ug)	Anterior Pituitary RIA (ug)	Protein (ug)
Intact	7	177 ± 2	60.9 ± 3.1	320.7 ± 26.5	20.81 ± 4.47	104.71 ± 8.21	724.40 ± 89.59
DES	9	150 ± 4[a]	52.4 ± 3.7	912.7 ± 44.0[a]	274.31 ± 34.59[a]	548.06 ± 47.39[a]	2216 ± 340.06[a]
BA-DES	7	153 ± 2[a]	63.0 ± 4.5	941.9 ± 111.0[a]	163.39 ± 21.52[ax]	336.20 ± 27.43[ax]	1093.83 ± 97.06[x]

a, $p < 0.05$ vs Intact
x, $p < 0.05$ vs DES

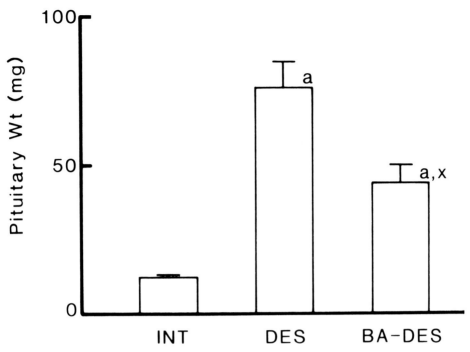

Figure 1. The effects of blinding and anosmia (BA) on diethylstilbestrol (DES)-induced changes in anterior pituitary weight in adult Fisher 344 rats. Combined blinding and olfactory bulbectomy were performed two weeks prior to implantation of 5 mg DES capsules, the animals were killed eight weeks later. There were 7-9 animals in each group. a, $p < 0.05$ vs intact (INT) controls; x, $p < 0.05$ vs DES animals.

weight was increased 5-fold over Sham animals (Fig. 1). This increase in weight was largely due to hyperplasia of pituitary cells as evidenced by the 13-fold increase in pituitary DNA content (Table 1). There was also an accompanying increase in RNA and protein content within the pituitaries of Sham-DES animals (Table 1). These findings agree well with those of Wiklund et al. (16) and demonstrate the potent effects of DES on the pituitaries of this strain of rats. DES also caused a decrease in body weight and a massive hypertrophy of the uteri of these animals (Table 1).

Of utmost importance for the present study was the finding that combined blinding and olfactory bulbectomy inhibited the DES-induced increases in pituitary weight (Fig. 1) and pituitary DNA content (Table 1) by 41% ($p < 0.01$) and 40% ($p < 0.01$), respectively. Similar differences were also evident for the pituitary content of both RNA and protein (Table 1). These data indicate a potent inhibition of DES-induced pituitary tumor induction and/or growth in blind-anosmic female rats. The similarity in the percentage of reduction of tumor weight and DNA content suggests that the primary effect of this dual-sensory deprivation is an inhibition of pituitary cell hyperplasia rather than strictly a hypotrophy of the cells.

Evidence that these effects of both DES and combined blinding and anosmia involve the prolactin cell population is that the changes in prolactin synthesis, storage, and release parallel the alterations in pituitary tumor size. Serum prolactin levels were increased 75-fold in Sham-DES versus Sham animals (Fig. 2), an increase that was attenuated by 47% (p<0.01) in BA-DES rats. Likewise prolactin synthesis, as measured by the incorporation of [³H]-leucine *in vitro*, was increased 7-fold in Sham-DES animals over that in the Sham group (Fig. 3). Once again, combined blinding and anosmia resulted in a 43% (p<0.01) reduction in the effects of DES on prolactin synthesis. Finally, blinding and olfactory bulbectomy resulted in a reduction in the high levels of total immunoreactive prolactin *in vitro* found in the Sham-DES group (Fig. 4). Interestingly, when the immunoreactive prolactin data were expressed in terms of pituitary weight there was a reduction in the concentration of immunoreactive prolactin in the Sham-DES group compared to the Sham animals; blinding and anosmia did not affect this decrease (Fig. 4).

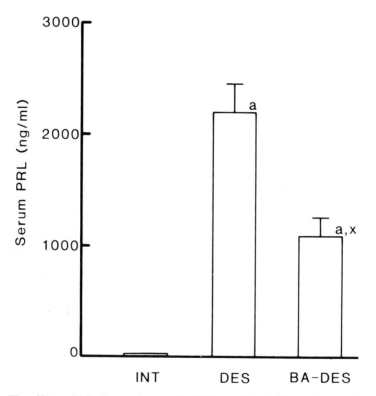

Figure 2. The effects of blinding and anosmia (BA) on diethylstilbestrol (DES)-induced alterations in serum prolactin levels of F344 rats eight weeks after implantation of DES capsules. Data are expressed in units of standard rat prolactin RP-3. See Figure 1 for more detail. a, p < 0.05 vs intact (INT) controls; x, p < 0.05 vs DES animals.

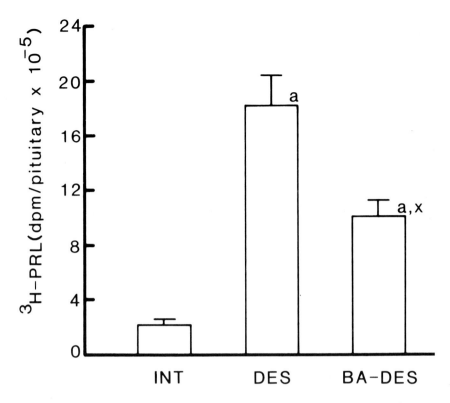

Figure 3. The effects of combined blinding and anosmia (BA) on the incorporation of [³H]-leucine into prolactin *in vitro* by pituitaries from diethylstilbestrol (DES)-treated rats. See Figure 1 for more details. a, $p < 0.05$ vs intact (INT) controls; x, $p < 0.05$ vs DES animals.

These data on mammotroph activity indicate that the increases in pituitary weight and DNA content in DES-treated rats can be largely accounted for by an increase in the activity of prolactin cells. This supports the findings of others (13-16) that the DES-induced pituitary tumors in F344 rats are composed principally of hyperactive prolactin cells. These data also support the conclusion that the inhibition of tumor growth in blind-anosmic rats is predominantly a product of the inhibition of mammotroph activity and perhaps prolactin cell proliferation in that in dual-sensory deprived animals all parameters of prolactinoma development tested here were attenuated to approximately the same extent as that seen for the inhibition of tumor weight and DNA content (i.e. 40-47%).

Though this evidence strongly indicates primary involvement of the prolactin cell population in the inhibition of tumor growth in BA rats, other pituitary cell populations may still be involved. Blinding and anosmia have been shown to affect pituitary levels of several anterior pituitary hormones including luteinizing hormone (LH), follicle stimulating hormone (FSH), and growth hormone (GH) (27-29). It is not probable that the gonadotroph population is involved in these effects in that chronic treatment

662

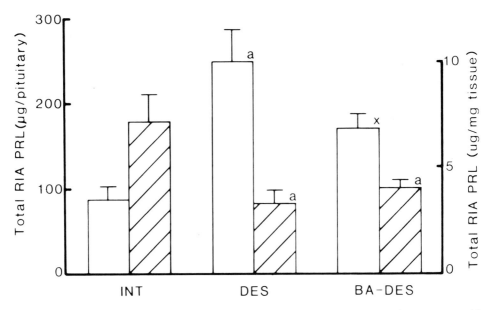

Figure 4. The effects of blinding and anosmia (BA) on the total amount of radioimmunoassayable prolactin *in vitro* in pituitaries from diethylstilbestrol (DES)-treated rats. See Figure 1 for more details. a, $p < 0.05$ vs intact (INT) controls; x, $p < 0.05$ vs DES animals.

with DES should produce an inhibition of both LH and FSH due to the negative feedback effects of estrogens on these hormones (30). Indeed, in the present study circulating levels of LH were reduced in Sham-DES animals compared to sham-implanted controls (Table 2); this effect was not altered in BA-DES animals. Similarly it is unlikely that the somatotroph population or alterations in circulating GH would be involved in the reduction of tumor size due to the fact that DES inhibits somatotroph activity (15,17,31) rather than causing a proliferation of these cells. In support of such an effect, body weights were reduced in DES-treated rats (Table 1) and this was not altered in BA-DES animals. This latter finding might at first seem to be at odds with previously published reports that combined blinding and anosmia causes a retardation of somatic growth by an apparent inhibition of GH (28). However, it is likely that DES-treatment masks any further reductions that may be caused by combined blinding and anosmia.

Table 2. *The effects of blinding and anosmia (BA) on diethylstilbestrol (DES)-induced alterations in serum luteinizing hormone (LH) levels.*

Treatment	Serum LH (ng/ml)
Intact	0.305 ± 0.042
DES	0.122 ± 0.008[a]
BA-DES	0.122 ± 0.012[a]

Serum LH values were determined by radioimmunoassay using reagents supplied by the National Pituitary Program. Hormone levels are expressed in units of RP-2 rat LH standard.

[a] $p < 0.05$ vs Intact

The mechanisms by which combined blinding and anosmia may affect prolactinoma development are currently being investigated in this laboratory. The most likely mediator of these effects in blind-anosmic rats is the pineal gland. Previous data from this lab (5-8) and others (2) indicate that the pineal is primarily responsible for the neuroendocrine-reproductive effects of combined blinding and olfactory bulbectomy.

The pineal might affect mammotrophs in several ways. First, pineal hormones may work through the hypothalamus by altering the secretion of controlling factors. In support of such a conclusion, the hypothalamic content of prolactin-inhibiting and prolactin-releasing factor activities are altered in BA rats (32,33). Recently, several studies have demonstrated that hypothalamic dopamine content and turnover can be affected by photoperiod through the pineal (34-38). Steger et al. (34,36) have found a diminution of dopamine turnover in the medial basal hypothalami of male hamsters exposed to short photoperiod for 10-12 weeks. Similarly, hypothalamic tyrosine hydroxylase activity was found to be decreased in blind-anosmic female rats thirty days after surgery (37). These authors concluded that the activity of tuberoinfundibular dopamine neurons is reduced in blind-anosmic rats. In contrast, Kumar et al. (38) found an increase in medial basal hypothalamic dopamine turnover in female hamsters exposed to constant darkness for 10 weeks. The resolution of these discrepancies must await studies that attempt to define the detailed time course of photoperiod-induced changes in dopamine turnover and correlate these changes with alterations in mammotroph activity. Importantly, it has been demonstrated previously that the prolactin-inhibiting effects of daily afternoon melatonin injections in anosmic male rats can be blocked by the administration of the dopamine receptor antagonist pimozide (39). Overall, these studies suggest that the pineal might affect pituitary prolactin secretion by altering the secretion of hypothalamic dopamine.

A second way in which the pineal might affect prolactin is via a direct effect of pineal hormones on the mammotrophs. The pineal is known to contain both prolactin releasing and prolactin-inhibiting factors (40,41). In this regard, arginine vasotocin and melatonin have been shown to directly stimulate and inhibit, respectively, the secretion of prolactin in vitro (42,43). Another possible direct action of the pineal hormones on prolactin cells is that these substances could interact with the dopaminergic control of mammotrophs. We have previously observed (unpublished observations) that eight weeks after combined blinding and anosmia in male Sprague-Dawley rats, the prolactin-inhibitory effect of 10 uM dopamine in vitro was significantly increased over that seen in control animals. Pinealectomy significantly prevented this increase in dopamine sensitivity. These findings are similar to that found in male hamsters exposed to short-photoperiod (35). Such an increase in sensitivity indicates two possibilities: first, that pineal hormones directly increase dopamine sensitivity, or second, that the changes in sensitivity are a result of some pineal-induced alteration of dopamine secretion from the hypothalamus.

Though the pineal gland is the probable mediator of the effects of blinding and anosmia, there is some evidence to suggest that not all of the effects of this dual-sensory deprivation can be prevented by pinealectomy. We have previously seen that though pinealectomy largely prevents the reduction in anterior pituitary weight in blind-anosmic rats, it is not a complete reversal (5-8). An intriguing possibility for pineal-independent effects of light-deprivation is that there are now recognized to be other sources of melatonin besides the pineal gland; these include the brain, retina, harderian gland, and gut (44-46). These alternate sources of melatonin might play a role in the photoperiodic control of reproduction and, hence, might affect the hypothalamus or pituitary.

In conclusion, the findings of the present study indicate that combined blinding and anosmia result in an inhibition of estrogen-induced prolactinoma development. The mechanism of this effect is currently unknown but these findings present the intriguing possibility that pineal-mediated events may, someday, be used in the clinical management of prolactinomas. Particularly in view of the possible interactions of pineal hormones with the dopaminergic control of mammotrophs, it could be envisaged that administration of such compounds may activate endogenous dopamine neuron activity and/or sensitize the prolactinomas to the effects of either endogenous dopamine or exogenously administered bromocriptine.

REFERENCES

1. Reiter RJ. (1980): Endocrine Review 2:109
2. Reiter RJ. (1974): In: Knobil E, Sawyer C (eds) Handbook of Physiology, Endocrinology, Vol IV, Part 2. American Physiological Society, Washington, DC, p 219
3. Tamarkin L, Westrom WK, Hamill AI, Goldman BD. (1976): Endocrinology 99:1534
4. Blask DE, Nodelman J. (1979): Neuroendocrinology 17:362
5. Leadem CA, Blask DE. (1981): Neuroendocrinology 33:268
6. Leadem CA, Blask DE. (1982): Biol Reprod 26:413
7. Leadem CA, Blask DE. (1982): Neuroendocrinology 35:133
8. Leadem CA, Blask DE. (1982): Cell Tiss Res 227:343
9. Donofrio RJ, Reiter RJ. (1972): J Reprod Fertil 31:159
10. Leadem CA, Blask DE. J Pineal Res, in press
11. Sasaki F, Sano M. (1980): J Endocrinol 85:283
12. Dunning WF, Curtis MR, Segaloff A. (1947): Cancer Res 7:511
13. Clifton KH, Meyer RK. (1956): Anat Rec 125:65
14. DeNicola AF, Von Lawzewitsh I, Kaplan SE, Libertun C. (1978): J Natl Cancer Inst 61:753
15. Kaplan SE, DeNicola AF. (1976): J Natl Cancer Inst 56:37
16. Wiklund J, Wertz N, Gorski J. (1981): Endocrinology 109:1700
17. Wiklund J, Gorski J. (1982): Endocrinology 111:1140
18. Phelps C, Hymer WC. (1983): Neuroendocrinology 37:23
19. Davies C, Jacobi J, Lloyd HM, Meares JD. (1974): J Endocrinol 61:411
20. Gala RR, Boss RS. (1975): Proc Soc Exp Biol Med 149:330
21. Kalbermann LE, Machiavelli GA, DeNicola AF, Weissenberg LS, Burdman JA. (1980): J Endocrinol 87:221
22. Raymond V, Bealieu M, Labrie F, Boissier J. (1978): Science 200:1171
23. West B, Dannies PS. (1980): Endocrinology 106:1108
24. Casanueva F, Cocchi D, Locatelli V, Flauto C, Zambotti F, Bestetti GL, Muller E. (1982): Endocrinology 110:590
25. Fine SA, Frohman LA. (1978): J Clin Inves 61:973
26. Lawson GM, Tsai M, Tsai SY, Minghetti PP, McClure ME, O'Malley B. (1982): In: Schrader WT, O'Malley BW (eds) Laboratory Methods Manual for Hormone Action and Molecular Endocrinology. Dept Cell Biology, Baylor College of Medicine.

27. Johnson LY, Reiter RJ. (1978): Prog Reprod Biol 4:116
28. Sorrentino S, Reiter RJ, Schlach DS, Donofrio RJ. (1971): Neuroendocrinology 8:116
29. Johnson LY. (1982): In: Reiter RJ (ed) The Pineal Gland, Vol III-Extra-Reproductive Effects. CRC Press, Boca Raton, p 107
30. Kalra SP. (1983): Endocrine Reviews 4:311
31. Reichlin S. (1974): In: Knobil E, Sawyer C (eds) Handbook of Physiology, Endocrinology, Vol IV, Part 2. American Physiological Society, Washington, DC, p 405
32. Blask DE, Reiter RJ. (1975): Neuroendocrinology 17:362
33. Blask DE, Reiter RJ. (1978): Mol Cell Endocrinol 11:243
34. Steger RW, Bartke A, Goldman BD. (1982): Biol Reprod 26:437
35. Steger RW, Bartke A, Goldman BD, Soares MJ, Talamantes F. (1983): Biol Reprod 29:872
36. Steger RW, Reiter RJ, Siler-Krodr TM. (1984): Neuroendocrinology 38:158
37. Morgan WM, Reiter RJ. (1982): In: Reiter RJ (ed) The Pineal and Its Hormones. Alan Liss, New York, p 243
38. Kumar MSA, Chen CL, Besch EL, Simpkins JW, Estes KS. (1982): Brain Res Bull 8:33
39. Blask DE, Nodelman J, Leadem CA. (1980): Experientia 36:1008
40. Blask DE, Vaughan MK, Reiter RJ, Johnson LY, Vaughan GM. (1976): Endocrinology 99:152
41. Chang N, Ebels I, Benson B. (1979): J Neural Trans 46:139
42. Vaughan MK, Blask DE. (1978): Prog Reprod Biol 4:90
43. Hanew K, Shiino M, Rennels EG. (1980): Proc Soc Exp Biol Med 164:257
44. Yu HS, Pang SF, Pang PL, Brown GM. (1981): Neuroendocrinology 32:262
45. Pang SF, Brown GM, Grota LJ, Chambers JW, Rodman RL. (1977): Neuroendocrinology 23:1
46. Bubenick GA. (1980): Horm Res 12:313

Prolactin. Basic and clinical correlates
R.M. MacLeod, M.O. Thorner and U. Scapagnini (eds.),
Fidia Research Series, vol. I,
Liviana Press, Padova © 1985

VARIABILITY OF STRUCTURE AND FUNCTION
IN PROLACTINOMAS

Alex M. Landolt

Department of Neurosurgery, University of Zurich
CH-8091 Zurich, Switzerland

The pathologist classifies tumors by forming groups of tumors that bear common morphologic characteristics. Specimens within individual tumor groups are not necessarily identical and when morphologic variations occur their importance must not be overestimated or used to create new subgroups without evidence of biological differences (1). In practice, clinicians frequently request that pathologists relate tumor morphology to biological behavior in order to determine prognosis and selection of postoperative treatment. Difficulties are inherent in answering this request, however, since the morphology of a tumor may vary under treatment without a concomitant change in its nature. We will demonstrate in the following paragraphs that drugs may change the structure, ultrastructure, and secretory function of prolactinomas and that these changes persist only as long as the drug is used.

Comparison of the ultrastructure of biopsy specimens with patients' hormone levels allows, to some extent, an understanding of their relationship (2-4). Such an analysis shows that secretory activity is affected by the relative size of the nucleus and nucleolus, the size and differentiation of the rough surfaced endoplasmic reticulum (RER), and the size of the Golgi apparatus. Other influential factors include the occurrence of oncocytic mitochondria, a sign of cellular degeneration, and the number and size of secretory granules stored, as well as the number of lysosomes engaged in crinophagy. The amount of hormone released by an adenoma cell is the net result of the function of these positive and negative factors and cannot be judged on the basis of only one factor (e.g. size of secretory granules).

It is possible to modify the size, numerical density, and differentiation of every cell organelle participating in hormone synthesis from gene translation to messenger RNA (mRNA) in the nucleolus, ribosomes attached to the RER, the RER, Golgi apparatus, secretory granules and their release at the cell surface (4). Such modifications, caused by hormonal and pharmacologic factors, can change the cell ultrastructure and its function simultaneously. That both occur rapidly demonstrates the flexibility of normal and neoplastic pituitary cells.

668

The evaluation of treatment-induced changes of cell structure in pituitary adenomas is difficult because of the naturally occurring variability of individual specimens within one group of adenomas. Interpreting findings in single cases of treated and untreated adenomas is therefore hazardous. Examination of individual adenomas before and after use of a drug can be done in experimental animals but is only rarely possible in humans (5). Transplantation of adenomas into thymus-dysgenetic "nude" mice followed by examination of the original adenoma, the transplanted control, and the transplanted adenoma after drug therapy demonstrates that the transplantation alone causes tissue degeneration that may interfere with evaluation of drug effect (6). The same may be true in some adenomas explanted in vitro (7,8). Morphometric examination of pituitary adenomas offers a different solution to the problem. The measurement of morphologic tumor characteristics (cell size, nucleus size, surface of RER, etc.) demonstrates that these parameters of individual adenomas show a normal distribution (Fig. 1). This allows a comparison between groups of treated and untreated adenomas using statistical methods. The results of such quantitative studies follow, together with results of qualitative examinations.

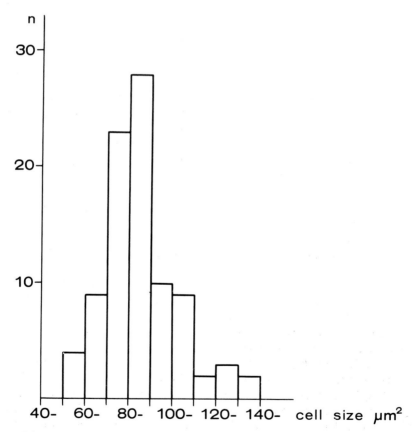

Figure 1. Histogram of average cell size found in 90 prolactinomas. Mean value 85.3 um², minimum 55.4 um², maximum 134.5 um², standard deviation 16.7 um².

STRUCTURE AND ULTRASTRUCTURE OF THE PROLACTINOMA

Only a short description of the structure and ultrastructure of the typical prolactinoma will be given because this topic is presented in detail by K. Kovacs in this volume.

The typical prolactinoma cell is round, oval, or polygonal and has an average section area of 85 um^2 (Figs. 1, 2a). The shape of the nucleus varies according to the tissue fixation technique used. It is round or oval in unfixed tissue culture material, supravital cytological smear preparations, and osmium-fixed, plastic-embedded tissue specimens (3,7,9-11). The polymorphic, indented shape observed after the glutaraldehyde fixation commonly used in electron microscopy must be judged to be an artifact. The nucleus occupies 35-48% of the cell section area (12-14). The nucleolus is usually prominent. Electron microscopy demonstrates that in the majority of cases the cytoplasm contains large RER complexes and prominent cisterns of the Golgi apparatus engaged in the formation of secretory granules (Fig. 3a). Mitochondria are usually inconspicuous. Secretory granules are 100-300 nm in diameter, and few remain stored in the cytoplasm of the usual sparsely granulated prolactinoma. Ongoing granule release can be observed along the entire cell circumference in about 60% of the biopsy specimens (15). Usually only one granule is released per secretory pit. Simultaneous release of two or more

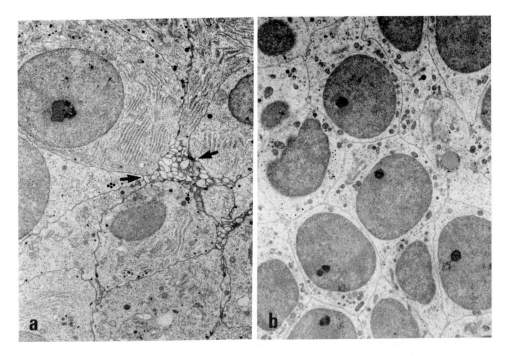

Figure 2. Low-power magnification electron micrograph of prolactinomas. (a) Untreated control adenoma. Note large areas of cytoplasm containing complexes of the rough-surfaced endoplasmic reticulum, Golgi cisterns bearing slender cell processes (arrows). (b) Bromocriptine-treated (six weeks, 7.5 mg/day) adenoma. The areas of cytoplasm are shrunken, contain few organelles and bear only few processes. Osmium fixation, magnification x3250.

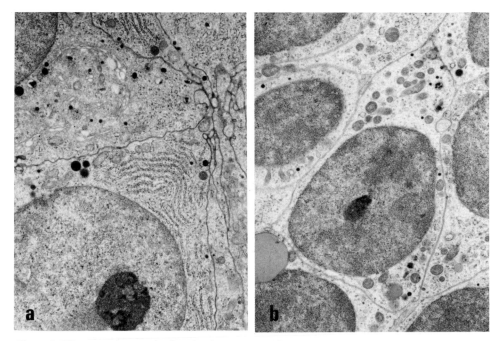

Figure 3. Electron micrograph of prolactinomas, at a higher magnification. Same biopsy specimens as in Figure 2. (a) Untreated control with differentiated cell organelles. Note cell processes. (b) Bromocriptine-treated biopsy specimen with reduced rough-surfaced endoplasmic reticulum and lipid bodies. Osmium fixation, magnification x6800.

granules into one pit is rare. A few prolactinomas show a dense accumulation of larger secretory granules with diameters of 600 nm and more (1,3,9,16,27). Occasionally, a few densely granulated cells can be found in otherwise sparsely granulated prolactinomas.

ESTROGEN-INDUCED CHANGES

It is well known that estrogens raise the plasma prolactin concentration in patients with prolactinomas (18). Parenteral estrogen administration to patients with invasive prolactinomas can cause a swelling of the tumors and lead to acute cranial nerve compression (19). The increased estrogen secretion during pregnancy can also cause an enlargement of prolactinomas with signs of tumor pressure (20-22). Histologic and ultrastructural examination of eight estrogen-treated prolactinomas revealed signs of tumor proliferation with increased numbers of mitoses, nuclear and nucleolar abnormalities, and interstitial hemorrhages (23). However, *in vitro* treatment of prolactinoma tissue cultures with estradiol (0.1-0.001 ug/ml tissue culture fluid) failed to increase the secretion rate of prolactin in experiments lasting four days (7). This contradicts the finding of a greater frequency and higher activity of estrogen receptors in prolactinomas than in other types of pituitary adenoma (24). A comparison of estrogen treated with untreated prolactinoma tissue cultures demonstrated the presence of many electron-dense inclusion bodies and lysosomes in the treatment group (7), however, no studies with quantitative determination of estrogen-induced cell changes are available.

BROMOCRIPTINE-INDUCED CHANGES

Light microscopic and low-power electron microscopic examination of prolactinomas treated at least four to six weeks with bromocriptine show a pronounced reduction in cytoplasm and a diminution of the nucleoli compared to untreated controls. The nuclei shrink less (Fig. 2a, b). The nuclear-cytoplasmic ratio increases from 0.92 to 1.11 (13), causing the nuclei to become densely accumulated and surrounded by narrow rims of cytoplasm. Cell necrosis is rarely seen (Fig. 4) (25). Treatment of three months or more causes an increase in the amount of perivascular fibrous tissue (26).

Electron microscopy at higher magnification demonstrates that the previously large complexes of RER are reduced to single dispersed tubules and vesicles (Fig. 3b). The area occupied by Golgi cisterns is reduced. Secretory granules are still present in a number equal to or larger than that in control biopsy specimens. The same is true of lysosomes and lipid bodies (14,27).

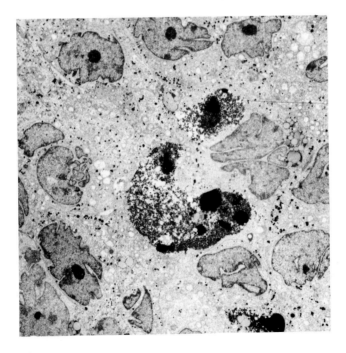

Figure 4. Short-term (7 days) bromocriptine-treated prolactinoma with few scattered, necrotic cells. Note deformation of cell nuclei caused by glutaraldehyde prefixation. Glutaraldehyde-osmium fixation, magnification x1800.

The immunohistochemical reaction with anti-prolactin causes positive staining in 93-100% of untreated prolactinomas (25,28,29). This quantitative procedure

Table 1. *Immunohistochemical staining with anti-prolactin of untreated and bromocriptine-treated prolactinomas*

		Immunostaining			Total number of cases
	+++	+	+	−	
Controls	3	5	0	0	8
Acute treatment (7 days)	1	3	2	0	6
Chronic treatment (4-6 weeks)	2	1	4	1	8

The control cases were selected randomly from a series of 32 immunostained, untreated adenomas.
+ + + : More than 50% immunoreactive cells
+ + : About 1/3 immunoreactive cells
+ : Few immunoreactive cells
0 : No immunoreactive cells
All reactions were done with the peroxidase-antiperoxidase (PAP) method of Sternberger (30) with formaldehyde-fixed, paraffin-embedded material. The anti-prolactin antibody (dilution 1:750) was kindly provided by the Hormone Distribution Officer of the National Pituitary Agency, Bethesda, Maryland.

reflects only the number of reacting cells and not qualitative differences in the amount of stored hormone. Reported results of immunostaining are inconclusive. One study compared nine patients treated with six weeks of bromocriptine to eight controls and found staining to be unchanged or slightly increased in the tumor group (12). On the other hand, some studies have suggested reduced staining after long-term bromocriptine. These include three patients treated for six weeks (5,14) as well as the current group of six patients receiving a week of intramuscular depot bromocriptine (acute parenteral treatment, see below) compared with eight controls and another eight patients given daily oral doses of 7.5 mg bromocriptine for four to six weeks (Table 1). The differences are not significant, although this may change when the number of cases is increased.

Results of morphometric analyses in the literature are presented in Table 2. The difference between the cell size of adenomas treated with bromocriptine for four to six weeks and that of untreated controls is due primarily to shrinking of the cytoplasm, with the nuclei shrinking less. The difference in the size of cells and cytoplasm between our patients and other reported control groups is difficult to explain. No difference is apparent in reported cell nuclei sizes or the parameters measured in cells from treated adenomas. This may be due in part to the fact that we use a semiautomatic particle size analyzer (MOP 2, Kontron Messgerate GmbH Munich, Germany) that also measures small cell processes. Point counting, a method used by other authors, neglects them. Since small cell processes are less numerous in bromocriptine-treated adenomas (Fig. 3a, b) their omission has less effect on measurement of cell size.

Clinical experience demonstrates that within a week after discontinuation of bromocriptine, prolactinomas can reenlarge and cause local pressure symptoms to reappear (31). Similarly, morphometric examination shows rapid reenlargement of the prolactinoma cells within the same time period (13). The ultrastructure resumes the appearance of that in untreated prolactinoma cells (14). Therefore, only adenomas treated until the eve of surgery must be used for examination of cytological changes caused by bromocriptine.

The size of the nucleolus, the surface of the RER and Golgi apparatus, and the number of ribosomes fixed to the membranes of the RER undergo more extensive reduction (46-82%) than the volume of cytoplasm (33%)(Table 3). The end point of shrinkage is reached after four to six weeks of treatment and no further reduction in cell size has been noted after treatment periods up to one year (12). Electron micrographs obtained from adenomas after four to six weeks of bromocriptine therapy, however, do not reveal the mechanism of removal of the different cell organelles. Recently this problem has

Table 2. *Average area of cells, cytoplasm, nucleus, and nucleolus in bromocriptine-treated (4 weeks or more) and untreated control prolactinomas as reported in published studies*

	Tindall et al. 1982	Bassetti et al. 1984	Landolt et al. 1983	Landolt et al. 1984
Controls				
No. of cases	2	8	67	10
Cell size (um²)	172	141	86	92
Cytoplasm (um²)	118	91	47	51
Nucleus (um²)	55	49	42	39
Nucleolus (um²)	3.5	—	2.5	2.4
Bromocriptine-treated adenomas				
No. of cases	2	9	5	8
Cell size (um²)	64	77	66	68
Cytoplasm (um²)	32	40	32	34
Nucleus (um²)	32	36	34	35
Nucleolus (um²)	1.5	—	1.3	1.3

been examined in a series of biopsy specimens obtained from patients seven days after intramuscular injection of depot bromocriptine (32).

Adenoma shrinking, with improvement of visual symptoms and the fall of serum prolactin levels, occurs some days after beginning bromocriptine treatment (19,33,34). However, technical difficulties have made an examination of acute morphological changes difficult. Part of the problem is that bromocriptine often must be given in slowly increasing doses because of the unpleasant side effects seen when it is started at the usual daily dose of 7.5 mg. This difficulty can be overcome with a new injectable form of long-acting bromocriptine that ensures a therapeutic and sustained plasma level within hours after injection (36). During removal of prolactinomas performed one week following a single treatment with this new drug form, the tumors have been found to be very soft and easily removable (37).

Morphometric examination of biopsy specimens obtained after short-term bromocriptine treatment, compared to data from untreated adenomas and adenomas treated four to six weeks with equivalent doses, shows that the major reduction in the

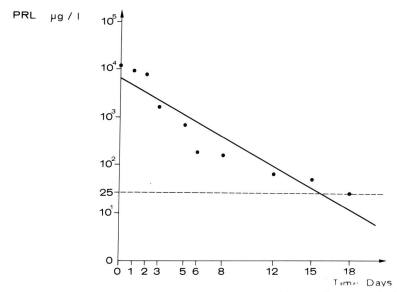

Figure 5. Exponential decrease of plasma prolactin levels observed in a patient treated with injectable bromocriptine-retard. Correlation coefficient r = 0.94. Data from Landolt and collaborators (19).

Table 3. *Changes in cytological parameters during bromocriptine treatment of prolactinomas**

	Untreated adenomas n = 10	Short-term treatment n = 6	Chronic treatment n = 8	H-Test p <	$T_{1/2}$ days
Cell volume (um²)	92.4 (100%)	71.0 (77%)	68.3 (74%)	0.05	2.2
Cytoplasm volume (um²)	51.3 (100%)	31.1 (61%)	34.3 (67%)	0.05	—
Nucleus volume (um²)	38.7 (100%)	41.0 (106%)	35.0 (90%)	— —	— —
Nucleolus volume (um²)	2.4 (100%)	1.6 (67%)	1.3 (54%)	0.1	3.7
RER surface/cell (um)	189 (100%)	113 (69%)	97 (51%)	0.01	2.7
RER ribosomes/cell	2267 (100%)	824 (36%)	420 (18%)	0.001	3.2
Ribosomes/mm membrane	10406 (100%)	8003 (77%)	5034 (48%)	0.001	8.2
Golgi surface/cell (um)	60 (100%)	32 (53%)	25 (42%)	0.1	3.0

Note: All results are shown as measured in thin sections of the average adenoma cell and *not* as partial volumes or volume densities.
$T_{1/2}$: half-life
* Data from Landolt and collaborators (32)

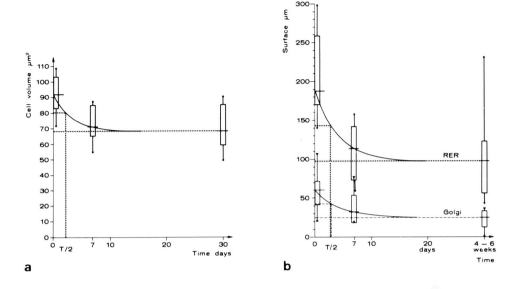

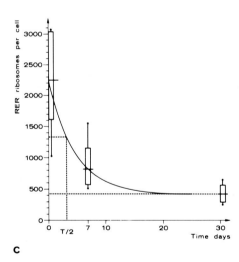

Figure 6. Shrinkage of cell volume (a), RER and Golgi cistern surface (b), and number of RER-fixed ribosomes (c) caused by bromocriptine. The horizontal bar shows the median value, the box shows the 25th and 75th percentiles, and the vertical line connects the minimum and maximum values.

676

size of cells, cytoplasm, nucleolus, RER surface, Golgi cistern surface, and the number of membrane-fixed ribosomes occurs within one week (Table 3) (32). Since bromocriptine decreases plasma prolactin concentration exponentially (Fig. 5) we can estimate that the half-life of observed reduction in cell size, nucleolus volume, RER surface, Golgi cistern surface, and number of RER ribosomes is two to four days. This assumes that the shrinkage of these structures also follows an exponential curve towards the baseline represented by adenomas treated for four to six weeks (Table 3, Fig. 6a-c).

Sequential analysis of the processes leading to adenoma shrinkage suggest the following: bromocriptine blocks the DNA to mRNA transcription of the prolactin gene. The fall of the mRNA production occurs within one hour after beginning treatment (38). This leads to an immediate fall in the prolactin synthesis and secretion (39,40). The half-life of prolactin synthesis calculated from the data of Maurer (39) is 0.8 days. A rapid reduction of RER-fixed ribosomes (polysomes, rRNA) engaged in prolactin synthesis is a further consequence of the fall of mRNA production. However, this process occurs at a slower speed than the reduction of prolactin synthesis. Its half-life is 3.2 days. Renewal of RER membranes is reduced or stopped as a direct or indirect consequence of the reduction of rRNA. It is apparent, however, that bromocriptine also increases the rate of flow of RER-membrane material along the secretory pathway to

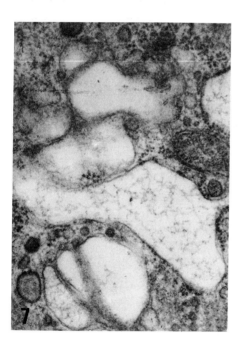 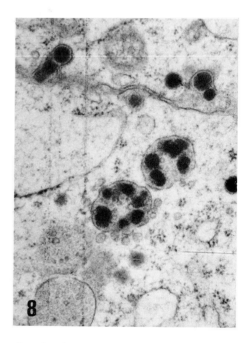

Figure 7. Electron micrograph of membrane formation showing characteristics of both RER and Golgi cisterns in an adenoma treated with bromocriptine for seven days. Osmium fixation, magnification x31300.

Figure 8. Lysosomal destruction of secretory granules in a prolactinoma after short-term treatment with bromocriptine. Electron micrograph, osmium fixation, magnification x31300.

the Golgi apparatus, secretory granules, lysosomal digestion, and cell surface. It has been suggested that this membrane transport occurs in the normal turnover of endoplasmic membranes (41-43). But its increased rate is demonstrated by several observations: there exist membrane formations that bear characteristics of the RER and of the Golgi apparatus (Fig. 7). These formations are not seen in untreated prolactinomas and suggest a rapid transformation of RER into Golgi membranes. Quantitative data do not show that the surface of the Golgi apparatus increases during the phase of rapid RER shrinkage. To the contrary, its surface shrinks with a speed similar to that of the RER surface (Fig. 6b, Table 3).

There are no lysosomes engaged in autophagy of membrane material as in phenobarbital-treated rat hepatocytes (44), so membrane material must pass through the stage of the Golgi cisterns to form membranes of secretory granules. The secretory granules are then processed in two ways: 1) Some are destroyed by crinophagy. Qualitative picture analysis suggests the presence of a larger number of autophagic vacuoles engaged in digestion of secretory granules (Fig. 8). This is supported by the prolactin determinations in bromocriptine-treated cell cultures of rat pituitary cells that demonstrate increased prolactin destruction (40). Lysosomes may be transformed into the lipid bodies seen more frequently in bromocriptine-treated prolactinomas (Figs. 2a, b, 3a, b). Others spill their contents into the intercellular space (Fig. 9) which is particularly enlarged around capillaries (37). 2) Other secretory granules are released at a higher than normal speed. This activated granule release is illustrated by frequent pictures showing simultaneous

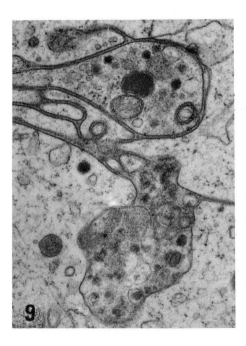

Figure 9. Release of the contents of a lysosome into the intercelluar space in a prolactinoma exposed to bromocriptine for seven days. Electron micrograph, osmium fixation, magnification x31300.

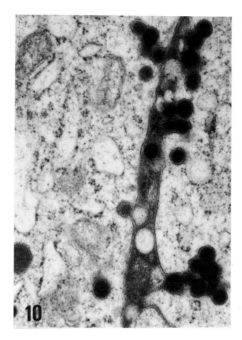

Figure 10. Rapid release of secretory granules in a prolactinoma treated with bromocriptine for seven days. Note the simultaneous release of several secretory granules into one secretory pit. Electron micrograph, osmium fixation, magnification x31300.

release of several granules into one secretory pit of the cell membrane similar to what is seen in stimulated rat prolactin cells during lactation (Fig. 10)(45). Rapid granule release is present only in prolactinomas removed after a short-term treatment with bromocriptine, never in prolactinomas following chronic (four to six weeks) treatment, and only rarely in untreated control specimens.

Since plasma prolactin levels decrease rapidly during the first days of bromocriptine treatment in patients with prolactinomas (Fig. 5) (19,31,35), the simultaneous release of an increased number of secretory granules suggests that these granules contain less prolactin than granules secreted during normal conditions. The fall in prolactin synthesis is more rapid than shrinking of the endoplasmic membrane system.

The rapid cell shrinkage with spilling of secretory products and lysosome contents into the intercellular space creates intratumoral clefts in the vicinity of blood vessels (37). This cleft formation after short-term treatment softens the tumor and facilitates adenoma extirpation (46-48). Later, however, collagen fibers are formed in these spaces leading to perivascular fibrosis which increases the consistency of the adenomas and makes radical removal more difficult (47). The amount of fibrous area surrounding intratumoral blood vessels in relation to the cross-sectional area of the vessels is significantly higher in prolactinomas treated with bromocriptine for periods of three months or more compared to untreated controls (26). There is no significant difference in blood vessel diameter between biopsy specimens of treated adenomas and controls.

The average blood vessel cross-sectional area in 21 untreated controls was 303 um^2 (s.d. = 114 um^2), and it was 366 um^2 (s.d. = 153 um^2) in biopsy specimens of 20 adenomas treated with bromocriptine for three months or more. The amount of perivascular fibrous tissue does not depend on the total amount of bromocriptine used.

Structure, ultrastructure, and secretory function of prolactinomas are not necessarily stable but may be changed by hormones and drugs. It is difficult to estimate which of these changes are caused because of a naturally-occurring variability in the structure of individual adenomas. Measurement of cytological parameters and statistical comparison of groups of treated and untreated adenomas represent the only approach to this problem.

Estrogens lead to enlargement of prolactinomas because of cell proliferation and intratumoral hemorrhage. This can produce complications.

In summary, bromocriptine blocks the DNA to mRNA transcription of the prolactin gene. Prolactin synthesis decreases within hours after beginning treatment. The size of the nucleolus, the number of RER-fixed ribosomes, the surface of the RER, the surface of the Golgi apparatus, and the cell size are reduced with a half life of two to four days. Reduction of the RER membranes and Golgi apparatus occurs by faster transport of the membrane material from the RER to the Golgi apparatus and secretory granules. The granules are then either released faster than usual or destroyed by autophagy. The rapid fall of the plasma prolactin level in spite of the release of an increased number of secretory granules suggests that the granules contain less prolactin than under normal conditions. Lysosomes may spill their contents into the intercellular space. Cell shrinkage together with the release of intracellular material causes an enlargement of intercellular spaces. Initially this produces a softening of the tumor, but later perivascular fibrosis occurs as a result of collagen deposition.

ACKNOWLEDGMENTS

The author thanks Dr. William J. Morris, U.S. Army Medical Center, Landstuhl, Germany, for assistance in editing the manuscript, Verena Osterwalder and Peter Roth, Department of Neurosurgery, University of Zurich for photography and art work, and the EMDO Foundation Zurich and the Sandoz Foundation Basle for financial support.

REFERENCES

1. Horvath E, Kovacs K. (1980) In: Erzin C, Horvath E, Kaufman B, Kovacs K, Weiss MH (eds) Pituitary Diseases. CRC Press, Boca Raton, Florida, p 1
2. Dingemans KP, Assies J, Jansen N, Diegenbach PC. (1982): Virchows Arch [Pathol Anat] 396:167
3. Landolt AM. (1975): Acta Neurochir (Wien) Suppl 22:1
4. Landolt AM. (1984) In: Camanni F, Muller EE (eds) Pituitary Hyperfunction. Raven Press, New York, p 135
5. Rengachari SS, Tomita T, Jeffries DF, Watanabe I. (1982): Neurosurgery 10:242
6. Landolt AM, Kistler GS, Barker M, Deen D, Wilson CB. (1980) In: Derome PJ, Jedynak CP, Peillon F (eds) Pituitary Adenomas. Asclepios Publishers, France, (1980):, p 49

7. Anniko M, Werner S, Wersall J. (1981): Acta Otolaryngol (Stockh) 92:343
8. Peillon F, Cesselin F, Brandi A-M. (1980): In: Derome PJ, Jedynak CP, Peillon F (eds) Pituitary Adenomas. Asclepios Publishers, France, p 71
9. Landolt AM. (1978): In: Krayenbuhl H (ed) Advances and Technical Standards in Neurosurgery. 5:3
10. Landolt AM, Krayenbuhl H. (1972): J Neurosurg 37:289
11. Scheithauer B. (1982): In: Laws ER, Randall RV, Kern EB, Abboud CF (eds) Management of Pituitary Adenomas and Related Lesions. Appleton-Century-Crofts, New York, p 129
12. Bassetti M, Spada A, Pezzo G, Giannattasio G. (1984): J Clin Endocrinol Metab 58:268
13. Landolt AM, Minder H, Osterwalder V, Landolt TA. (1983): Experientia 39:625
14. Tindall GT, Kovacs K, Horvath E, Thorner MO. (1982): J Clin Endocrinol Metab 55:1178
15. Robert F. (1981): Neurochirurgie 27, Suppl 1:61
16. Peake GT, McKeel DW, Jaratt HL, Daughaday WH. (1969): J Clin Endocrinol Metab 29:1385
17. Yaghmai F. (1977): In: Allen MB, Mahesh VB (eds) The Pituitary -- a Current Review. Academic Press, New York, p 373
18. White MC, Anapliotou M, Rosenstock J, Mashiter K, Joplin GF. (1981): Lancet II:1394
19. Landolt AM, del Pozo E, Hayek J. (1984): Lancet (in press)
20. Gemzell C, Wang CF. (1979): Fertil Steril 31:363
21. Magyar DM, Marshall JR. (1978): Am J Obstet Gynecol 132:739
22. Nillius SJ, Bergh T, Larsson S-G. (1980): In: Derome PJ, Jedynak CP, Peillon F (eds) Pituitary Adenomas. Asclepios Publishers, France, p 103
23. Peillon F, Vila-Porcile E, Olivier L, Racadot J. (1970): Ann Endocrinol (Paris) 31:259
24. Pichon M-F, Bression D, Peillon F, Milgrom E. (1980): J Clin Endocrinol Metab 51: 897
25. Gen M, Uozumi T, Shinohara S, Naito M, Ito A, Mori S, Kajiawara H. (1983): Neurol Med-Chir 23:61
26. Landolt AM, Osterwalder V. (1984): J Clin Endocrinol Metab 58:1179
27. Anniko M, Wersall J. (1981): Acta Pathol Microbiol Scand [A] 89:41
28. Girod C, Mazzuca M, Trouillas J, Tramu G, Lheritier M, Beauvillain J-C, Claustrat B, Dubois M-P. (1980): In: Derome PJ, Jedynak CP, Peillon F (eds) Pituitary Adenomas. Asclepios Publishers, France, p 3
29. Landolt AM. (1984): In: Lamberts SWJ, Assies J, Tilders FJH, van der Veen EA (eds) Proceedings of the 3rd European Symposium on Pituitary Adenomas, Amsterdam, (1983): (in press)
30. Sternberger LA: Immunocytochemistry. (1979): John Wiley & Sons, New York, ed 2, p 122
31. Thorner MO, Perryman RC, Rogol AD, Conway BP, MacLeod RM, Login IS, Morris JL. (1981): J Clin Endocrinol Metab 53:480
32. Landolt AM, Osterwalder V, Landolt TA. (1984): Experientia (in press)
33. Landolt AM. (1982): Neurosurgery 11:395
34. Thorner MO, Schran HF, Evans WS, Rogol AD, Morris JL, MacLeod RM. (1980): J Clin Endocrinol Metab 50:1026
35. Woodhouse NJY, Khouqueer F, Sieck JO. (1981): Horm Res 14:141
36. Portmann L, Felber JP, Maeder E, Lancranjan I. (1983): Endocrinology 112: suppl, abstr 524
37. Landolt AM. (1984): In: Martin JB, Zervas NT, Ridgway EC, Black PM (eds) International Symposium on Pituitary Tumors, Boston, (1983): (in press)
38. Maurer RA. (1981): Nature 294:94
39. Maurer RA. (1980): J Biol Chem 255:8092
40. Dannies PS, Rudnick MS. (1980): J Biol Chem 255:2776
41. Bergmann JE, Tokuyasu KT, Singer SJ. (1971): Proc Natl Acad Sci USA 78:1746
42. Franke WW, Morre DJ, Deumling B, Cheetham RD, Kartenbeck J, Jarasch E-D, Zentgraf H-W. (1971): Z Naturforsch 26B:1031

43. Morre DJ. (1977): In: Brinkley BR, Porter KR (eds) International Cell Biology (1976-1977). Rockefeller University Press, New York, p 293
44. Bolender RP, Weibel ER. (1973): J Cell Biol 56:746
45. Farquhar MG (1971) In: Heller H, Lederis K (eds) Subcellular Organization and Function in Endocrine Tissues. Cambridge University Press, Cambridge, p 79
46. Barrow DL, Tindall GT, Kovacs K, Thorner MO, Hovath E, Hoffman JC. (1984): J Neurosurg 60:1
47. Landolt AM, Keller PJ, Froesch ER, Muller J. (1982): Lancet I:657
48. Weiss MH, Wycoff RR, Yadley R, Gott P, Feldon S. (1983): Neurosurgery 12:640

Prolactin. Basic and clinical correlates
R.M. MacLeod, M.O. Thorner and U. Scapagnini (eds.),
Fidia Research Series, vol. I,
Liviana Press, Padova © 1985

PROLACTIN-PRODUCING TUMORS OF THE HUMAN PITUITARY: MORPHOLOGIC FEATURES

Kalman Kovacs

Department of Pathology, St. Michael's Hospital
University of Toronto, Toronto, Ont. M5B 1W8 Canada

Prolactin-producing tumors are the most frequently occurring neoplasms in the human pituitary. Their existence was first suggested by Forbes and her associates (1) in 1954. These authors presented the findings in 15 non-acromegalic women with amenorrhea, persistent lactation, and low urinary FSH excretion. Seven patients had a pituitary tumor, and it was proposed that all of them had overproduction of prolactin by the pituitary gland. The morphologic features of a prolactin-secreting tumor were first reported by Herlant and his associates (2) in 1965. They found that a pituitary chromophobic adenoma, removed by surgery from a 37-year old female patient with amenorrhea and galactorrhea, was composed of prolactin cells.

Progress in biochemical and imaging techniques allowed for earlier and more accurate diagnosis of pituitary neoplasms. Advancement in microsurgical methods made it possible to safely remove pituitary adenomas even if they were small. The morphologic study of surgical specimens permitted a deeper insight into the structural features of pituitary tumors. Application of sophisticated morphologic techniques, such as immunocytology, transmission electron miscroscopy, scanning electron miscroscopy, immunoelectron miscroscopy, and morphometry, led to a new pituitary adenoma classification (3-7). Based on extensive morphologic studies, pituitary adenomas were divided on the grounds of hormone content, ultrastructural features, cellular composition, and cytogenesis. A better understanding of pituitary cytopathology emerged from these studies and pituitary tumors, capable of producing prolactin, became better known and were convincingly defined.

This review focuses on the morphologic features of prolactin-producing pituitary tumors. It deals only with human material and does not include findings on animal pituitaries. Although marked progress was made in the morphologic investigation of pituitary tumors harvested from various animals, there are substantial species differences, and results found in animal pituitaries cannot be conclusively extrapolated to the human gland. In the last decade, numerous works concentrating on the prolactin problem were reported; it is obvious that every publication discussing morphology, clinical and biochemical manifestations, surgical techniques, and medication cannot be covered here. Only a few recent papers are quoted, mainly those that examine primarily the morphology of prolactin-producing pituitary adenomas (8-53).

We have studied close to 1,000 surgically-removed pituitary adenomas by histology, immunocytology, and transmission electron microscopy. In selected cases, immunoelectron microscopy was also performed. The patients were men and women of various ages, with various clinical and biochemical findings. Additional material obtained from autopsies consisted of 150 pituitary adenomas and approximately 2000 nontumorous adenohypophyses harvested from male and female subjects of various ages, dying of different diseases.

Tissue for conventional histology and immunocytology was fixed in 10% buffered formalin and embedded in paraffin. Sections were stained with hematoxylin-eosin (HE), hematoxylin-phloxin-saffron (HPS), the periodic acid-Schiff (PAS) method and, in some cases, with orange G, light green, aniline blue, aldehyde fuchsin, aldehyde thionin, lead hematoxylin, Herlant's erythrosin, and Brookes' carmoisin techniques. For assessment of the reticulin fiber network, the Gordon-Sweet silver method was applied. For the demonstration of GH, PRL, ACTH, endorphins, beta-LPH, TSH, FSH, LH, and alpha-subunit of glycoprotein hormones, the immunoperoxidase technique was used as described in detail in previous publications (32,33).

For electron microscopy, tissue was fixed in 2.5% glutaraldehyde, postfixed in 1% osmium tetroxide, dehydrated in graded ethanol, processed through propylene oxide, and embedded in epoxy resin. Semithin sections were stained with toluidine blue and examined with a light microscope to select appropriate areas for the electron microscopic investigation. Ultrathin sections were stained with uranyl acetate and lead citrate and studied with a Philips 300 electron microscope.

From the practical point of view, neoplastic transformation is the most important abnormality of lactotrophs, also called prolactin cells. The structural features of adenomatous lactotrophs will be described in the following pages.

Lactotrophs can undergo neoplastic transformation and give rise to adenoma. Progress in clinical medicine, biochemistry, imaging techniques, surgery, and advancement in morphology established that prolactin-producing adenomas are the most commonly occurring tumors in the human pituitary. They vary considerably in size and are either microadenomas, which remain intrasellar and can be diagnosed by serum prolactin measurements and sophisticated imaging methods, or are rapidly growing macroadenomas that spread outside the sella turcica and invade adjacent tissues, such as the sphenoid sinus, optic nerve, or hypothalamus. The differences in their pace of growth are not invariably evident from their structural features, thus no definite conclusions can be drawn from their morphologic appearances as to their biologic behavior.

The clinical manifestations of prolactin-producing adenoma are amenorrhea, galactorrhea, infertility, decreased libido, and impotence. The clinical symptoms are not conspicuous in every patient, and can be absent in men and postmenopausal women. In patients with large adenoma, local symptoms such as visual disturbances, nausea, vomiting, and headaches may predominate. Patients may die secondary to elevated intracranial pressure or invasion of the hypothalamus. Occasional cases of prolactin-producing tumor give rise to distant metastases. These tumors are termed prolactin-producing tumor give rise to distant metastases. These tumors are termed prolactin-producing carcinomas. In patients with microadenoma, imaging techniques may fail to show changes in the sella turcica. Great caution is required in the assessment of findings, since minute radiological changes may be overemphasized and the adenoma diagnosis cannot be confirmed by morphologic examination.

Biochemically, in patients with prolactin-secreting tumors, the most consistent finding is the rise in serum prolactin concentrations. High serum prolactin levels do not prove the diagnosis of prolactin-producing adenoma, since hyperprolactinemia may occur in patients with other lesions of the sella region. In these cases, injury of the hypothalamus or hypophysial stalk blocks the production, release, or adenohypophysial transport of dopamine and other possible prolactin-inhibiting factors, and alleviation from inhibition causes increased prolactin secretion from nontumorous lactotrophs, resulting in hyperprolactinemia. Many lesions can lead to an increase in serum prolactin concentrations: craniopharyngioma, pituitary oncocytoma, null cell adenoma, metastatic carcinoma, sarcoidosis, lymphocytic hypophysitis, or injury or section of the the pituitary stalk. Some cases of ACTH-secreting microadenoma are associated with a rise in serum prolactin levels. The mechanism of hyperprolactinemia in these patients is obscure; it cannot be interpreted as a stalk section effect, since the adenomas are small and no suprasellar extension or damage of the pituitary stalk can be demonstrated. It is well known that pregnancy, lactation, stress, and various drugs such as estrogens and antidopaminergic compounds are accompanied by hyperprolactinemia.

In patients with hyperprolactinemia due to conditions other than prolactin-secreting adenoma, serum prolactin concentrations do not exceed 200 ng/ml. Hence, if serum prolactin levels are higher than 200 ng/ml the diagnosis of prolactin-secreting adenoma is justified. A correlation exists between adenoma size and serum prolactin concentrations; large tumors are associated with more marked hyperprolactinemia. However, in patients with large acidophil stem cell adenoma, a rise in serum prolactin concentrations may be unexpectedly moderate or slight.

Seven tumor types can produce prolactin in the human pituitary: 1) densely granulated prolactin cell adenoma; 2) sparsely granulated prolactin cell adenoma; 3) mixed growth hormone cell-prolactin cell adenoma; 4) acidophil stem cell adenoma; 5) mammosomatotroph cell adenoma; 6) prolactin cell carcinoma; 7) plurihormonal adenoma with prolactin component. In the following pages, the structural characteristics of these tumor types will be discussed.

Densely granulated prolactin cell adenomas are uncommon tumors. By light microscopy, the adenoma cells are acidophilic. The cytoplasmic granules are coarse and numerous, and stain with acid dyes, such as eosin, phloxin, orange G, and light green, as well as with Herlant's erythrosin and Brookes' carmoisin. The staining methods, however, are not reliable and should be replaced by sensitive and specific immunocytologic procedures which demonstrate prolactin in the cytoplasm of adenoma cells. Ultrastructural examination reveals that the adenoma cells resemble nontumorous lactotrophs in the storage phase. They are oval or irregular, with spherical or oval, slightly eccentric nuclei and dense nucleoli. The well developed cytoplasm contains moderately conspicuous RER membranes, prominent Golgi complexes, and a few rod-shaped mitochondria. The secretory granules are numerous, spherical, oval or slightly irregular, evenly electron dense, and measure 400-800 nm. Exocytoses, on the capillary and lateral cell surfaces, are apparent.

The sparsely granulated prolactin cell adenoma is the most often occurring tumor type in the human pituitary. Whereas a female preponderance is noted among the surgically-removed tumors, it is evident, based on an immunocytologic study of unselected autopsy material, that prolactin-containing tumors are equally frequent in men. By light microscopy, the adenoma cells are chromophobic or slightly acidophilic, PAS as well as lead hematoxylin negative and exhibit positive staining with Herlant's erythrosin or Brookes' carmoisin. The immunoperoxidase method conclusively demonstrates the presence of prolactin in the cytoplasm of adenoma cells localized in the secretory granules and the conspicuous Golgi complexes.

Under the light microscope, sparsely granulated prolactin cell adenomas show diffuse, trabecular, or papillary patterns. The diffuse pattern is found in most of the surgically-removed adenomas, whereas the papillary pattern predominates among the small incidental adenomas revealed at unselected autopsies. The histologic difference raises the question of whether diffuse adenomas are more active endocrinologically and have a faster growth rate than papillary adenomas.

By electron microscopy, sparsely granulated prolactin cell adenomas possess characteristic features and can be diagnosed conclusively. The ultrastructural appearance of sparsely granulated adenomatous prolactin cells resembles that of nontumorous, actively-secreting lactotrophs seen in the pituitary after estrogen stimulation; they are polyhedral or elongated with long cytoplasmic processes and interdigitating plasma membranes. The nuclei are large, spherical, oval or slightly irregular, the nucleoli are dense and prominent. The abundant cytoplasm contains well developed RER membranes consisting of long-parallel cisternae or short, slightly dilated, slim stacks, studded with ribosomes on their external aspects. Nebenkerns, i.e. concentric whorls of RER membranes, are seen in the cytoplasm of many adenoma cells. The Golgi apparatus, composed of several moderately dilated sacculi and vesivles, and dense, irregular, forming secretory granules, is conspicuous. The mitochondria are oval or elongated and have lamellar or tubular transverse cristae and moderately electron dense matrix. The secretory granules are sparse, spherical, oval or irregular, evenly electron dense, measure 150-300 nm, and are randomly distributed in the cytoplasm. Exocytosis is a characteristic feature of adenomatous prolactin cells. Granule extrusion can be seen on the capillary and lateral cell surfaces. The term "misplaced exocytosis" is used when secretory granules are extruded on the lateral cell surface, distant from the capillaries and intercellular extensions of the basement membranes. Misplaced exocytosis occurs only in prolactin-secreting cells and is regarded as a diagnostic marker of this cell type. Although it is reasonable to assume that the number of exocytoses depends on the rate of hormone discharge, no close correlation can be established between the number of granule extrusion sites and serum prolactin concentrations. The volume densities of various cytoplasmic organelles and size, number, and volume densities of secretory granules do not correlate with the magnitude of hyperprolactinemia. However, a relationship exists between adenoma size evaluated by various imaging methods and serum prolactin levels. Although abundance of mitochondria may be apparent in the cytoplasm of a few adenoma cells, oncocytic change is not characteristic of sparsely granulated prolactin cell adenomas. Large lysosomes and uptake of secretory granules by lysosomes may be noticeable in some adenoma cells. The latter change is called crinophagy and may represent degradation of unused secretory material by a lysosomal mechanism.

Deposition of endocrine amyloid may be noted in some sparsely granulated prolactin cell adenomas. Amyloid fibers are located intracellularly in the dilated RER cisternae or in large extracellular aggregates. Their fine structure differs from that of immune amyloid. Compared with other adenoma types, calcification is seen most commonly in sparsely granulated prolactin cell adenomas. The first step of calcification occurs intracellularly in the internal compartments of mitochondria. The process continues and additional calcification leads to the development of large, extracellular, amorphous calcium apatite deposits and psammoma bodies which can be recognized by light microscopy.

No major clinical or biochemical differences can be established in patients harboring densely or sparsely granulated prolactin cell adenomas.

Medication with dopaminergic agonists, such as bromocriptine, causes regression of prolactin-producing tumors. This effect is reversible and the tumor regrows after discontinuation of the treatment. Clinically, amenorrhea and lactation cease, and women may become pregnant. In men, potency and libido improve substantially. The clinical amelioration is accompanied by a decrease of serum prolactin levels and reduction of tumor size, leading to correction of local symptoms. Morphologically, the most important change is reduction of cell size, reduction of nuclear, nucleolar, and cytoplasmic volume, increase of nuclear/cytoplasmic ratio, and reduction of volume densities of RER and Golgi complexes. There is no change in mitochondrial and lysosomal volume densities and some increase may be found in secretory granule number, size, and volume densities. The morphometric changes are reversible and the adenoma cells enlarge after withdrawal of dopaminergic agonists.

Mixed growth hormone cell-prolactin cell adenomas consist of two distinct cell types, growth hormone cells and prolactin cells, and produce two hormones, growth hormone and prolactin. Hence, they are bimorphous, bihormonal tumors. By light microscopy, the adenoma cells are acidophilic or chromophobic. By the immunoperoxidase method, growth hormone and prolactin are demonstrated in two separate cell types. Electron microscopy detects two cell populations, densely or sparsely granulated growth hormone cells and prolactin cells, and the ultrastructural appearances of adenoma cells are similar to those found in pure growth hormone cell adenomas or prolactin cell adenomas. The two cell types may occur singly or in small groups. In some adenomas, especially in those of children and adolescents, bihormonal cells containing growth hormone and prolactin may be noted.

Clinically, mixed growth hormone cell-prolactin cell adenomas are accompanied by acromegaly or gigantism, amenorrhea, galactorrhea, infertility, decreased libido, and impotence. The majority of tumors show a slow pace of growth, although suprasellar extension and local symptoms such as visual disturbances and headache may be evident. By radioimmunoassay, serum growth hormone concentrations are high and serum prolactin levels are elevated or within the normal range. In patients with normal serum prolactin levels, prolactin is not released from the adenoma cells in sufficient amounts to result in hyperprolactinemia.

Acidophil stem cell adenomas consist of one cell type, assumed to represent the common precursor of growth hormone cells and prolactin cells, termed acidophil stem cell. Hence, these tumors are monomorphous and bihormonal.

By light microscopy, acidophil stem cell adenomas are chromophobic or slightly acidophilic, and PAS and lead hematoxylin negative, and may show some staining with Herlant's erythrosin and Brookes' carmoisin. The immunoperoxidase technique reveals growth hormone and prolactin in the cytoplasm of the same adenoma cells. Immunostaining for prolactin is predominant; immunocytologic procedures for growth hormone may yield weak or negative results. In some areas, groups of adenoma cells contain only prolactin or growth hormone, suggesting differentiation toward a mature monohormonal cell line.

By electron microscopy, the adenoma cells are enlongated or irregular with large, oblong nuclei. The cytoplasm is well developed and contains short, ribosome-studded RER profiles or long parallel RER cisternae, or concentric RER whorls. The RER is somewhat less organized and the Golgi complexes are less conspicuous than in well differentiated, sparsely granulated prolactin cell adenomas. Fibrous bodies, aggregates of type II microfilaments, smooth-walled tubules, as well as numerous centrioles, characteristic features of sparsely granulated adenomatous growth hormone cells, may be noted. Free ribosomes and polysomes, as well as mitochondria, may be apparent in large numbers; oncocytic transformation occurs in the majority of tumors. Some mitochondria exhibit rarefaction, loss of cristae, ballooning, and gigantism. The secretory granules are sparse, spherical, oval or irregular, evenly electron dense, and measure 150-300 nm. Misplaced exocytoses are evident.

Clinically, patients with acidophil stem cell adenoma have increased serum prolactin levels, but the degree of hyperprolactinemia is less, in many cases, than one would anticipate on the grounds of tumor size. Amenorrhea, galactorrhea, infertility, loss of libido, and impotence may be noted; however, often local symptoms prevail. Serum growth hormone concentrations are, in most cases, within the normal range. Acromegalic features may be evident, suggesting the production of an abnormal growth hormone by the adenoma cells which may be biologically active but cannot be measured by radiommunoassay. The distinction of acidophil stem cell adenoma is important, since these tumors are often rapidly growing and prone to recur. They often spread outside the sella and invade neighboring tissues and their complete surgical removal is very difficult. Acidophil stem cell adenomas respond to dopaminergic agonist therapy. Bromocriptine medication suppresses tumor growth and causes a reduction in adenoma size.

Mammosomatotroph cell adenomas consist of well-differentiated cells which, by electron microscopy, show the combined features of growth hormone cells and prolactin cells. They are rare tumors, containing both growth hormone and prolactin, as shown by the immunoperoxidase technique; hence, they are monomorphous and bihormonal, The two hormones are produced by a single cell type, termed mammosomatotroph cell.

By light microscopy, mammosomatotroph cell adenomas are acidophilic, PAS as well as lead hematoxylin negative. The immunoperoxidase technique may reveal the presence of prolactin and growth hormone in the cytoplasm of the same adenoma cells.

By electron microscopy, mammosomatotroph cell adenomas are composed of spherical or oval cells with large nuclei and conspicuous nucleoli. The well developed cytoplasm contains several parallel arrays of RER membranes. The Golgi complexes are prominent and consist of several dilated sacculi and vesicles. The mitochondria are rod-shaped with transverse lamellar cristae and moderately electron dense matrix. The secretory granules are numerous, spherical, oval or pleomorphic, and measure 200-2000 nm. Extrusion of secretory granules may be noted. A characteristic feature of this adenoma type is the presence of large extracellular deposits of secretory material which may exhibit growth hormone immunoreactivity.

Clinically, mammosomatotroph cell adenomas are often intrasellar tumors with a slow growth rate and a long history of acromegaly. Serum growth hormone levels are elevated. Serum prolactin concentrations are increased or within the normal range. The prognosis of mammosomatotroph cell adenoma is, in the majority of patients, good and surgery often leads to a complete cure.

Prolactin cell carcinomas are exceptionally rare. Their diagnosis is justified in patients with documented distant metastases. The tumor cells produce prolactin which can be demonstrated in their cytoplasm by the immunoperoxidase technique. The ultrastructural features of prolactin cell carcinoma are not characteristic. The tumor cells can be so anaplastic that even detailed electron microscopic studies fail to establish their derivation.

The clinical manifestations of prolactin cell carcinoma are not well defined, and more cases must be examined before the clinical correlations become evident. The patients may show marked hyperprolactinemia. Amenorrhea, galactorrhea, infertility, decreased libido, and impotence may be apparent. The most frequent symptoms are local and are due to tumor invasion. The tumors may show a rapid growth rate, spread outside the sella turcica and invade and destroy neighboring tissues, such as the sphenoid or cavernous sinus, the optic nerve or other cranial nerves, and the hypothalamus. Visual disturbances, headache, nausea, pain, or increased intracranial pressure may be manifest. The clinical presentation hinges on the location and extent of tumor invasion and subsequent tissue compression, damage, and destruction. Distant metastases, depending on their location, may lead to additional symptoms.

Plurihormonal adenomas arising in the anterior pituitary produce two or more hormones, different in chemical composition, immunoreactivity and biologic action. These tumors are monomorphous or plurimorphous, and their cytogenesis has yet to be clarified.

Monomorphous adenomas are composed of one cell type and two or more hormones are present in the same population of cells, as shown by the immunoperoxidase technique. Ultrastructural examination discloses one cell type which differs from cells seen in nontumorous adenohypophyses or adenomas secreting only one hormone.

Plurimorphous adenomas consist of two or more cell populations. These tumors are mixed adenomas, since each cell contains only one hormone, by the immunoperoxidase technique, and show resemblance in ultrastructural features to their nontumorous counterparts.

Mixed growth hormone cell-prolactin cell adenomas, acidophil stem cell adenomas, and mammosomatotroph cell adenomas are plurihormonal adenomas, since they produce growth hormone and prolactin; these three types were dealt with above. They originate in the acidophil cell line, i.e. somatotrophs, lactotrophs, or the common progenitor of somatotrophs and lactotrophs, and differ in the degree and direction of differentiation.

Other plurihormonal adenomas produce unusual combinations of adenohypophysial hormones, such as prolactin and TSH or prolactin, growth hormone and TSH or prolactin, growth hormone and ACTH, or prolactin and alpha-subunit, etc. They are uncommon adenomas; the monomorphous forms may derive from an uncommitted stem cell, whereas the plurimorphous variants may originate in two or more well-differentiated cell types. The endocrine activity of plurihormonal adenomas cannot be explained on the basis of the one cell-one hormone theory. It remains to be elucidated whether plurihormonal clones, capable of synthesizing more than one hormone, exist in the human adenohypophysis. These cells are apparently dormant under normal conditions, but in the course of neoplastic transformation or subsequent cellular proliferation, they may acquire the ability to produce two or more different hormones.

Clinically, plurihormonal adenomas can lead to different symptoms depending on which hormones are secreted in excess. Discrepancies may be evident among clinical symptoms, serum hormone levels, and immunocytologic findings, since some hormones may be synthesized by the adenoma cells but are not discharged into the circulation in such quantities as to cause clinical abnormalities and elevation of serum hormone levels. Hence, immunocytochemistry is of profound importance in demonstrating hormone content of the tumor cells.

Histologically, plurihormonal adenomas producing prolactin and some other hormone or hormones are chromophobic, acidophilic, or consist of an admixture of chromophobic and acidophilic cells. The presence of prolactin can be demonstrated in the cytoplasm of some adenoma cells by the immunoperoxidase technique. In monomorphous adenomas, the ultrastructural investigation discloses one cell type which cannot be classified. In plurimorphous adenomas, the prolactin component is represented by well-differentiated, bihormonal mammosomatotroph cells or sparsely granulated prolactin cells. In patients with increased prolactin secretion, amenorrhea, galactorrhea, infertility, decreased libido, and impotence may be noted.

In summary, this review deals with the morphologic features of prolactin-producing tumors, the most commonly-occurring neoplasms of the human pituitary. They range from sharply demarcated, slowly expanding microadenomas to more rapidly growing macroadenomas, spreading outside the sella turcica and invading adjacent tissues. Among surgically removed prolactin-secreting pituitary adenomas, a female preponderance is evident, whereas in autopsy material, prolactin cell adenomas are at least as frequent in men as in women. Prolactin-producing tumors vary in morphology and can be divided into seven different types. Their separation is useful, since they differ in clinical presentation, hormone production, and biologic behavior. Densely granulated prolactin cell adenomas are rare. Sparsely granulated prolactin cell adenomas represent the most often occurring morphologic variant. These two types are associated with varying degrees of hyperprolactinemia and, in most cases, with amenorrhea, galactorrhea, infertility, decreased libido, and impotence. Large tumors are accompanied by local symptoms, such as visual disturbances and headache. Mixed growth hormone cell-prolactin cell adenomas produce growth hormone and prolactin and are composed of two different cell types. Acidophil stem cell adenomas are monomorphous tumors and usually show more rapid growth than the other variants. Mammosomatotroph cell adenomas are uncommon, slowly growing monomorphous tumors associated with acromegaly and hyperprolactinemia. Prolactin cell carcinomas are pleomorphic, rapidly proliferating tumors, which give rise to distant metastases and are capable of secreting prolactin. Some pituitary adenomas secrete not only prolactin but other adenohypophysial hormones as well, and two or more hormones different in chemical composition, immunoreactivity, and biologic action can be revealed in the cytoplasm of adenoma cells. These plurihormonal adenomas may be monomorphous, consisting of one cell type, or plurimorphous, composed of more than one cell population.

The last two decades witnessed extraordinary progress in the understanding of structure-function correlations of endocrine glands, including the pituitary. Despite substantial advances, more studies are required to elucidate the pathogenesis of prolactin-producing adenomas and their responsiveness to treatment. Long-term follow-up of patients is needed to obtain a deeper insight as to why some neoplasms have a rapid growth rate, while others remain small. Morphology, at present, cannot conclusively distinguish between proliferating and nonproliferating tumors. Extensive work should be directed to clarify the regulation of adenomatous lactotrophs and the role of dopaminergic receptors in the suppression of their proliferation. Bromocriptine, a dopaminergic agonist, ameliorates the clinical symptoms, decreases serum prolactin levels, and causes regression of prolactin-secreting pituitary adenomas. The main effect of dopaminergic agonist medication is the reversible reduction in cell size; the tumors regrow and serum prolactin levels rise after withdrawal of treatment. It is expected that the next decade will continue to bring important discoveries and will satisfy the curiosity of researchers in this exciting field.

ACKNOWLEDGMENTS

This work was supported in part by Grant MA-6349 of the Medical Research Council of Canada. The author is greatly indebted to Dr. E. Horvath, Mrs. Gezina Ilse, Mrs. Noemi Losinski, Miss Donn McComb, and Mrs. Nancy Ryan for their invaluable contribution throughout this study, and to Mrs. Wanda Wlodarski for excellent secretarial work.

REFERENCES

1. Forbes AP, Henneman PH, Griswold GC, Albright F. (1954): J Clin Endocrinol Metab 14:265
2. Herlant M, Laine E, Fossati P, Linquette M. (1965): Ann Endocrin (Paris) 26:65
3. Horvath E, Kovacs K. (1976): Can J Neurol Sci 3:9
4. Horvath E, Kovacs K. (1980). In: Pituitary Diseases. CRC Press, Boca Raton, p 1
5. Kovacs K, Horvath E. (1982). In: Hormone Secreting Pituitary Tumors. Year Book Med Publ., Chicago, p 97
6. Kovacs K, Horvath E, Ezrin C. (1977): Pathol Annu 12(2):341
7. Kovacs K, McComb DJ, Horvath E. (1983): Neuroendocr Perspect 2:251
8. Barrow DL, Tindall GT. (1983): J Clin Neuro-ophthalmol 3:229
9. Barrow DL, Tindall GT, Kovacs K, Thorner MO, Horvath E, Hoffman JC Jr. (1984): J Neurosurg 60:1
10. Bassetti M, Spada A, Pezzo G, Giannattasio G. (1984): J Clin Endocrinol Metab 58:268
11. Burrow GN, Wortzman G, Rewcastle NB, Holgate RC, Kovacs K. (1981): New Engl J Med 304:156
12. Cohen DL, Diengdoh JV, Thomas DGT, Himsworth RL. (1983): Clin Endocrinol 18:259
13. Corenblum B, Sirek AMT, Horvath E, Kovacs K, Ezrin C. (1976): J Clin Endocrinol Metab 42:857

14. Delafontaine P, Ochsner F, Pizzolato GP. (1982): Acta Neuropathol 57:81
15. Esiri MM, Adams CBT, Burke C, Underdown R. (1983): Acta Neuropathol 62:1
16. Faria MA Jr, Tindall GT. (1982): J Neurosurg 56:33
17. Guyda H, Robert F, Collu E, Hardy J. (1973): J Clin Endocrinol Metab 36:531
18. Halmi NS: (1982): Virchows Arch A Pathol Anat 398:19
19. Halmi NS, Duello T. (1976): Arch Pathol Lab Med 100:346
20. Heitz PU. (1979): Hormone Res 10:1
21. Horvath E, Kovacs K. (1974): Arch Pathol 97:221
22. Horvath E, Kovacs K, Killinger DW, Smyth HS, Platts ME, Weiss MH, Erzin C. (1983): Virchows Arch A Pathol Anat 398:277
23. Horvath E, Kovacs K, Scheithauer BW, Randall RV, Laws ER Jr, Thorner MO, Tindall GT, Barrow DL. (1983): Ultrastruct Path 5:175
24. Horvath E, Kovacs K, Singer W, Ezrin C, Kerenyi NA. (1977): Arch Pathol Lab Med 101:594
25. Horvath E, Kovacs K, Singer W, Smyth HS, Killinger DW, Ezrin C, Weiss MH. (1981): Cancer 47:761
26. Ishikawa H, Nogami H, Kamio M, Suzuki T. (1983): Virchows Arch A Pathol Anat 399:221
27. Kameya T, Tsumuraya M, Adachi I, Abe K, Ichikizaki K, Toya S, Demura R. (1980): Virchows Arch A Pathol Anat 387:31
28. Kleinberg DL, Boyd AE III, Wardlow S, Frantz AG, George A, Bryan N, Hilal S, Greising J, Hamilton D, Seltzer T, Sommers CJ. (1983): New Engl J Med 309:704
29. Kovacs K, Horvath E. (1979). In: Clinical Neuroendocrinology. A Pathophysiological Approach. Raven Press, New York, p 366
30. Kovacs K, Horvath E, Corenblum B, Sirek AMT, Penz G, Ezrin C. (1975): Virchows Arch A Pathol Anat 366:113
31. Kovacs K, Horvath E, Ezrin C, Weiss MH. (1982): Virchows Arch A Pathol Anat 395:59
32. Kovacs K, Horvath E, Ryan N. (1981). In: Diagnostic immunohistochemistry. Masson, New York, p 17
33. Kovacs K, Horvath E, Thorner MO, Rogol AD. (1984): Virchows Arch A Pathol Anat 403:77
34. Landolt AM. (1975): Acta Neurochir Suppl 22:1
35. Lipper S, Insenberg HD, Kahn LB. (1984): Arch Pathol Lab Med 108:31
36. Lloyd RV, Gikes PW, Chandler WF. (1983): Am J Surg Path 7:251
37. Martin NW, Hales M, Wilson CB. (1981): J Neurosurg 55:615
38. Martinez AJ, Lee A, Moossy J, Maroon JC. (1980): Ann Neurol 7:24
39. MCCarty KS Jr., Dobson CE II. (1980): Clin Obstet Gynecol 23:367
40. McComb DJ, Bayley TA, Horvath E, Kovacs K, Kourides IA. (1984): Cancer 53:1538
41. McComb DJ, Ryan N, Horvath E, Kovacs K. (1983): Arch Pathol Lab Med 107:488
42. Nissim M, Ambrosi B, Bernasconi V, Giannatasio G, Giovanelli MA, Bassetti M, Vaccari U, Moriondo P, Spada A, Travaglini P, Faglia G. (1982): J Endocrinol Invest 5:409
43. Peake GT, McKeel DW, Jarrett L, Daughaday WH. (1969): J Clin Endocrinol Metab 29:1383
44. Randall RV, Laws ER Jr, Abboud CF, Ebersold MJ, Kao PC, Scheithauer BW. (1983): Mayo Clin Proc 58:108
45. Rilliet B, Mohr G, Robert F, Hardy J. (1981): Surg Neurol 15:249
46. Robert F, Hardy J. (1975): Arch Pathol 99:625
47. Sang H, Johnson C. (1984): Human Path 15:94
48. Scheithauer BW. (1982). In: Management of Pituitary Adenomas and Related Lesions with Emphasis on Transsphenoidal Microsurgery. Appleton-Century-Crofts, New York, p 129
49. Spark RF, Baker R, Bienfang DC, Bergland R. (1982): J Am Med Assoc 247: 311
50. Tindall GT, Kovacs K, Horvath E, Thorner MO. (1982): J Clin Endocrinol Metab 55:1178
51. Vance ML, Evans WS, Thorner MO. (1984): Ann Intern Med 100:78
52. Weiss MH, Wycoff RR, Yadley R, Gott P, Feldon S. (1983): Neurosurgery 12:640
53. Zimmerman EA, Defendini R, Frantz AG. (1974): J Clin Endocrinol Metab 38:577

Prolactin. Basic and clinical correlates
R.M. MacLeod, M.O. Thorner and U. Scapagnini (eds.),
Fidia Research Series, vol. I,
Liviana Press, Padova © 1985

FUNCTIONAL HETEROGENEITY OF HUMAN PROLACTIN-PRODUCING PITUITARY ADENOMA CELLS

Miyuki Ishibashi and Tohru Yamaji

Third Department of Internal Medicine, Faculty of Medicine,
University of Tokyo, Hongo, Tokyo 113, Japan

Prolactinoma is the most frequently diagnosed functioning pituitary tumor and may account for approximately 30% of all pituitary tumors. In addition, the existence of mixed growth hormone (GH)-prolactin adenomas is known in a substantial number of patients with acromegaly (1,2). We have recently shown that the concomitant production and secretion of prolactin from human corticotroph adenomas is not unusual and could occur in patients with Cushing's disease whose serum prolactin levels are slightly elevated or even in subjects without hyperprolactinemia (3). Thus almost all functioning pituitary adenomas are composed of, or at least contain, prolactin cells.

While morphological characteristics of prolactin cell pituitary adenomas have been extensively studied by several investigators (4-6), the functional aspects of these tumors are not well understood. The present study was undertaken to examine the *in vitro* responses of prolactin cell adenomas to secretagogues to determine whether functional heterogeneity exists among these adenomas and to elucidate the origin of prolactin cells in the adenomas.

MONOLAYER CULTURE OF PITUITARY ADENOMA CELLS

Pituitary adenoma tissues were obtained by transsphenoidal adenomectomy from 12 patients with prolactinoma, 20 patients with acromegaly, one patient with Cushing's disease and one patient with Nelson's syndrome (Table 1). In all of the adenomas, the presence of prolactin cells was demonstrated by immunohistochemistry. The method for the monolayer culture of pituitary cells has been previously described in detail (7,8). In brief, pituitary adenomas were cut into small pieces and dispersed by incubation with trypsin-collagenase solution at 37 C. A 2-ml aliquot containing 2-8 x 10^5 dissociated cells was planted in plastic Petri dishes (35 x 10 mm) and incubated at 37 C in a humidified atmosphere of 95% air-5% CO_2. The culture medium consisted of

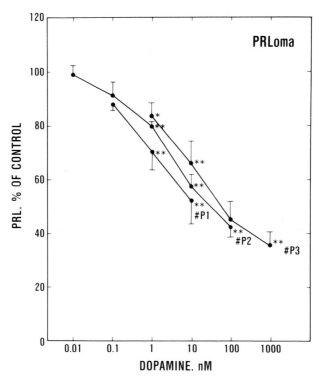

Figure 1. Effect of varying concentrations of dopamine on prolactin secretion by cultured pituitary adenoma cells taken from 3 patients with prolactinoma. *, $p < 0.05$ vs. controls; **, $p < 0.01$ vs. controls.

Eagle's Minimum Essential Medium in Earle's solution including 10% fetal calf serum, 100 U/ml penicillin and 10 ug/ml streptomycin sulfate. Plating efficiencies of cells varied from tissue to tissue and were generally higher for pituitary adenoma cells from acromegalic patients (20-55%) than for prolactinoma cells or corticotroph adenoma cells (4-14%). Pituitary cells actively secreted prolactin into the media and the responses

Table 1. *Patients with pituitary adenomas*

	Number of patients	Age (yrs)	Serum hormone levels		
			PRL (ng/ml)	GH (ng/ml)	ACTH (pg/ml)
Prolactinoma	12	21-47	115-16,400	—	—
Acromegaly	20	24-59	7-58	8-370	—
Cushing's disease and Nelson's syndrome	2	39,43	76,293	—	180,615

DOPAMINE (DA)

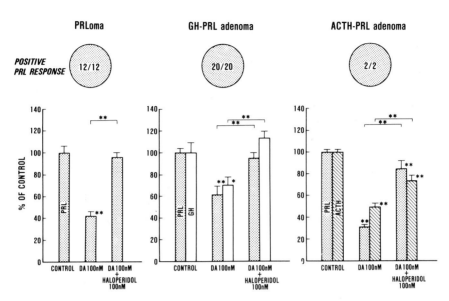

Figure 2. Effect of dopamine alone or in combination with haloperidol on prolactin, GH, and ACTH secretion by cultured adenoma cells. *, $p < 0.05$ vs. controls; **, $p < 0.01$ vs. controls.

to secretagogues were satisfactorily maintained for as long as one month by changing medium at 2-4 day intervals, although a gradual decline in prolactin release was seen when the culture was continued (7).

Incubation studies, started after the cells formed a monolayer, were performed at intervals of at least two days. Individual cultures were randomly allocated for each experiment. Four or more cultures were used for the control and variables and run simultaneously. On the day of the experiment, the medium was replaced by 2 ml of Eagle's Minimum Essential Medium in Earle's solution containing 0.5% human serum albumin instead of fetal calf serum. Cells were incubated for 1 h at 37 C in a humidified atmosphere of 95% air and 5% CO_2. The medium was then removed and cells were further incubated for 2 h in 2 ml of fresh medium with or without test materials. After incubation, the medium was centrifuged and the supernate was stored at -20 C until assayed.

Prolactin, GH, and ACTH concentrations in the medium of both preincubation and experimental incubation were determined by radioimmunoassays as previously described (7-10). Immunological materials for the radioimmunoassay were kindly donated by the National Hormone and Pituitary Program and the National Institute of Arthritis, Diabetes, Digestive and Kidney Diseases, U. S. Public Health Service. Results are expressed as the percentage of hormones secreted in the experimental incubation compared with those secreted during the preincubation for individual cultures. For comparison, the mean values obtained in the control study were designated as 100%. Values in figures are the mean ± SEM. The significance of difference was calculated using Student's t-test and analysis of variance.

PROLACTIN RESPONSES TO DOPAMINE AND SOMATOSTATIN

Figure 1 shows the effect of varying concentrations of dopamine on prolactin secretion by cultured adenoma cells taken from 3 patients with prolactinoma. Dopamine at a concentration as low as 1 nM significantly decreased prolactin secretion in all experiments and a parallel dose-response relationship was obtained between prolactin secretion and dopamine concentrations.

The effect of dopamine on prolactin secretion was then compared in 3 different groups of prolactin cell adenomas, i.e., pure prolactinomas, mixed GH-prolactin adenomas and mixed ACTH-prolactin adenomas. As shown in Figure 2, dopamine consistently inhibited both GH and prolactin secretion by mixed GH-prolactin adenomas obtained from 20 patients with acromegaly. The result is in accordance with our earlier observation that bromocriptine does reduce the secretion rates of GH and prolactin from pituitary adenoma tissues of acromegaly in a perifusion system (11). Similarly, both ACTH and prolactin secretion from mixed ACTH-prolactin adenomas were

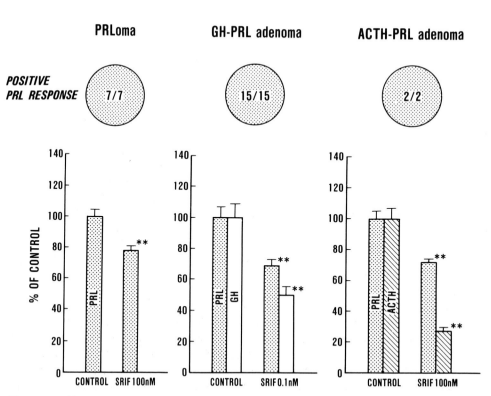

Figure 3. Effect of somatostatin on prolactin, GH and ACTH secretion by cultured adenoma cells. *,p < 0.05 vs. controls; **, p < 0.01 vs. controls.

THYROTROPIN-RELEASING HORMONE (TRH)

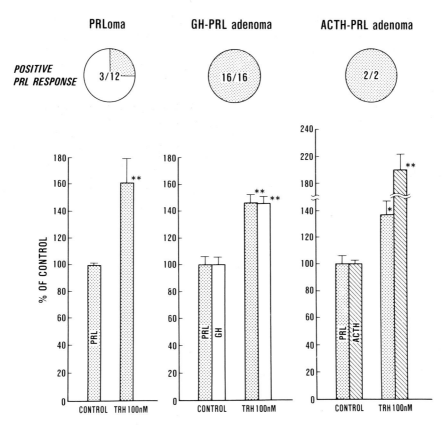

Figure 4. Effect of TRH on prolactin, GH and ACTH secretion by cultured adenoma cells. *, p<0.05 vs. controls; **, p<0.01 vs. controls.

significantly decreased by dopamine. When a dopamine antagonist, haloperidol, was added to the incubation media, the inhibitory action of dopamine on hormone release was blocked suggesting that the effect of dopamine was occasioned through a specific dopaminergic receptor activation.

Addition of somatostatin to the media clearly suppressed, in a manner similar that of dopamine, prolactin secretion from cultured adenoma cells of all three groups (Fig. 3). Although the effect of somatostatin on prolactin secretion in men is controversial, the result clearly indicates that somatostatin acts on pituitary adenoma cells to inhibit prolactin secretion. In one mixed ACTH-prolactin adenoma, ACTH secretion was also suppressed by somatostatin. Of further interest is the response of mixed GH-prolactin adenomas. In this group of adenomas, secretion of both GH and prolactin was supersensitive and responded to a picomolar concentration of somatostatin.

698

The foregoing results have shown that dopamine as well as somatostatin unequivocally inhibits prolactin secretion from pituitary adenoma cells of all three groups and further suggest that GH cells and ACTH cells coexisting in prolactin cell adenomas respond to dopamine and somatostatin in a qualitatively similar fashion.

PROLACTIN RESPONSES TO TRH, GRF, AND CRF

To clarify whether a difference may exist in prolactin responses to secretagogues among different groups of prolactin cell adenomas, we then tested the effects of thyrotropin-releasing hormone (TRH), human growth hormone-releasing factor (GRF), and ovine corticotropin-releasing-factor (CRF) on prolactin secretion from cultured pituitary adenoma cells. Figure 4 illustrates the prolactin responses to TRH. In mixed GH-prolactin adenomas, TRH significantly increased the secretion rates of both hor-

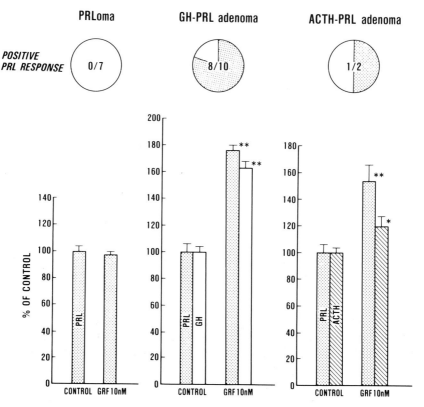

Figure 5. Effect of GRF on prolactin, GH and ACTH secretion by cultured adenoma cells. *,p < 0.05 vs. controls; **, p < 0.01 vs. controls.

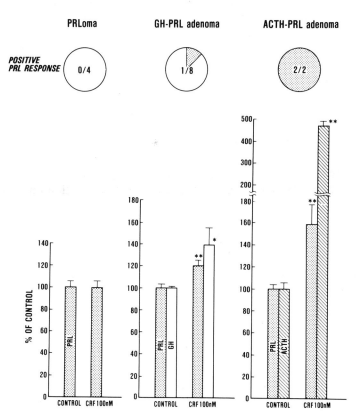

Figure 6. Effect of CRF on prolactin, GH and ACTH secretion by cultured adenoma cells. *, p < 0.05 vs. controls; **, p < 0.01 vs. controls.

mones in all the experiments. TRH likewise induced ACTH and prolactin release from 2 mixed ACTH-prolactin adenomas. In contrast, the positive prolactin response to TRH was observed in only one-fourth of the prolactinomas. Since normal human pituitary prolactin cells respond to TRH to secrete prolactin (7), the result suggests a possible alteration of TRH receptor on prolactinoma cells.

When hGRF (1-44) was added to the incubation media, GH secretion was significantly increased in mixed GH-prolactin adenomas (Fig. 5). Moreover, prolactin secretion also was enhanced by GRF in approximately 80% of this type of pituitary adenoma. In sharp contrast, none of the 7 prolactinomas studied responded to GRF. In one mixed ACTH-prolactin adenoma, GRF increased both ACTH and prolactin secretion.

Figure 6 depicts the effect of ovine CRF on prolactin secretion from pituitary adenoma cells of three different groups. In 2 mixed ACTH-prolactin adenomas, CRF

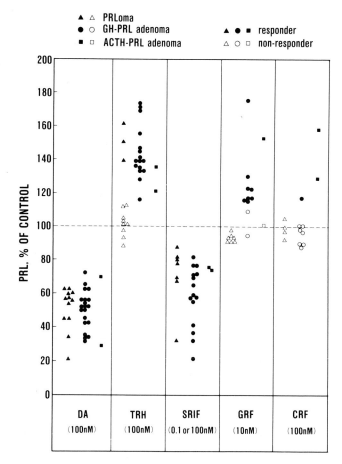

Figure 7. *In vitro* prolactin responses to various secretagogues in prolactinomas, mixed GH-prolactin adenomas, and mixed ACTH-prolactin adenomas.

elicited a significant increase in the release of both hormones and this stimulatory effect of CRF was blocked by coincubation of the cells with hydrocortisone. Although one out of 8 mixed GH-prolactin adenomas responded to CRF with a modest rise in GH and prolactin levels, the remainder did not respond. Similarly, CRF was ineffective in triggering prolactin secretion from prolactinoma cells in all experiments.

FUNCTIONAL HETEROGENEITY OF HUMAN PROLACTIN-PRODUCING PITUITARY ADENOMA CELLS AND ITS SIGNIFICANCE

Figure 7 summarizes the prolactin responses to various stimuli in pure prolactinomas, mixed GH-prolactin adenomas, and mixed ACTH-prolactin adenomas. Dopamine and somatostatin uniformly inhibited prolactin secretion in all groups of

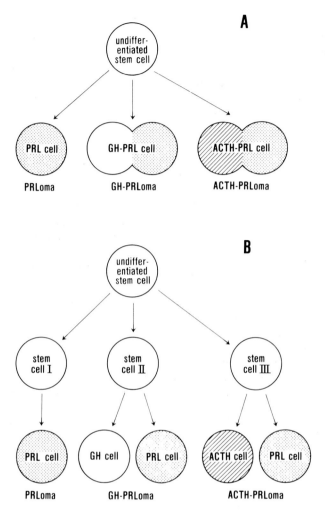

Figure 8. Development of human prolactin-producing pituitary adenomas.

pituitary adenomas. TRH, on the other hand, induced prolactin release in mixed GH-prolactin adenomas and in mixed ACTH-prolactin adenomas, however, most prolactinomas did not respond to TRH. Although GRF triggered prolactin secretion from many GH-prolactin-producing adenomas and from one mixed ACTH-prolactin adenoma, none of the pure prolactinomas responded. In 2 mixed ACTH-prolactin adenomas, prolactin secretion was increased in response to CRF, whereas no stimulatory effect of CRF was observed in most adenomas in the remaining groups. These results clearly show that functional heterogeneity exists in human prolactin-producing pituitary adenomas.

What then is responsible for the functional heterogeneity of prolactin-producing adenomas? At least two formulations should be considered in this context. First, in mixed adenomas, a single cell may produce and secrete both hormones as in postulation A in Figure 8. Second, in mixed adenomas, two hormones may be derived from separate cells as in postulation B. Since no definitive evidence has been obtained, on a morphological basis, for a single pituitary adenoma cell to produce two separate hormones (1,2,4,5,12,13), postulation B may be more likely. If this assumption is correct, then it may be concluded that, in mixed pituitary adenomas, prolactin cells and GH or ACTH cells arise from a common ancestor.

REFERENCES

1. Guyda H, Robert F, Colle E, Hardy J. (1973): J Clin Endocrinol Metab 36:531
2. Zimmerman AE, Diffendini R, Frantz AG. (1974): J Clin Endocrinol Metab 38:577
3. Yamaji T, Ishibashi M, Teramoto A, Fukushima T. (1984): J Clin Endocrinol Metab 58:790
4. Horvath E, Kovacs K. (1976): Canad J Neurol Sci 3:9
5. Kovacs K, Horvath E. (1979): In: Tolis G, Labrie F, Martin JB, Naftolin F (eds) Clinical Neuroendocrinology. Raven Press, New York, p 367
6. Robert F. (1983): In: Tolis G, Stefanis C, Mountokalakis T, Labrie F (eds) Prolactin and Prolactinoma. Raven Press, New York, p 339
7. Ishibashi M, Yamaji T. (1984): J Clin Invest 73:66
8. Ishibashi M, Yamaji T. (1981): J Clin Invest 68:1018
9. Yamaji T. (1974): Metabolism 23:745
10. Ishibashi M, Yamaji T, Kosaka K. (1977): J Clin Endocrinol Metab 45:275
11. Ishibashi M, Yamaji T. (1978): J Clin Endocrinol Metab 47:1251
12. Corenblum B, Sirek AMT, Horvath E, Kovacs K, Ezrin C. (1976): J Clin Endocrinol Metab 42:857
13. Sherry SH, Guay AT, Lee AK, Hedley-Whyte ET, Federman M, Freidberg SR, Woolf PD. (1982): J Clin Endocrinol Metab 55:947

Prolactin. Basic and clinical correlates
R.M. MacLeod, M.O. Thorner and U. Scapagnini (eds.),
Fidia Research Series, vol. I,
Liviana Press, Padova © 1985

Section XI
Clinical and therapeutic
aspects of hyperprolactinemia

ETIOLOGY OF PROLACTINOMAS: AN OVERVIEW

Steven W. J. Lamberts and Michael O. Thorner

Depts. of Internal Medicine
Erasmus University, Rotterdam, The Netherlands
and University of Virginia Charlottesville, Virginia

Studies on the pathogenesis of prolactinomas and clinical and therapeutic aspects of hyperprolactinemia continue to be topics of immense importance. Weiner et al. proposed an attractive hypothesis to explain the etiology of prolactin secreting adenomas in animals and humans. This is based on the observation that an anomalous direct arterial blood supply to a region of the anterior pituitary exists in a percentage of the human population rather than a local response to estrogenic stimulation. In the rat, however, Leadem presented data demonstrating the importance of estrogens in prolactinoma development but presented evidence that the pineal gland may also have a moderating effect on this process. Translation of these two important presentations into a clinical setting is awaited in the future. Drs. Landolt and Kovacs discussed the morphological aspects of human prolactinomas. There is still major controversy as to whether the amount of fibrosis in prolactinomas is increased by bromocriptine treatment. Dr. Landolt agreed that there was no increase in fibrosis in non-prolactinomas treated with bromocriptine. Dr. Kovacs pointed out, however, that fibrosis in the pituitary is very common and therefore it is very difficult to be dogmatic as to whether the amount of fibrosis seen in some patients who have been treated with bromocriptine is indeed increased over that of non-bromocriptine treated prolactinomas. The question of the mammosomatotroph was again discussed in the light not only of the histological and immunocytochemical findings but also of functional studies performed *in vitro*. This was particularly emphasized in the studies of Drs. Ishibashi and Yamaji who investigated the effects of dopamine, GRF, and CRF in primary cultures of human pituitary tumors removed at the time of surgery.

The diagnosis and management of hyperprolactinemia was discussed in detail. Dr. Malarkey presented data on patients with mild hyperprolactinemia pointing out that some of them demonstrate a reduction in prolactin over time and very few of these tumors continue to expand while being followed over a number of years. Drs. Molitch and Reichlin discussed the characteristics of prolactin secretion in response to various stimuli including the administration of L-dopa and carbidopa in patients with hypothalamic disease. However, the responses were very variable and it was extremely difficult to come to any conclusions. A new method for demonstrating pituitary tumors was described by Dr. Muhr using positron emission tomography with the aid of [^{11}C]-bromocriptine. However, these studies appear to be preliminary at the present time and their role in diagnosis is still open to question. The experiences that have been encountered by many investigators in their research using newer dopamine agonists were presented.

Finally Drs. Besser and Laws summarized the dilemmas of clinicians in their treatment of patients with prolactinomas. In contrast to previous Congresses, there appears to be much greater agreement about the merits of medical therapy and surgery between physicians and surgeons. Dr. Laws presented data that appears to be representative of that found by many different centers now that there is an incidence of recurrence of hyperprolactinemia in approximately a quarter of patients successfully treated by surgery. Dr. Besser discussed his approach to the treatment of hyperprolactinemia emphasizing not only medical treatment but also radiotherapy. However, he did stress that the method of administration of external pituitary radiation is extremely important and radiotherapy between medical centers cannot be compared in the same way that surgical results cannot be compared, as they are highly dependent upon the radiotherapeutic and surgical technique and the skill of the individual who performs them.

Prolactin. Basic and clinical correlates
R.M. MacLeod, M.O. Thorner and U. Scapagnini (eds.),
Fidia Research Series, vol. I,
Liviana Press, Padova © 1985

Section XI
Clinical and therapeutic
aspects of hyperprolactinemia

PATIENTS WITH IDIOPATHIC HYPERPROLACTINEMIA INFREQUENTLY DEVELOP PITUITARY TUMORS

William B. Malarkey, Tammy L. Martin, and Moon Kim

Department of Medicine and Obstetrics and Gynecology,
The Ohio State University Hospitals
Columbus, Ohio 43210

Hyperprolactinemia is a common clinical disorder and has been found in up to 25% of patients with secondary amenorrhea (1,2). Idiopathic hyperprolactinemia (IH) can be defined as the presence of elevated serum prolactin levels in a patient in the absence of demonstrable pituitary or CNS disease and of any other recognized cause of increased prolactin secretion.

Before the diagnosis of IH can be accepted, the presence of a microadenoma of the pituitary has to be excluded. The presence of a normal brain CT scan assists in establishing the diagnosis of IH, however, many physicians have assumed that numerous patients with IH harbor microadenomas not seen by CT scan evaluations.

The purpose of this study was to evaluate the long term clinical outcome of 41 patients initially diagnosed as having IH. The initial mean ± SE serum prolactin level of these patients was 57 ± 6 ng/ml and all had galactorrhea and/or amenorrhea. Their skull x-rays and/or CT scans were normal. Their mean followup period was 5.5 years with a range of 2 to 11 years. Twenty subjects were followed more than 5 years and 21 patients were reevaluated 2 to 5 years after their initial visit. All of the serum prolactin levels were measured in the same laboratory where the potency of various NIH standards has been evaluated and appropriate corrections to the original VLS #1 standard have been made periodically. All of the patients were reevaluated during the last 6 months of 1983. At this time their mean ± SE serum prolactin level remained the same, decreased, and returned to normal in 34 of the 41 subjects (Fig. 1). A change of 50% from the initial prolactin level was considered a significant change. This definition was used because in our experience with 24 hour blood sampling in patients with IH we rarely saw two daytime serum prolactin levels that varied from one another by more than 50% (3).

Six of nine patients whose initial serum prolactin levels were less than 40 ng/ml returned into the normal range during the followup period while 2 remained the same and one increased (Fig. 1). Eight of 24 patients whose initial serum prolactin level was

706

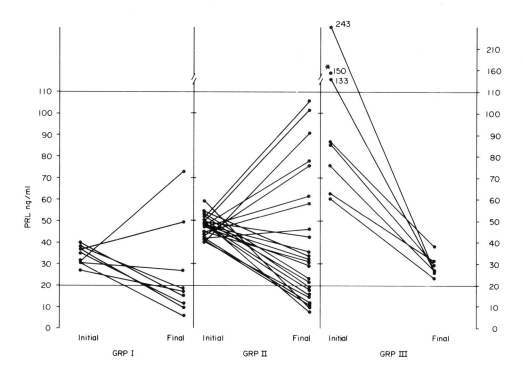

Figure 1. Patients with idiopathic hyperprolactinemia whose initial prolactin levels were < 40 ng/ml (Group I), 40-60 ng/ml (Group II), and > 60 ng/ml (Group III). One subject (*) in Group III subsequently developed a pituitary tumor. Note the frequent decrease in final serum prolactin levels obtained 2 to 11 years (mean 5.5) following the initial determination. Fourteen subjects had followup serum prolactin levels which decreased into the normal range (< 20 ng/ml).

between 40 and 60 ng/ml returned to normal while 2 decreased, 9 remained the same, and 5 increased (Fig. 1). In the group of eight patients whose initial serum prolactin level was greater than 60 ng/ml, seven had prolactin levels which decreased and one which increased (Fig. 1). This latter patient's initial serum prolactin level was 150 ng/ml and was the only subject who developed a clinically detectable pituitary tumor 9 years following her initial evaluation. No patient demonstrated a worsening of signs or symptoms at the followup evaluation, at which time 7 patients had no further amenorrhea or galactorrhea. Six of the patients, however, with normal serum prolactin levels still had galactorrhea. This latter finding suggests that following an initial elevation in serum prolactin levels lactation can be maintained with a normal serum prolactin concentration.

CT scans performed on all patients who had a significant increase in serum prolactin levels at followup evaluation did not reveal any evidence of a pituitary tumor except in the previously mentioned subject.

All of these women were in their reproductive years although not all were sexually active. Nine pregnancies, however, occurred spontaneously without drug treatment and 18 pregnancies occurred following the short term use (<5 months) of bromocriptine. All of these women delivered normal infants and none developed signs or symptoms of pituitary tumor during or following these pregnancies.

In summary: 1) If a tumor is not present in a patient with hyperprolactinemia when she is initially evaluated, it is unlikely that she will develop this lesion over the next 5 to 6 years; 2) patients with IH whose initial serum prolactin levels are less than 40 ng/ml will usually decrease into the normal range; 3) also, patients whose initial prolactin levels are less than 100 ng/ml will usually decrease or remain the same on later evaluations; 4) Successful induction of pregnancy and a normal gestation and delivery are to be expected in IH patients; and 5) our data does not support the use of ablative pituitary therapy in patients with idiopathic hyperprolactinemia.

REFERENCES

1. Frank S, Murray MAF, Jequier AM, Steele SJ, Nabarro JDN, Jacobs HS. (1975): Clin Endocrinol (Oxf) 4:597
2. Pepperell RJ. (1981): Fertil Steril 35:267
3. Malarkey WB. (1975): J Clin Endocrinol Metab 40:198

Prolactin. Basic and clinical correlates
R.M. MacLeod, M.O. Thorner and U. Scapagnini (eds.),
Fidia Research Series, vol. I,
Liviana Press, Padova © 1985

Section XI
Clinical and therapeutic
aspects of hyperprolactinemia

HYPOTHALAMIC HYPERPROLACTINEMIA: NEUROENDOCRINE REGULATION OF PROLACTIN SECRETION IN PATIENTS WITH LESIONS OF THE HYPOTHALAMUS AND PITUITARY STALK

Mark E. Molitch[1] and Seymour Reichlin

Division of Endocrinology and Metabolism, Department of Medicine
Tufts University School of Medicine, New England Medical Center
Boston, Massachusetts 02111

Hyperprolactinemia caused by lesions of the hypothalamus and of the pituitary stalk is due to disturbance of the neuroendocrine mechanisms that control prolactin secretion. Extensive experimental study in animals has demonstrated that prolactin secretion is under tonic inhibitory control by one or more prolactin inhibitory factors (PIF), the most important of which is dopamine. Several hypothalamic factors with prolactin releasing activity have also been identified, but their physiological roles in prolactin regulation are uncertain. It has been assumed for many years that the hyperprolactinemia observed in patients with hypothalamic-stalk disease can be regarded as a manifestation of a "pituitary isolation syndrome" due to disinhibition of tonic PIF acting at the level of the pituitary lactotrophs (1). To test this hypothesis we have characterized in detail a number of aspects of neuroendocrine regulation of prolactin secretion in a group of patients in whom hyperprolactinemia was attributed to PIF deficiency, and have compared the incidence of hyperprolactinemia with other aspects of anterior pituitary function.

PATIENTS

Included in this series are 6 patients with lesions of the hypothalamus and/or pituitary stalk region, 8 patients with large "non-functioning" pituitary adenomas with moderate to marked extrasellar extension that was presumed to have deformed the

---

[1] Present address: Center for Endocrinology, Metabolism and Nutrition, Northwestern University Medical School, 303 E. Chicago Ave., Chicago, IL 60611

Table 1 Case Descriptions

Case No.	Age	Sex	Diagnosis	Basal PRL (ng/ml)	Pituitary Status				Post-operative PRL (ng/ml)	Comments
					GH	ACTH	TSH	ADH		
1	26	F	Craniopharyngioma	50.5	D[1]	N[2]	N	N	55.9	Postop DI, Panhypopit.
2	29	F	Craniopharyngioma (Rathke's cleft cyst)	122.0	D	N	N	N	27.6	Postop DI, Panhypopit.
3	32	F	Postop. for Rathke's cleft cyst	58.9	D	D	D	D		Postop DI, Panhypopit. Preop. PRL 3.0 ng/ml
4	23	F	Postop. for craniopharyngioma	30.8	D	D	D	D		Postop DI, Panhypopit. Preop PRL 12-18 ng/ml
5	20	F	Eosinophilic granuloma	20.0	N	N	D	D		PRL levels 10-30 ng/ml
6	77	M	Ectatic basilar artery	40.2	−[3]	D	D	D		↑ PRL after L-thyroxine Rx
7	54	F	Non-secreting adenoma	47.6	D	N	−	N	18.2	On L-thyroxine Rx for 1 hypothyroidism
8	66	M	Non-secreting adenoma	36.5	D	D	D	D	24.0	
9	62	M	Non-secreting	34.9	D	N	D	N	8.0	Delayed TSH response to TRH at 60' from <2.5 to 7.1 T_4 5.4, T_3 70
10	56	F	Non-secreting adenoma	75.3	D	D	N	N	28.2	↑ PRL after L-thyroxine Rx

Table 1 Case Descriptions Continued

Case No.	Age	Sex	Diagnosis	Basal PRL (ng/ml)	Pituitary Status GH	ACTH	TSH	ADH	Post-operative PRL (ng/ml)	Comments
11	37	F	Non-secreting adenoma	38.0	D	D	D	N	14.9	Delayed TSH response to TRH at 60' from <2.5 to 10.2, T_4 3.1
12	71	F	Non-secreting adenoma	38.4	D	D	D	N	<2.5	Delayed TSH response to TRH at 60' from <2.5 to 12.5
13	33	F	Non-secreting adenoma	86.9	N	N	N	N	33	
14	61	F	Non-secreting adenoma	98.4	-	N	N	N	<2.5	
15	27	F	Empty sella (PEG)[4]	63.8	N	N	N	N		
16		F	Empty sella (PEG, CT)	77.5	N	N	N	N		
17	35	F	Empty sella (CT)	28.8	-	N	N	N		
18	43	M	Empty sella (CT)	76.8	N	N	N	N		
19	26	F	Empty sella (PEG)	33.2	N	N	N	N		
20		M	Empty sella (CT)	42.3	N	N	N	N		
21	43	F	Empty sella (CT)	67.0	N	N	N	N		Chronic hypothyroidism on L-thyroxine replacement

----

[1] D - Decreased function; [2] N - Normal function; [3] (-) - Not tested; [4] Radiologic study used: PEG - pneumocephalogram; CT - computed tomography

pituitary stalk, and 7 patients with the empty sella syndrome. Cases 1, 2 and 4 have been published previously (2). The diagnosis and clinical features are summarized in Table 1.

TESTING PROCEDURES

TRH was administered as an intravenous bolus in a dose of 500 ug. Hypoglycemia was achieved by intravenous injection of a bolus of regular insulin (0.15 u/kg). For the L-dopa test, 500 mg of L-dopa (Larodopa, Roche) was administered orally. In the carbidopa/L-dopa test, carbidopa (3,4) was administered orally in a dose of 50 mg every 6 hours for 24 hours before the administration of 100 mg of L-dopa. To test for the presence of partial ADH deficiency, patients underwent an overnight dehydration test (5).

BASAL PROLACTIN LEVELS

Basal prolactin levels are listed in Table 1. All patients but 1 had a prolactin level < 100 ng/ml. In case 2, preoperative prolactin levels ranged between 93 and 148 ng/ml. Following transsphenoidal resection of a Rathke's cleft cyst with resultant development of diabetes insipidus and panhypopituitarism indicating high stalk section, prolactin levels fell to 25-28 ng/ml.

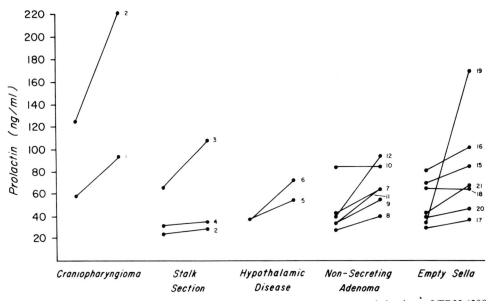

Figure 1. Basal and peak prolactin levels in response to the intravenous injection of TRH (500 ug). The case numbers correspond to the cases described in Table 1.

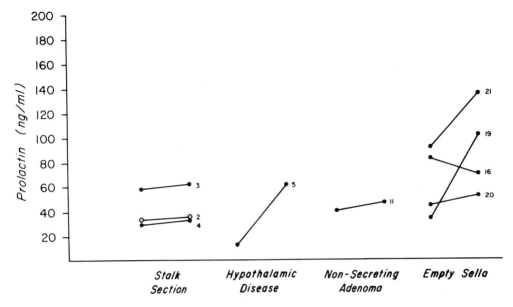

Figure 2. Basal and peak prolactin levels in response to insulin-induced hypoglycemia. Case numbers as in Table 1.

RESPONSE TO TRH

TRH tests were performed to assess the pituitary lactotroph response to direct stimulation (Fig. 1). All patients tested had blunted (increment < 100% above basal) prolactin responses to TRH except one woman with a non-secreting adenoma (Case 12) and another (Case 16) with an empty sella syndrome both of whom had a normal response.

RESPONSE TO HYPOGLYCEMIA

Hypoglycemia was induced to assess the overall integrated hypothalamic control of prolactin secretion (Fig. 2). Tests were not performed in older patients or those with lesions that might have served as seizure foci. Blunted responses (increment < 100% above basal) were found in the three tested patients with stalk section, the tested patient with a non-secreting adenoma, and three of the four tested patients with the empty sella syndrome. Normal responses were seen in the patient with eosinophilic granuloma (Case 5) and the one tested patient with the empty sella syndrome who had a normal response to TRH (Case 16).

RESPONSE TO L-DOPA AND CARBIDOPA/L-DOPA

Of the two patients with hypothalamic/stalk tumors (Cases 1 and 2), prolactin levels in one were suppressed normally by L-dopa whereas the other had a blunted response (Fig. 3). Following surgical treatment (including stalk section) their responses were qualitatively similar. The prolactin levels of the other patients with stalk section were suppressed normally by L-dopa. The patient with the eosinophilic granuloma (Case 5) was normoprolactinemic on the day she was tested and suppressed normally. Of the five patients with non-secreting adenomas three suppressed normally (Cases 8, 9, 11) but the other two (Cases 7, 10) had blunted responses. Of the five patients with empty sellas tested, only two (Cases 15, 17) were suppressed normally by L-dopa.

When stalk sectioned patients are given L-dopa, it is presumed that inhibition of prolactin secretion is brought about by stimulation of dopamine receptors of the lactotrophs, and that inhibition of dopa decarboxylase by the peripherally active inhibitor carbidopa would abolish this response. What was observed was that carbidopa significantly blunted the response to L-dopa in seven patients with either stalk section or large non-functioning tumors, but did not abolish the response in any patient and in one case was completely without effect in modifying the inhibitory response to L-dopa (Case 5). The studies of the patient with eosinophilic granuloma (Case 5) were inconclusive because her prolactin levels were normal on the days of the tests. In the

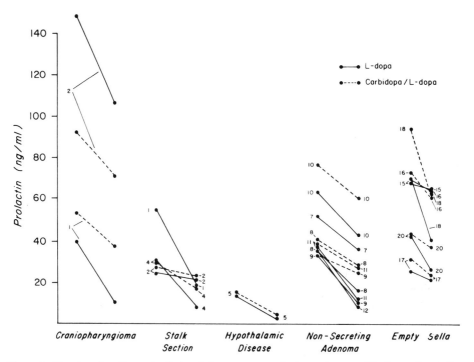

Figure 3. Basal and nadir prolactin levels in response to L-dopa alone and L-dopa after 24 hours of pretreatment with the decarboxylase inhibitor carbidopa. Case numbers as in Table I.

other 5 cases, L-dopa did not lower prolactin levels and hence the carbidopa effect could not be evaluated. Thus, all seven of the cases that could be evaluated showed persistent inhibitory responses, albeit blunted, to L-dopa even when peripheral conversion was blocked. This implies either incomplete stalk section in these patients or incomplete blockade of peripheral dopa decarboxylation by carbidopa in the dose administered.

OTHER ANTERIOR AND POSTERIOR PITUITARY FUNCTION

These patients had varying degrees of anterior pituitary dysfunction (Table 1). Data on gonadotropin/gonadal function are not presented because it is difficult in these cases to know whether loss of function is due to hypothalamic disease, pituitary disease, or the effects of hyperprolactinemia. GH deficiency was documented in each of the eleven patients with structural disease who were tested using the response to hypoglycemia or L-dopa. However, GH testing was not repeated in most cases after sex hormone replacement; this has been shown to be necessary for accurate documentation of GH deficiency in patients with hypogonadism (6). Therefore, these results with respect to GH are inconclusive. Only one patient with an empty sella had decreased GH response to stimulation. ACTH deficiency was documented by metyrapone testing or hypoglycemia stimulation in seven of the fourteen patients with structural disease. TSH adequacy in these patients was variable. One patient (Case 7) had chronic primary hypothyroidism and had undetectable TSH levels even after TRH stimulation (while taking thyroxine). Eight patients had normal thyroid function and TSH responses to TRH. Six patients -- the four with postoperative stalk section, one with eosinophilic granuloma (Case 5), and one with ectatic basilar artery (Case 6) -- had hypothyroidism associated with low serum T_4 and T_3 levels and absent TSH responses to TRH. Three cases with non-secreting adenomas (Cases 9, 11 and 12) had mild hypothyroidism with delayed increments of TSH from 2.5 to 7.1 uU/ml, 10.2, and 12.5 uU/ml, respectively, at 60 min after TRH. All patients with empty sellas had normal ACTH and TSH function.

The four patients with postoperative stalk section and the patients with eosinophilic granuloma (Case 5) and ectatic basilar artery (Case 6) had diabetes insipidus. None of the patients with non-secreting tumors or empty sellas had this finding.

DISCUSSION

Transection of the pituitary stalk by a surgical section is the model of pituitary isolation to which the other cases of hypothalamic hyperprolactinemia may be compared. With stalk transection the hypothalamic-pituitary portal vessels are severed, causing cessation of transmission of release and inhibitory factors to the pituitary. However, pituitary tissue in the posteromedial portion of the gland is preserved, presumably because it receives blood from the short hypophysial portal vessels which are supplied by the inferior hypophysial arteries (7). The degree of hyperprolactinemia found in patients with stalk section is relatively modest (27-56 ng/ml in Cases 1-4) in this study. Three additional patients have been reported in the literature in whom pituitary stalk section was performed as palliative therapy for cancer (8,9). They also had only modest elevation of prolactin levels (27-36 ng/ml). The prolactin responses to TRH in our three cases were blunted as was also true for two of the three patients reported by others (8,9).

One possible explanation for the blunting of TRH-induced responses is that stalk section-induced prolactin hypersecretion is associated with a smaller, more rapidly turning over pool, and a smaller readily releasable pool (10-12). The possible effects of stalk section on TRH receptors has not been determined.

Stimulation of prolactin secretion by hypoglycemia is probably mediated via the hypothalamus. As predicted, our three patients with stalk section had no significant elevation of prolactin in response to hypoglycemia, compatible with complete stalk section.

Direct stimulation of lactotroph dopamine receptors by dopamine (after conversion from L-dopa) in stalk sectioned patients caused a normal fall in prolactin levels in three of four such patients (Cases 2 and 4 from our series and Case 22 from the literature). However, when the conversion from L-dopa to dopamine in the periphery was blocked by carbidopa the fall in prolactin was only blunted and not abolished. Because these patients had other evidence of complete stalk section (panhypopituitarism and diabetes insipidus), we conclude that carbidopa in the doses used does not cause complete blockade of peripheral dopa decarboxylation.

Patients with true stalk section, therefore, have prolactin levels that basally are modestly elevated (27-56 ng/ml), that respond poorly to the direct stimulus of TRH, that do not respond to a stimulus mediated by the hypothalamus, i.e. hypoglycemia, and that respond normally to L-dopa.

The group of patients with mass lesions causing hypoprolactinemia (Cases 1, 2, 6-14) consisted of two patients with craniopharyngiomas, 8 patients with non-secreting pituitary adenomas and a patient with an ectatic basilar artery compressing the hypothalamus. These non-secreting adenomas were all chromophobic by conventional staining and did not stain positively for any hormone using immunohistochemical techniques. Hyperprolactinemia due to the suprasellar extension of immunohistochemically negative adenomas has been reported only once previously by Arafah et al (13) in 5 patients. Hyperprolactinemia has been documented in a number of patients with mass lesions of the hypothalamus in the literature. The prolactin responses to TRH were blunted in 7 of our 9 tested patients and in 24 of 32 similar cases in the literature (13-24). In our patients, responses to L-dopa were normal in seven of ten and these normal responses became blunted, but not completely abolished, after pretreatment with carbidopa in six of these seven. A similar blunting of the L-dopa suppression by carbidopa was seen in one of two similarly tested patients with hypothalamic lesions studied by Ferrari et al (25). This blunting of the L-dopa response to carbidopa is similar to what is seen in patients with prolactinomas (4,26).

The blunting but not complete abolition of prolactin response to L-dopa/carbidopa suggests that there is continued hypothalamic dopamine transmission to the pituitary in these patients with hypothalamic tumors. This may be explained by 3 possibilities: (1) there is only a partial disruption of hypothalamic/stalk function; (2) activation of prolactin releasing factors may also be involved; or (3) carbidopa, in the dose used, does not cause complete decarboxylase inhibition.

In our patients with mass lesions and infiltrative disease of the hypothalamus, as well as those similar cases reported by others, function of the other pituitary hormones was variable. In very few patients could it be said that there was the precise equivalent of stalk section.

It has been speculated that the prolactin elevation seen in patients with the empty sella syndrome is due to "pressure on the pituitary stalk which may interrupt prolactin inhibitory factor transport in a fashion similar to that of stalk section" (27). In the seven patients with hyperprolactinemia and an empty sella, other anterior pituitary functions were normal except for decreased GH reserve in one case, implying that the stalk itself was intact. In our series 6 or 7 patients had blunted prolactin responses to TRH and 3 of 4 had blunted responses to hypoglycemia. Thus these patients with partially empty sellas respond in a fashion similar to other patients with hypothalamic disease. It is possible that the empty sella is associated with distortion of the hypothalamic architecture rather than distortion of stalk architecture, resulting in selective hypothalamic dysfunction.

Although the majority of patients with hypothalamic or stalk lesion have prolactin levels that are only moderately elevated, a few exceptionally high values have been reported in some cases. In addition to Case 2 whose values were 122 ng/ml, 14 cases have been reported by others with values between 104 and 219 ng/ml (17,19,23,24,28-33) and this is strikingly higher than levels in patients with simple stalk section. In Case 2 basal levels were around 120 ng/ml with otherwise normal pituitary function except for decreased GH reserve. Following surgery, during which she underwent stalk section (as evidenced by the development of panhypopituitarism and diabetes insipidus), her prolactin levels fell to the 25-30 ng/ml range.

In this review of our own data and that of the literature on patients with hypothalamic hyperprolactinemia we have examined the hypothesis that the hyperprolactinemia is due to stalk dysfunction and resultant dopamine deficiency and have found this hypothesis wanting. Some patients do indeed behave as if they had a classical stalk section. In most, however, anterior pituitary function is otherwise relatively normal, implying that the stalk was functioning normally. This selectivity of the defect, resulting in hyperprolactinemia, argues for a true hypothalamic lesion which may be fixed or alterable, as in patients with non-secreting tumors whose hyperprolactinemia resolved when the suprasellar component was resected. Such selective hormone responses to hypothalamic lesions have been reported in many animal studies (cf. 34,35).

On the basis of the data presented and this review of the neuroendocrine regulation of prolactin secretion we can postulate several possible mechanisms for the hyperprolactinemia found in patients with hypothalamic disease

(1) Loss of PIF and PRF activity. Because PIF activity predominates in the basal state, loss of both PIF and PRF results in hyperprolactinemia. This is the equivalent of stalk section, giving rise to prolactin levels in the 25-60 ng/ml range in conjunction with panhypopituitarism. Anatomically such lesions could be within the stalk itself or in the medial basal hypothalamus in a position to disrupt all of the peptidergic and aminergic pathways converging on the median eminence. The blunted response to TRH in such patients may be due to the effects of chronic decreased exposure to TRH and this may be improved by more prolonged administration of TRH. Alternatively, the basal turnover of prolactin may cause a depletion of a rapidly releasable pool (10-12) that otherwise would be responsive to TRH.

718

(2) Selective loss of PIF activity with retained and unopposed PRF activity. Midline lesions could potentially cause distortion of the tuberoinfundibular dopaminergic pathways while sparing PRF pathways that arise anteriorly, possibly from the suprachiasmatic and preoptic areas. Selective loss of PIF with retention of some PRF activity would be expected to cause higher prolactin levels than stalk section with loss of both PIF and PRF. A number of patients were described who had prolactin levels ranging from 100-200 ng/ml and in Case 2 removal of a Rathke's cleft cyst, which had caused selective hyperprolactinemia in the range of 120-140 ng/ml, resulted in stalk section with diabetes insipidus, panhypopituitarism, and a fall in prolactin levels to the 25-30 ng/ml range. These cases likely fall into this category.

(3) Increased PRF activity with preserved PIF activity. Anterior hypothalamic lesions that are irritative could potentially stimulate PRF pathways, similar to findings in experimental animals (36,37). The finding of a normal carbidopa/L-dopa test in one patient with hypothalamic hyperprolactinemia and one patient with an empty sella suggests that dopaminergic control mechanisms were normal and their hyperprolactinemia may be due to increased PRF.

(4) Combination of loss of PIF activity and increased PRF activity. This combination, while possible, would be hard to prove. Possibly some of the cases cited with the highest prolactin levels had this combination.

REFERENCES

1. Boyd AE III, Reichlin S. (1978): Psychoneuroendocrinology 3:113
2. Kapcala LP, Molitch ME, Post KD, Biller BJ, Prager RJ, Jackson IMD, Reichlin S. (1980): J Clin Endocrinol Metab 51:798
3. Frantz AG, Suh HK, Noel GL. (1973): In Usdin E, Snyder S (eds) Frontiers in Catecholamine Research. Pergamon Press, Oxford, p 843
4. Fine SA, Frohman LA. (1978): J Clin Invest 61:973
5. Miller M, Dalakos T, Moses AM, Fellerman H, Streeten DHP. (1970): Ann Intern Med 73:721
6. Lippe B, Wong SL, Kaplan SA. (1971): J Clin Endocrinol Metab 33:949
7. Daniel FM, Prichard MML, Schurr PH. (1958): Lancet 1:1101
8. Woolf PD, Schlach DS. (1973): Ann Intern Med 78:88
9. Lister RC, Underwood LE, Marshall RN, Friesen HG, Van Wyk JJ. (1974): J Clin Endocrinol Metab 39:1148
10. Nicoll CS, Swearinger KC. (1970): In: Martini L, Motta M, Fraschina F (eds) The Hypothalamus. Academic Press, New York, p 449
11. Swearingen KC, Nicoll C. (1971): J Endocrinol 53:1
12. Stachura ME. (1982): Endocrinology 111:1769
13. Arafah BM, Brodkey JS, Manni A, Velasco ME, Kaufman B, Pearson DH. (1982): Clin Endocrinol (Oxf) 17:213
14. Tolis G, Goldstein M, Friesen HG. (1973): J Clin Invest 52:785
15. Judd SJ, Lazarus L. (1976): Aust NZ J Med 6:30
16. Jenkins JS, Gilbert CJ, Ang V. (1976): J Clin Endocrinol Metab 43:394
17. Woolf PD, Lee LA, Leebaw WF. (1978): Metabolism 27:869
18. Turpin G, Metzger J, Gataini J, DeGennes JL. (1979): Ann d'Endocrinol (Paris) 40:371
19. Nakasu Y, Nakasu S, Handa J, Takeuchi J. (1980): Surg Neurol 13:154
20. Shah RP, Leavens ME, Samaan NA. (1980): Arch Intern Med 140:1608

21. Valenta LJ, DeFeo DR. (1980): Am J Med 68:614
22. Klijn JG, Lamberts SWJ, DeJong FH, Birkenhager JC. (1981): Fertil Steril 35:155
23. Leramo OB, Booth JD, Zinman B, Bergeron C, Sima AAF, Morley TP. (1981): Neurosurgery 8:477
24. Maira G, DiRocco C, Anile C, Roselli R. (1982): Child's Brain 9:205
25. Ferrari C, Rampini P, Benco R, Caldara R, Scarduelli C, Crosignani PG. (1982): J Clin Endocrinol Metab 55:897
26. Molitch ME, Goodman RH, Post KD, Biller BJ, Moses AC, King LW, Feldman ZT, Reichlin S. (1982): J Clin Endocrinol Metab 55:1118
27. Haney AF, Kramer RS, Wiebe RH, Hammond CB. (1979): Am J Obstet Gynecol 134:917
28. Snyder PJ, Jacobs LS, Rabello MM, Sterling FH, Shore RN, Utiger RD, Daughaday WH. (1974): Ann Intern Med 81:751
29. Spiegel AM, DiChiro G, Gorden P, Ommaya AK, Kolins J, Pomeroy TC. (1976): Ann Intern Med 85:290
30. Laws ER Jr. (1981): Neurosurgery 8:480
31. Kamoi K, Tchuchida I, Sato H, Tanaka R, Ishiguro T, Kaneko K, Iwasaki Y, Shibata A. (1981): J Clin Endocrinol Metab 53:1285
32. Robinson AG, Verbalis JG, Nelson PB. (1981): Program 63rd Ann Meeting Endo Soc (Cincinnati) 364 (abst. #1126)
33. Page RB, Plourde PV, Coldwell D, Heald JI, Weinstein J. (1983): J Neurosurg 58:766
34. Brown GM, Schalch DS, Reichlin S. (1971): Endocrinology 89:694
35. Willoughby JO, Terry LC, Brazeau P, Martin JB. (1977): Brain Res 127:137
36. Tindall JS, Knaggs GS. (1977): Brain Res 119:211
37. Malven PV. (1975): Neuroendocrinology 18:65

Prolactin. Basic and clinical correlates
R.M. MacLeod, M.O. Thorner and U. Scapagnini (eds.),
Fidia Research Series, vol. I,
Liviana Press, Padova © 1985

Section XI
Clinical and therapeutic
aspects of hyperprolactinemia

PROLACTIN AND SEX STEROID CONCENTRATIONS IN FOLLICULAR FLUID FOLLOWING DIFFERENT OVARIAN STIMULATION METHODS FOR *IN VITRO* FERTILIZATION

H. G. Bohnet and V. Baukloh

Institute for Hormone and Fertility Disorders,
2000 Hamburg 50, Federal Republic of Germany

For *in vitro* fertilization programs in the human, optimal ovarian stimulation for development of multiple follicles with oocytes of good quality is essential. Different regimens have been applied, resulting in variable success rates (1,2). In order to assess the influence of ovarian stimulation on follicular growth, prolactin and sex steroids were measured in follicular fluids following four different regimens of clomiphene and/or hMG/hCG administration.

A. Clomiphene/hCG: Clomiphene was given from day 5 to 9 of the menstrual cycle (100 mg per day); follicle puncture was timed 36 h after an hCG injection (5000 IU) based on the ultrasonographic diameter of the dominant follicle (≥ 20 mm) and serum estradiol-17 beta (E_2) levels (≥ 300 pg/ml per follicle) (3).

B. Clomiphene plus hMG/hCG (rigid schedule): Clomiphene was given as outlined in A with additional injections of hMG (150-225 IU per day) on days 6, 8, and 10 of the menstrual cycle; hCG was given according to the same criteria as described above (4).

C. Clomiphene plus hMG/hCG (individualized schedule): Clomiphene was given as outlined in A up to day 9 of the cycle. From day 10 onwards hMG was injected daily until the patient exhibited an E_2 plateau and the diameter of the leading follicle was around 20 mm. hCG was given 24-36 h after discontinuation of hMG. (5)

D. hMG/hCG (150 IU per day) was given from day 3 up to day 8 on average; ultrasonographic monitoring of follicular development and measurement of serum E_2 were used for determining hMG dosage. The injections were continued until at least one follicle reached 16 mm diameter and serum E_2 concentrations exceeded 300 pg/ml; hCG (5000 IU) was administered approximately 50 hours after the last hMG injection. (6)

In retrieved follicular fluids, prolactin and the steroid hormones testosterone (T), estradiol (E_2), and progesterone (P) were measured using commercial radioimmunoassay kits. Maturity of obtained oocytes was graded according to morphological appearance of the cumulus oophorus and the corona radiata.

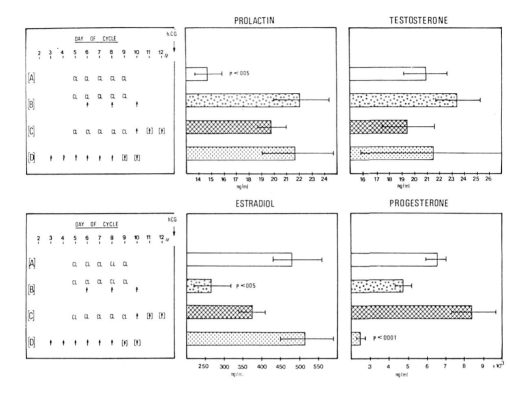

Figure 1. Follicular prolactin and sex steroid concentrations after four different methods of ovarian hyperstimulation (mean ± standard error).

Oocyte recovery and fertilization rates after the four different ovarian stimulation methods are given in Table I. In A the highest recovery rate was observed. There was no statistically significant difference between methods.

In groups A and C three pregnancies occurred. The follicular hormonal milieu was markedly different following the various stimulation regimens (Fig. 1). In A, lowest follicular prolactin concentrations were observed when compared to C or D. E_2 levels were lowest in group B. hMG/hCG stimulation (D) resulted in follicular P concentrations significantly lower than those seen following all other treatment schedules. T levels were not significantly different following the stimulation methods applied.

Linear regression analysis revealed positive correlations between follicular prolactin and T concentrations for type A and B follicles (Table II) and negative correlations between prolactin and E_2 for type A, as well as between prolactin and P for type A and B follicles. T and E_2 concentrations were positively correlated in type D follicles only. Positive regression lines were obtained between follicular E_2 and P concentrations after stimulation methods A and B while there was no statistical significance following stimulation methods C and D.

Table 1. *Oocyte Recovery and Fertilization Rate in IVF-Patients After Four Different Methods of Ovarian Hyperstimulation*

Stimulation Method	No. of Punctures	No. of Follicles	No. of Retrieved Oocytes	Recovery Rate	No. of Fertilized Oocytes	Fertili- zation Rate
A Clompiphene/hCG	26	42	38	90%	27	71%
B Clompiphene + hMG/ hCG, rigid schedule	11	21	17	81%	10	59%
C Clomiphene + hMG/ hCG, individualized schedule	24	50	31	62%	23	74%
D hMG/hCG	7	18	13	72%	8	62%

Morphologic grading of oocyte maturity showed differing distribution of oocyte qualities among the four stimulation methods (Fig. 2); 50% of oocytes obtained from type A follicles were judged to be mature (+ + +) because of expanded silky cumulus and dispersed corona cells (7). The majority of oocytes collected following methods B, C, and D were classified as intermediate (+ +) or immature (+) (B: 65%, C: 100%,

Table II. *Linear Correlations Between Hormone Concentrations In Follicular Fluids Obtained after Different Methods of Ovarian Hyperstimulation (For explanation see Table 1).*

		T		E_2		P	
		Slope	P	Slope	P	Slope	P
prolactin	A	+0.75	0.01	−14.27	0.05	−122.47	0.05
	B	+0.50	0.05	N.S.		− 98.28	0.05
	C	N.S.		N.S.		N.S.	
	D	N.S.		N.S.		N.S.	
T	A			N.S.		N.S.	
	B			N.S.		N.S.	
	C			N.S.		N.S.	
	D			+ 9.89	0.01	N.S.	
E_2	A					+ 4.74	0.001
	B					+ 1.33	0.05
	C					(+ 4.39	0.10)
	D					(+ 0.21	0.10)

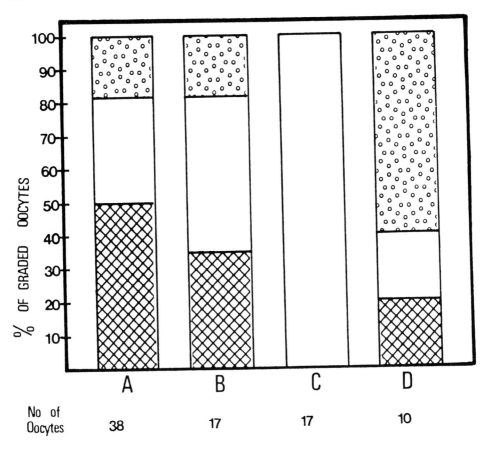

Figure 2. Distribution of oocyte maturity grades in follicles of *in vitro* fertilization patients after different methods of ovarian hyperstimulation.

[dotted]	+ + +	- oocytes mature
[blank]	+ +	- oocytes intermediate
[triangle]	+	- oocytes immature

D: 80% of oocytes). However, fertilization rates of (+ +)- and (+)-grades oocyte (Fig. 3) were in the same range or better than those of (+ + +)-oocytes from type A follicles.

All follicles following the different stimulation methods were grouped according to whether an oocyte was obtained and whether the oocyte was fertilized. The corresponding hormone concentrations were compared (Fig. 4). In stimulation methods A, B, and C higher prolactin levels (not statistically significant) were observed in follicles not yielding oocytes. There were no follicles without ova in stimulation type D. The follicular fluids also exhibited significantly ($p < 0.05$) lower E_2 and P concentrations than fluids from follicles yielding fertilizable ova. There were no statistical differences between follicular hormone concentrations of fertilized and unfertilized oocytes.

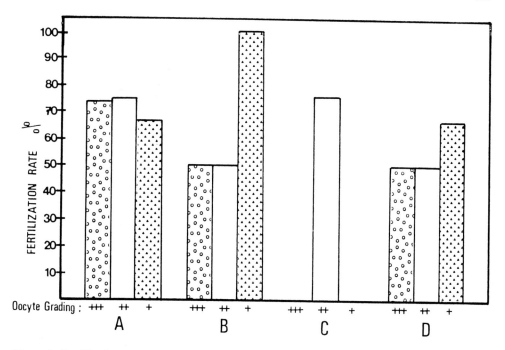

Figure 3. Fertilization rates of oocytes graded in maturity according to morphological appearance after different methods of ovarian hyperstimulation.

When the hormonal milieus of follicles following the different types of ovarian stimulation are compared to those reported by Testart et al. (8) for the spontaneous cycle (T < 13, E_2 > 100, P > 6000 ng/ml) it is obvious that all methods resulted in higher than natural T but E_2 concentrations similar to the natural situation. In stimulations B (clomiphene plus hMG/hCG, rigid schedule) and D (hMG/hCG) significantly lower follicular P concentrations were observed than in spontaneously developing follicles. This is in agreement with the higher percentage of intermediate and immature oocytes retrieved in these cycles when compared to A. Thus morphological appearance of cumulus and corona cells appears to be not a fully reliable criterion, as oocytes derived from hMG/hCG-stimulated ovaries exhibited fertilization rates similar to those of stimulation methods A, B, and C.

Follicular prolactin concentrations in natural cycles have been reported by NcNatty et al. (9) to reach a nadir of 14 ng/ml just prior to ovulation. The only stimulation method resulting in a comparably low preovulatory prolactin level in this study was A (clomiphene/hCG). In the follicular fluids significant linear correlations were calculated between prolactin and T (positive) and E_2 and P (negative), respectively. Similar correlations were shown in type B follicles, except the prolactin-E_2 correlation, with flatter slopes of the regression lines. In type C and D follicles no linear correlations between prolactin and sex steroid concentrations were observed. Inhibiting ef-

726

fects of high prolactin concentrations on P production by granulosa cells *in vitro* were also reported by McNatty and co-workers. (10).

Recently Carson et al. (11) reported low follicular E_2 and P concentrations in follicles from which no oocytes were retrieved. The same situation was observed in the present study for stimulation methods A, B, and C. Additionally, there was a tendency towards higher prolactin levels in these follicles than in those yielding oocytes.

Although stimulation with clomiphene/hCG resulted in follicles which closely resembled spontaneously maturing follicles, stimulation with clomiphene plus hMG/hCG, applied in an individualized manner, seems to be preferable since more oocytes per patient were obtained than following clomiphene stimulation. In type D-treated cycles follicular prolactin concentrations appeared to have no critical effect on sex steroid production. A possible inhibitory effect of prolactin on oocyte maturation as suggested by Channing et al. (12) may be overcome by IVF culture methods.

Hopefully, improvements in stimulation methods will lead to increased pregnancy rates by furnishing us with a larger number of embryos to transfer.

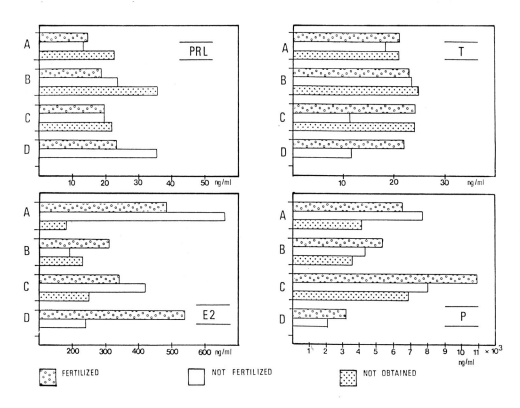

Figure 4. Comparison of prolactin and sex steroid concentrations in follicles yielding fertilized and not fertilized oocytes and those from which no ova were retrieved within four types of ovarian hyperstimulation.

REFERENCES

1. Mandelbaum J, Plachot M, Cohen J, Junca A-M, Debache C. (1983). In: Beier, Lindner (eds) Fertilization of the Human Egg *in vitro*. Springer-Verlag Berlin, p 123
2. Seegar Jones G. (1983). In: Acosta (ed) Infertility 6. Marcel Dekker, New York, p 11
3. Trounson AO, Leeton JF. (1982). In: Edwards, Purdy (eds) Human Conception *in vitro*. Academic Press, London, p 51
4. Frydman R, Testart J, Giacomini P, Imbert MC, Martin E, Nahoul K. (1982): Fertil. Steril. 38:312
5. McBain JC, Trounson A. (1984). In: Wood, Trounson (eds) Clinical *in vitro* Fertilization. Springer Verlag, Berlin, p 49
6. Seegar Jones G. (1984): Endocrine Reviews 5:62
7. Mohr L, Trounson A. (1984). In: Wood, Trounson (eds) Clinical *in vitro* Fertilization. Springer Verlag, Berlin, p 99
8. Testart J, Frydman R, Castanier M, Lasalle B, Belaisch J. (1983). In: Beier, Lindner (eds) Fertilization of the Human Egg *in vitro*. Springer-Verlag, Berlin, p 73
9. McNatty KP, Hunter WM, McNeilly AS, Sawers RS. (1975): J Endocrinol 64:555
10. McNatty KP, Sawers RS, McNeilly AS (1974): Nature 250:653
11. Carson RS, Trounson AO, Findlay JK. (1982): J Clin Endocrinol Metab 55:798
12. Channing CP, Evans VW. (1982): Endocrinology 111:1746

Prolactin. Basic and clinical correlates
R.M. MacLeod, M.O. Thorner and U. Scapagnini (eds.),
Fidia Research Series, vol. I,
Liviana Press, Padova © 1985

Section XI
Clinical and therapeutic
aspects of hyperprolactinemia

[11]C-BROMOCRIPTINE UPTAKE IN PITUITARY ADENOMAS

C. Muhr, P.O. Lundberg, G. Antoni, K. Bergstrom, P. Hartvig, H. Lundqvist, B. Langstrom, and C. G. Stalnacke

Department of Neurology, University Hospital and other institutions, Uppsala University, Uppsala, Sweden

Recent years' development in neuroendocrinology has led to new concepts concerning pituitary adenomas. Classifications based on this new knowledge are being established. Dopamine-agonistic drugs have meant a new and very important treatment alternative. There are, however, several still unsolved questions and there is an urge for further knowledge and understanding of the characteristics of pituitary adenomas.

Positron emission tomography (PET) is a unique method that makes possible an *in vivo* dynamic autoradiography. This means that the uptake and elimination of different labelled substances can be studied selectively in an organ. For example, the amino acid metabolism can be examined with labelled methionine and pharmaceutical agents can be studied directly within the effector organ. Especially concerning the pituitary, and probably also pituitary adenomas, with its many regulation mechanisms it should be of value to perform *in vivo* examinations. The experimental methodology work preceding the present study has been carried out on rhesus monkeys (1,2). A preliminary report on the PET technique on human pituitary tumors was presented at the Third European Workshop on Pituitary Adenomas (3).

The positron emission tomography was carried out in a model PC 384-3B, Instrument AB Scanditronix, Uppsala, Sweden. The PET-camera was built up of two rings; within each ring were 96 BGO detectors. Three adjacent slices are produced of approximately 13 mm thickness (FWHM) and with an in-plane resolution of 8 mm. Coincidental detection was used to avoid secondary and unspecific radiation. The radioactivity was continuously measured within the examined organs and the data were stored in a computer. The radioactive uptake could be displayed as tomograms on TV monitors. By use of so-called regions of interests (ROI) any selected area could be marked out, for example the pituitary tumor, and the radioactive uptake within this region selectively calculated and the dynamic curves studied (Fig. 1). This made it possible to compare the uptake and dynamic curves within different regions and also to compare different labelled substances within the same region.

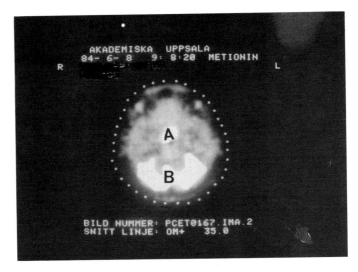

Figure 1. PET-scan with regions of interest (ROI) marked out of the pituitary tumor (a) and cerebellum (b).

For each patient a special helmet was produced and a fixation system, including a coordinate system, was used to permit an exact and reproducible position at each PET and CT examination (4,5).

Each patient was examined in the PET-camera with [^{68}Ga]-EDTA which will correlate to the blood volume within the examined organ, the labelled amino acid [^{11}C]-L-methionine and [^{11}C]-bromocriptine labelled as marked*.

The radioactive substance was administered intravenously in a dose of 35-200 MBq. The measurement of the radioactive uptake in the head started at the time of injection and was continued for up to 90 minutes. Venous blood samples were taken at special time intervals for measurement of the radioactivity in the blood.

The formula: [^{11}C]-substance tumor $- \dfrac{[^{68}\text{Ga}]\text{-EDTA tumor}}{[^{68}\text{Ga}]\text{-EDTA blood}}$ x [^{11}C]-substance blood

was used to correct and subtract for the blood content of the labelled substance.

The patients were examined clinically including perimetry as described by Goldmann. Hormonal evaluation of hypothalamo-pituitary functions, including the thyroid, adrenals, and gonads, was performed including basal levels of prolactin, follicle stimulating hormone (FSH), luteinizing hormone (LH), estradiol, testosterone, growth hormone (GH), cortisol, thyroid stimulating hormone (TSH), thyroxine, thyroid globulin as well as 24 hour cortisol profile, urine-cortisol, TRH-LH-RH test, L-dopa test, and 24 hour GH profile in acromegalic patients.

Roentgenography included plain sellar films in anterior-posterior and lateral pro-

(Fig. 2.a)

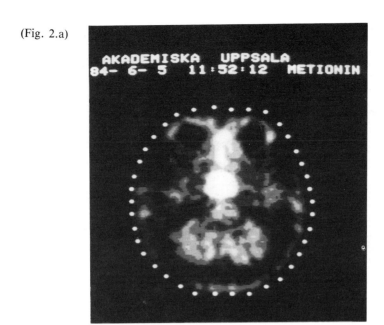

Figure 2. PET-scan from a 65-year-old female demonstrating a high uptake in the pituitary adenoma. (a) [^{11}C]-methionine, (b) [^{11}C]-bromocriptine.

(Fig. 2.b)

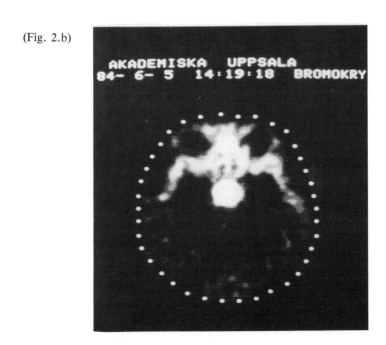

(Fig. 3.a)

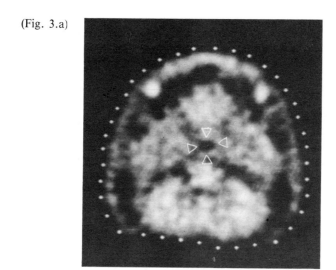

Figure 3. PET-scan of a 47-year-old male with a partially cystic pituitary adenoma showing low uptake in the center of the tumor of (a) [^{11}C]-methionine, (b) [^{11}C]-bromocriptine.

(Fig. 3.b)

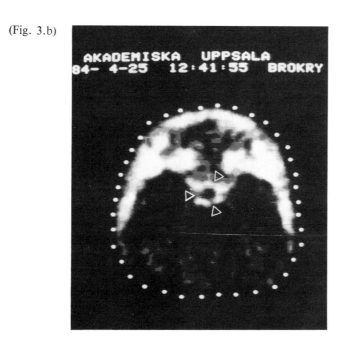

jections and computed tomography before and after contrast injection and, most often, coronal projections.

Routine histological examinations and immunocytochemistry (prolactin, GH, ACTH, LH, beta-endorphin and meth- and leu-enkephalin) were made. Nuclear DNA content was determined in tumor tissue from the patients who were operated on and also, if possible, in the material obtained by fine needle biopsy.

Fifteen patients with pituitary adenoma were studied. There were 9 females and 6 males. Their age range was 26-80 years, mean 55 years. Two patients had acromegaly, one of these had an invasive adenoma. Five patients had hyperprolactinemia, one of these had an invasive adenoma with a serum prolactin of 4,200 ug/L (normal less than 20 ug/L). The other 4 patients with raised serum prolactin had levels between 25-59 ug/L.

Ten patients had visual field defects with partial or complete bitemporal hemianopsia. Two other patients had ocular motor nerve palsies. Roentgen examination showed in all patients a considerably enlarged sella turcica. Three patients had no suprasellar tumor extension; two of these had acromegaly of which one was invasive. The remaining 12 patients had suprasellar tumor extension. All tumors showed contrast enhancement. CT showed a partial cystic tumor in 5 of the patients.

Eight patients had no clinical or laboratory signs of hormonal hypersecretion. Five patients had secondary thyroidal and adrenal insufficiency requiring substitution and 8 patients had secondary gonadal insufficiency.

The uptake of [^{11}C]-L-methionine was the same or up to 3 times higher in the pituitary tumors than in the cerebellum. Eight patients had relatively higher and 7 patients lower uptake (Fig. 2,3)

In the patients with a cystic portion of the tumor the uptake was in all cases lower within the cystic parts. The dynamic curves in most adenomas showed, within a short time after injection, a rise of activity to a level that remained the same throughout the study (Fig. 4). When the values were corrected and subtracted for blood content according to the above-mentioned formula, a slow increase in the uptake could be seen (Fig. 5).

[^{11}C]-methionine is metabolized into [^{11}C]-serine that contributes to the protein synthesis as methionine does (6). From studies on patients with malignant glioma it has been shown that the uptake of [^{11}C]-L-methionine is of value to differentiate the grade of malignancy within these tumors. The more malignant tumors have higher uptake of [^{11}C]-L-methionine (7). No method is yet available to determine how active a pituitary adenoma is as regards growth. Determination of the DNA content within the tumor is probably of value (8,9). The uptake of [^{11}C]-L-methionine within the tumor reflects the amino acid metabolism and could thus be expected to correlate to the activity of the tumor. The pituitary adenomas so far examined have shown different levels of [^{11}C]-L-methionine and it will be of great interest to follow these patients to evaluate the use of this information.

The uptake of [^{11}C]-bromocriptine was 2-10 times higher in the pituitary adenomas than in cerebellum. Six patients showed relatively higher and 9 patients relatively lower uptake (Fig. 2,3). The dynamic studies showed varying patterns: in some tumors the uptake rose within a short time and then remained fairly stable during the examination, while in other patients the uptake also increased to a high level but then decreased with time (Fig. 6 a, b). Using the same formula as mentioned above for correction and

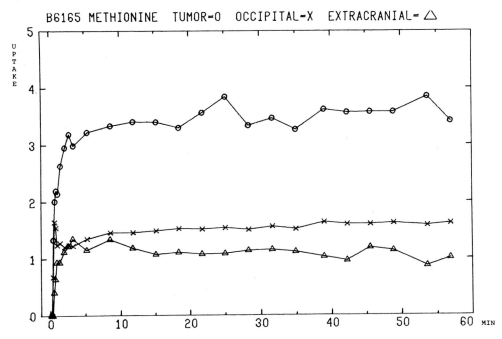

Figure 4. A dynamic curve of the uptake of [11C]-methionine demonstrating the typical pattern.

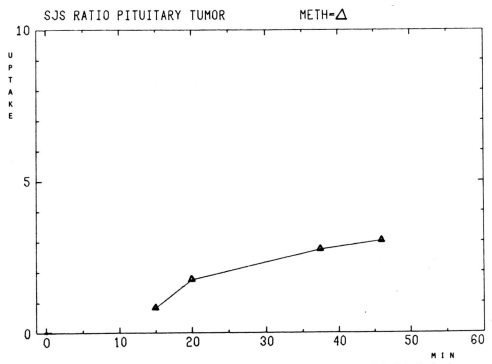

Figure 5. A dynamic curve with correction made for the blood content of the labelled substance showing a slow increase with time of [¹¹C]-methionine in the adenoma (△).

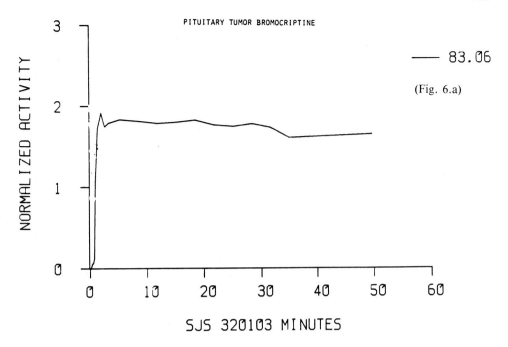

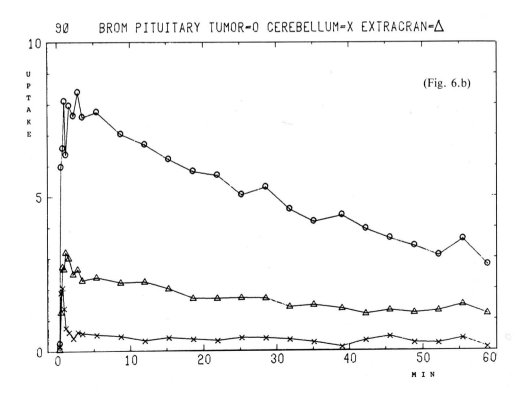

Figure 6. The dynamic curve of the uptake of [^{11}C]-bromocriptine within the pituitary adenoma demonstrating (a) a fairly stable level and (b) uptake decreasing with time.

736

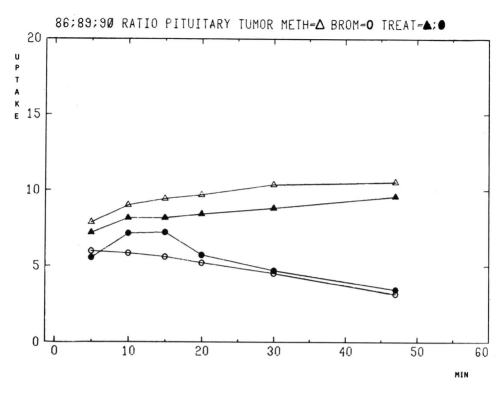

Figure 7. The dynamic curves showing an almost identical uptake in a pituitary adenoma of [^{11}C]-methionine (△) and [^{11}C]-bromocriptine (○) before (○, △) and during (●, ▲) bromocriptine treatment.

subtraction for blood content of labelled substance, the dynamic in some patients showed a more stable level of the uptake of [^{11}C]-bromocriptine while in other tumors the level decreased with time. These interesting variations in the uptake and dynamics of [^{11}C]-bromocriptine might mean that in some tumors, the ones with the more stable levels, an entrapment of bromocriptine takes place within the tumor. Bromocriptine has been shown to act through the dopamine receptors within the pituitary adenoma (10).

There is, however, no method to tell which adenomas will respond to bromocriptine treatment. Hyperprolactinemia with highly elevated serum prolactin indicates a prolactin-producing adenoma but for moderately elevated serum prolactin this might depend on a loss of inhibition from hypothalamus (1). The findings from the PET studies with signs of entrapment of [^{11}C]-bromocriptine in some of the adenomas might prove to be of value in the choice of treatment. Longer follow-up of the patients in the present study might clarify this.

Three patients were studied with PET both before and during bromocriptine treatment. In all these patients the dynamic curves showed an almost identical uptake of [^{11}C]-L-methionine and [^{11}C]-bromocriptine within the tumor and also within the compared area in cerebellum (Fig. 7). None of these patients seemed to respond to the bromocriptine medication. It will be of interest will be to do the same study on a patient who responds to bromocriptine.

REFERENCES

1. Lundberg PO, Muhr C, Hartvig P, Bergstrom K, Lindberg B, Jung B, Lundqvist H, Langstrom B, Stalnacke CG. (1983): In Advance abstracts of papers XIV Endocrinologia Congress, suppl 256 acc, vol 103, p 85. Stockholm: Burson-Marsteller AB
2. Lundberg PO, Muhr C, Antoni G, Bergstrom K, Hartvig P, Lindberg B, Lundqvist H, Langstrom B, Stalnacke CG. (1984): First Symposium of the European Neuroendocrine Association, Basel
3. Muhr C, Lundberg PO, Bergstrom K, Hartvig P, Lundqvist H, Langstrom B, Stalnacke DG. (1983): Third European Workshop on Pituitary Adenomas, Amsterdam
4. Greitz T, Bergstrom M, Boethius J, Kingsley D, Ribbe T. (1980): Neuroradiology 19:1
5. Bergstrom M, Boethius J, Eriksson L, Greitz T, Ribbe T, Widen L. (1981): J Computer Assisted Tomography 5:136
6. Lundqvist H, Stalnacke CG, Langstrom B, Jones B. (1984): In: L. Widen (ed) The Metabolism of the Human Brain Studied by Positron Emission Tomography. Raven Press, New York, in press
7. Lilja A, Bergstrom K, Spannare B, Halldin C, Langstrom B, Lundqvist H. (1983): Amer J Neuroradiology 4:1139
8. Muhr C, Lundberg PO, Bergstrom K, Grimelius L, Hugosson R, Olsson Y, Stahle J, Wide L. (1982): Acta Neurol Scand 65, suppl 90:103
9. Lundberg PO, Muhr C, Bergstrom K, Grimelius L, Hugosson R, Olsson Y, Stahle J, Wide L. (1984): International Symposium on Prolactinomas, Graz,
10. Lundberg PO, Osterman PO, Wide L. (1981): J Neurosurg 55:194

Prolactin. Basic and clinical correlates
R.M. MacLeod, M.O. Thorner and U. Scapagnini (eds.),
Fidia Research Series, vol. I,
Liviana Press, Padova © 1985

Section XI
Clinical and therapeutic
aspects of hyperprolactinemia

DOPAMINE RECEPTORS IN HUMAN PITUITARY ADENOMAS

M.C. Rubio[1], V. Rettori[2], A. Seilicovich[3], E. Pardal[3], I. Molocznik[3]

[1]Instituto de Investigaciones Farmacologicas (CONICET); [2]Centro de Investigaciones en Reproduccion, UBA; [3]Instituto de Neurocirugia "Costa Buero", UBA. Buenos Aires, Argentina

The tonic hypothalamic inhibitory control of prolactin secretion by dopamine has been well estabished (1). Dopamine is released by neurons in the hypothalamus into the portal vessels (2), and interacts with specific receptors located on lactotrophs. These receptors have been studied in several species including the rat (3), monkey (4), porcine (5), and bovine (6). The presence of dopaminergic receptors in the human pituitary has also been reported (7,8).

The existence of several types of dopaminergic receptors in the brain, with different affinities for agonists and antagonists (9,10), has been postulated. Since the characterization of dopaminergic receptors in the human pituitary is incomplete, the present study was undertaken to characterize the receptor in the normal human pituitary and in prolactinomas using [^{3}H]-dopamine as the radioligand.

Nine human prolactin-secreting or growth hormone-secreting pituitary adenomas and one chromophobe pituitary adenoma were surgically removed. The age of patients ranged from 21 to 52 years. The pituitaries were collected soon after accidental death of young subjects, with one being obtained from a patient bearing prostatic carcinoma. The tissue was immediately frozen. Before surgery, all patients were free of treatment for at least one month. Presurgical prolactin levels were determined to be in the normal range (1-20 ng/ml) by radioimmunoassay. The mean serum prolactin levels of patients with prolactinomas were 282.5 ± 50.4 ng/ml. Serum prolactin levels of acromegalic patients were slightly above the upper limit of the normal range while the patient with the chromophobe adenoma presented a value within the normal range (Table 1).

Dopamine receptors were studied according to the method of Bacopoulus (11). The tissue was homogenized (1:50 W/V) in 20 mM Tris-HCl buffer (pH 7.4), and centrifuged at 20,000 x g for 15 min. The pellet was resuspended in the same proportion in fresh buffer and centrifuged again. The pellet was resuspended in the same buffer and incubated at 37 C for 15 min in order to destroy endogenous dopamine. After centrifugation the supernatant was discarded and the pellet was resuspended in the incubation

Table 1. *[³H]-dopamine binding to control and adenomatous tissue of human anterior pituitary*

Patient No.	Age (yrs)	Sex		Prolactin (ng/ml)	[³H]-DA binding (fmoles/mg protein)
1	33	F	Prolactinoma	320	425
2	21	F	Prolactinoma	320	392
3	25	F	Prolactinoma	65	452
4	36	F	Prolactinoma	300	438
5	23	F	Prolactinoma	250	385
6	26	F	Prolactinoma	440	352
7	25	M	Acromegalic	25	ND
8	52	M	Acromegalic	36	25
9	46	F	Chromophobe adenoma	18	61
10	—		Prostatic carcinoma (normal)	—	131
11	—		Normal	—	120
12	—		Normal	—	165

ND: non detectable.

medium (2 mg protein/ml). The incubation medium consisted of 20 mM Tris-HCl buffer (pH 7.4), 5 mM EDTA, 1.1 mM ascorbic acid, 15 mM pargyline, 0.1 mM 3,4- dihydroxybenzoic acid (as COMT inhibitor) and 2-40 nM [³H]-dopamine (34 Ci/mmol, New England Nuclear). After 10 min of incubation at room temperature (25 C) the mixture was quickly passed through glass fiber (Whatman GF/B) filter under vacuum. The filters were washed with 15 ml of 20 mM Tris-HCl buffer (pH 7.4) containing 5 mM EDTA, 15 uM pargyline, and 100 uM 3,4-dihydroxybenzoic acid. The filters were placed in vials containing 10 ml of scintillation solution [POPOP 100 mg, PO 5 g, toluene (600 ml), Triton X-100 (300 ml), ethanol (100 ml)]. After 24 h the vials were counted in a scintillation counter.

Specific binding was obtained by subtracting non specific binding from the total counts. Non specific binding was determined in the presence of 10 mM spiroperidol. A Scatchard plot was used to calculate the dissociation constant (K_D) and maximal number of binding sites (Bmax) (12).

In some competition experiments 0.1 mM guanyl-5' yl imidodiphosphate (Gpp(NH)p) was added to the incubation medium. In these experiments separation of bound from free ligand was performed by centrifugation at 45,000 x g for 10 min. Proteins were determined by the method of Lowry et al. (13).

The specific binding of [³H]-dopamine (40 nM) in the pituitary gland was approximately 40% of the total binding (Fig. 1). Nonspecific binding was about 60% of the total binding and was similar to that when cold dopamine (10 uM) or spiperone (10 uM) was used as competitive inhibitor.

The maximal number of binding sites obtained with 40 nM [³H]-dopamine in prolactinomas (407 ± 15 pmoles/mg protein) was four times higher than that of normal

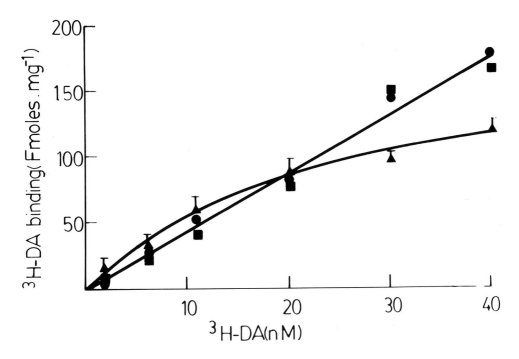

Figure 1. Saturation plot of [³H]-dopamine binding to normal human pituitary.
● Nonspecific binding in the presence of 10 uM dopamine
■ Nonspecific binding in the presence of 10 uM spiroperidol
▲ specific binding for [³H]-dopamine. Shown are mean values ± S.E.M.

pituitaries (139 ± 13 pmoles/mg protein, $p < 0.001$). Acromegalic adenomas presented undetectable or very low number of binding sites (Table 1).

Three different Scatchard analyses were performed using pools of tissue obtained from patients 1-4, 2-3, and 5-6. The K_D in prolactinomas (9.7 ± 1.7 nM) was similar to that in normal pituitaries (7.1 ± 1.0) ($p < 0.2$). Bmax was significantly ($p < 0.001$) higher in prolactinomas (419 ± 21 fmol/pg protein) than in normal tissue (139 ± 10.7). Figure 2 shows the kinetic analysis determined in pool of patients 1-4.

The IC_{50} for spiperone was determined by competition experiments in the pool of patients 5-6. Similar inhibitory potency of this antagonist was obtained in prolactinomas (4 nM) and normal pituitaries (6.3 nM) (Fig. 3).

In some experiments [³H]-dopamine was displaced by cold dopamine in the presence of 0.1 mM Gpp(NH)p in order to stabilize the low affinity (for the agonist) form of receptors. Figure 4 shows the competition study performed in the pool of patients 2-3 and normal pituitaries. The IC_{50} was very similar (approximately 250 nM) in both tissues, corresponding to a K_D for [³H]-dopamine of 210 nM.

The present study revealed the presence of a single class of dopamine binding sites in the human pituitary tissue. The characterization of dopaminergic receptors in the

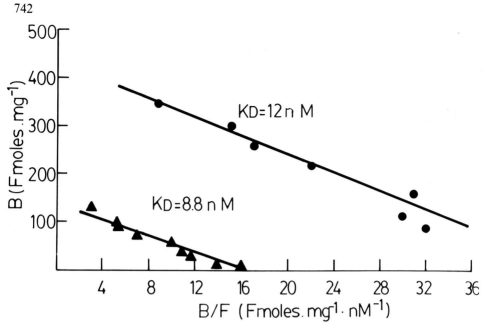

Figure 2. Scatchard plot of [³H]-dopamine binding to normal human pituitary (▲) or to prolactin-secreting adenomas (●). Each point represents the mean of triplicate samples.

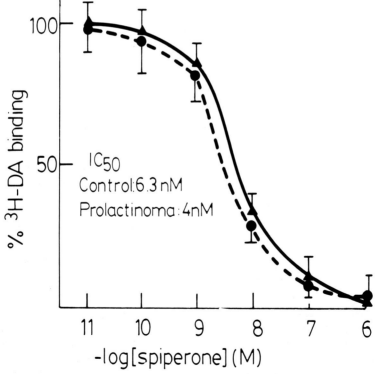

Figure 3. Curves for a spiroperidol/[³H]-dopamine competition experiment in normal human pituitary (▲) or in prolactin-secreting adenomas (●). Shown are mean values ± S.E.M. of three experiments. IC_{50} was calculated by probit.

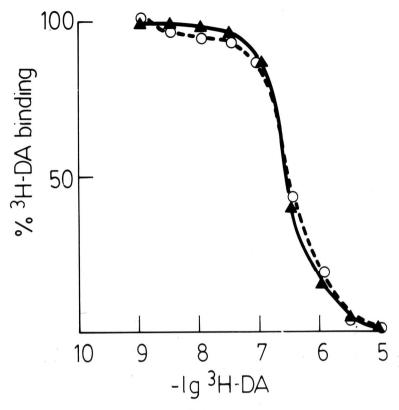

Figure 4. Curves for a dopamine/[³H]-dopamine competition experiments in normal human pituitary (▲) and prolactin-secreting adenomas (○). The experiment was performed in the presence of Gpp(NH)$_p$: 0.1 mM. Each point represents the mean of triplicate samples.

pituitary gland indicated that these receptors may correspond to the classical description of D$_2$ type receptors (10). D$_2$ type receptors are characterized by two conformational forms, one having high affinity for agonists and antagonists (type D$_4$ according to Seeman (9)), and the other having a low affinity for the agonist. Our results demonstrate that pituitary receptors have high affinity for both [³H]-dopamine and spiroperidol while in the presence of GTP analog (Gpp(NH)p) the affinity for [³H]-dopamine decreased. These results are compatible with the existence of an equilibrium between RH and RL forms of D$_2$ receptors (10). Several lines of evidence indicate that the D$_2$ is the type of dopaminergic receptor present in the pituitary of many species (9).

No differences in affinity for [³H]-dopamine and spiroperidol were detected between normal pituitaries and prolactinomas. Nevertheless, prolactinomas showed an almost four times higher number of binding sites than normal tissue.

These results confirm the data presented by Cronin et al. (7) using [³H]-spiroperidol as radioligand, demonstrating an increase in the number of binding sites in prolactinomas. In contrast, Bression et al. (8) detected two classes of binding sites with different affinities in human pituitary membranes using [^{3}H]-domperidone as radioligand. These authors did not observe differences between receptors of normal tissue and those of prolactin-secreting adenomas. The sensitivity of pituitary dopaminergic receptors agrees with the physiologically relevant concentrations of this amine in the pituitary stalk plasma (14,15).

The presence of dopaminergic receptors in adenomas of acromegalic patients confirms previous reports (7,16). The number of binding sites for [^{3}H]- dopamine seemed to be lower in these adenomas as compared to normal pituitaries.

The high number of dopaminergic receptors in prolactinomas could be the consequence of an actual increase in the number of binding sites caused by a deficiency in the concentration of dopamine reaching the pituitary lactotrophs. Alternatively, it could be the result of a relative increase in the number of prolactin cells within the heterogeneous population of cells in the pituitary, as has been discussed by other authors (7,8). The finding that dopaminergic receptors are increased in prolactinomas suggests that the low sensitivity of these tumors to dopamine (17) may be related to a defect beyond the dopamine receptor.

REFERENCES

1. McCann SM, Lumpkin MD, Mizunuma H, Khorram O, Ottlecz A, Samson WK. (1984): Trends in Neuroscience 7:127
2. Ben-Jonathan M, Porter JC. (1976): Endocrinology 98:1497
3. Bremmer RM, Greengrass PM, Morville M, Blackburn K. (1978): J Pharm Pharmacol 30:388
4. Brown G, Seeman P, Lee T. (1976): Endocrinology 99:1407
5. DeLean A, Kilpatrick BF, Caron MG. (1982): Mol Pharmacol 22:290
6. Cresse I, Schneider R, Snyder SH. (1977): Eur J Pharmacol 46:377
7. Cronin MJ, Cheung CY, Wilson CB, Jaffe RB, Weiner RI. (1980): J Clin Endocrinol Metab 50:387
8. Bression D, Brandi AM, Martres MP, Nousbaum A, Cesselin F, Racadot J, Peillon F. (1980): J Clin Endocrinol Metab 51:1037
9. Seeman P. (1980): Pharmacol Rev 32:229
10. Cresse I. (1982): Trends in Neuroscience 5:40
11. Bacopoulus NG. (1981): Biochem Pharmacol 30:2037
12. Scatchard B. (1949): Ann NY Acad Sci 51:660
13. Lowry OH, Rosebrough NJ, Farr AL, Randall RS. (1951): J Biol Chem 193:265
14. DeGreef WJ, Neill JD. (1979): Endocrinology 105:1093
15. Gudelsky GA, Porter JC. (1980): Endocrinology 106:526
16. Serri O, Marchisio AM, Collu R, Hardy J, Somma M. (1984): Horm Res 19:97
17. Serri O, Kuehel O, Buu NT, Somma M. (1983): J Clin Endocrinol Metab 56:255

Prolactin. Basic and clinical correlates
R.M. MacLeod, M.O. Thorner and U. Scapagnini (eds.),
Fidia Research Series, vol. I,
Liviana Press, Padova © 1985

Section XI
Clinical and therapeutic
aspects of hyperprolactinemia

MALE HYPOGONADISM AND PROLACTIN SECRETING PITUITARY ADENOMAS

R. F. A. Weber, S. W. J. Lamberts, J. T. M. Vreeburg*, and J. C. Birkenhager

Depts. of Internal Medicine III and Clinical Endocrinology, *Endocrinology, Growth and Reproduction, Erasmus University, Rotterdam, The Netherlands

Hyperprolactinemia, whether due to hypothalamic-pituitary disorders, drug use, hypothyroidism, renal failure or other diseases, has been associated with reproductive dysfunctions in women and men. For many years hyperprolactinemia in women has

Table 1. *Clinical features of untreated men with prolactinomas*

number of patients	diminution or loss of libido %	impotence %	gynecomastia[1]/ galactorrhea[2] %[1]	%[2]	reference		
22	91	91	14	14	Buvat et al.,	1978	(1)
8	75	100	50	38	Carter et al.	1978	(2)
21	76	76					
8[a]	75	75	10	10	Franks et al.	1978	(3)
10	n.m.	68	n.m.	28	Thorner & Besser	1978	(4)
15[a]							
30	80	80	33	30	Derome et al.	1979	(5)
25	n.m.	88	40	20	Peillon et al.	1979	(6)
22	95	n.m.	27	18	Grisoli et al.	1980	(7)
15	80	80	27	20	Serri et al.	1980	(8)
57	98	98	28	14	Eversmann et al.	1981	(9)
24[b]							
8	n.m.	87	12	12	Prescott et al.	1982	(10)
26	100	100	n.m	n.m.	Spark et al.	1982	(11)

n.m., not mentioned
[a] acromegaly
[b] after surgery

been regarded as a cause of menstrual irregularities. Hyperprolactinemia in men does not cause "typical" manifestations and may not be recognized by the patient or his physician. Nevertheless, impotence, loss of libido, hypogonadism, and less frequently gynecomastia and galactorrhea are regarded as prominent features in the majority of men with an untreated prolactin-secreting pituitary adenoma (Table 1) and may be present for a long time.

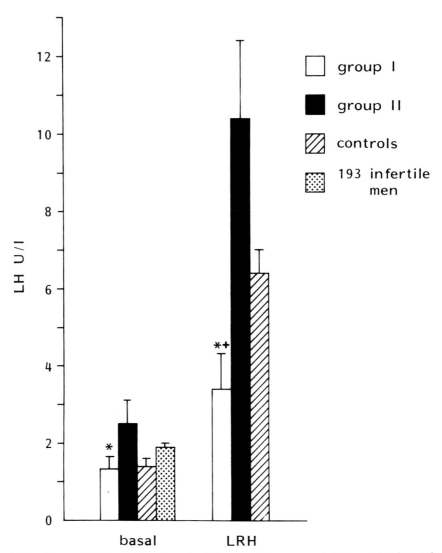

Figure 1. Basal serum levels of LH and maximal increment in response to 100 ug LRH i.v. Values are given as mean ± SEM. * $p < 0.05$ group I vs group II. + $p < 0.05$ group I vs controls

Most of the male patients with a prolactinoma present with headache, disturbed vision, and visual field defects due to intra-, supra- and parasellar extension of tumor mass. Surprisingly, impotence and loss of libido do not prompt the patient to seek medical advice. Hyperprolactinemia seems to be a minor cause of impotence, loss of libido and other reproductive dysfunctions (Table 2). The incidence of hyperprolactinemia among 598 infertile men in our clinic was 2%.

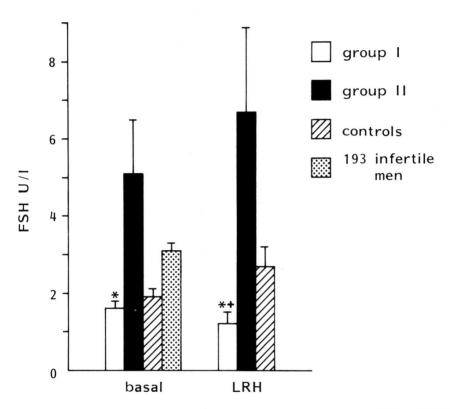

Figure 2. Basal serum levels of FSH and maximal increment in response to 100 ug LRH i.v. Values are given as mean ± SEM * p < 0.05 group I vs group II + p < 0.05 group I vs controls

The mechanisms by which hyperprolactinemia leads to reproductive dysfunctions have not yet been elucidated. Moreover, most of the men with prolactinomas described in the literature have macroadenomas (2,5,9). Therefore, the data of the majority of hyperprolactinemic men must be explained not only by the elevated serum prolactin levels but by local compression or destruction of normal pituitary tissue due to the tumor mass.

Table 2. *Incidence of hyperprolactinemia in men with reproductive dysfunctions syndrome*

	number of patients	incidence %	reference	
infertility	235	9	Roulier et al.,	1978 (12)
	50		Masala et al.,	1979 (13)
	171	4	Segal et al.,	1979 (14)
	208	1	Hargreave et al.,	1977 (15)
	39	< 1	Blacker et al.,	1977 (16)
	151		Pierrepoint et al.,	1978 (17)
	103		Rjosk & Schill,	1979 (18)
	142		Abyholm & Molne,	1980 (19)
	205		Gray et al.,	1980 (20)
	300		Laufer et al.,	1981 (21)
impotence	134	16	Ambrosi et al.,	1980 (22)
	105	7	Spark et al.,	1980 (23)
	53	< 1	Rjosk & Schill,	1979 (18)
	30		Miller et al.,	1980 (24)

In order to study the role of prolactin in hyperprolactinemic states we compared the clinical features of 19 men with a prolactin-secreting macroadenoma (group I) with those of 13 hyperprolactinemic men with infertility (group II). All the patients of group I presented with local tumor symptoms. Headache was present in 10 patients, visual impairment in 8 patients, and symptoms of panhypopituitarism in 4. Patients of group II were referred because semen abnormalities were suggested to be the cause of their infertility. In none of the patients of group II was the presence of a pituitary tumor suspected. Prolactin levels in group I were 982 ± 294 ug/l (mean ± SEM) and 42 ± 8 ug/l in group II. All patients underwent plain skull radiography, polytomography, and CAT scanning or pneumonencephalography when indicated to visualize supra- and parasellar extension of the pituitary tumor. Ophthalmic evaluation comprised visual fields, visual acuity, and fundoscopy. All patients in group I had a macroadenoma. The diagnosis of microadenoma (tumor less than 1 cm in diameter; sella described as not enlarged) was suspected in 11 patients of group II: two patients had a macroadenoma. Retrospectively, complaints of impotence and loss of libido were most conspicuous in the majority of patients in group I, as mentioned in the literature (Table 1). Gynecomastia and galactorrhea were observed in 2 patients of each group. Two patients of group II suffered from diminished libido.

GONADOTROPHINS

In 1974 Thorner et al. (25) observed normal basal gonadotropins and a normal response to LRH in 4 hyperprolactinemic men. Other investigators confirmed this finding: many studies of untreated hyperprolactinemic men (most of them with a macroadenoma) indicate that basal levels of LH and FSH are normal in 80% of the patients. However, the response of serum gonadotropins to LRH is blunted for LH in 70% and for FSH in 75% of the investigated patients. In our patients with a macroadenoma (group I) basal levels of LH and FSH were not significantly different from those of a control group, but after administration of LRH the absolute maximal increment of LH and FSH was decreased (Fig. 1, 2).

For comparison with the 13 infertile men with hyperprolactinemia, the mean serum levels of LH and FSH of men visiting our department of male infertility are given. LH and FSH levels in our 13 infertile men with hyperprolactinemia were not different from those of infertile men without hyperprolactinemia. In addition, although prolactin levels in patients of group II were clearly elevated, no suppression of either basal or LRH-stimulated levels of serum gonadotrophins was observed.

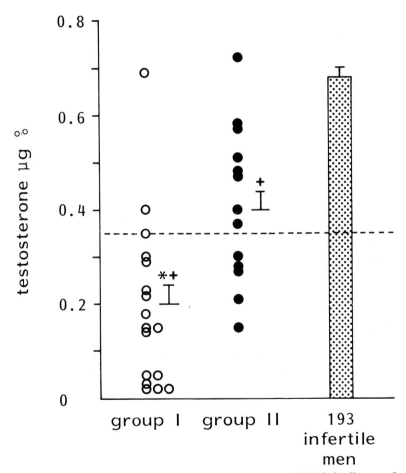

Figure 3. Basal serum testosterone levels in group I, group II and 193 infertile men. Individual values and means ± SEM are given. Broken line represents lower limit of normal value * p < 0.005 group I vs group II + p < 0.001 vs 193 infertile men

TESTOSTERONE

In many hyperprolactinemic male patients serum testosterone levels have been reported to be low. In our study serum testosterone levels were considerably decreased in patients with a macroadenoma and high prolactin levels (group I) (Fig. 3).

Also, in patients with microadenoma serum testosterone levels (0.40 ± 0.04 ug%) were statistically different from those of infertile controls (0.68 ± 0.02 ug%), whereas in 5 out of 13 patients serum testosterone levels were below the normal range. The finding that in hyperprolactinemic patients serum testosterone levels are decreased, combined with the observation that serum gonadotropins are normal, suggests that an inhibitory effect of hyperprolactinemia on the hypothalamus and the Leydig cells might be involved. An alternative explanation might be that the pulsatile pattern of LH secretion is impaired in hyperprolactinemic patients, leading to a relative testicular insensitivity to LH (26).

Finally, in contrast to group II patients, patients with a macroadenoma had several disturbed anterior pituitary functions: the pituitary-adrenal axis, tested by measuring serum 11-deoxycortisol after the administration of metyrapone, and the pituitary-thyroidal axis measured by serum T_4 levels and TRH stimulated TSH levels, were insufficient in the majority of patients of group I. These findings are comparable with those in patients with pituitary adenomas, regardless of their hormonal production (27). Since tumor size not only correlates with serum prolactin levels but also with pituitary dysfunction due to destruction or compression, it is unclear whether in men with prolactin-secreting macroadenomas prolactin is the major factor in the development of hypogonadism.

REFERENCES

1. Buvat J, Asfour M, Buvat-Herbaut M, Fossati P. (1978): In: Robijn C, Harper M. (eds) Progress in Prolactin Physiology and Pathology. Elsevier/North Holland Biomedical Press, Amsterdam, p 317
2. Carter JN, Tyson JE, Tollis G, van Vliet S, Faiman C, Friesen HG. (1978): N Engl J Med 299:847
3. Franks S, Jacobs HS, Martin N, Nabarro JDN. (1978): Clin Endocrinol 8:277
4. Thorner MO, Besser GM. (1978): Acta Endocrinol 88, suppl 216:131
5. Derome PJ, Peillon F, Bard RH, Jedynak CP, Racadot J, Guiot G. (1979): Nouv Presse Med 8:577
6. Peillon F, Bard H, Mowszowicz I, Cesselin F, Lagoguey M, Boyet F. (1979): Ann Endocrinol (Paris) 40:73
7. Grisoli F, Vincentelli F, Jaquet P, Guibot M, Hassoun J, Farnarier P. (1980): Surg Neurol 13:241
8. Serri O, Somma M, Rasio E, Beaurgard H, Hardy J. (1980): Can Med Assoc J 122:1007
9. Eversmann T, Eichinger R, Fahlbusch R, Rjosk HK, von Weder K. (1981): Schweiz Med Wochenschr 111:1782
10. Prescott RWG, Johnston DG, Kendall-Taylor P, Crombie A, Hall K, McGregor A, Hall R. (1982): Lancet i:245
11. Spark RF, Wills CA, O'Reilly GO, Ransil BJ, Bergland BJ. (1982): Lancet ii:129

12. Roulieer R, Mattei A, Franchimont P. (1978): In: Robijn C, Harper M. (eds) Progress in Prolactin Physiology and Pathology. Elsevier/North Holland Biomedical Press, Amsterdam, p 305
13. Masala A, Delitala G, Alagna S, Devilla L, Rovasio PP, Lott G. (1979): Fertil Steril 31:63
14. Segal S, Yaffe H, Laufer N, Ben-David M. (1979): Fertil Steril 32:556
15. Hargreave TB, Kyle KF, Kelly AM, England P. (1977: Br J Urol 49:747
16. Blacker C, Asfour M, Boutemy J-J, Gasnault J-P, Fossati P, L'Hermite M. (1977): Nouv Presse Med 42:3979
17. Pierrepoint CG, John BM, Groom GV, Wilson DW, Gow JG. (1978): J Endocrinol 76:171
18. Rjosk H-K, Schill W-B. (1979): Andrologia 11:297
19. Abyholm T, Molne K. (1980): Int J Androl 3:229
20. Gray P, Franken DR, Slabber CF, Potgieter GM. (1980): Andrologia 13:127
21. Laufer N, Yaffe H, Margalioth EJ, Livshin J, Ben-David M, Schenker JG. (1981): Arch Androl 6:343
22. Ambrosi B, Gaggini M, Moriondo P, Faglia G. (1980): JAMA 244:2608
23. Spark RF, White RA, Conolly PB. (1980): JAMA 243:750
24. Miller JB, Howard SS, MacLeod RM. (1980): J Urol 123:862
25. Thorner MO, McNeilly AS, Hagan C, Besser GM (1974): Br Med J 2:419
26. Boyar RM, Kapen S, Finkelstein JW, Perlow M, Sassin JF, Fukushima DK, Weitzman ED, Hellman L. (1974): J Clin Invest 53:1588
27. Snyder PF, Bigdeli H, Gardner DF, Mihailovic V, Rudenstein RS, Sterling FH, Utiger RD. (1979): J Clin Endocrinol Metab 48:309

Prolactin. Basic and clinical correlates
R.M. MacLeod, M.O. Thorner and U. Scapagnini (eds.),
Fidia Research Series, vol. I,
Liviana Press, Padova © 1985

Section XI
Clinical and therapeutic
aspects of hyperprolactinemia

THE INFLUENCE OF ESTROGENS ON THE SENSITIVITY OF PROLACTIN, TSH, AND LH TO THE INHIBITORY ACTIONS OF DOPAMINE IN HYPERPROLACTINEMIC PATIENTS

P. E. Harris, R. Valcavi*, C. Artioli*, P. Casoli*, S. M. Foord, C. Dieguez, J. R. Peters, R. Hall, and M. F. Scanlon

Neuroendocrine Unit, Department of Medicine, Welsh National School
of Medicine, Heath Park, Cardiff, S. Wales
*Sezione Endocrino Metabolica, 2a Div. Medica,
Ospedale, S. Maria Nuova, 42100 Reggio Emilia, Italy

It has generally been considered that estrogens and dopamine are antagonistic with respect to lactotroph function. Histologically, it is well established that estrogens stimulate lactotroph hypertrophy and mitosis in the rat (1). At the functional level, estrogens stimulate the synthesis of prolactin mRNA (2) and in the rat, they antagonize the effects of dopamine directly at the level of the lactotroph (3), leading ultimately to sustained hyperprolactinemia and prolactinoma formation (4). This estrogen effect is thought to cause pituitary gland enlargement during pregnancy. Although there is no clear evidence in man that estrogen-containing compounds lead to prolactinoma formation (5,6), it is generally felt that estrogens should be used with caution in patients with pathological hyperprolactinemia.

In ovariectomized, stalk-sectioned rhesus monkeys, hyperprolactinemia occurs because of the disruption of normal inhibitory hypothalamic-pituitary dopaminergic connections. In these animals, prolactin sensitivity to the inhibitory effect of infused dopamine is increased by estrogen replacement therapy (7). In normal human females, prolactin sensitivity to the inhibitory effects of dopamine is maximal at mid-cycle, following the preovulatory estradiol surge (8), and the administration of estrogen to agonadal women increases the dopaminergic inhibition of prolactin to the pattern of response seen on day 2 of normally cycling women (9). These data suggest that in primates and humans, estrogens may sensitize the lactotroph to the inhibitory actions of dopamine.

Dopamine has a known inhibitory action on TSH release both *in vivo* and *in vitro* (10-12) and this inhibitory action is increased in patients with hyperprolactinemia (13-15). Dopamine has also been implicated in the inhibitory control of gonadotrophin release in man (5,15). In particular, Quigley and Yen (16) have reported that patients

754

with pathological hyperprolactinemia show an exaggerated LH release following intravenous administration of the central dopamine receptor blocking drug metoclopramide, although others have failed to confirm these findings (17). Recent work using the dopamine antagonist domperidone has failed to demonstrate any change in LH release following peripheral receptor blockade.

The aim of this study was to test the hypothesis that estrogens increase prolactin sensitivity to dopamine in pathological hyperprolactinemia, by studying the effect of short term low dose estrogen pretreatment and antiestrogen pretreatment with tamoxifen (TAM) in the prolactin response to low dose dopamine infusion.

Table 1. *Mean sum of decrements in serum prolactin, LH, and TSH following dopamine infusion.*

	DA	DA + E$_2$	DA + TAM
PRL (mU/L)	8013 ± 1902	10988 ± 2489**	11697 ± 2611*
LH (U/L)	12.3 ± 5.1	57.3 ± 13.4*	24.0 ± 11.0
TSH (mU/L)	4.65 ± 1.23	8.1 ± 1.58**+	4.38 ± 0.41+

Results are expressed as Mean ± SEM
PRL/TSH N = 7, LH N = 5
Data analyzed by multiple analysis of variance (ANOVA). *P<0.05, **P<0.02, +P<0.05 between E$_2$ and TAM treatment.

Table 2. *Correlation between incremental increase in basal prolactin/LH levels after E$_2$/TAM pretreatment with increased decremental change in prolactin/LH levels in E$_2$TAM primed dopamine infusions.*

	PRL (DA + E$_2$)	PRL (DA + TAM)	LH (DA + E$_2$)
r	0.93	0.83	0.94
	p < 0.001	p < 0.005	p < 0.01

r = Correlation coefficient

In view of the role of dopamine in the inhibitory control of TSH and LH release, we have also studied the responses of these trophic hormones to the same experimental manipulations.

Seven female patients (aged 22-57 years) with hyperprolactinemia due to presumed prolactin-secreting microadenomas and otherwise intact pituitary function were studied. Three patients who subsequently underwent transethmoidal exploration of the anterior pituitary had the presence of a prolactin-secreting pituitary adenoma confirmed histologically and immunohistochemically; two patients had abnormal pituitary fossae on plain skull x-ray, and CAT scanning in the remaining two patients failed to reveal any radiological change. All patients however, had reduced or absent prolactin responses (rise < 200% of basal levels) to TRH administration (200 ug intravenously) consistent with the diagnosis of prolactinoma (14,18). The two patients with radiologically normal fossae showed exaggerated TSH responses to domperidone, which is also consisa solid phase, two site immunoradiometric assay, with intra- and interassay coefficients of variation of 3.3% and 7.8% respectively, at a standard dose of 7.8 mU/L. The sensitivity was 0.5 mU/L. LH wasmeasured by double antibody radioimmunoassay, with intra- and interassay coefficients of variation of 10% and 6.8% respectively at a standard dose of 23 mU/L.

Changes in prolactin, LH, and TSH levels have been expressed both as absolute changes and as decremental changes from basal levels (mean ± SE); the integrated changes in serum prolactin, LH, and TSH levels were assessed by calculation of the sum of prolactin, LH, and TSH decrements from the baseline values over the 3 hour infusion period. Statistical analysis was by paired Student's 't' test, and by multiple analysis of variance (ANOVA).

Ethinyl estradiol (E_2) pretreatment stimulated a rise in basal prolactin levels in all subjects (mean ± SE, mU/L; 2903 ± 761 vs 2293 ± 684, $p < 0.05$), while TAM produced a higher but more variable increase in basal prolactin levels (mean ± SE, mU/L; 3402 ± 757, p = n.s.). The serum prolactin levels fell during dopamine infusion, both in the unprimed state and following E_2/TAM treatment (Fig. 1a,b). During dopamine

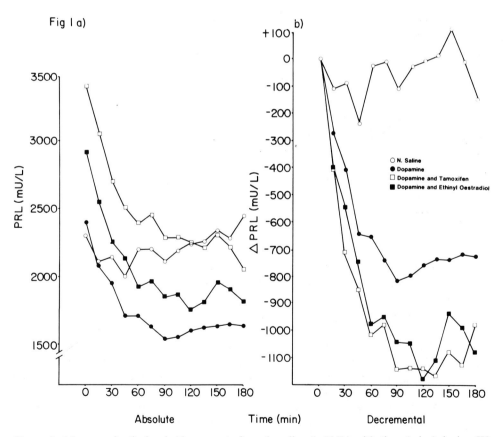

Figure 1. Mean prolactin levels/decrements from baseline (mU/L) with time (mins) during IV dopamine infusion (0.06 ug/kg/min).

756

a solid phase, two site immunoradiometric assay, with intra- and interassay coefficients of variation of 3.3% and 7.8% respectively, at a standard dose of 7.8 mU/L. The sensitivity was 0.5 mU/L. LH wasmeasured by double antibody radioimmunoassay, with intra- and interassay coefficients of variation of 10% and 6.8% respectively at a standard dose of 23 mU/L.

Changes in prolactin, LH, and TSH levels have been expressed both as absolute changes and as decremental changes from basal levels (mean ± SE); the integrated changes in serum prolactin, LH, and TSH levels were assessed by calculation of the sum of prolactin, LH, and TSH decrements from the baseline values over the 3 hour infusion period. Statistical analysis was by paired Student's 't' test, and by multiple analysis of variance (ANOVA).

Ethinyl estradiol (E_2) pretreatment stimulated a rise in basal prolactin levels in all subjects (mean ± SE, mU/L; 2903 ± 761 vs 2293 ± 684, $p < 0.05$), while TAM produced a higher but more variable increase in basal prolactin levels (mean ± SE, mU/L; 3402 ± 757, p / n.s.). The serum prolactin levels fell during dopamine infusion, both in the unprimed state and following E_2/TAM treatment (Fig. 1a,b). During dopamine

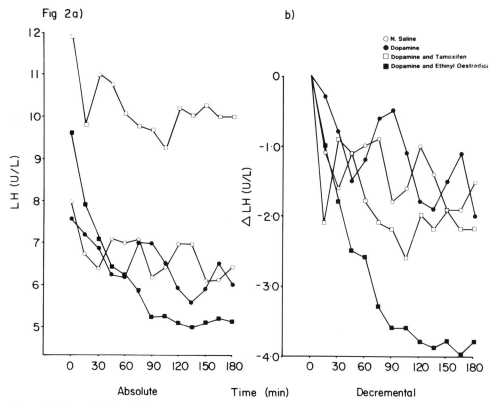

Figure 2. Mean LH levels/decrements from baseline (U/L) with time (mins) during IV dopamine infusion (0.06 ug/kg/min).

infusion, the decrement in prolactin levels was significantly greater following E_2 pretreatment (sum of decrements, mean ± SE, mU/L; 10988 ± 2489 vs 8013 ± 1902, p < 0.02) and TAM pretreatment (sum of decrements, mean ± SE mU/L; 11697 ± 2611, p < 0.05) (Table 1). The individual increments in basal prolactin levels both after E_2 and TAM pretreatment showed a positive correlation with the greater decrement in prolactin levels during E_2 and TAM primed dopamine infusions (E_2, r = 0.93, p < 0.01; TAM, r = 0.83, p < 0.05) (Table 2).

E_2 pretreatment produced a rise in basal LH levels in 5/7 patients, and during dopamine infusion, there was a fall in LH levels in all 5 patients who showed this change (Fig. 2, a,b). The decremental fall in LH levels was significantly greater following E_2 pretreatment (sum of decrements, mean ± SE U/L; 57.7 ± 13.4 vs 12.3 ± 5.1, p < 0.05) (Table 1). As with prolactin, when these subjects were analyzed, there was a significant positive correlation between the rise in basal LH levels after E_2 and the greater decremental change in LH levels in E_2-primed dopamine infusion (r = 0.94, p < 0.01) (Table 2). TAM pretreatment produced a rise in basal LH levels, with no response to dopamine infusion (Fig. 2a,b).

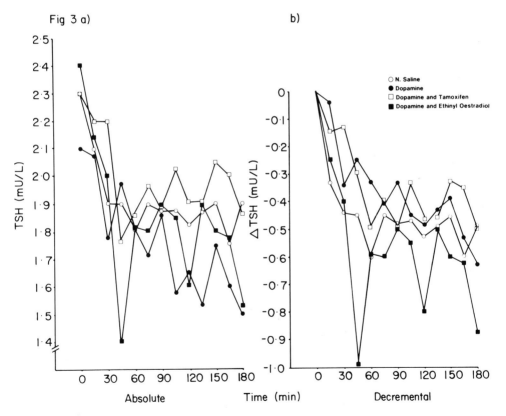

Figure 3. Mean TSH levels/decrements from baseline (mU/L) with time (mins) during IV dopamine infusion (0.06 ug/kg/min).

Basal TSH levels were unaffected in E_2-primed individuals (Fig. 3a,b), with a significantly increased decremental change (sum of decrements, mean ± SE mU/L; 8.1 ± 1.58 vs 4.65 ± 1.23, p < 0.02) (Table 1). A significantly greater decremental effect was also noted between E_2 and TAM pretreatment following dopamine infusion (sum of decrements, mean ± SE, mU/L; E_2, 8.1 ± 1.58 vs TAM, 4.38 ± 0.41, p < 0.05) (Table 1).

Estrogen treatment in hyperprolactinemic patients caused a variable rise in serum prolactin and LH levels. The decremental fall in prolactin and LH levels during dopamine infusion in these subjects was greater following E_2 pretreatment, although there was a considerable interindividual variation. Although E_2 priming had no effect on basal TSH levels, there was a significantly increased decremental change following dopamine infusion. TAM treatment produced a similar effect to E_2 on basal prolactin and LH levels. The decremental changes seen during dopamine infusion following TAM pretreatment were similar to the effects of E_2 as regards the dopaminergic inhibition of prolactin, but no change was seen as regards the dopaminergic inhibition of LH. TAM treatment was without effect both on the basal TSH levels and on the decremental changes during dopamine infusion.

In normal females, only minimal hyperprolactinemia may occasionally be seen following estrogen treatment (22), and indeed a lowering of basal prolactin levels has been reported in some women treated with 17-beta estradiol (23). It is possible that prolactin levels in such estrogen treated normal subjects are controlled by activation of the short loop feedback of prolactin on hypothalamic dopaminergic activity. By contrast, in hyperprolactinemic patients who show evidence of reduced dopaminergic inhibition of prolactin release at the lactotroph level (11,14,15), the more striking and significant rise in prolactin levels which follows estrogen pretreatment may be facilitated by this reduced dopaminergic activity. It should be noted that a similar effect on basal LH levels was seen in 5/7 patients treated with E_2, but in two patients, the basal LH levels actually fell. No striking E_2 effect was noted on basal TSH levels. In addition to these effects, we have found that estrogen priming over this short period of time incrased prolactin, LH, and TSH sensitivity to the inhibitory actions of dopamine. Furthermore, the degree of increase in the dopaminergic inhibition of prolactin and LH was directly related to the degree of rise in basal levels inducted by estrogen.

TAM is a well-known anti-estrogen that has been suggested to be a useful adjunct to dopamine agonist therapy in some resistant hyperprolactinemic patients (24). The results of TAM pretreatment in this study, however, were conflicting. Unlike E_2 pretreatment, TAM pretreatment had no effect on the decremental changes in LH/TSH levels during dopamine infusion, and indeed, the absolute changes of LH during dopamine infusion appear to be reversed following TAM priming (Fig. 2a). Paradoxically however, TAM and E_2 pretreatments both had similar effects on basal prolactin levels and decremental prolactin changes during dopamine infusion. In vitro, TAM has been shown to sensitize prolactinoma cells to the inhibitory actions of bromocriptine (25). Furthermore, TAM and 17-beta estradiol induce similar changes in circulating prolactin levels when administered separately to post-menopausal women (22). These data suggest that TAM might also possess intrinsic estrogen agonist actions, in addition to its known antiestrogen actions. Such intrinsic agonist/antagonist actions may explain the results obtained in this study, TAM having predominantly estrogen agonist actions on the lactotroph, and antagonist actions on the thyrotroph and gonadotroph.

In summary, these data provide evidence that in prolactinoma patients, estrogens may have a dual action on the lactotroph: to stimulate synthesis and release of prolactin and to increase the sensitivity of the lactotroph to the inhibitory actions of dopamine. The similar increased response of LH and TSH to the inhibitory actions of dopamine suggests that estrogens may have a more general effect, acting to increase sensitivity to the inhibitory actions of dopamine of a variety of anterior pituitary cell types. The mechanism on varying this alteration in dopaminergic function is unknown at present. It should be emphasized that the duration of E_2/TAM treatment was short in this study. This may account for the considerable interindividual variation in responses. It should also be noted that although the decremental changes in prolactin, LH and TSH were increased during dopamine infusion following estrogen priming, the absolute final values achieved were not lower than during dopamine infusion in the unprimed state. It is possible that longer periods of estrogen/TAM treatment may produce a greater uniformity of response and further increases in trophic hormone sensitivity to the inhibitory actions of dopamine.

REFERENCES

1. Lloyd HM, Meares JD, Jacobi J. (1973): J Endocrinol 58:227
2. Lieberman ME, Maurer RA, Gorski J. (1978): J Proc Natl Acad Sci USA 12:5946
3. Raymond V, Beaulieu M, Labrie F, Boissiez J. (1978): Science 200:1173
4. Furth J, Clifton KH. (1966): In: The Pituitary Gland. Butterworth, London, Vol 2:460
5. Hulting AL, Werner S, Hagenfeldt K. (1983): Contraception 27:69
6. Shy KK, McTiernan AM, Darling JR, Weiss NS. (1983): J Am Med Assoc 249:2204
7. Neill JD, Frawley LS, Plotsky PM, Tindall FT. (1981): Endocrinol 108:489
8. Judd SJ, Rakoff JS, Yen SSC. (1978): J Clin Endocrinol Metab 47:494
9. Yen SSC. (1979): In: Fuxe K, Hokfeldt T, Tuft R (eds) Central Regulation of the Endocrine System. Plenum Press, New York, p 387
10. Burrow GN, May PB, Spaulding SW, Donabeslan RK. (1977): J Clin Endocrinol Metab 45:65
11. Scanlon MF, Weightman DR, Shale DJ, Mora B, Heath M, Snow MH, Lewis M, Hall R. (1979): Clin Endocrinol 10:7
12. Foord SM, Peters JR, Dieguez C, Scanlon MF, Hall R. (1977): Endocrinol 94:1077
13. Scanlon MF, Pourmand M, McGregor AM. (1979): J Clin Endocrinol Invest 2:307
14. Scanlon MF, Rodriguez-Arnao MD, McGregor AM. (1981): Clin Endocrinol 2:133
15. Quigley ME, Judd SJ, Gilliland GB, Yen SSC. (1979): J Clin Endocrinol Metab 48:718
16. Quigley ME, Yen SSC. (1980): Am J Obstet Gynaecol 137:653
17. Elli R, Scaperotta RC, Travaglini P. (1983): In: 3rd International Workshop on Pituitary Adenomas, Amsterdam (abstract)
18. Cowden ES, Ratcliffe JG, Thomson JA, MacPherson P, Doyle D, Teasdale GM. (1979): Lancet i:1155
19. Rodriguez-Arnao MD, Peters JR, Foord SM. (1983): J Clin Endocrinol Metab 57:975
20. Massara F, Cassanni F, Martra M. (1983): Clin Endocrinol 18:103
21. Connell JMC, Padfield PL, Bunting EA, Ball SG, Inglis GC Beastall GH, Teasdale GH, Davies DL. (1983): Clin Endocrinol 18:527
22. Yen SSC, Ehara Y, Siler TM. (1974): J Clin Invest 53:652

23. Hegalson S, Wieking N, Carlstrom K, Dambern G, Von Schonetz B. (1982): J Clin Endocrinol Metab 54:404
24. Volker W, Gehrug WG, Berning R, Schmidt RC, Schneider J, Von Zur Muhlen A. (1982): Acta Endocrinol 101:491
25. De Quijada M, Timmermans HAT, Lamberts SWJ, MacLeod RM. (1980): Endocrinol 106:702

Prolactin. Basic and clinical correlates
R.M. MacLeod, M.O. Thorner and U. Scapagnini (eds.),
Fidia Research Series, vol. I,
Liviana Press, Padova © 1985

Section XI
Clinical and therapeutic
aspects of hyperprolactinemia

ENDOCRINE EFFECTS OF THE DOPAMINE AGONIST LISURIDE IN PATIENTS WITH CHRONIC RENAL FAILURE ON LONG-TERM HEMODIALYSIS

U. Desaga*, E. Reich-Schulze*, K-J Graf**, R. Dorow***, and H. Frahm*

*Second Medical Clinic, Hamburg-Eppendorf; **Dept. Internal Medicine, Klinikum Charlottenburg, Free University Berlin; ***Research Laboratories Schering AG, Berlin (West), FRG

It has been postulated that a number of symptoms observed in male patients, such as hypogonadism, loss of libido, impotence, impaired spermatogenesis, gynecomastia, and galactorrhea can in some cases be related to hyperprolactinemia and low testosterone levels (for reviews see 1, 2). Frequent observation of most of these symptoms in patients with chronic renal failure (RF) and reports of concomitant hyperprolactinemia in patients of both sexes with RF seem to support this postulation (3). However, the mechanism by which prolactin is assumed to affect gonadal function in humans has not yet been fully established.

In several reports on disturbances of thyroid function in patients with RF, authors found lowered levels of T_3, T_4 and FT_4, but elevated rT_3 levels, and an impaired TSH response to TRH stimulation. However, others describe normal thyroid function in patients with RF without nephrosis both under conservative therapy and under chronic hemodialysis (4).

The various endocrine disturbances observed in patients with RF have been linked with changes in central dopaminergic mechanisms. This assumption prompted us to reevaluate several endocrinological findings in male and female patients with chronic RF before and during treatment with the potent dopamine agonist lisuride (LIS).

In order to evaluate the incidence of hyperprolactinemia in patients with RF undergoing chronic hemodialysis, blood samples were collected from 317 patients immediately after dialysis. The influence of hemodialysis on elevated levels of prolactin (prolactin $\geq$ 30 ng/ml) was investigated in 27 patients by measuring prolactin at the beginning and end of a single hemodialysis.

Thirty hyperprolactinemic patients (21 female and 9 male) and 10 male normoprolactinemic RF patients complaining about disturbed sexual function were treated

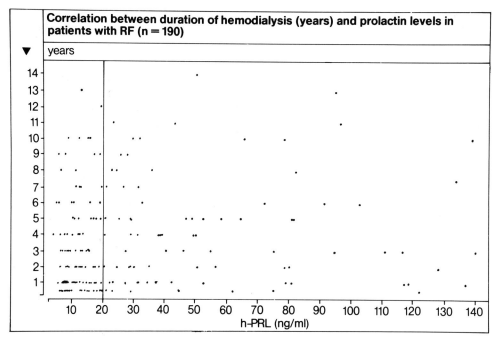

Figure 1. Correlation between duration of hemodialysis (years) and prolactin levels in patients with RF (n = 190).

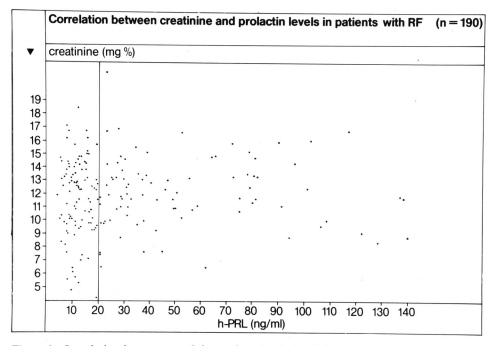

Figure 2. Correlation between creatinine and prolactin levels in patients with RF (n = 190).

with the potent dopamine agonist LIS. LIS was given for at least 3 months in a dosage of 0.075 mg/d (0.025 mg t.i.d.). From the 6th week of treatment onwards the LIS dosage was increased up to 0.15 mg/d in 10 out of the 40 patients. All patients had given their informed consent for this therapy.

Endocrinological parameters were investigated as follows: basal and TRH/LH-RH (TRH: 400 ug i.v.; LH-RH: 100 ug i.v.) stimulated concentrations of prolactin, TSH, LH, and FSH were measured prior to LIS treatment as well as at the end of treatment in the 10th or 12th week. Basal serum levels of prolactin, testosterone, LH, FSH TSH, T_3, T_4, FT_4, and rT_3 were monitored at 2-week intervals.

PROLACTIN

28% of male and female patients with RF (90 out of 317) exhibited basal plasma prolactin levels higher than 30 ng/ml after hemodialysis (range: 30 - 386). Only two male patients with prolactin levels higher than 30 ng/ml exhibited slight gynecomastia. Whereas all female patients were amenorrheic except one, none of the patients presented with galactorrhea.

There was no apparent correlation between basal prolactin concentrations and the levels of serum creatinine, age of patients, and years on hemodialysis (Figs. 1-3). Basal prolactin fell by 28% in 70% of patients after a single hemodialysis, while 30% of pa-

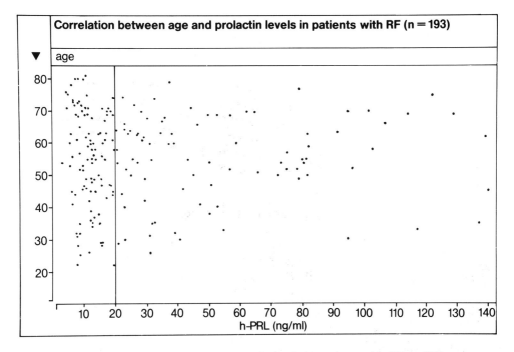

Figure 3. Correlation between age and prolactin levels in patients with RF (n-193).

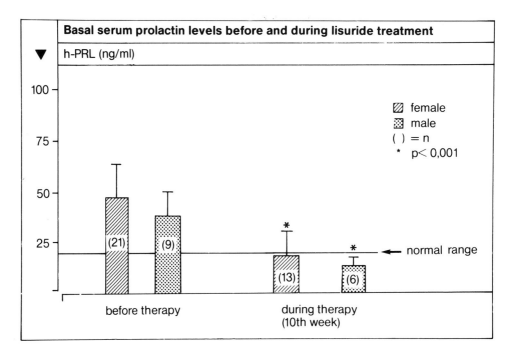

Figure 4. Basal serum prolactin levels before and during lisuride treatment.

tients showed a 15% increase in prolactin. In 21 female and 9 male patients, who subsequently were to receive LIS therapy, basal prolactin was 46.7 ± 21.6 and 36.2 ± 10.5, ($\bar{x}$ ± SD), respectively (Fig. 4). Prior to treatment all patients showed impaired release of prolactin after TRH, i.e. 41% of male and 46.7% of female patients (Fig. 5). The concentration of prolactin was lowered significantly in all patients after 3 months therapy with LIS (female: 17.2 ± 12.9; male: 12 ± 5.6 ng/ml, $\bar{x}$ ± SD). The response of prolactin to TRH increased during treatment (male, 82.6%; female, 79%) (Fig. 5).

THYROID HORMONES

None of the investigated patients showed clinical signs of a disturbed thyroid function. Table 1 offers a summary of the results of T_3, T_4 and rT_3. The table distinguishes between patients with elevated and those with normal prolaction concentrations and gives results from functional tests (TRH/LH-RH) before and during LIS therapy. A comparison of results of T_3, T_4, and rT_3 prior to and during LIS therapy reveals no apparent difference between normo- and hyperprolactinemic patients. Furthermore, there was no difference in basal or stimulated TSH in either group before and during LIS treatment (Table 2). Before therapy, FT_4 levels were significantly lowered only in hyperprolactinemic patients. During treatment with LIS the FT_4 levels increased slightly

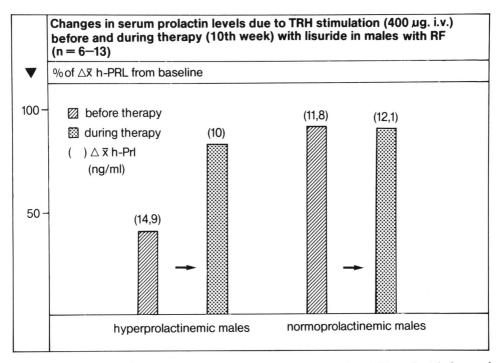

Figure 5. Changes in serum prolactin levels due to TRH stimulation (400 ug. i.v.) before and during therapy (10th week) with lisuride in males with RF (n = 6-13).

and returned to within the normal range; there was no longer a difference between those levels observed in normoprolactinemic patients before and during LIS therapy (Fig. 6).

Table 1. *Thyroid hormones before (A) and during (B) LIS treatment (10th - 12th weeks)*

		T_3		T_4		rT_3	
		A	B	A	B	A	B
Hyperprolactinemic	n	21	21	21	21	21	21
patients	$\bar{x}$	1.2	1.3	74.1	77.4	0.13	0.14
	SD	0.4	0.4	21.4	19.2	0.04	0.03
Normoprolactinemic	n	9	8	9	8	9	8
patients	$\bar{x}$	1.2	1.1	74.7	84.5	0.13	0.15
	SD	0.5	0.3	18.6	29.4	0.05	0.06
Normal range	(ug/l)	(0.8 - 1.8)		(45 - 120)		(0.09 - 0.35)	

Table 2. *TSH values before and during LIS treatment (10th - 12th week)*

| | | TSH before LIS | | TSH during LIS | |
		A	B	A	B
Hyperprolactinemic patients	n	30	30	22	22
	x̄	1.7	5.2	1.8	5.1
	SD	0.8	2.4	1.1	3.6
Normoprolactinemic patients	n	13	13	9	9
	x̄	2.1	5.9	1.8	4.8
	SD	1.7	3.6	1.2	1.9

Normal range for TSH: basal < 4uU/ml

TRH-stimulated < 24uU/ml

A = basal TSH; B = TRH-stimulated TSH

TESTOSTERONE, LH, AND FSH

The levels of basal serum LH and FSH were found to be elevated in all 19 male patients prior to treatment, whereas only 9 out of the 19 patients (45%) exhibited distinctly lowered ($\leq$ 3.5 ng/ml) basal serum testosterone levels (Figs. 7 and 8). There was no correlation between lowered serum testosterone levels and hyperprolactinemia in these patients. Throughout treatment with LIS no major changes were apparent as regards testosterone, LH, and FSH levels independent of the lowering effect of LIS on basal serum prolactin levels as found in all patients. There was also no difference in the LH and FSH response to LH-RH stimulation when the tests prior to treatment are compared compared with the results of the tests in the 10th or 12th week of treatment.

DISCUSSION

Different sources estimate that the incidence of hyperprolactinemia varies between 37% and 76% in patients with chronic RF. In our study 28% of the patients with RF showed prolactin levels higher than 30 ng/ml, the increase being greater in female than in male patients. This difference could be due to estrogens (5).

The genesis of hyperprolactinemic states in patients with RF remains unclear, however. There is obviously no correlation between increased concentrations of prolactin, the patients' age, the level of serum creatinine, and the number of years the patients were on hemodialysis (Fig. 1-3). With respect to hyperprolactinemia in patients with RF it should be taken into account that the metabolic clearance rate (MCR) of [131]J-prolactin has been reported as being reduced by about 30% (6). It is assumed that this is primarily a consequence of the cessation of glomerular filtration as demonstrated in animal experiments (7). Our findings indicate that the reduced MCR obviously cannot be of major importance, since prolactin levels decreased slightly in only 70% of

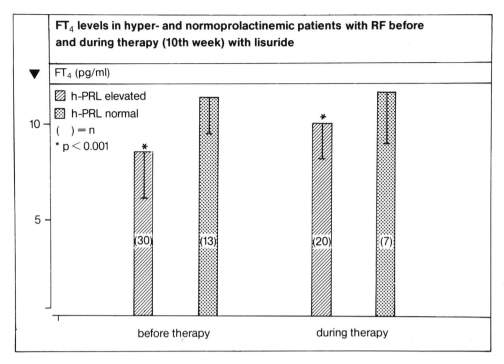

Figure 6. FT₄ levels in hyper- and normoprolactinemic patients with RF before and during therapy (10th week) with lisuride.

the patients, while the remaining 30% of patients even exhibited a 15% increase in prolactin levels, when the levels before and after dialysis are compared. As another possible cause for hyperprolactinemia an increased secretion rate for prolactin has been discussed (6).

However, despite the various assumptions made it is interesting that during treatment with even very low doses of LIS (0.025 mg t.i.d.) serum prolactin levels decreased in all patients with RF. Although severe side effects were not observed after LIS, more than 50% of the patients discontinued the therapy, indicating low compliance. With respect to long-term dopamine agonist treatment, bromocriptine has also been reported to lower prolactin levels; however, bromocriptine had to be withdrawn due to severe side effects (8). The high incidence of side effects observed with bromocriptine (particularly emesis and hypotension) indicates a hypersensitivity of patients with RF to dopamine agonists, since similar dosages (2.5 mg t.i.d.) are normally well tolerated in the treatment of pituitary tumors or in the inhibition of lactation. In our study we therefore used a very low dosage of LIS, which normally is recommended for the prevention of migraine attacks.

Since LIS lowers basal (elevated and normal) serum prolactin levels and restores the impaired response of prolactin due to TRH these results confirm the supposition of a high sensitivity of RF patients towards dopamine agonists. It therefore seems likely that in patients with chronic RF, hyperprolactinemia might be caused by central disturbances in the dopaminergic control of prolactin.

None of our patients exhibited increased prolactin levels due to hypothyroidism. In agreement with other authors (4) we found no major disturbances of thyroid function in patients with RF except for slightly lowered FT_4 levels prior to LIS treatment, primarily in the group of hyperprolactinemic patients with RF. In our study mean FT_4 levels rose to normal during LIS treatment. As we have not yet investigated thyroxin binding globuline (TBG) and FT_3 levels, we cannot decide whether the change in FT_4 levels is due to a decrease in TBG concentrations or to an altered conversion of T_4 to R_3 (9).

Various reports suggest that hyperprolactinemia affects gonadal function, possibly interacting with gonadotrophic secretion (e.g. feed-back control and pulsatile release) which in turn leads to disturbances of the gonadal function and spermatogenesis. However, conflicting results have been published on this topic (1, 2, 10-12).

On the basis of the hypothesis that there is a causal interaction between elevated prolactin secretion and gonadal dysfunction, a number of studies have attempted to restore the gonadal function by decreasing prolactin levels with dopamine agonists such as bromocriptine and LIS (10). These studies have rendered divergent results with respect to the effectiveness of dopamine agonists in restoring gonadal function. Only limited data are available relative to long-term treatment with dopamine agonists on gonadal dysfunction in RF patients (8). However, there are various reports indicating an im-

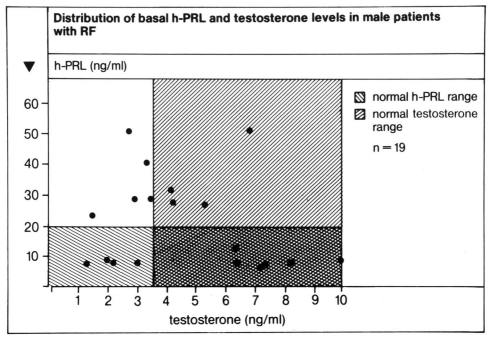

Figure 7. Distribution of basal h-prolactin and testosterone levels in male patients with RF.

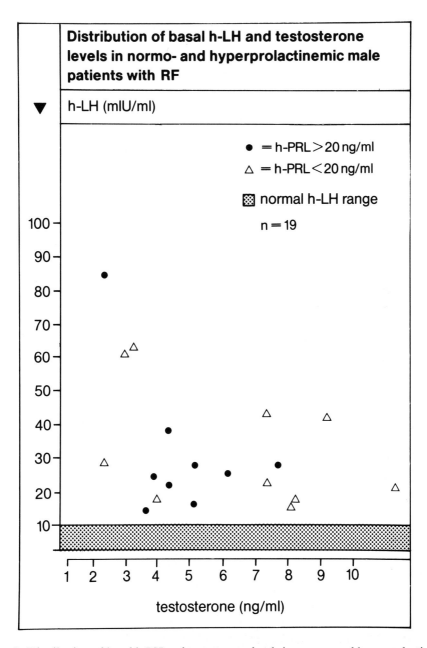

Figure 8. Distribution of basal h-LH and testosterone levels in normo- and hyperprolactinemic male patients with RF.

provement of sexual function and spermatogenesis in these patients after treatment with the dopamine agonist LIS (13). In a long-term study in healthy male volunteers it was found that LIS had no effect on the response of TSH, LH, FSH, and testosterone to TRH/LH-RH stimulation (10).

The data of the present study support previous findings in that no correlation is found between elevated prolactin levels and lowered or subnormal testosterone levels in RF patients. Throughout the treatment with LIS testosterone, LH and FSH levels of all groups remained in the range of the pretreatment phase. In particular, it should be emphasized that there was no correlation between the increase in the LH and FSH levels and serum prolactin and/or testosterone concentrations prior to and during LIS treatment. These findings may indicate that increase in the secretion of LH and FSH concentrations in serum precedes disturbances of the gonadal androgen production. However, the cause of this change in gonadotrophic hormone secretion, and its relevance for endocrine gonadal function, requires further detailed evaluation.

The data obtained by this study permit us to conclude that: 1) The incidence of prolactin levels higher than 30 ng/ml is about 30% in patients with RF; a single hemodialysis lowered the prolactin levels by 30% in 70% of patients, whereas in 30% of patients prolactin levels were increased (by 15%) after dialysis. 2) There is no correlation between elevated prolactin levels and levels of serum creatinine, the age of the patients, and the number of years the patients were on hemodialysis. 3) Basal as well as elevated serum prolactin levels were attenuated in all RF patients after very low doses of LIS, indicating a hypersensitivity of RF patients to dopamine agonists. 4) The degree of prolactin stimulated by TRH is decreased in hyperprolactinemic patients with RF and increased after prolactin normalization due to LIS treatment. 5) TSH and thyroid hormones (T_4, T_3, rT_3) are within the normal range. Only FT_4 is lowered in hyperprolactinemic patients with RF, but rises to normal values during LIS therapy. 6) There is no correlation between elevated prolactin levels and lowered or subnormal testosterone levels in male patients with RF. 7) Elevated basal levels of LH and FSH were observed in all male patients with RF, probably as a consequence of primarily disturbed gonadal function or due to direct disturbances in central mechanisms unknown at present. 8) There is no correlation between the LIS-induced lowering of serum prolactin levels and the follow-up data for serum testosterone, LH, and FSH levels; throughout treatment they all remained within the range of pretreatment levels. 9) No severe side effects were apparent in this study following LIS treatment.

ACKNOWLEDGMENTS

The investigations were carried out in patients of the 'Dialysezentrum Alter Teichweg' and 'Dialysezentrum Eppendorf', Hamburg. Our thanks are due to the medical staff for all their assistance. We also would like to thank Mrs. I. Kutren, Klinikum Charlottenburg, Berlin, for her skillful technical assistance.

REFERENCES

1. Hermans U, Hafez ESE. (1981): Arch Androl 6:95
2. Fluckiger E, del Pozo E, Von Werder K. (1982): Prolactin, Physiology, Pharmacology and

Clinical Findings Springer-Verlag, Berlin, p 224

3. Cowden EA, Ratcliffe WA, Ratcliffe JG, Kennedy AC. (1981): Acta Endocrinol 98:488
4. Rudorff KH, Schmitz B, Jahnke K. (1982): Akt Endokr Stoffw 3:55
5. Kokot F. (1983): In: Tolis et al (eds) Prolactin and Prolactinomas. Raven Press, New York, p 249
6. Sievertsen GD, Lim VS, Nakawatase C, Frohman LA. (1980): J Clin Endocrinol Metab 50:846
7. Emmanouel DS, Fang VS, Katz AJ. (1981): Am J Physiol 240:437
8. Bommer J, Ritz E, del Pozo E, Bommer G, Andrassy K. (1979): Nierenund Hochdruck-krankh 18:220
9. Wolfson M, Raouf A, O'Gorman P, Marsden P. (1981): Clin Endocrinol 15:579
10. Graf K-J, Schmidt-Gollwitzer M, Horowski R, Dorow R. (1982): Clin Endocrinol 17:243
11. Magrini G, Ebiner JR, Burckhardt P, Felber JP. (1976): J Clin Endocrinol Metab 43:944
12. Hrubesch M, Wagner H, Loew H, Hauss WH. (1975): Mat Med Nordm 27:304
13. Ruilope L, Garcia-Robles R, Paya C, de Villa LF, Morales JM, Parada J, Sancho J, Rodicio JL. (1984): Kidney, in press

Prolactin. Basic and clinical correlates
R.M. MacLeod, M.O. Thorner and U. Scapagnini (eds.),
Fidia Research Series, vol. I,
Liviana Press, Padova © 1985

Section XI
Clinical and therapeutic
aspects of hyperprolactinemia

BIOACTIVITY OF CIRCULATING PROLACTIN DURING THE MENSTRUAL CYCLES OF ASYMPTOMATIC HYPERPROLACTINEMIC AND NORMOPROLACTINEMIC WOMEN

Michael S. Blank and Maria L. Dufau

Section on Molecular Endocrinology, Endocrinology and Reproduction Research Branch, National Institute of Child Health and Human Development, National Institute of Health, Bethesda, MD USA 20205

Hyperprolactinemia without accompanying symptoms such as amenorrhea or galactorrhea is now more widely recognized (1-4). Before cases of asymptomatic hyperprolactinemia were identified, elevated circulating levels of prolactin were usually associated with infertility (5). One explanation for the lack of symptoms in these individuals is an over-abundance of larger molecular weight forms of prolactin (2,3). The larger forms of prolactin may not pass readily from the circulation, thus having difficulty in effecting a full end-organ response. Other possible explanations for lack of symptoms include diminished target organ responsiveness, bioinactive circulating forms of prolactin, or deranged secretory patterns. We have examined the latter two possibilities in an asymptomatic hyperprolactinemic subject compared with normoprolactinemic women during the menstrual cycle. The detailed investigation of menstrual cycle patterns of prolactin bioactivity was simplified by the availability of an *in vitro* replication bioassay (6).

An asymptomatic hyperprolactinemic (AHPr) woman and three normoprolactinemic (NPr) women were studied. All patients showed signs of at least 3 regular menstrual periods before entry into the study and exhibited normal levels of ovarian steroids during the phases of the menstrual cycle which were under study. Serial blood samples were withdrawn from each patient through an indwelling venous catheter at 10 or 15 min intervals for up to 480 min. Plasma samples (50 ul or less) were assayed for immunoactivity by homologous radioimmunoassay for human prolactin (hPRL) and for bioactivity by Nb2 rat lymphoma cell bioassay (6). The hPRL standard used in both assays was AFP 2312C. Radioimmunoassay and bioassay data were reduced by computer programs. Bioassay samples were analyzed at a minimum of three dose levels and checked for parallelism with the standard curve. The minimal detectable dose of the RIA and bioassay was approximately 1 ng hPRL/ml serum. All samples from individual patients were analyzed within the same assay.

To test for the presence of factors in serum which could synergize with prolactin in stimulating Nb2 lymphoma growth, dilutions of serum (5-100 equivalents) from each subject were incubated with cells in the presence or absence of 250 pg hPRL (equivalent to 5 ng hPRL/ml). Potency estimates obtained with and without prolactin were compared. Analysis of the profiles of plasma prolactin pulses was conducted using a computerized cycle detection program based on a threshold method (7). Isolated, large prolactin pulses which exceeded other pulses by at least 50% in amplitude were omitted from analyses and the data re-scanned to prevent missing actual pulses among the remaining data (8).

Levels of prolactin in the AHPr subject ranged from 36 to 79 ng/ml RIA and from 44 to 97 ng/ml by bioassay. B:I ratios fell between 0.84 and 1.77. In three NPr women, RIA values ranged from 5.2 to 43 ng/ml and bioassay values from 3.5-35 ng/ml. B:I ratios in NPr women ranged from 0.33 to 1.37. Mean prolactin levels and B:I ratios by phase of the menstrual cycle are listed in Tables 1 and 2. Levels of prolactin and B:I ratios in the AHPr were consistently higher during each stage of the menstrual cycle.

Table 1. *Mean prolactin B:I ratios during the menstrual cycle*

Patient	Phase of menstrual cycle		
	Follicular	Midcycle	Luteal
AHPr[a]	1.25 ± 0.02[c](33)[d]	1.02 ± 0.02 (37)	1.16 ± 0.03 (27)
NPr1[b]	0.61 ± 0.02 (33)	0.76 ± 0.02 (37)	0.69 ± 0.02 (33)
NPr2	0.39 ± 0.02 (11)	0.63 ± 0.02 (37)	0.93 ± 0.03 (33)
NPr3	0.70 ± 0.27 (28)	0.63 ± 0.34 (22)	—

[a] asymptomatic hyperprolactinemic; [b] normoprolactinemics; [c] mean ± SE; [d] number of samples

Table 2. *Mean prolactin levels (ng/ml) during the menstrual cycle*

Condition	Phase of menstrual cycle					
	Follicular		Midcycle		Luteal	
	BIO	RIA	BIO	RIA	BIO	RIA
AHPr	68.5	54.9	49.2	49.0	64.7	55.7
NPr	13.7[a]	17.3	10.8	16.9	8.2	9.9
	(6.5,20.8)[b]	(10.8-29.9)	(5.4-16.1)	(7.2-25.7)	(5.4,10.9)	(7.9,11.8)

[a] mean of means; [b] range

The patterns of plasma prolactin immuno- and bioactivity and B:I ratio in the AHPr subject are shown in Figure 1. It is readily apparent that few biological and no immunological prolactin pulses are detected. It can be seen also that increases in B:I ratio in this subject are related more to relative decreases in RIA values than to increases in bioactivity (Fig. 1). In most instances when an increase occurred in the B:I ratio of a NPr individual, it was due to an augmentation of bioactivity; however, there were clear instances in which an isolated decrease in immunoactivity accounted for the increase in B:I ratio. The latter situation predominated in the AHPr woman during the follicular and midcycle stages.

In normoprolactinemic women (Fig. 2) several instances were noted (NPr1: follicular and luteal phases; NPr2: midcycle phase) in which transient secretory episodes were superimposed on the decay phase of a bioactive prolactin peak. These fluctuations were not identified as pulses and sometimes they were associated with immunoactivity (e.g. NPr1: follicular phase). Pulse signal-to-noise ratios (SNR) were lowest in the AHPr patient (0.4-1.6). The ranges of SNR's in the three normoprolactinemic women were: NPr1, 1.4-2.8; NPr2, 2.6-3.5; NPr3, 2.3-3.3. A SNR of > 2 is recommended for enhanced reliability of the cycle detection program (7) with the number of samples collected in the present study. When this criterion was relaxed to 1.6 for the AHPr subject (this would result in an over-estimation of the number of pulses), only one biological pulse in the follicular phase, four biological pulses in the luteal phase, and no RIA pulses were identified (Table 3). In contrast, an average of 3.3-4.0 biological and 3.5-5.3 RIA prolactin pulses were identified in NPr subjects (Table 3).

Sixty-nine percent of 29 immunoassay pulses and 70% of the 30 bioactive pulses analyzed were concordant. Thus, discordant pulses (pulses occurring alone) accounted for approximately 30% of the total pulses examined. No evidence was found for a synergistic circulating factor in NPr subjects with the usual amounts of serum used for assay (50 ul or less). That is, differences in cell growth stimulated by serum with or without added prolactin (250 pg) were accounted for entirely by the added prolactin. However, stimulation of cell replication consistent with the addition of an additional 250 pg prolactin was obtained with serum from the AHPr subject.

The computerized threshold method (7) detected pulsations of circulating prolactin immuno- and bioactivity in all stages of the menstrual cycle in normoprolactinemic

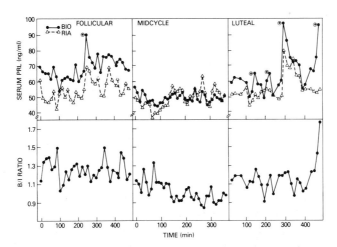

Figure 1. Circulating prolactin bioactivity (BIO) and immunoactivity (RIA) (upper panel) and bioactivity:immunoactivity ratios (lower panel) in an asymptomatic hyperprolactinemic during three stages of the menstrual cycle. Asterisks denote pulses identified by cycle detection (7): (★) = bioactive peaks, ★ = immunoactive peaks. Note break in ordinate scale.

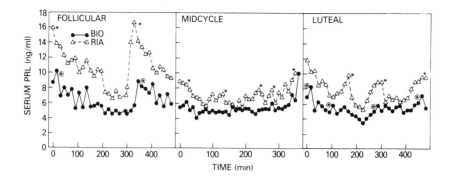

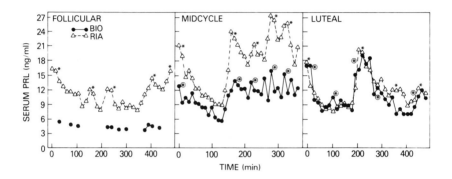

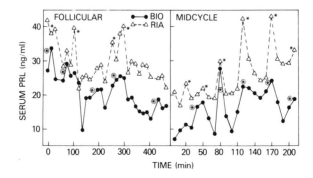

Figure 2. Circulating prolactin bioactivity (BIO) and immunoactivity (RIA) in three normoprolactinemic women (NPr1, upper; NPr2 middle; NPr3, lower) during different stages of the menstrual cycle. Asterisks denote pulses identified by cycle detection (7): (★) = bioactive peaks, ★ = immunoactive peaks.

women. This finding contrasts with previous studies in which no consistent patterns of prolactin secretion during the menstrual cycle were found (9,10). The use of a systematic, iterative method for detecting pulsations in sequential, biological data may be responsible for these differences.

Table 3. *Numbers of prolactin pulses detected during menstrual cycle*

Phase of cycle	Condition	BIO	RIA
Follicular	AHPr	1	0
	NPr	3.5[a]	3.7
		(2,5)[b]	(2-5)
Midcycle	AHPr	0	0
	NPr	3.3	5.3
		(0-5)	(5-6)
Luteal	AHPr	4	0
	NPr	4	3.5
		(3,5)	(3,4)

[a] mean; [b] range

The results of this investigation indicate that despite normal bioactivity, prolactin secretion profiles are altered in a woman who exibits elevated prolactin levels but no symptoms. Specifically, an AHPr woman demonstrated a lack of bioactive prolactin peaks relative to NPr subjects during the follicular and midcycle phases and a signal-to-noise ratio for immunoactivity which was near unity throughout the menstrual cycle. Although the B:I ratios showed fluctuations in this individual, they were probably due to decreases in immunoactivity since a high degree of concordance was observed between decreases in immunoactivity and elevations of the B:I ratio. Furthermore, while the overall concordance between biological and immunological prolactin pulses was approximately 70 percent, the AHPr woman exhibited no concordance of biological pulses during the menstrual cycle. In contrast, NPr subjects had 84% concordance of bioactive pulses. Despite these marked differences in patterns of bioactive prolactin secretion the overall mean B:I ratios in the AHPr woman were the highest observed. This is not consistent with the presence of bioinactive forms of prolactin in the circulation of this individual.

Evidence presented here for the presence of a bioactive synergistic mitogen (11) in the serum of the AHPr subject may explain the higher B:I ration relative to NPr women studied. However, it will be necessary to obtain prolactin bioassay values from a larger number of normoprolactinemics to make a definite statement regarding the status of this AHPr subject relative to the normal B:I range.

In previous studies it was found that prolactin secretion during the menstrual cycle was higher at midcycle and during the luteral phase (9,12) but this was not a consistent finding (10). In the present study mean prolactin levels were higher during the luteal or midcycle phases of three NPr women while levels in the AHPr women were lowest at midcycle. However, mean peak amplitudes were higher during the luteal phase of the AHPr and of one NPr woman while no differences were noted in the remaining women. Thus, patterns rather than absolute levels of prolactin bioactivity may be more helpful in ascertaining the physiological status of prolactin secretion in any one individual.

We did not test for the presence of large molecular forms of prolactin in the APHr woman and this remains a possibility in explaining her lack of symptoms (13). Some authors have speculated that these larger forms may exibit slow or negligible egress from the capillaries (3). This phenomenon could also explain the somewhat longer than half-time disappearance rate of endogenous prolactin pulses in the luteal phase of the AHPr woman. Another speculation to consider in explaining the lack of amenorrhea in the AHPr subject is the requirement which target organs have for pulsatile stimulation in order to maintain maximal responsiveness (14). Perhaps elevated, unchanging levels of prolactin in this woman can desensitize the ovary and prevent the adverse effects of overstimulation. Of course, primary target organ insensitivity should also be considered.

ACKNOWLEDGMENTS

We thank the National Hormone and Pituitary Program for hPRL standard; Drs. C.T. Beer and H.G. Friesen for Nb2 rat lymphoma cells; Drs. T.C. Hamilton and R. Ozols for the use of a Coulter cell counter; and Drs. R.A. Steiner and D.K. Clifton for providing a computer program for analyses of prolactin pulses.

REFERENCES

1. Tambascia M, Bahamondes L, Pinotti J, Collier AM, Dachs JL, Faundes A. (1980): Fertil Steril 34:282
2. Whittaker PG, Wilcox T, Lind T. (1981): J Clin Endocrinol Metab 53:863
3. Andersen AN, Pedersen H, Djursing H, Andersen BV, Friesen HG. (1982): Fertil Steril 38:625
4. Lindstedt G, Lundberg P-A, Bengtsson C, Nystrom E, Bjurstam N, Leman J and Rybo G. (1984): Clin Chem 30:165
5. Bohnet HG, Dahlen HG, Wuttke W, Schneider HPG. (1976): J Clin Endocrinol Metab 42:132
6. Tanaka T, Shiu RPC, Gout PW, Beer CT, Noble RL, Friesen HG. (1980): J Clin Endocrinol Metab 51:1058
7. Clifton DK, Steiner RA. (1983): Endocrinology 112:1057
8. Dufau ML, Veldhuis JD, Fraioli F, Johnson ML, Beitins IL. (1983): J Clin Endocrinol Metab 57:993
9. Ehara Y, Siler T, VandenBerg G, Sinha YH, Yen SSC. (1973): Am J Obstet Gynecol 117:962
10. McNeilly AS, Chard T. (1974): Clin Endocrinol 3:105
11. Nicoll CS, Herbert N, Steiney S, Delidow B. (1983): Am Zool 23:899
12. Vekemans M, Delvoye P, L'Hermite M, Robyn C. (1977): J Clin Endocrinol Metab 44:989
13. Jackson RD, Wortsman J, Malarkey WB. (1983): Clin Res 31:273A
14. Knobil E. (1981): Biol Reprod 24:44

Prolactin. Basic and clinical correlates
R.M. MacLeod, M.O. Thorner and U. Scapagnini (eds.),
Fidia Research Series, vol. I,
Liviana Press, Padova © 1985

Section XI
Clinical and therapeutic
aspects of hyperprolactinemia

TERGURIDE (9-10 TRANSDIHYDROLISURIDE) IN THE TREATMENT OF HYPERPROLACTINEMIA AND ACROMEGALY

J. Marek, J. Sramkova, J. Bauer, and K. Rezabek

3rd Dept. of Medicine and Dept. of Neurology, Charles University
and Research Institute for Pharmacy and Biochemistry
Prague, Czechoslovakia

The effectiveness of dopaminergic drugs in lowering prolactin in pathological hyperprolactinemic states and growth hormone (GH) in acromegaly is well documented. At present, bromocriptine is the most widely used dopamine agonist in the long-term treatment of these conditions. More recently lisuride was proved to be as active as bromocriptine in reducing prolactin and GH levels (1,2).

Ergoline derivatives as ergotamine and ergotoxine are known to yield derivatives with more suitable properties by their hydrogenation in position 9-10. Terguride: N-(D-6-methyl-8-isoergolin-l-yl)-N',N-diethylcarbamide hydrogen maleate, a dihydroderivative of lisuride, was synthetized by Zikan et al. and proved in rats to suppress effectively the lactation (3), to reduce growth of mammary carcinomas (4), to decrease the content of the adenohypophysial prolactin (5), to decrease the weight of prostate while a simultaneous administration of prolactin prevented this effect (6), to inhibit serum prolactin in female rats treated with reserpine and to lower prolactin levels in human volunteers (7).

In the present study terguride was used on long-term basis (3-24 months) in the treatment of clinical manifestations of hyperprolactinemia in pituitary adenomas (22 patients) and in acromegaly (9 patients). Prolactin, growth hormone and testosterone were measured by radioimmunoassay. The following standards were used: MRC 75/504 Mill Hill, London, for prolactin and GH Greenwood batch 6.I.C.Rf for growth hormone. Testosterone was determined with commercial kits. Normal values were: prolactin 2-25 ug/l in women, 2-20 ug/l in men, basal GH below 3 ug/l, testosterone 11-44 nmol/l in men.

TERGURIDE IN PROLACTINOMAS

There have been more reasons for the treatment of patients with prolactinomas: 1) to normalize hyperprolactinemia and thus enable pregnancy, 2) to normalize hyperprolactinemia and thus restore regular menstrual cycle, 3) to reduce the size of prolactinoma, and 4) to prevent the regrowth of large invasive prolactinomas incompletely removed by surgery.

TREATMENT OF STERILITY

Seven women (age 21-32 years) with prolactinomas desiring pregnancy were treated with terguride 3-24 months. In one woman the therapy was withdrawn after 3 months because of side effects. All but one of the other women conceived within 3 weeks to 4 months. In one woman with macroadenoma prolonged therapy was necessary for resumption of menstrual cycle (13 months) and conception (22 months). Terguride treatment was stopped after the confirmation of pregnancy in the 2nd or 3rd month after conception. Up to now one woman has given birth to a healthy child after uncomplicated pregnancy. Data of individual patients are given in Table I.

Table I. *Terguride therapy of sterility*

Patient	Age	Duration of treatment (months)	Daily dose of terguride (mg)	Prolactin ug/l Before	On	Pregnancy
1.	31	6	1.5	110	14	yes
2.	36	24	3.0	1300	4	yes
3.	33	5	4.5	200	35	yes
4.	29	5	6.0	580	20	yes
5.	31	3	1.0	53	2	yes
6.	28	5	3.0	360	34	yes
7.	29	3	3.0	590	12	no

TREATMENT OF AMENORRHEA

Treatment of amenorrhea is asked by women not desiring pregnancy mostly from psychological reasons. However, hyperprolactinemic amenorrhea was shown to be joined with osteoporosis (8) and the resumption of menstrual cycle may prevent the bone changes. Therefore the treatment of amenorrhea caused by hyperprolactinemia seems to be indicated even in the absence of other reasons for treatment (e.g. sterility, tumorous extension).

Four women (aged 23 - 33 years) in this group were treated with relatively low doses of terguride (1.0 to 1.5 mg daily) and resumed regular menstrual cycle after 3 - 6 weeks. Individual data are shown in Table 2.

Table 2. *Terguride therapy of amenorrhea*

Patient	Age	Duration of treatment (months)	Daily dose of terguride (mg)	Prolactin ug/l Before	On	Time interval to resumption of menses weeks
1.	23	3	1.5	110	2.5	3
2.	33	6	1.5	114	2.5	6
3.	23	5	1.0	50	4.0	6
4.	30	6	1.5	36	1.7	5

TREATMENT OF TUMOR ENLARGEMENT

An attempt to reduce tumor size is indicated in macroadenomas, especially in those with extrasellar extension, where the adenomatous growth endangers pituitary function and the optic nerve and can even spread intracerebrally. Ergoline derivatives were shown to cause shrinkage of prolactinomas in some patients and sometimes even their complete disappearance (9-11). The partial effect of ergoline derivatives can be completed by radiotherapy or surgery. Shrinkage of the tumor makes its excision easier and more certain (12).

We have treated 8 patients, 5 women and 3 men, aged 16 - 51 years, with macroprolactinomas. Six of them had extrasellar extension. Clinical data and the effects of therapy on prolactin and testosterone levels are given in Table 3. Prolactin levels fell in all patients, however normalization was not achieved in two of them. In these two patients increased terguride dosage had no additive effect on prolactin levels. In all treated males a rise in plasma testosterone levels was observed during the therapy.

Table 3. *Terguride therapy of tumor enlargement*

Patient	Sex and Age	Duration of treatment (months)	Daily dose of terguride (mg)	Prolactin ug/l Before	On	Testosterone mm/l of Before	On
1.	m,32	8	4.0	7000	13	0.6	7.9
2.	f,35	24	3.0	1300	4		
3.	f,37	12	2.0	855	6		
4.	f,16	6	2.0	3000	16		
5.	f,27	6	6.0	1880	195		
6.	f,32	6	1.5	136	16		
7.	m,51	24	6.0	1200	115	7.3	16.5
8.	m,22	6	3.0	346	2	6.6	50.0

The size-reducing effects of terguride in prolactinomas are given in Table 4. The size of prolactinomas was measured by CT (Siretom 2000 E, Siemens) before and after

5 months of treatment. Terguride was without size reducing effect in one patient, however, even in this patient degenerative changes in the tumor were disclosed after therapy. In one patient there was complete disappearence of the tumor, both in intrasellar and suprasellar portions. In three other patients only the suprasellar portion disappeared with reduction of the intrasellar part. In the remaining two patients there was a partial reduction of intrasellar or suprasellar portion.

Table 4. *Size reduction of prolactinomas with terguride*

| Patient | Size of adenoma | | | | Degenerative changes on treatment |
| | Within sella | | Suprasel. ext. | | |
	Before	On	Before	On	
1.	+ + +	+ +	+ + +	+	Present
2.	+ + +	+ +	+ +	0	Present
3.	+ + +	+ +	0	0	Present
4.	+ +	+	+ +	0	Absent
5.	+ +	+	+	0	Present
6.	+ +	+ +	+ +	+	Absent
7.	+ +	+ +	0	0	Present
8.	+	0	+	0	Absent

Diameter:　+, 1 cm;　+ +, 1-2 cm;　+ + +, 3 cm

PREVENTION OF PROLACTINOMA REGROWTH

In patients with prolactin secreting macroadenomas surgery often fails to normalize prolactin levels signaling remaining adenomatous tissue (13). The recurrence of invasively growing adenomas is frequent. Consequently, an attempt to prevent the regrowth of prolactinomas by ergoline derivatives seems to be indicated. With terguride we have normalized prolactin levels in three patients with prolactinomas with residual prolactin hypersecretion after surgery. However, all patients were treated only for short periods. More long-standing experience is necessary to confirm the benefit of terguride in this indication.

Table 5. *Prevention of prolactinoma recurrence with terguride*

| Patient | Sex and age | Duration of treatment (months) | Daily dose of terguride (mg) | Prolactin ug/1 | |
				Before	On
1.	m,22	6	1.5	148	4.0
2.	m,32	7	1.0	210	1.6
3.	f,36	6	1.5	3000	5.5

TERGURIDE IN ACROMEGALY

In acromegaly removal of the pituitary adenoma is the treatment of choice. In some patients, however, surgery is contraindicated while in others even repeated surgical interventions do not restore normal GH levels. This is especially so in extensive tumors, where adenoma cells tend to infiltrate structures adjoining the hypophysis including the spenoid bone. In these patients alternative methods of treatment are required. Radiotherapy, whether conventional external irradiation, proton beam or ^{90}Y implantation, has been used with some success but suffers from the disadvantage of delayed effect. Ergoline derivatives which cause a paradoxical reduction of GH in some acromegalic patients can be very useful in this situation. However, they are less efficacious in the management of acromegaly than in hyperprolactinemia. There are considerable differences in data about the percentage of responsive acromegalic patients. With bromocriptine a high number of successfully treated patients (79- 90%) has been reported by some authors (14,15), while others have demonstrated rather disappointing results with less than 25% of responsive acromegalics (16,17). Lindholm et al. (18) considered bromocriptine wholly inefficacious. Similar results as with bromocriptine were obtained with lisuride (1,2) and pergolide (19). With all these drugs there can be troublesome side effects that prompted us to evaluate the therapeutic effect of terguride in acromegaly.

Terguride was given to 9 patients with active acromegaly, 5 women and 4 men, aged 28 - 54 years (Table 6). Seven of them experienced residual GH hypersecretion after pituitary surgery. In one patient the surgery was contraindicated because of heart disease and one patient refused the operation. With one exception patients were given 2 mg terguride daily for 3 months and as the effect was not complete, the dose was then increased to 3 - 4 mg daily. The duration of treatment was 3 - 24 (mean 8.2) months.

Table 6. *Clinical data of acromegalics treated with terguride*

Patient	Sex and age	Previous surgery and time interval to terguride (years)		Duration of treatment (months)	Maximum daily dose of terguride (mg)
1.	f,28	yes	(3)	24	4
2.	m,50	yes	(1/2)	6	4
3.	f,51	yes	(10)	12	1.5
4.	m,36	yes	(2)	8	4
5.	m,36	yes	(1/2)	6	4
6.	f,31	yes	(1/2)	3	2
7.	m,54	no		3	2
8.	f,36	no		8	3
9.	f,30	yes	(1/2)	4	4

The results of the treatment are shown in table 7. As an index of daily GH secretion a profile was obtained from 7-9 samples. In the table GH means and ranges before the treatment are compared with those on the therapy. Glucose supression test was performed with 100 g glucose load and the blood for GH estimation was obtained at 30, 0, 60 and 120 min.. TRH test was performed with 200 ug TRH i.v. with sampling for GH at 30, 0, 20 and 60 min.. GH response was defined as present when the doubling of basal GH levels was recorded. The following criteria were adopted for the assessment of effectiveness of therapy. Full response: 1) all or most values of multiple sampling being 5 ug/1 or less; 2) Suppression of GH by glucose load to 3 ug/l or less; 3) absent TRH stimulation of GH secretion. Partial response: GH values 50% or less of pretreatment levels without the criteria of full normalization.

In only one patient the full response to the terguride therapy was achieved with all GH values below 4.0 ug/l, suppression of GH after glucose load to 2 ug/l and no stimulation of GH secretion after TRH. In 6 patients partial response was obtained in laboratory data together with the clinical improvement. As anticipated, prolactin secretion responded to terguride in all 3 hyperprolactinemic acromegalics as well as in 6 who were normoprolactinemic.

Table 7. *Laboratory data in acromegalics treated with terguride*

Patient			Growth hormone profile ug/1 (mean and range)		GH after glucose (ug/l)		GH after TRH (ug/l)		PRL (ug/l)	
	Before		On		Bef.	On	Bef.	On	Bef.	On
1.	16.7	(13-23)	2.8	(2-3.5)	5	2	16	4	15	2
2.	67.6	(41-84)	7.9	(5-10)	125	14	420	400	80	13
3.	9.9	(4-16)	3.5	(2-5)	—	5	48	8	3	1
4.	187.5	(150-230)	84.4	(66-106)	—	170	—	120	10	2
5.	110.3	(90-135)	55.4	(45-65)	55	33	104	63	64	5
6.	13.6	(5-20)	5.6	(5-7)	8	3	20	—	4	1
7.	73.1	(30-110)	16.7	(12-27)	70	—	570	—	300	3
8.	27.0	(18-42)	24.5	(17-24)	—	—	—	26	4	2
9.	8.1	(4-15)	7.9	(5-10)	5	4	25	24	7	2

SIDE EFFECTS OF TERGURIDE TREATMENT

Selection of patients for terguride treatment was not at random because the therapy was preferentially given to patients with previous lisuride intolerance. In 16 of 31 patients treated with terguride, lisuride was previously withdrawn because of side effects. Only 4 of these 16 patients had side effects also with terguride (twice slight, twice important).

Side effects with terguride were seen in 10 patients (9 with prolactinoma, 1 with acromegaly), i.e. in 32%. They are summarized in Table 8. In only 3 patients (10%) the side effects were important and the treatment had to be withdrawn. In others side effects were slight and/or transient and the treatment could be continued.

Table 8. *Side-effects with terguride*

Symptoms:	No. of affected patients
Nausea, epigastric discomfort	5
General weakness, fatigue, somnolence	6
Disturbed thermoregulation (acrohypothermia, chills, perspiration, increase of temperature, heat intolerance)	4
Physical disturbance (depression, anxiousness, disturbed concentration, sleeplessness)	4
Headaches	3
Weight loss	2
Appetite stimulation	1
Aggravation of hypertension	1
Ptyalism	1

There were no orthostatic collapses and fainting even in the beginning of therapy though the treatment was usually started with 0.5 mg t.i.d.. Orthostatic blood pressure (BP) reduction was minimal even after a single initial dose of 1.0 mg as measured in 9 patients: For systolic BP (mean and range) 4.4 (0 - 15) mmHg, for diastolic BP 7.8 (0 -15) mmHg. No BP reduction was seen with long-term medication of terguride.

Incidence of nausea was reduced when terguride was taken with meals as in other ergoline derivatives. Similar to fatigue, nausea was mostly pronounced between 60 and 90 minutes after terguride ingestion. Both side effects were lessened by drinking coffee and in one patient even with beer. Anxiousness could be successfully treated with anxiolytics (dosulepin, medazepam).

CONCLUSIONS

Terguride was shown to have a potent prolactin-lowering effect enabling resumption of menstrual cycle and pregnancy in women and increase of plasma testosterone in men. It caused shrinkage or even disappearance of prolactinomas in most patients. These effects are fully comparable with other ergoline derivatives. Terguride was well-tolerated in 75% of patients with previous lisuride intolerance. The absence of important blood pressure reduction and fainting even with high terguride doses is of special interest. Some side-effects uncommon with other ergoline derivatives suggest specific central action of terguride and require further investigation.

REFERENCES

1. Liuzzi A, Chiodini PG, Oppizzi G, Botalla L, Verde G, De Stefano L, Colusi G, Graf KJ, Horowski R. (1978): J Clin Endocrinol Metab 46:196

2. Marek J, Sramkova J, Schullerova M, Stephan J, Schreiberova O. (1981): Endokrinologie 78:175
3. Auskova M, Rezabek K, Marhan O, Zikan V, Semonsky M. (1979): Endocr. Experim 13:171
4. Teller MN, Stock CC, Hellman L, Mountain IM, Bowie M, Rosenberg BJ, Boyar RM, Budinger JM. (1977): Cancer Res 37:3932
5. Krejci P, Auskova M, Rezabek K, Bilek J, Semonsky M. (1975): Endocr Experim 9:175
6. Auskova M, Rezabek K, Marhan O, Zikan V, Semonsky M. (1979): Endocr. Experim 13:171
7. Wachtel H, Dorow R. (1983): Life Sci 32:421
8. Klibanski A, Neer RM, Beitinis IZ, Ridgway EC, Zervas NT, McArthur JW. (1980): N Engl J Med 303:1511
9. Chiodini P, Liuzzi A, Cozzi R, Verde G, Oppizzi G, Dallabonzana D, Sielta B, Silvestrini F, Borghi G, Luccarelli G, Rainer E, Horowski R. (1981): J Clin Endocr Metab 53:737
10. Ayers JWT. (1983): Fert Steril 40:6
11. Vance ML, Evans WS, Thorner MO. (1984): Ann Intern Med 100:78
12. Barrow DL, Tindall GT, Kovacs K, Thorner MO, Horvath E, Hoffman JC. (1984): J Neurosurg 60:1
13. Ciric I, Mikhael M, Stafford T, Lawson L, Garces R. (1983): J Neurosurg 59:395
14. Sachdev Y, Gomez-Pan A, Tunbridge WMG, Duns A, Weightman DR, Hall R. (1975): Lancet 2:1164
15. Wass JAH, Thorner MO, Morris DV, Rees LH, Stuart-Mason A, Jones AE, Besser GM. (1977): Brit Med J 1:875
16. Dunn PJ, Donald RA, Espiner EA. (1977): Clin Endocrinol (Oxf) 7:273
17. Werner S, Hall K, Sjoberg HE. (1978): Acta Endocrinol (Kbh) 88:190 Suppl 216
18. Lindholm J, Riishede J, Vestergaard S, Hummer L, Faber O, Hagen C. (1981): New Engl J Med 304:1450
19. Kendall-Taylor P, Upstill-Goddard G, Cook D. (1983): Clin Endocrinol (Oxf) 19:711

Prolactin. Basic and clinical correlates
R.M. MacLeod, M.O. Thorner and U. Scapagnini (eds.),
Fidia Research Series, vol. I,
Liviana Press, Padova © 1985

Section XI
Clinical and therapeutic
aspects of hyperprolactinemia

TREATMENT OF HYPERPROLACTINEMIA WITH THE NEW DOPAMINE AGONIST MESULERGIN (CU 32-085)

K. von Werder, R. Landgraf, O. A. Muller, H. K. Rjosk, and E. del Pozo

Department of Medicine Innenstadt, Univ. of Munich, FRG
and Women's Clinic, Basle, Switzerland

Ergot alkaloids with dopaminergic activity can be divided into three groups according to their structure (1). 2-brom-alpha-ergocryptine, bromocriptine, belongs to the lysergic acid amines and contains a tripeptide (2). The most important prolactin inhibitors of the clavines family are pergolide (3) and lergotrile (4). The use of the latter has been abandoned because of side effects. The most important dopaminergic compounds of the 8 alpha-aminoergolines are lisuride (5) and mesulergin (CU 32-085). Unfortunately this latter compound has also been withdrawn because of side effects.

All these substances lead to dopamine receptor stimulation and inhibition of prolactin secretion without uterotonic and vascular effects which are found in other ergot alkaloids (1,2). Most of our knowledge in medical therapy of hyperprolactinemia derives from experience with bromocriptine, which has been specifically developed as a prolactin inhibitor (2). Bromocriptine was introduced into clinical research soon after the establishment of human prolactin as a separate anterior pituitary hormone (1). The beneficial effect of bromocriptine in patients with prolactinomas has been widely documented though there are still patients who may not tolerate the drug because of side effects. These include hypotension and gastrointestinal disturbances. In addition, headaches and nasal stuffiness which are seldom severe and in most cases transitory may occur (2). Cold-sensitive digital vasospasms have been observed in up to 30% of acromegalic patients (2). These vasospasms resemble ergotism but never lead to ischemia and can be reversed by lowering the bromocriptine dosage.

Other symptoms like dyskinesia, psychiatric disorders, erythromelalgia, elevation of hepatic transaminases and cardiac arythmia are rarely observed in hyperprolactinemic patients, but more frequently in patients with Parkinson's disease who represent an older population with additional morbidity (2). So far no toxic or teratogenic effects of dopamine agonists in humans have been reported (1). There are no data showing

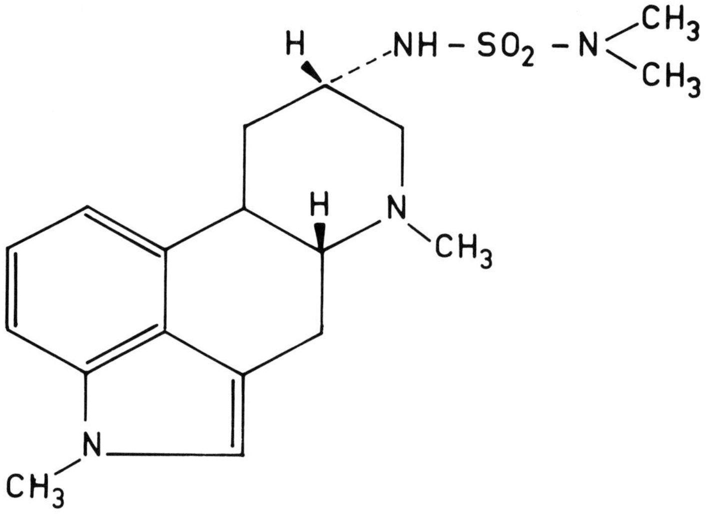

Figure 1. Mesulergin (CU 32-085) is an 8 alpha-aminoergoline (N-1,6-dimethyl-ergolin-8 alpha-yl-N', dimethylsulfamide-HCl).

that the more potent drugs like pergolide and lisuride have fewer side effects than bromocriptine in the same prolactin normalizing dosage. However, it has been shown

Table 1. *Response rate in inhibiting puerperal lactation in 84 females before milk let down and 34 females with established lactation.*

Indication	n	Responders	Non Responders	Rebound
Inhibition of lactation	84	81 (96.5)	3 (3.5)	4 (5)
Suppression of established lactation	34	32 (94)	2 (6)	0

Mesulergin was given in a dosage of 0.5 mg twice a day for 2 weeks.

in individual patients that switching from one drug to another may lead to better tolerance and to normalization of prolactin levels (6).

In the following study we report the results of tolerance and dose finding studies conducted with the new dopamine agonist mesulergin (CU 32-085, Sandoz, Basle, Switzerland). This compound is a 8 alpha-amino-ergoline with prolactin inhibiting properties via dopaminergic stimulation (Fig. 1).

Preliminary studies with mesulergin have shown that the drug possesses a high potency in inhibiting prolactin release with a low incidence of side effects (7, 8). This drug may therefore serve as an alternative to bromocriptine and lisuride in those patients who cannot tolerate the two established drugs.

Since dose finding studies conducted in 26 normal volunteers showed that 0.5 mg CU 32-085 led to a longer lasting decrease of prolactin secretion, capsules with 0.5 mg CU 32-085 were generally used.

In the post partum situation 0.5 mg CU 32-085 administered twice daily over 14 days revealed an overall response rate of 96.5% in inhibiting lactation. Only three cases out of 84 were treatment failures (Table 1). In 34 women with established lactation

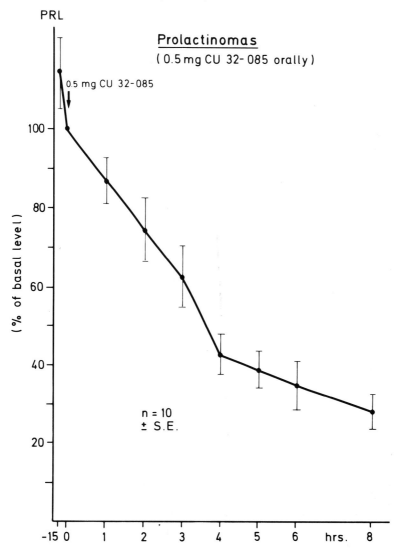

Figure 2. Prolactin levels in 10 patients with prolactinomas before and after oral administration of 0.5 mg mesulergin (CU 32-085). The drug was given at 0900 in the fasting state.

the latter could be suppressed in 94% whereas in two females no response was seen.

Ten patients with macroprolactinomas and prolactin levels ranging from 2680 to 320,400 uU/ml received 0.5 mg CU 32-085 orally in the fasting state. One h after administration of mesulergin prolactin levels were significantly lower compared to basal level (Fig. 2). In two patients prolactin levels were measured over a period of 24 hrs. At that time, prolactin levels were still lower compared to the basal level though there was already an increase of the prolactin level compared to the 8 respectively 12 h value (Fig. 3). There was no significant influence on growth hormone secretion or on any other anterior pituitary hormone level. In all patients, except one who showed a fall in blood pressure, the drug was well tolerated when given in the fasting state.

However, in one acromegalic female, who received 0.5 mg CU 32-085 in another study conducted in 10 acromegalic patients (8), severe hypotension occurred which responded only to the combined administration of intravenous metoclopramide and 50 ml of 20% human albumin.

Eleven patients with hyperprolactinemia, one female with a microprolactinoma, and 6 females and 4 males with macroprolactinomas were subjected to long term treatment with mesulergin. The time of treatment was one year, ranging from 4 to 32 months. The dosage ranged from 0.5 mg (female microprolactinoma patient) to 4.5 mg mesulergin per day. If the daily dosage was higher than 1.0 mg the latter was divided into 3 single

Prolactinomas

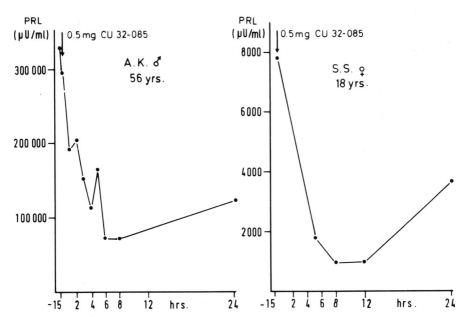

Figure 3. Prolactin levels in 2 patients with macroprolactinomas after oral administration of 0.5 mg mesulergin (CU 32-085). After 24 h prolactin is still lower compared to the basal level.

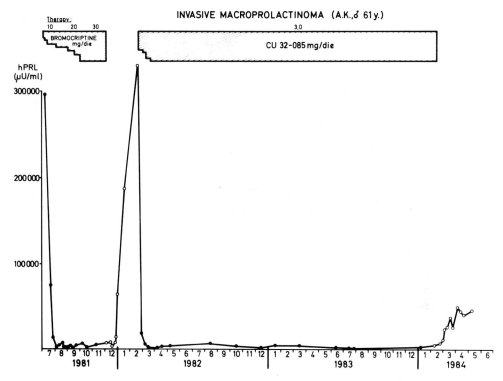

Figure 4. Dopamine agonist therapy in a patient with a macroprolactinoma. After bromocriptine withdrawal, a rapid increase of the prolactin levels within one month up to the level before therapy is observed. After the administration of CU 32-085 normalization of prolactin levels again is achieved. The second withdrawal of dopamine agonist treatment, which had been pursued for two years, leads to a less rapid increase of prolactin levels which do not reach the pretreatment range during the observation period. Tumor shrinkage and tumor expansion were parallel to the prolactin levels.

dosages, which were taken with a meal. The female with the microprolactinoma and 3 females and 3 males with macroprolactinomas had normal prolactin levels during mesulergin therapy. One female complained about hypotension after increasing the dosage to more than 1.5 mg/day; in two females side effects occurred when more than 3.0 mg/day, which had not normalized prolactin levels, was given. In one male 4.5 mg was unable to normalize prolactin levels; the dose was not increased though there was no evidence of intolerance. Hemoglobin, WBC, thrombocytes, and blood chemistry, ECG and chest x-ray (after 6 months) were regularly monitored. In none of the patients could any abnormalities be noted. Withdrawal of mesulergin after long term treatment was followed by persisting suppression of prolactin levels (Fig. 4) as seen after long term bromocriptine treatment (6).

However, in one female patient who had been previously treated with transsphenoidal surgery and radiotherapy for a large invasively growing macroprolactinoma, increasing dosages of bromocriptine and mesulergin did not lead to suppression of the prolactin levels. In this patient, who had no CT-evidence for pituitary tumor recurrence in the sella region, a spinal prolactinoma metastasis could be confirmed after laminectomy by immunohistochemistry (Fig. 5). Since this tumor could not be removed surgically she was irradiated and very high bromocriptine dosages were given, which had only a slight effect on prolactin levels. This indicated a loss of dopamine receptors of this tumor, which could also explain the inefficacy of mesulergin.

Tumor shrinkage was documented in one patient after 10 months of mesulergin treatment (Fig. 6). This has been reported already for this drug (9) and is seen in the majority of cases treated with other dopamine agonists (10,11).

In 10 of the hyperprolactinemic patients the efficacy of long term treatment with mesulergin was compared with the results obtained with long-term bromocriptine treatment (Table 2).

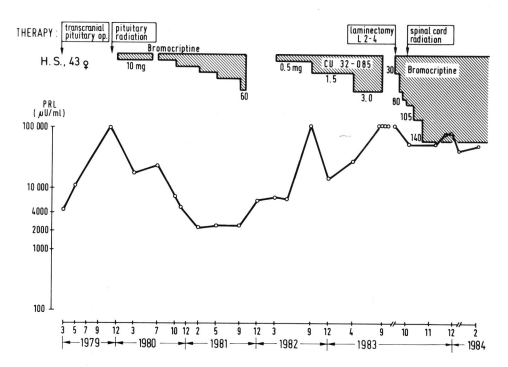

Figure 5. Spinal metastasis of a pituitary prolactinoma after previous surgery and radiotherapy. Despite high dosages of bromocriptine and CU 32-085 prolactin levels remained elevated indicating loss of dopamine receptors of the spinal tumor. The latter was shown to be a prolactinoma by immunohistochemistry. There was no adenoma recurrence detectable at cranial CT.

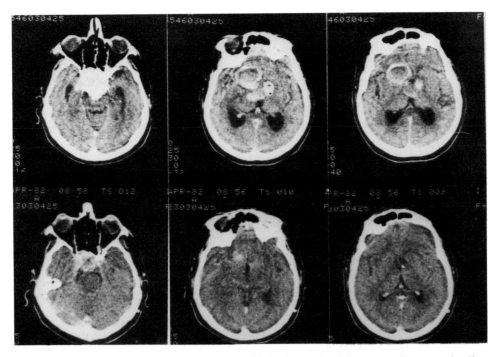

Figure 6. Shrinkage of a cystic prolactinoma which extends into the suprasellar space leading to Foramen Monroi blockade after long-term treatment with CU 32-085. Above before starting therapy, below after 10 month treatment with 3.0 mg CU 32-085 daily.

Table 2. *Long-term therapy with bromocriptine (BC) and mesulergin (CU 32-085). Human prolactin (hPRL) levels in 10 patients with hyperprolactinemia before and during bromocriptine therapy and during therapy with CU 32-085.*

Patient	sex and age	hPRL (uU/ml) before ther.	hPRL (uU/ml) BC-therapy	BC-dosage (mg/day)	hPRL (uU/ml) CU 32-085	CU 32-085 dosage (mg/day)
S.F.	f 29	3,370	not tolerated	—	175	0.5
F.H.	f 28	5,465	1,980	3.75	443	2.5
S.S.	f 31	436,000	not tolerated	—	9,212	1.5
R.K.	f 30	4,518	230	90.0	100	3.0
D.K.	f 31	20,000	2,637	60.0	1,428	3.0
H.K.	f 32	2,700	578	5.0	35	1.0
P.R.	m 35	41,000	876	10.0	114	1.5
A.K.	m 61	297,255	4,000	30.0	284	3.0
N.S.	m 60	30,289	237	10.0	92	0.5
H.R.	m 35	375,000	183,450	30.0	23,000	4.5

Both forms of treatment were pursued for at least 4 months. In all patients CU 32-085 treatment followed bromocriptine treatment. The values for hPRL represent the mean of at least 3 hPRL measurements before and during treatment with the dopamine agonists.

Two patients, who had not tolerated bromocriptine, had normal or clearly lowered prolactin levels after mesulergin. Four patients had normal prolactin levels during mesulergin therapy which could not be obtained by previous bromocriptine therapy in the maximally tolerated dosage (Table 2). In 4 patients prolactin levels were not normal during mesulergin treatment, though they were again lower compared to the prolactin levels during bromocriptine treatment.

In conclusion, mesulergin (CU 32-085) is a potent and usually well tolerated dopamine agonist. Though double-blind studies are still lacking comparing the results achieved with this compound with established dopamine agonists, it seems that mesulergin is an alternative to bromocriptine in the management of hyperprolactinemic patients who do not tolerate bromocriptine in prolactin normalizing dosages.

REFERENCES

1. Fluckiger F, del Pozo E, von Werder K. (1982): Prolactin-Physiology, Pharmacology and Clinical Findings. In: "Monographs in Endocrinology", vol 23, Springer-Verlag, Berlin
2. Thorner MO, Fluckiger E, Calne DB. (1980): Bromocriptine. Raven Press, New York
3. Franks S, Horrocks PM, Lynch SS, Butt WR, London DR. (1983): Brit Med J 286:1177
4. Cleary RE, Crabtree R, Lemberger L. (1975): J Clin Endocrinol 40:830
5. Liuzzi A, Chiodini PG, Oppizzi G, Botalla L, Verde G, De Stefano L, Colussi G, Graf KJ, Horowski R. (1978): J Clin Endocrinol 46:196
6. von Werder K, Eversmann T, Fahlbusch R, Rjosk HK. (1982): In: WF Ganong, L Martini (eds) Frontiers in Neuroendocrinology. Raven Press, New York, p 123
7. del Pozo E, Brownell J, Landgraf R, Sand M, von Werder K. (1983): Acta Endocr 102 Suppl 253:34
8. Sand M. (1983): Therapie der Hyperprolaktinamie und Akromegalie mit Mesulergin (CU 32-085). Doctoral thesis, Univ. of Munich
9. Wollesen F, Andersen T, Knigge U, Dissing I, Karle A. (1983): Acta Endocr (Kbh) 103 Suppl 256:85
10. Chiodini PG, Liuzzi A, Cozzi R, Verde G, Oppizzi G, Dallabonzana D, Spelta B, Silvestrini F, Borghi G, Luccarelli G, Rainer E, Horowski R. (1981): J Clin Endocr 53:737
11. del Pozo E, Gerber L, Hunziker S. (1983): In: Tolis G, Stefanis C, Mountokalakis T, Labrie F (eds) Prolactin and Prolactinomas. Raven Press, New York, p 403

Prolactin. Basic and clinical correlates
R.M. MacLeod, M.O. Thorner and U. Scapagnini (eds.),
Fidia Research Series, vol. I,
Liviana Press, Padova © 1985

Section XI
Clinical and therapeutic
aspects of hyperprolactinemia

SUCCESSFUL TREATMENT OF HYPERPROLACTINEMIA WITH A NEW DOPAMINERGIC AGENT, CU 32-085 (24 CASES)

Anne Caufriez, Georges Copinschi, Daniel Desir, Jean Mockel and Marc L'Hermite

University of Brussels, Belgium

The efficiency of bromocriptine treatment in hyperprolactinemia is now well recognized. Bromocriptine reduces the prolactin levels within one to seven hours after oral administration and for a period of 12 hours in normal subjects.

A small dose of bromocriptine (2.5 mg a day), three times a day, restores normal prolactin levels in 60% of hyperprolactinemic patients. With high doses it is possible to normalize prolactin levels in 95% of patients (1) but this reducing effect is accompanied by adverse side effects: patients are complaining of postural hypotension, dizziness, gastrointestinal symptoms as vomiting, nausea or bladder irritability (2). These adverse reactions may also lead the patients to stop the medication. Recently, a new dopaminergic agent, CU 32-085, has been synthesized. We studied the effects of this drug in 24 patients, 25-57 y.o. (3 males, 21 females), suffering from hyperprolactinemia with a duration of 4 mo. to 19 yr. (mean $\pm$ SE: 4 ± 1 y.).

Clinical data are summarized in Table 1. Two patients had macroprolactinomas, 17 had microprolactinomas, and 5 had functional hyperprolactinemia. Diagnosis was based on conventional X-rays and CT scans of the sella turcica and consistently elevated values (> 500 uU/mL) of serum prolactin. Eleven patients presented spontaneous and/or provoked galactorrhea. One women was taking an oral estro-progestative pill and another one was menopaused. In the other 19 women, 9 had amenorrhea, 2 had anovulatory cycles, 4 had luteal insufficiency, 4 had normal cycles; one patient was receiving IM progestagens. None of the patients received hyperprolactinemic drug. Eight patients never had previous treatment, 2 underwent surgery (1 with radiation therapy) and 15 patients were previously treated with bromocriptine (n = 13) or pergolide (n = 2) but were off therapy for at least 1 month.

Plasma prolactin levels were measured, in duplicate, on each sample using an homologous RIA and expressed in microunits of the pituitary research standard No 71/222 of the Medical Research Council, Great Britain; 1 uU of this standard is equivalent to 0.045 ng of the standard VLS (3). Basal prolactin levels averaged (apply-

Table 1. Individual data in patients on CU 32-085

Patient N°	Age yrs	Sex	Diagnosis	Basal PRL μU/ml	Treatment CU 32-085		Galactorrhea		Menstrual cycle		
					PRL μU/ml	Dose mg/d	B	T	B	T	
1	46	F	Functional	755	199	0.5	+	0	N	N	Pregnancy within 2 mo therapy
2	26	F	Microadenoma	1275	196	0.5	+	0	LI	N	Oral contraception
3	29	F	Microadenoma	928	112	0.2	0	0	/	/	
4	33	F	Functional	1536	32	0.5	0	0	LI	N	
5	27	F	Microadenoma	2013	486	1.0	+	0	LI	N	Stop for side effects
6	47	F	Microadenoma	4000	-	-	0	/	N	/	
7	43	M	Macroadenoma	37740	1043	1.0	0	0	/	/	
8	41	F	Functional	2269	< 100	1.0	+	0	Am	N	
9	37	F	Microadenoma	4000	197	0.5	+	0	Am	Am	
10	51	F	Microadenoma	3350	275	1.5	0	0	Am	N	Menopause
11	55	F	Microadenoma	1148	42	3.0	0	0	/	/	
12	32	F	Microadenoma	1802	146	0.75	++	0	Am	N	
13	39	F	Microadenoma	1893	300	1.25	++	0	Anov	N	
14	47	F	Microadenoma	910	171	1.0	0	0	Am	Anov	
15	25	F	Microadenoma	2347	1038	0.75	++	++	LI	LI	Progestogens IM
16	57	M	Microadenoma	1865	142	0.5	0	0	/	/	Stop for side effects
17	37	F	Microadenoma	770	185	0.5	++	0	N	N	
18	30	F	Functional	1880	55	0.1	0	0	N	N	
19	51	M	Macroadenoma	13000	459	2.0	0	0	/	/	
20	34	F	Microadenoma	1214	498	3.0	++	+	Am	Anov	
21	37	F	Microadenoma	1511	400	1.5	0	0	Anov	N	
22	35	F	Microadenoma	4022	138	1.0	++	0	Am	N	
23	18	F	Functional	1324	272	0.75	0	0	Am	N	
24	42	F	Microadenoma	2850	111	1.0	0	0	Am	Am	

N : normal; LI : luteal insufficiency; Anov : anovulation; Am : amenorrhea

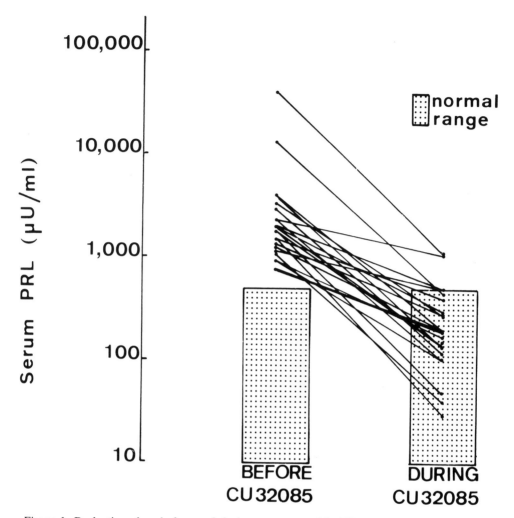

Figure 1. Prolactin values before and during treatment with CU 32-085.

ing a log transformation) 2158 uU/ml (902-5305) (mean ± SD), ranging from 755 to 37740 uU/ml.

Oral CU 32-085 treatment was initiated using a single dose of 0.1 mg bedtime and increased progressively thereafter according to prolactin values (measured at weekly intervals for 6 weeks and subsequently at monthly intervals) for a period of 2 to 12 months. Individual daily CU 32-085 requirements ranged from 0.1 to 3.0 mg divided in one, two or three doses.

Clinical and hormonal results are shown in Table 1 and Fig. 1. Prolactin values were normalized in 15 patients within 2 months therapy and in 6 additional patients within 6 months. Prolactin response to therapy was not related to initial hormonal level.

CU 32-085 had to be stopped in two patients (numbers 6 and 15) because of adverse side effects (nausea, lipothymia, headache) before normalization of prolactin levels and one macroprolactinoma was operated after prolactin levels had been reduced from 37740 to 1043 uU/ml with 1.0 mg CU 32-085 per day.

When initially present, galactorrhea disappeared under treatment in all patients but two; in these last two patients prolactin values under treatment were 498 and 1038 uU/ml. CU 32-085 treatment improved menstrual disturbances in all patients but two (including one who stopped the medication for side effects). One patient became pregnant within 2 months therapy.

Most patients reported minor side effects, including headache, nausea, lipothymia, postural hypotension, dizziness, which disappeared after 2 months even if increasing the dose.

In conclusion, CU 32-085 appears to be a good alternative to conventional medical therapy of hyperprolactinemia.

ACKNOWLEDGMENTS

This work was supported in part by the Belgian Fonds de la Recherche Scientifique Medicale. We are indebted to Sandoz Laboratories for the supply of CU 32-085.

REFERENCES

1. Crosignani PG, Ferrari C, Liuzzi A, Benco R, Mattei A, Rampini P, Dellabonzana D, Scarduelli C, Spelta B. (1982): Fertil Steril 37:61
2. Barbieri RL, Ryan KJ. (1983): Fertil Steril 39:727
3. Badawi M, Bila S, L'Hermite M, Perez-Lopez FR, Robyn C. (1974): In: Radioimmunoassay and Related Procedures in Medicine. International Atomic Energy Agency, Wien, vol 1:411

Prolactin. Basic and clinical correlates
R.M. MacLeod, M.O. Thorner and U. Scapagnini (eds.),
Fidia Research Series, vol. I,
Liviana Press, Padova © 1985

Section XI
Clinical and therapeutic
aspects of hyperprolactinemia

PHARMACOKINETIC PARAMETERS AND EFFECTS ON ANTERIOR PITUITARY FUNCTION OF CU 32-085, A NOVEL DOPAMINE AGONIST IN NORMAL MEN[+]

Joao L.C. Borges, William S. Evans, Horst F. Schran[*], Alan D. Rogol, Donald L. Kaiser, Robert M. MacLeod, Lance Boyett, Richard L. Elton[*], and Michael O. Thorner

Departments of Internal Medicine, Pediatrics, and Pharmacology,
University of Virginia School of Medicine, Charlottesville, VA 22908
and *Pharmaceutical Research and Development, Sandoz, Inc.,
East Hanover, NJ 07936

CU 32-085 is a new synthetic 8-amino-ergoline N-(1,6-dimethylergolin-8 alpha-yl)-N', N'-dimethylsulfamide-HCl which has recently been developed as a therapeutic alternative to the dopamine agonists which are currently available. Since data concerning the effects of this dopamine agonist on circulating pituitary hormone levels are limited, we examined the effects of single doses of CU 32-085 on both basal and thyrotropin-releasing hormone (TRH)-stimulated levels of several anterior pituitary hormones in normal men. Our experimental design included TRH-stimulation in order to avoid potential difficulties in interpretation of results which are related to the well established circadian rhythm of prolactin, i.e., it is well documented that serum prolactin falls progressively from relatively high levels during the night to low levels during the morning. Since such low concentrations are often at or below the level of detectability of currently available radioimmunoassays, TRH was used to raise circulating levels of prolactin into an easily radioimmunoassayable range. It has been previously demonstrated that prolactin stimulation via this mechanism lends itself to inhibition by dopaminergic agents (1,2). We report, in addition, on both the plasma levels achieved after administration of and the bioavailability parameters associated with this dopamine agonist and also compare the effects of CU 32-085 on serum prolactin to those of a single 2.5 mg dose of bromocriptine.

[+] This is an abbreviated report of that published in Clinical Pharmacology and Therapeutics.

STUDY DESIGN

Six healthy men (mean age 29 years, range 22-34) participated in this study having provided written informed consent. The following doses of CU 32-085 were administered to each subject during the three initial study periods (I-III) in a random order: 1) 0.1 mg CU 32-085 (one 0.1 mg capsule plus one placebo capsule); 2) 0.35 mg CU 32-085 (one 0.1 mg capsule plus one 0.25 mg capsule); and 3) two placebo capsules. The subjects were recalled after the completion of period III for testing with a single dose of 0.5 mg CU 32-085 (two 0.25 mg capsules; period IV). To compare the effects of CU 32-085 on serum prolactin levels with those after 2.5 mg bromocriptine, the volunteers returned for a final study period (period V). In each case the study periods were separated by at least 14 days.

After an overnight fast, during each of the five study periods, a dopamine agonist or placebo was administered at 0800 h (day 1) with 60 ml of water. Standardized meals were served at 1200 h , 1800 h, and 0900 h (day 2). Although water was available *ad libitum*, no additional ingestion was allowed. At 0630 h on day I a venous cannula (heparin lock) was placed in the forearm vein. Blood samples were obtained at fixed intervals prior to drug/placebo administration and for 24 h thereafter. Serum was stored at -20 C until assayed for prolactin, growth hormone (GH), luteinizing hormone (LH), follicle stimulating hormone (FSH), thyroid-stimulating hormone (TSH), and cortisol (as an index of corticotroph secretion). In addition, plasma was obtained for measurement of CU 32-085 concentrations. During period IV, blood samples were obtained only for measurement of prolactin, GH, TSH, and CU 32-085 concentrations. During period V only serum prolactin was measured. After drug administration intravenous (iv) boluses of 25 ug synthetic TRH were given at 2, 5, 12, and 24 h. Radial pulse and blood pressure were monitored at fixed intervals both with the subject in the supine position and after 3 minutes in the upright position.

Plasma levels of CU 32-085 were measured using RIA developed by J. Rosenthaler and H. Munzer, Biopharmaceutical Department of Sandoz, Ltd. (Switzerland). The sensitivity of the assay was 8 pg/tube and the intra- and inter-assay coefficients variation were 2.6% and 5.3% at 10 ng/ml. The samples were assayed in triplicate on two separate occasions and these six concentration estimates averaged.

DATA AND STATISTICAL ANALYSIS

A. Anterior pituitary hormones

The secretion of all anterior pituitary hormones and cortisol was expressed as integrated serum levels per hour. Secretory rates were calculated for the interval prior to (0730-0800 h; basal secretion rate) and for several intervals after administration of drugs/placebo at 0800 h. Each secretory rate after drugs/placebo was adjusted by subtracting the basal secretory rate in order to represent changes in integrated levels from pre-drug/placebo administration levels. Changes in hormone secretion during selected intervals after placebo were compared with those after the various doses of CU 32-085 and after the dose of bromocriptine using analysis of variance with Duncan's Multiple

Range Test. In addition, the probability of a dose response relationship existing between hormone secretion and the doses of CU 32-085 was assessed using linear regression.

B. Pharmacokinetic parameters

Peak concentration (C_{max}), time to peak concentration (t_{max}), area under the concentration/time curve (AUC), apparent rate constants (M_1 = constant of absorption, M_2 = constant of elimination), and lag time to absorption (LT) were calculated for the circulating plasma-drug concentration data and analyzed employing statistical methods. C_{max} was defined as the highest measured concentration, t_{max} as the time interval from drug administration to the highest measured value, and AUC was obtained by addition of the trapezoids formed by the plasma concentrations and the time intervals from 0 to 25 h. A least squares curve fitting algorithm was used to fit the individual plasma concentrations of CU 32-085 in order to obtain pharmacokinetic parameters which were less affected by analytical variation of concentration estimates than those derived directly from the raw data. Curve fitting provided the apparent rate constants, LT, and AUC (0-infinity). For the pharmacokinetics parameters C_{max} and AUC, regression through the origin was employed to establish the relationship with the dose. The appropriateness of the mathematical function fitted was determined by performing a test for a lack of fit (3). Confidence limits (95%) for the regression coefficients of the dose parameters function were computed according to Snedecor and Cochran (4).

In order to compare the dose levels, analysis of variance was performed. Pair-wise comparisons between dose levels were made using the residual error term. The techniques were applied to each of the bioavailability parameters and the natural logarithmic transforms (univariate ANOVA).

RESULTS

Serum prolactin

In Figure 1 are presented the dynamic changes caused by TRH on serum prolactin during placebo or CU 32-085 treatment. Prolactin secretory rates were calculated: 1. for the interval following drug/placebo administration and prior to the first challenge with TRH (i.e., 0800-1000 h; defined as "unstimulated" release); 2. for the 60 minute periods following administration of TRH (i.e., 1000-1100 h, 1300-1400 h, and 2000-2100 h on Day 1 and 0800-0900 h on Day 2; defined as "TRH stimulated release"); and 3. for the 0800-2000 h (Day 1) and 2000-0900 h (Day 2) intervals. Visual inspection of the data suggested that the changes noted with lower doses of the drug were brief and were masked when the entire 0800 (Day 1)-0900 h was analyzed, thus accounting for selection of the latter time intervals for analysis. Unstimulated (0800-1000 h) prolactin secretory rates (ng/ml/h; mean ± SEM) after placebo (-1.05 ± 1.00), 0.1 mg (-1.75 ± 2.00), 0.35 mg (1.28 ± 1.42) and 0.5 mg (-2.6 ± 1.56) CU 32-085 were no different. No inhibition of TRH-stimulated prolactin secretion occurred after 0.1 mg CU 32-085. Both the 0.35 mg and 0.5 mg doses of CU 32-085 inhibited prolactin secre-

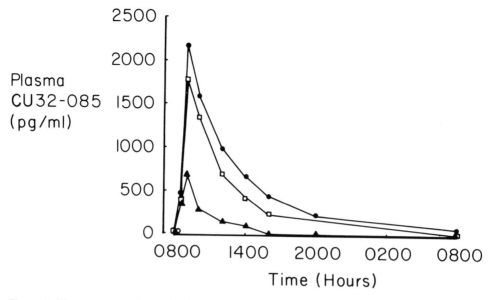

Figure 1. Mean serum prolactin in six normal men after placebo, CU 32-085 or bromocriptine, with administration of TRH (25 ug i.v.) at l000 h, 1300 h, 2000 h and 0800 h. Placebo (△); CU 32-085 0.1 mg (▲); CU 32-085 0.35 mg (□); CU 32-085 0.5 mg (●) and bromocriptine 2.4 (○).

tion in response to TRH given at l000 and 1300 h (p = 0.02 and 0.03, respectively) but not at 2000 or 0800 h (Day 2). Prolactin secretion after 0.1 mg and 0.35 mg CU 32-085 was no different from that following placebo during either 0800-2000 h or 2000-0900 h intervals, but was supressed after the 0.5 mg dose during both the 0800-2000 h (p = 0.0009) and 2000-0900 h (p = 0.04) intervals. Although there was a lack of significant inhibition of prolactin after the 0.1 and 0.35 mg doses, significant dose response relationships were found between the CU 32-085 doses and prolactin secretion during both the 0800-2000 h (R^2 = 0.27, p = 0.009) and 2000 - 0900 h (R^2 = 0.18, p = 0.04) intervals.

When compared to placebo, bromocriptine did not lower unstimulated (0800 - 1000 h) prolactin secretion (-1.05 ± 1.00 vs 2.35 ± 1.39; P > 0.05). However, bromocriptine did inhibit prolactin secretion in response to TRH given at 1000, 1300, and 2000 h. Bromocriptine also lowered prolactin secretion during both the 0800-2000 h and 2000-0900 h intervals (p < 0.05).

Serum GH

GH secretion after 0.1 and 0.35 mg of CU 32-085 was no different from that after placebo during either interval. After the 0.5 mg dose of CU 32-085, GH secretion was

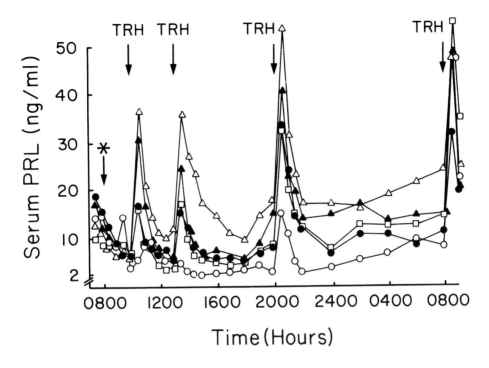

∗ DA Agonist or Placebo

Figure 2. Mean plasma concentration of immunoreactive CU 32-085 (plus metabolites) after oral administration at 0800 h, CU 32-085 0.1 mg (▲), CU 32-085 0.35 mg (□) and CU 32-085 0.5 mg (●).

Reproduced with permission from Editor, Clinical Pharmacology and Therapeutics.

increased during both the 0800-2000 h and 2000-0900 h intervals (p > 0.05). Although there was no significant change in serum GH levels after 0.1 mg or 0.35 mg of CU 32-085, dose response relationships were documented between CU 32-085 doses and GH secretion during both the 0800-2000 h (R^2 = 0.28, p = 0.002) and 2000-0900 h (R^2 = 0.37, p = 0.001) intervals.

Serum TSH

TRH-stimulated TSH secretion was not affected by any dose of CU 32-085.

Serum cortisol and gonadotropins

When compared to placebo, secretory rates of cortisol, LH, and FSH were not different after 0.1 or 0.35 mg CU 32-085.

Pharmacokinetic parameters

In Figure 2 are shown the mean CU 32-085 plus metabolite plasma concentrations after administration of 0.1, 0.35, and 0.5 mg CU 32-085. Increasing the dose of CU 32-085 from 0.1 mg to 0.5 mg resulted in a significant increase for the AUC and C_{max} parameters. The parameters M_1, M_2, and LT were independent of the dose.

The functional relationship of C_{max} or AUC and the dose (including the origin) was best expressed by a straight line, y (where y is either C_{max} or AUC) = slope x dose. All slopes were positive, with the difference from zero slope being highly significant (p = 0.0001). The data show that the hypothesis of a straight line through the origin for the parameters-dose relationship is tenable.

Clinical effects

In Table 1 are shown the clinical effects after administration of placebo, the three doses of CU 32-085, or 2.5 mg bromocriptine. Orthostatic symptoms, including dizziness and postural hypotension, were most frequently encountered. One subject fainted while standing when vital signs were being recorded prior to drug administration. Adverse effects were seen between 1 and 8 h after CU 32-085 administration. There were no statistically significant changes in either systolic or diastolic blood pressure or in pulse rate after CU 32-085 or bromocriptine in the recumbent position. Vital signs in the standing position could not be recorded due to orthostatic symptoms on 7 and 5 occasions after administration of 0.35 or 0.5 mg CU 32-085, respectively, and on 9 occasions after 2.5 mg of bromocriptine. Thus, statistical analysis of standing vital signs (i.e. from the residual subjects) would be meaningless.

Table 1. *Frequency of Adverse Effects*

Dose	Placebo	CU 32-085 Dose (mg)			Bromocriptine (mg)
		0.10	0.35	0.50	2.5
Orthostatic Symptoms	—	17%	50%	33%	83%
Nasal Congestion	—	17%	17%	17%	17%
Headaches	—	17%	17%	17%	17%
Nausea	—	—	17%	—	33%
Sleepiness	—	—	—	17%	—
Dry Mouth	—	17%	—	—	—

DISCUSSION

Our results indicate that in normal men CU 32-085 inhibits circulating prolactin in a dose-related manner and the duration of such inhibition appears related to the RIA plasma drug concentrations. These plasma concentrations showed a linear dose proportionality in the 0-0.5 mg dose range. Peak plasma levels of CU 32-085 (plus metabolites) of 4-5 ng/ml/mg dose are considerably above those achieved with bromocriptine (approximately 0.2 ng/ml/mg) (5), suggesting the equivalence of 0.1 mg CU 32-085 with 2.5 mg bromocriptine on a pharmacokinetic basis. The higher plasma levels of CU 32-085 may be accounted for by a greater degree of absorption and differences in the elimination rate ($t_{1/2}$ CU 32-085: alpha phase 2 h, beta phase 10 h; $t_{1/2}$ bromocriptine: 4-5h).

CU 32-085 has been developed as a therapeutic alternative to the currently available dopamine agonists. While 2.5 mg of bromocriptine is more potent in blunting TRH-stimulated prolactin secretion, 0.5 mg of CU 32-085 is equally potent in inhibiting the overall prolactin release during both the initial 12 h and the subsequent 13 h period after administration of the drug. Recently, del Pozo et al. (6) reported that the prolactin-lowering effect of CU 32-085 is five-fold greater (on a per milligram oral dose basis) than that of bromocriptine when given chronically to patients with prolactinomas. This group also reported that once a serum prolactin nadir was obtained, a single daily dose of CU 32-085 was able to maintain this effect for 24 h and, moreover, the patients who had shown poor tolerance to bromocriptine showed a better response rate to CU 32-085.

We detected no change in TRH-stimulated TSH secretion after administration of CU 32-085 when compared to placebo. Our results suggest that, although TSH secretion is modulated by dopamine (7,8), release of this hormone is not as sensitive to CU 32-085 as is prolactin. Moreover, no significant change in gonadotropin levels was seen after CU 32-085 administration. While these data appear to distinguish CU 32-085 from other dopamine agonists which have been shown to inhibit LH secretion (1), our results may be due to the relatively low doses of CU 32-085 used. The effects of CU 32-085 on GH levels were similar to those expected of a dopamine agonist. Serum GH levels were noted to be elevated in a dose-dependent manner after CU 32-085 administration. The initial growth hormone peak was similar to that seen with other dopamine agonists (2,6,8) and measurement over the 24 h study period showed continued enhancement of GH release. It is well known, however, that long term bromocriptine therapy does not lead to chronic elevation of serum GH levels.

The adverse effects, including orthostatic symptoms, headaches, nasal congestion, and nausea, are commonly seen upon initiation of dopamine agonist therapy. However, the frequency of orthostasis and nausea was higher after 2.5 mg bromocriptine and the volunteers reported that the symptoms were less tolerable than those felt with CU 32-085 at all doses. Del Pozo et al. (6) reported that doses of CU 32-085 similar to those used by us did not result in changes in blood pressure in normal volunteers. While the reason for the descrepancy between their report and ours is unclear, the more pronounced side effects documented in our study could be due in part to the administration of CU 32-085 after a 14 h period of fasting, since it is well known that absorption of ergot drugs is slowed when administered orally with food (9).

In summary, it appears that CU 32-085 is a potent dopamine agonist which is effective in lower doses than bromocriptine. CU 32-085 has several potential advantages when compared to other dopamine agonists which have been used as medical therpay for hyperprolactinemia. First, CU 32-085 appears to be associated with less intense side-effects when compared to bromocriptine. Secondly, the prolonged duration of a dose such as 0.5 mg given in a chronic fashion may allow single daily administration of the medication to be effective in hyperprolactinemic states. However, it is clear that clinical studies involving a large population of patients will be required to ascertain whether or not these potential advantages of CU 32-085 will be realized.

[Note added in proof: CU 32-085 has been withdrawn worldwide due to animal toxicity. It is believed that this may be related to the strain of rats used for the long term toxicological studies.]

ACKNOWLEDGMENTS

These studies were supported by NICHAD grant HD13197; General Clinical Research Grant RR 0847, and a Research Grant from Sandoz, Inc., East Hanover, N.J. We thank Mrs. Ina Hofland and Mrs. Donna Harris for help with the preparation of this manuscript.

REFERENCES

1. Perryman RL, Rogol AD, Kaiser DL, MacLeod RM, Thorner MO. (1981): J Clin Endocrinol Metab 53:772
2. Thorner MO, Ryan SM, Wass AH, Johns A, Bouloux P, Williams S, Besser GM. (1978): J Clin Endocrinol Metab 47:372
3. Daper N. (1981): In: Smith H (ed) Applied Regression Analysis. J Wiley and Sons, Inc., New York
4. Snedecor GW, Cochran WG. (1967): Multiple regression. In: Snedecor GW, Cochran WG, (eds) Statistical methods, Sixth Ed, The Iowa State Press
5. Schran HF, Bhuta Sl, Schwarz HT, Thorner MO. (1980): Adv Biochem Psychopharmacol 23:125
6. Del Pozo E, Brownell J, Landgraf R, Sand M, Von Werder K. (1983): Acta Endocrinol (Suppl 252) 102:34
7. Leebaw WF, lee LA, Woolf PD. (1978): J Clin Endocrinol Metab 47:480
8. Burrow GN, Many PB, Spaulding SW, Donabedian RK. (1977): J Clin Endocrinol Metab 45:65
9. Thorner MO, Schran HF, Evans WS, Rogol AD, Morris JL, MacLeod RM. (1980): J Clin Endocrinol Metab 50:1026

Prolactin. Basic and clinical correlates
R.M. MacLeod, M.O. Thorner and U. Scapagnini (eds.),
Fidia Research Series, vol. I,
Liviana Press, Padova © 1985

Section XI
Clinical and therapeutic
aspects of hyperprolactinemia

CU 32085 (MESULERGIN) IN THE TREATMENT OF HYPERPROLACTINEMIA

D. Dewailly, P. Thomas, J. Buvat, J. L. Wemeau, J. C. Fourlinnie, and P. Fossati

Department of Endocrinology and Diabetology, Centre Hospitalier Régional, 59037 Lille Cédex, France

Bromocriptine has now been used successfully for more than 15 years in the treatment of hyperprolactinemia. This ergot alkaloid belongs to the family of the lysergic acid amides and is highly efficient in lowering plasma prolactin levels, in both normal and hyperprolactinemic subjects. More recently, with the advent of computerized tomographic scans, bromocriptine has been shown to induce shrinkage of macroprolactinomas in about 60-80% of cases. In most patients, the usual dosage of 2.5 mg twice a day is enough to normalize the prolactin level. However, some patients need higher doses, 60 mg/day in some cases; moreover, the prolactin cannot be normalized in about 5-10% of patients who are resistant to bromocriptine or who do not tolerate the efficient dose. Side effects are generally acceptable with doses less than 10 mg/day but become troublesome at higher doses. Furthermore, some patients do not tolerate even the usual doses.

For these reasons other compounds are currently under investigation, such as lisuride, pergolide, or CU 32085 (mesulergin). The latter belongs to the family of the synthetic 8 alpha amino ergolines. It has, *in vitro*, a very high potency to inhibit the binding of [³H]-dopamine in calf caudate. In rats, *in vivo*, it displays biphasic effects, acting first as a dopamine antagonist within the first 2-3 hours after its ingestion and then as a potent and long-lasting dopamine agonist. It is likely that this second effect is linked to its transformation to a major metabolite (1,20-N,N-bidemethylated) which can be extracted from urine (2).

So far, the effects of CU 32085 have not been studied extensively in humans. In an open trial with bromocriptine and CU 32085 in the treatment of Parkinsonism (3), both drugs were equally tolerated but the latter was shown to have a more rapid and stronger effect on tremor, bradykinesia, fluctuations, and "on-off" effects than bromocriptine. In the treatment of hyperprolactinemia, previous reports from ourselves (4) and others (5,6) on limited series of patients have shown that CU 32085 has the same efficiency as bromocriptine with 5-fold lower doses. However, these preliminary data needed to be more extensively documented, especially regarding duration of action, tolerance, and anti-tumoral effect of the drug.

KINETICS OF PROLACTIN SUPPRESSION BY CU 32085

We administered orally 2.5 mg of bromocriptine at 8 a.m. and, 48 hours later, 0.5 mg CU 32085 to 10 previously untreated hyperprolactinemic patients (prolactin ranging from 28 to 3,250 ng/ml). According to the duration of action of bromocriptine which is less than 48 hours, the prolactin returned to its initial level in all patients before receiving CU 32085. Figure 1 shows that CU 32085 had a more lengthened effect than bromocriptine with a 5 fold lower dose (18 vs 12 h), the difference being statistically significant by variance analysis.

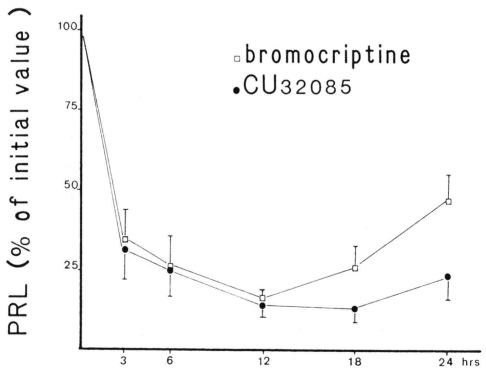

Figure 1. Kinetics of prolactin suppression after acute oral administration of 0.5 mg of CU 32085 or 2.5 mg bromocriptine (each point represents the mean ± SEM of 10 hyperprolactinemic patients).

THERAPEUTIC EFFECTIVENESS OF CU 32085

More than 40 of our hyperprolactinemic patients have been treated for at least 3 months with CU 32085, at doses ranging from 0.5 to 5 mg/day. 3 criteria must be used to assess the effectiveness of a prolactin suppressive agent (7): 1) normalization of prolactin level, 2) recovery of normal gonadal functions, and 3) shrinkage of the prolactinoma, if it is apparent on CT scans.

Normalization of prolactin

Figure 2A shows that for 24 out of 37 patients (65%) treated with CU 32085 (0.5 mg twice a day) over at least 3 months, the prolactin returned to normal values (i.e., <20 ng/ml). The best results were obtained in patients with microadenomas (n = 11) and with idiopathic hyperprolactinemia (n = 6) rather than in those with macroprolactinoma, operated on (n = 12) or not (n = 8). Out of the 24 patients whose prolactin was normalized, 16 maintained their prolactin levels within the normal range while receiving only 0.5 mg once a day, even 24 hours after ingestion of the drug.

On the other hand, 10 patients needed doses higher than 1 mg/day and 4 of them did not normalize their prolactin, even at doses as high as 5 mg/day for one patient.

In comparison, bromocriptine (2.5 mg twice a day) had the same efficiency in our series of 83 patients (7), in 62 of whom (75%) prolactin returned to normal levels (Fig. 2B). The frequency of resistance to CU 32085 was not statistically lower than with bromocriptine (10.8 vs 18%). Two patients previously resistant to bromocriptine were not improved when placed on CU 32085.

The percentages of prolactin normalization and of prolactin suppression by both drugs were not statistically different (Fig. 3).

Recovery of normal gonadal functions

Table I shows that CU 32085 and bromocriptine had similar effects upon clinical symptoms in both men and women. Three pregnancies occurred with CU 32085 and were uneventful. The drug was immediately discontinued as soon as the pregnancy was known.

Table I. *Effect of bromocriptine (1) or CU 32085 (2) on clinical symptoms in hyperprolactinemic subjects*

Number of Patients and Etiology		WOMEN		MEN	
		Recovery of Menses	Cessation of Galactorrhea	Number of Patients	Improvement of Impotence
(1) Idiopathic	= 20	95%			
Microprol.	= 16	94%			
Macroprol.	= 26	69%			
Total	= 62	84%	77%	21	73%
(2) Idiopathic	= 6	100%			
Microprol.	= 10	90%			
Macroprol.	= 10	40%			
Total	= 26	73%	42%	11	45.4%

810

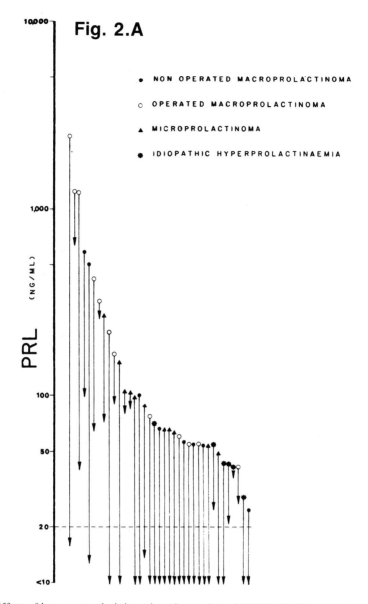

Figure 2. Effect of long-term administration (3 months) of CU 32085 (0.5 mg twice a day) (A), and of bromocriptine (2.5 mg twice a day) (B), in populations of 37 and 83 hyperprolactinemic subjects, respectively.

Shrinkage of prolactinomas

So far, we have been able to investigate the anti-tumoral effect of CU 32085 in only 5 macroprolactinomas. CT scans were performed before and after 3 months of treatment and were carefully reviewed by two neuroradiologists in a single session. Obser-

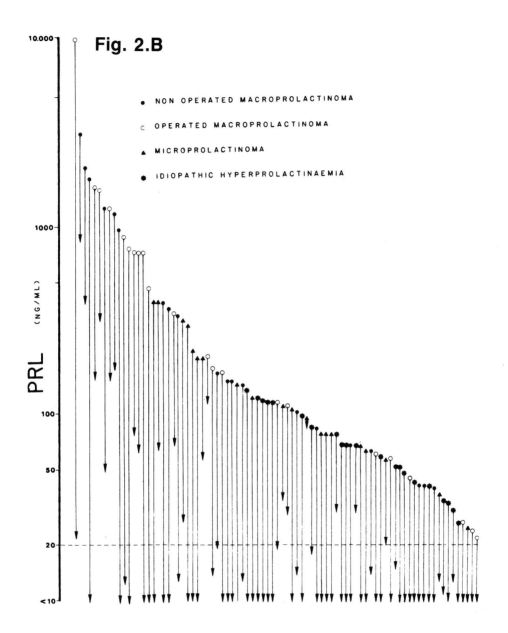

Figure 2. Effect of long-term administration (3 months) of CU 32085 (0.5 mg twice a day) (A), and of bromocriptine (2.5 mg twice a day) (B), in populations of 37 and 83 hyperprolactinemic subjects, respectively.

vations with non-comparable data were discarded. Partial shrinkage was ascertained in 2 out of the 5 observations (Fig. 4). It must be stressed that in the other 3 cases, 2 had received bromocriptine previously and that this drug induced no shrinkage either. Therefore, our small series is unsuitable for statistical comparison with bromocriptine which, in our experience, induced definite shrinkage in 10 out of 17 (58.7%) macroprolactinomas (7), when judged with the same criteria as above. Others (5,6) have also reported some cases of shrinkage of prolactinomas under CU 32085, but no statistical comparison with bromocriptine or other dopamine agonists is available so far in the literature.

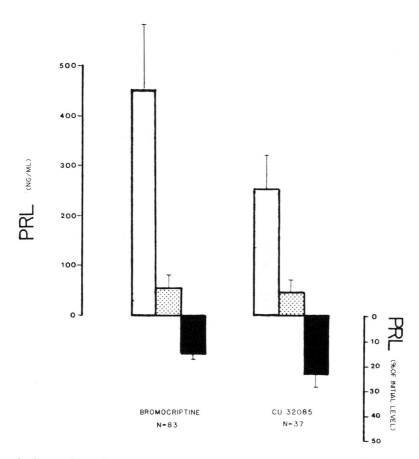

Figure 3. Comparison of CU 32085 (0.5 mg twice a day) and bromocriptine (2.5 mg twice a day) in the treatment of hyperprolactinemia. The left bars indicate the mean (± SEM) of the pre-treatment prolactin values in each group. The middle bars indicate the mean (± SEM) of the prolactin values under treatment. The right bars indicate the mean (± SEM) of the suppressive effect of each drug on prolactin levels.

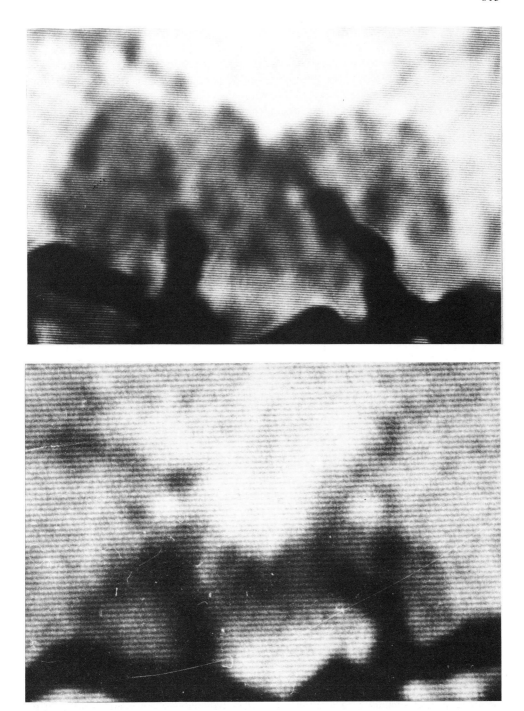

Figure 4. CT scans of a 17-year-old woman with macroprolactinoma before treatment with CU 32085 (top) and after 4 months of treatment (bottom).

SIDE EFFECTS OF CU 32085

Although some patients claimed to tolerate CU 32085 better than bromocriptine, the contrary was also true. Side effects were similar in nature and frequency to those induced by bromocriptine. They were more frequently mild and transient, such as nausea and dizziness. In one instance, CU 32085 induced severe hypotension with marked bradykardia and loss of consciousness. This occurred after administration of 0.5 mg at once, which should be avoided since we have observed other severe side effects in some patients. Hypotensive reactions have also been reported by others (6) in 2 out of 16 patients after oral administration of 0.5 mg CU 32085.

Therefore, it must be stressed that initiating a treatment with CU 32085 requires the same progressive increase of doses as with bromocriptine. In that way, 0.1 mg tablets are useful and allow a more precise fitting of the efficient and well tolerated dose in a given patient.

No abnormality of liver tests and blood cell analysis was observed under CU 32085 treatment.

To our knowledge, no documented trial of CU 32085 on the treatment of hyperprolactinemia has so far been available in literature. Some preliminary reports (4-6) have shown that it is as efficient as bromocriptine with 5 fold lower doses. The present study confirms these findings and provides further information such as its anti-tumoral effect and the duration of the maximal prolactin suppressive effect of the drug which is 18 hours. This is in agreement with the fact that 0.5 mg CU 32085 once a day is enough to maintain the prolactin of most patients within the normal range. However, although smaller doses of CU 32085 than of bromocriptine are needed, the side effects appeared to us similar in nature and frequency to those induced by bromocriptine. Therefore, we recommend the same prudence as with bromocriptine when initiating treatment with CU 32085.

ACKNOWLEDGMENTS

We are greatly indebted to the Laboratoires Sandoz for providing CU 32085 and to Mrs. S. Lefevre and N. Gantois for their expert secretarial assistance.

REFERENCES

1. Enz A. (1981): Life Sci 29:2227
2. Fluckiger E, Briner U, Enz A, Markstein R, Vigouret JM. (1983) In: Calne DB, Horowski R, McDonald RJ, Wuttke W (eds) Lisuride and Other Dopamine Agonists. Raven Press, New York, p 1
3. Jellinger K. (1982): J Neurol 227:75
4. Dewailly D, Cordonnier M, Buvat J, Wemeau JL, Fourlinnie JC, Bourdelle-Hego MF, Fossati P. (1983): Ann Endocrinol (Paris) 44:162
5. Oppermann D, Schaffner U, del Pozo E. (1984): Acta Endocrinol (Kbh) 105 (suppl) 264:136

6. VonWerder K, Fahlbusch R, Rjosk HK. (1983): In: Calne DB, Horowski R, McDonald RJ, Wuttke W (eds) Lisuride and Other Dopamine Agonists. Raven Press, New York, p 263
7. Fossati P, Dewailly D, Thomas-Desrousseaux P, Buvat J, Fermon C, Lemaire A, Bourdelle-Hego MF, Pouyol-Motte H, Lemaitre G, Clarisse J, Christiaens JL, Mazzuca M. Hormone Res, in press

Prolactin. Basic and clinical correlates
R.M. MacLeod, M.O. Thorner and U. Scapagnini (eds.),
Fidia Research Series, vol. I,
Liviana Press, Padova © 1985

Section XI
Clinical and therapeutic
aspects of hyperprolactinemia

PERSISTING NORMOPROLACTINEMIA AFTER WITHDRAWAL OF BROMOCRIPTINE LONG-TERM THERAPY IN PATIENTS WITH PROLACTINOMAS

W. Winkelmann, B. Allolio, U. Deuss, D. Heesen, and D. Kaulen

Department of Internal Medicine II, University of Köln, FRG.

Bromocriptine and other dopamine agonists are successfully used to normalize serum prolactin concentrations in patients with prolactinoma (1-4) thereby restoring normal gonadal function, libido, and fertility. There is now also impressive evidence that during therapy with dopamine agonists many prolactinomas shrink (5). This raises the question whether some prolactinomas could be cured by drug therapy alone. If this is the case, withdrawal of bromocriptine after a sufficiently long period of treatment should not lead to recurrence of hyperprolactinemia but to persistent normoprolactinemia and a normal prolactin response to provocative tests. Unfortunately so far the results of bromocriptine withdrawal have been disappointing, as prolactin levels almost invariably rose above the normal range indicating persistence of prolactin secreting pituitary tumor cells and a need for further therapy. However, in many patients the increase of serum prolactin after bromocriptine withdrawal did not reach pretreatment levels (4) suggesting that some permanent reduction of tumor mass had occurred. One could speculate that the duration of treatment had been too short to eradicate the tumor completely. We therefore investigated the effect of bromocriptine withdrawal in patients with prolactinoma receiving drug therapy for a minimum of 4 years.

A total of 44 patients with prolactinoma (23 females and 21 males) were evaluated. According to skull x-rays, CT scans, and serum prolactin concentrations the patients were divided into 5 patients with microprolactinoma (minute changes of the sella turcica, serum prolactin below 250 ng/ml) and 39 patients with macroprolactinoma. Twenty-eight patients with macroprolactinoma had been operated on prior to bromocriptine therapy. Initially the dose of bromocriptine was increased stepwise until normalization of serum prolactin was induced (maximum dose 60 mg/day, range 5-60 mg/day). As soon as normal prolactin levels had been achieved, bromocriptine was gradually reduced to the minimum dose necessary to maintain normoprolactinemia. After drug-induced normoprolactinemia had lasted 2 to 3 years bromocriptine therapy was interrupted for 4 weeks. If normoprolactinemia did not persist, drug therapy was resumed

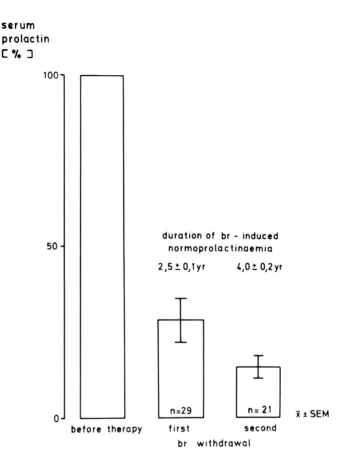

Figure 1. Serum prolactin after withdrawal of bromocriptine therapy in patients with macroprolactinomas (pretreatment values = 100%).

and again interrupted after 1 to 2 years. Serum prolactin was measured by RIA using commercially available reagents (Serono/Biodata).

In 2 female and 2 male patients with macroprolactinoma long term therapy with high dose bromocriptine (60 mg/day) failed to induce normoprolactinemia, although prolactin levels decreased significantly. In all other patients normal prolactin levels were induced by bromocriptine (Table 1). The time necessary to reach normoprolactinemia varied considerably (1 to 35 months) in this group. In 7 patients (17.5%, 3 out of 5 with microprolactinoma, 4 out of 35 patients with macroprolactinoma) we found persisting (> 6 months) normal basal prolactin levels (< 25 ng/ml) after bromocriptine withdrawal. In the majority serum prolactin levels rose above the normal range after cessation of drug therapy, but pretreatment concentrations were not reached (Fig. 1). After a second withdrawal period (1-2 years later) the prolactin increase was even smaller (15.1 ± 3.3 vs $27.7 \pm 5.4\%$ of pretreatment values, mean $\pm$ SEM, $p < 0.02$) indicating that the reincrease of prolactin after interruption of bromocriptine therapy depends on the duration of drug induced normoprolactinemia. The data of the 7 patients with peristent normoprolactinemia are given in Table 2 and Figure 2. The mean duration of bromocriptine therapy was 4.8 ± 0.5 years and thus not significantly different from the duration of treatment in the remaining patients. However, the dose necessary to induce normoprolactinemia tended to be smaller in patients with persistent normoprolactinemia and could be reduced even further during therapy. CT scans revealed evidence of tumor shrinkage and cystic regression in 4 of the patients. The follow up periods now range from 6-37 months. So far no clinical or radiological evidence of tumor growth has been observed after cessation of bromocriptine therapy.

Table 1. *Long-term treatment (> 4 years) with bromocriptine in patients with prolactinoma*

	n	%	duration of treatment	prolactinoma macro f	macro m	micro f	micro m
whole group	44		5.2 ± 0.9	19	20	4	1
persisting hyperprolactinemia during treatment	4		5.6 ± 1.3	2	2	0	0
normoprolactinemia during treatment	40	100	5.2 ± 0.9	17	18	4	1
persisting normoprolactinemia after br withdrawal	7	17.5	4.8 ± 0.5	2	2	3	0
persisting partial suppression of prolactin after br withdrawal	33	82.5	5.3 ± 0.9	15	16	1	1

To assess the regulation of prolactin secretion in these patients we examined prolactin responses to TRH (0.4 mg i.v.) and metoclopramide (MCP, 10 mg orally) after a minimum of 6 months after drug withdrawal. Compared with healthy subjects, only two patients showed a normal response to TRH and only one of these two patients exhibited a normal increase of serum prolactin after MCP (Fig. 3). In the rest of the patients the prolactin response to TRH or MCP was diminished or blunted.

Our study shows that in some patients with prolactinoma bromocriptine therapy can be safely withheld after a treatment period of at least 4 years. Up to now no recurrence of hyperprolactinemia or tumor expansion has been observed in our patients with persistent normoprolactinemia, although the follow up period may still be too short. These findings are at variance with a report by Ambrosi et al., who found an increase of prolactin to pretreatment levels after withdrawal of bromocriptine (6). Others have found that after interruption of therapy prolactin levels were persistently suppressed below pretreatment values, but still clearly above the normal range (3,4). However, in these studies the duration of therapy was shorter and in agreement with Eversmann et al., we found that the degree of suppression of prolactin after drug withdrawal correlates with the duration of treatment (4). Recently Moriondo et al. have also reported

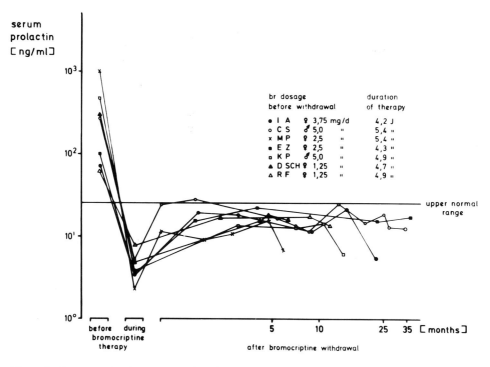

Figure 2. Serum prolactin concentrations in 7 patients with persisting normoprolactinemia after withdrawal of bromocriptine therapy in comparison to prolactin levels during and before therapy.

Table 2. *Patients with persistent normoprolactinemia after bromocriptine withdrawal*

	age (yr)	mean serum prl before treatment (ng/ml)	operation before br treatment	duration of withdrawal (months)	tumor shrinkage
R.F.*	34	61.0 ± 1.0	0	18.5	0
I.A.*	49	71.1 ± 3.2	0	22.5	+
E.Z.*	41	99.0 ± 2.9	0	37.0	0
C.S.**	48	272 ± 15	0	34.0	+
D.S.**	39	297 ± 55	+	15.5	+
K.P.**	57	466 ±144	0	17.0	+
M.P.**	35	995 ± 44	+	6.0	0

* microprolactinoma
** macroprolactinoma

persisting normoprolactinemia after bromocriptine withdrawal in 5 out of 30 patients with microprolactinoma (7).

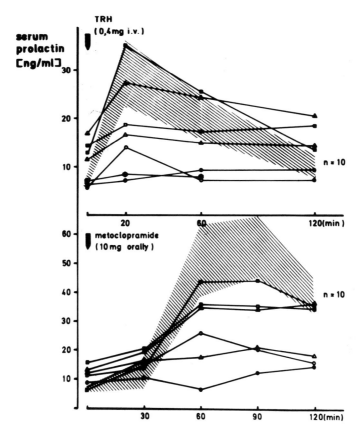

Figure 3. Serum prolactin after TRH and metoclopramide in patients with persisting normoprolactinemia after withdrawal of bromocriptine in comparison to normal persons (shaded areas).

Patients with prolactin-secreting pituitary tumors have diminished prolactin responses after administration of TRH and MCP. It is unclear whether this alteration is related to an underlying defect in prolactin regulation, to hyperprolactinemia itself, or to an inability of the tumor cells to increase prolactin secretion beyond a presumed maximum level. Successful surgery of prolactin-secreting tumors usually restores a normal response to TRH and MCP within 6 months, although persistent defects in prolactin secretion in response to hypoglycemia and chlorpromazine have been described (8). In contrast, only one out of 7 patients with persistently normal basal prolactin after bromocriptine withdrawal exhibited a normal response to TRH and MCP, indicating profound disturbances in the regulation of prolactin in the majority of these patients. There are several possible explanations for these results. The circulating prolactin may be secreted by remnants of pituitary tumor tissue and not by normal lactotropes. In this case the impaired response to TRH and MCP reflects the abnormality of the tumor cells. On the other hand long-term treatment with bromocriptine may also alter the regulation of normal lactotropes, leading to a diminished or even absent prolactin increase after administration of TRH or MCP. Thus further long-term follow-up is necessary to decide if this defect in prolactin secretion will persist.

Our results suggest that termination of bromocriptine therapy is feasible in some patients with macroprolactinomas as well as microprolactinomas. Further long-term follow-up studies are necessary in patients with persisting normoprolactinemia to decide if some of them are cured.

REFERENCES

1. Besser GM, Park L, Edwards CRW, Forsyth IA, McNeilly AS. (1972): Br Med J 3:669
2. Thorner MO, McNeilly AS, Hagan C, Besser GM. (1974): Br Med J 2:419
3. von Werder K, Eversmann T, Rjosk H-K, Fahlbusch R. (1982): In: Ganong WF, Martini L (eds.) Frontiers in Neuroendocrinology. Raven Press, New York, 7:123
4. Eversmann T, Fahlbusch R, Rjosk H-K, von Werder K. (1979): Acta Endocrinol (Copenh) 92:413
5. McGregor AM, Scanlon MF, Hall R, Hall K (1972): Br Med J 2:700
6. Ambrosi B, Travaglini P, Moriondo P, Nissim M, Nava C, Bochicchio D, Faglia G (1982): Acta Endocrinol (Copenh) 100:10
7. Moriondo P, Travaglini P, Nava C, Giovanelli M, Faglia G. (1983): Acta Endocrinol (Suppl 256) 103:84 (Abstract)
8. Tucker H St G, Lankford HV, Gardner DF, Blackard WG. (1980): J Clin Endocrinol Metab 51:968

Prolactin. Basic and clinical correlates
R.M. MacLeod, M.O. Thorner and U. Scapagnini (eds.),
Fidia Research Series, vol. I,
Liviana Press, Padova © 1985

Section XI
Clinical and therapeutic
aspects of hyperprolactinemia

EFFECTS OF CHRONIC BROMOCRIPTINE TREATMENT ON T AND B LYMPHOCYTES IN PATIENTS WITH MACROPROLACTINOMAS

V. Popovic, S. Crnogorac, D. Micic, M. Nesovic, P. Djordjevic, D. Manojlovic, J. Micic, D. Djuric, B. Pendic, and S. Brikic

Internal Clinic A, Dept. of Endocrinology and City Hospital Dept. of Immunology, School of Medicine, University of Belgrade
Koste Todorovic 26, 11000 Belgrade, Yugoslavia

The natural history of prolactinoma is not well defined. Whether it is a primary central hypothalamic defect in dopaminergic function or a primary pituitary lesion is still a matter of debate. Recent evidence from studies using specific dopamine receptor blocking drugs indicates increased dopaminergic tone due to raised plasma prolactin level (positive feedback) effects on tuberoinfundibular dopaminergic system (1).

The immune system is not as autonomous as once believed. Destructive lesions in the hypothalamus result in marked alterations of immune responsiveness such as diminished, delayed type hypersensitive reactivity abrogation of antibody formation (2), and inhibition of lymphocytic blastogenesis (3,4). Destruction of the tuberoinfundibular region of the hypothalamus in rodents leads to a significant increase in tumor growth (5,6). The possible link between the lesions and the mediators of immunity could be through the secretion of hormones. The functional significance of the relationship between concentrations of circulating hormones and immune responsiveness is not clear. Numerous reports suggest that immune surveillance for neoplastic disease is provided by either cytotoxic T lymphocytes or natural killer cell (NK) activity (4).

Assuming that the etiology of prolactinomas and results of experimental studies lend support to the theory that hormones, neurotransmitters, and neuropeptides modulate immune response, it seemed logical to compare the number of T and B lymphocytes both before and after chronic bromocriptine treatment was administered to patients with macroprolactinomas.

Six patients with macroprolactinomas, 4 female and 2 male were studied. They were 21-52 years old and not previously treated. Plasma prolactin profiles were taken at 8, 11, 13, and 19 h. Tumor size was estimated, using high resolution CT scan GE 8800, before and after treatment for at least three months. All patients had normal anterior pituitary reserve. Only patients who were bromocriptine responders and who had evident tumor shrinkage were included in this study. Prolactin (RIA) was determined using Biodata kits with a normal range of 5-25 ng/ml; and interassay CV = 9%. Test procedures for E rosettes (T lymphocytes), EA rosettes (subpopulation of B lymphocytes), and EAC rosettes (subpopulation of B lymphocytes) were performed by the method of Jondal (7). Results were expressed as a percentage of cells forming rosettes. From 12 healthy subjects, normal values for our laboratory were obtained. Test procedures for "active" E rosettes (subpopulation of T lymphocytes) were performed by the method of Wybran (8) and the results were expressed as the percentage of rosette forming cells. The tests were performed before and after treatment.

Basal prolactin in our patients with macroprolactinomas was 165 ± 20 ng/ml while after chronic bromocriptine treatment prolactin levels were normalized in all except one patient (Table 1). High resolution CT scan showed evident tumor shrinkage in all cases (two patients had suprasellar expansion).

The percentage of E rosettes from peripheral blood in 12 healthy controls ranged from 38-46%. Two patients (case 1 and 6) showed decreased E rosette formation before treatment (Table 1). After three months of treatment no significant change in the range of percentage of E rosette forming cells was found, although individual variations existed. The two patients who initially had low percentage showed an increase after treatment, while one patient (case 5) showed a decrease at three and six months of treatment. Values found in healthy subjects for "A" E rosettes ranged from 19-34%. Two patients (case 1 and 6) had decreased percentage initially. The range of percentage of "A" E rosette forming cells did not change significantly after treatment, although the two patients with low percentage increased, while one patient (case 5) decreased the percentage at three and six months of treatment. Normal values for EA rosette forming cells ranged from 9-20%. Initially one patient had a low normal value (case 2) while two patients had high values (case 4 and 5). After chronic treatment the range of percentage of EA rosette forming cells did not change. One patient (case 2) increased this percentage to over high-normal values after three months of treatment but showed, after twelve months of treatment, a normalized percentage of EA rosette forming cells. One patient (case 5) decreased the percentage after three months of treatment and the percentage remained decreased after six months as well. The normal values for EAC rosette forming cells were 6-18%. Initially one patient (case 2) had low values, but after chronic bromocriptine treatment (at three months and at one year) the percentage of EAC rosette forming cells normalized. In one patient (case 5) initially high values normalized at three and six months of treatment.

In our study we found that the range of percentage of rosette forming cells in patients with macroprolactinomas is very broad; the clinical significance of this finding is unclear. Normal adult values have also shown variability and the significance of the low- and high-normal values is not clear. We have thus interpreted our results on an individual basis since only six patients with macroprolactinomas met the established criteria. Two patients initially showed decreased values of E and "A" E rosette forming cells. One patient had normal EA rosette values and two had high values of EA and EAC rosettes. Further delineation of immune system derangement is difficult to define in terms of changes in populations of lymphocytes but our results point to a necessity for more specific immunologic data such as T helper/suppressor ratio and

NK cell activity in patients with prolactinomas. It is well known that patients harboring brain neoplasms, some of which are adjacent to the hypothalamus, are profoundly immunosuppressed (9).

Our patients were chronically treated with a high dose bromocriptine regimen. It is well known that macroprolactinomas are more sensitive to dopamine agonists and that most macroprolactinomas shrink (10). We have selected these patients for our study. Although there were individual variations, the range of rosette forming cells did not change after treatment.

Recently dopamine receptors have been demonstrated to exist on lymphocytes (11) and there is a change in dopamine activity in patients with prolactinomas (12). It has been observed that a significant decrease of [^{3}H]-spiroperidol binding in Parkinsonism exists and that chronic levodopa treatment causes an increase in the number of binding sites (13). The clinical significance of this is not clear, although animal experiments are in progress (14). Dopamine receptors on lactotrophs in patients with prolactinomas are intact.

In addition to catecholamine receptors, shown to exist on the lymphocyte, hormonal receptors are found as well. It is said that alterations in the hormone concentrations may be manifested by a qualitative and quantitative change in suppressor cell population or by changes in the migratory patterns of lymphocytes (4). An intact pituitary is necessary for maintenance of NK cell activity and hypophysectomy causes depressed NK activity.

Animal studies to date support the theory that hormones modulate immune response and further clinical studies are necessary.

REFERENCES

1. Spitz I, Haas M, Trestian S, Zylber Haran E, Shilo S. (1983): Clin Endocrinol (Oxf) 19:285
2. Tyrey L, Nalbandov A. (1972): Am J Physiol 222:179
3. Cross R, Mareksbery W, Brooks W, Roszman T. (1980): Brain Res 196:79
4. Cross R, Mareksbery W, Brooks W, Roszman T. (1984): Immunology 51:399
5. Bindoni M, Belluardo N, Licciardello S, Marchese A, Cicirata F. (1980): Neuroendocrinology 30:88
6. Forni G, Bindoni M, Santoni A, Belluarado N, Marchese A, Giovarelli M. (1983): Nature 306:183
7. Jondal M, Holm G, Wigzell H. (1972): J Exp Med 136:207
8. Wybran J, Carr M, Fudenberg H. (1972): J Clin Invest 51:2537
9. Cross R, Brooks W, Roszman T, Mareksbery W. (1982): J Neurol Sci 53:557
10. von Werder K, Eversman T, Rjosk H, Fahlbush R. (1984): In: International Symposium on Prolactinomas, Graz, p 111 (Abstract book)
11. Le Fur G, Meininger V, Phan T, Gerard A, Baulac M, Uzan A. (1980): Life Sci 27:1587
12. Bybee D, Nakawatase C, Szabo M, Frohman L. (1983): Neuroendocrinology 36:27
13. Le Fur G, Meininger V, Baulac M, Phan T, Uzan A. (1981): Rev Neurol (Paris) 137:89
14. Wilner K, Butler I, Seifert W, Clement-Cormier Y. (1980): Biochem Pharmacol 29:701

Prolactin. Basic and clinical correlates
R.M. MacLeod, M.O. Thorner and U. Scapagnini (eds.),
Fidia Research Series, vol. I,
Liviana Press, Padova © 1985

Section XI
Clinical and therapeutic
aspects of hyperprolactinemia

LONG TERM EFFECTS OF THE MEDICAL TREATMENT OF MACROPROLACTINOMAS

G. Oppizzi, D. Dallabonzana, G. Verde, M. T. Marsili*, G. Luccarelli**, P. G. Chiodini, and A. Liuzzi

Division of Endocrinology and *Ophthalmology, Ospedale Niguarda and **Neurological Institute, C. Besta, Milan, Italy

The effectiveness of the medical treatment of macroprolactinomas (MP) with dopaminergic drugs has been widely demonstrated (1-3); the data so far collected on hormonal and neuroradiological effects of the dopaminergic treatment of MP have not allowed to date any firm conclusion on the very prolonged periods and of eventually obtaining a cure of the disease. For these reasons we report here the results of a study performed on 26 out of our series of 57 patients with MP treated with dopaminergic drugs; these 26 patients were selected for having completed at least two years of treatment with normalization of their prolactin levels. In 20 of them a tumor size reduction was also documented.

The aim of this study was to assess the possibility of obtaining a satisfactory control of prolactin hypersecretion and of tumor growth in spite of a progressive reduction of the drug doses, i.e. to establish the minimal effective dose of the drugs. The clinical summaries of the patients are reported in Table 1. Before starting the treatment, all the patients underwent a computed tomography (CT), an ophthalmological investigation and determination of pretreatment prolactin levels by taking plasma samples four times a day on two different days.

The medical treatment with bromocriptine (Br; 22 patients) or lisuride (L; 4 patients) was started with slowly increasing drug doses in order to minimize side effects. The maintenance dose of the drug was established in the attempt to reduce not only prolactin levels but also tumor size. Plasma prolactin levels were determined monthly and visual fields at least once a year.

The pretreatment prolactin levels were 1893 ± 411 ng/ml (mean ± SE, range 100-6700), and fell within the normal range with doses of Br ranging between 7.5 and 20 mg/day or of L between 0.6 and 0.8 mg/day. The CT documented a shrinkage of the tumor in 20 out of 26 patients during the first year of treatment (Table 1).

Thus the results we have obtained during the first two years of follow up confirm those of previous studies (1-3) showing that dopamine agonists can reduce the tumor size in a consistent proportion of patients with MP. The progressive decrease of the

Table 1. *Clinical summaries of the 26 patients.*

Case no.	Age yrs	Sex	Treatment months	Drug dose mg/day*		PRL bas	(ng/ml) 24 month	tumor size	Visual fields
1	44	F	39	Br	10.0	6700	17	red	am
2	45	F	63	Br	7.5	1000	20	red	nor
3	41	F	57	L	0.8	3400	16	red	nrz
4	41	F	78	L	0.8	3000	30	red	nor
5	42	F	40	Br	10.0	270	12	red	nor
6	40	M	84	Br	7.5	2000	15	red	un
7	50	M	48	Br	5.0	700	1	un	un
8	23	F	43	Br	10.0	1000	38	un	nor
9	45	F	72	L	0.6	1300	11	un	un
10	57	M	54	Br	10.0	4000	1	red	am
11	28	F	49	Br	20.0	6000	19	red	nrz
12	57	M	56	Br	5.0	155	8	red	nrz
13	20	F	40	Br	15.0	5800	3	red	nor
14	50	M	72	Br	7.5	735	8	un	nor
15	43	M	42	Br	7.5	1200	7	red	nor
16	58	M	48	Br	15.0	3600	35	un	un
17	40	F	60	Br	7.5	170	23	red	nor
18	36	M	28	Br	7.5	110	37	un	am
19	46	M	36	Br	7.5	175	22	red	nor
20	70	M	38	Br	7.5	176	1	red	nor
21	55	M	72	Br	7.5	5100	4	red	un
22	41	M	56	Br	7.5	100	1	red	nor
23	36	M	84	Br	5.0	150	5	red	nor
24	23	F	72	L	0.4	100	10	red	nor
25	30	F	50	Br	5.0	1500	9	red	nrz
26	40	F	45	Br	7.5	800	12	red	nrz

* mean of the first two years of treatment

nor: normal; nrz: normalized; un: unchanged; red: reduced; am: ameliorated

maintenance dose was attempted in these selected patients from the third year of therapy. Drug dose was decreased at three- month intervals provided that prolactin levels were still near the normal range; should the drug reduction be followed by a rise of prolactin we would set the dosage at the preceding levels. Before starting the progressive reduction of the dose of the drug employed, plasma prolactin vaues were 14 ± 2 ng/ml (range

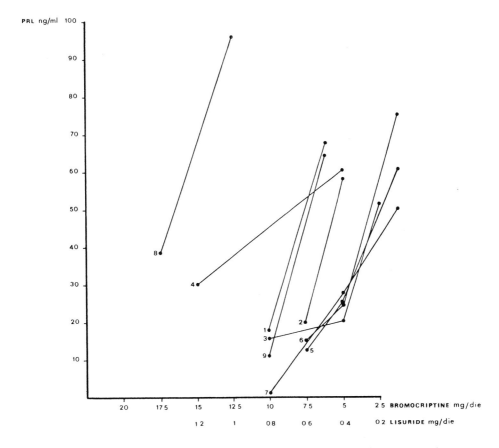

Figure 1. Plasma PRL levels vs drug doses in 9 patients after at least two years of treatment. Numbers indicate patients as reported in Table 1. ●—● : three month period.

1-38). In 9 out of the 26 patients the dose reduction was followed by a prompt rise of prolactin values (Fig. 1). In the remaining 17 it was possible to halve the dose without appreciable changes in prolactin levels and in 12 of these 17, prolactin levels remained within the normal range in spite of the administration of only 2.5 mg/day of Br or of 0.2 mg/day of L. In 5 out of these 12, drug doses as low as 0.625 mg/day of Br or equivalent doses of L kept prolactin levels constantly suppressed (Fig. 2). These minimal doses were withdrawn in the five patients and in only one of them did the prolactin levels remain normal over a 12 month follow up (Fig. 3). No tumor reenlargement was observed in any of these 26 patients during the trial; it is of special note that this event did not occur when very low drug dosages were given to 12 of the 26 patients. In one patient (no. 4) CT documented a further reduction of the adenoma size during the third and fourth year of treatment. In another patient (no. 3) the reduction of the adenoma was documented only after 3 years of uninterrupted treatment;

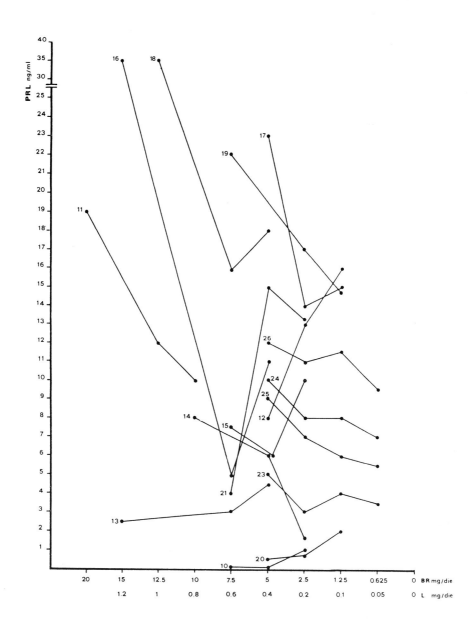

Figure 2. PRL levels vs drug doses in 16 patients after at least two years of treatment. Numbers indicate patients as reported in Table 1. ●——● : three month period. The last points indicate the minimal drug doses capable of maintaining suppressed PRL levels.

only in the patient whose prolactin levels remained normal after drug withdrawal did CT fail to evidence tumoral tissue even one year later.

Whether the medical teatment can cure these patients is still open to question; in any case should this treatment be indefinitely prolonged, it is of value to determine the lowest dose capable of controlling prolactin hypersecretion.

The reason why we planned to perform a progressive decrease of the dose rather than an abrupt drug withdrawal derives from analysis of the data of the literature showing that the latter strategy may be dangerous for the patient. In fact after short (4) or relatively short treatments (5), interruption of the therapy is always followed by a reexpansion of the tumor and worsening of the visual fields. More recently Nissim et al. (6) reported a persistent lowering of prolactin and the maintenance of tumor shrinkage in a few patients with MP after withdrawal of a 1-3 year treatment, whereas in others the tumor reenlarged. Our data show that in a consistent proportion of patients prolactin levels can be kept within the normal range with very low doses of Br or of L. However these minimal doses are necessary since prolactin levels rose in all but one patient after complete drug withdrawal.

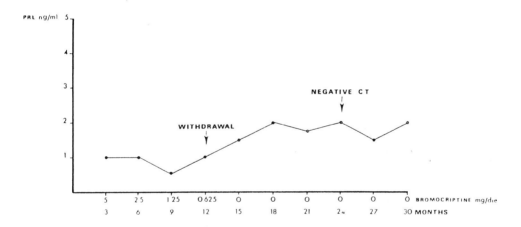

Figure 3. PRL levels in case No. 22 vs months of treatment and drug doses (1 month after drug stopping PRL levels are still within the normal range).

The attainment of prolactin suppression by low Br doses does not imply that the sensitivity of the lactotrophs to the drug is increasing with the duration of the treatment; indeed in 9 out of our 26 patients the reduction of the dose was followed by a rapid increase of plasma prolactin levels in spite of periods of treatment superimposable to those of the other 17 patients. The reason for the wide variability of the sensitivity to dopamine agonists even during very prolonged treatments is not easily explainable. It has been shown (7) that in the rat the pituitary clearance of L is markedly lower than the plasmatic one; thus it is possible that the maintenance dose could depend on the individual turnover rate of the drug at the pituitary level.

A meaningful result of this study is the demonstration that these minimal doses are capable of controlling not only prolactin hypersecretion over time but also tumor growth. In fact in none of our 17 patients was any tumor enlargement documented even when they were treated with 0.625 mg/day of Br or equivalent doses of L. The value of these observations is strengthened by the fact that surgery is often ineffective in obtaining a cure of MP and most of these patients still need medical treatment after adenomectomy owing to incomplete removal of the tumor.

In spite of these favorable results we have to stress that the cure by medical treatment of MP is also infrequent. In fact only in one of the 26 patients so far studied, has withdrawal of the drug been followed by the persistence of normal prolactin levels without evidence of tumor tissue even after one year of follow up.

In conclusion we propose that medical treatment may be considered as the basic approach to selected patients with MP; in particular it can be indefinitely prolonged when minimal doses of the drug can obtain both normalization of prolactin levels and persistent control of tumor growth.

ACKNOWLEDGMENTS

This study was supported by CNR, Special Project "Control of Neoplastic Growth" Grant no. 820033496.

REFERENCES

1. McGregor AM, Scanlon MF, Hall R, Hall K. (1979): Br Med J 2:700
2. Chiodini PG, Liuzzi A, Cozzi R, Verde G, Oppizzi G, Dallabonzana D, Spelta B, Silvestrini F, Borghi G, Luccarelli G, Rainer E, Horowski R. (1981): J Clin Endocrinol Metab 53:737
3. Wass JA, Williams J, Charlesworth M, Kindsley DPE, Halliday AM, Doniach I, Rees L, MacDonald VI, Besser GM. (1982): Br Med J 284:1908
4. Nissim M, Ambrosi B, Bernasconi V, Giannattasio G, Giovannelli MA, Bassetti M, Vaccari V, Moriondo P, Spada A, Travaglini P, Faglia G. (1982): J Endocrinol Invest 5:409
5. Thorner MO, Martin WH, Rogol AD, Morris JL, Perryman RL, Conway BP, Howards SS, Wolfman MG, MacLeod RM. (1980): J Clin Endocrinol Metab 51:438
6. Nissim M, Ambrosi B, Giovine C, Moriondo P, Travaglini P, Faglia G. (1983): Acta Endocrinol (Suppl 256) 103:86
7. Dorow R, Breitkopf M, Graf KJ, Horowski R. (1983): In: Calne DB, Horowski R, McDonald RJ, Wuttke W (eds). Lisuride and Other Dopamine Agonists, Raven Press, New York, p 161

Prolactin. Basic and clinical correlates
R.M. MacLeod, M.O. Thorner and U. Scapagnini (eds.),
Fidia Research Series, vol. I,
Liviana Press, Padova © 1985

Section XI
Clinical and therapeutic
aspects of hyperprolactinemia

CLINICAL AND THERAPEUTIC ASPECTS OF HYPERPROLACTINEMIA

G. M. Besser, J.A.H. Wass, A.Grossman, R. Ross, I. Doniach, A.E. Jones, and L.H. Rees.

St. Bartholomew's Hospital, London, ECIA 7BE, UK

In the 15 years since the establishment of prolactin as a distinct human pituitary hormone, hyperprolactinemia has been widely recognized as a frequent cause of reproductive dysfunction in women and rather less commonly of impotence in men. The availability of potent medical means of lowering pathologically elevated prolactin levels using the dopamine agonists related to the ergot alkaloids has not only provided an efficient, highly successful method for reversing the hypogonadism associated with hyperprolactinemia but also has led to a medical means of shrinking many pituitary tumors. During the studies involved in working out the details of the management of hyperprolactinemic patients using the dopamine agonists, much knowledge has accrued concerning the physiology of the hypothalamic-pituitary-gonadal axis in health and disease.

CLINICAL FEATURES AND CAUSES OF HYPERPROLACTINEMIA

The clinical features of the hyperprolactinemic syndromes are now well recognized. Galactorrhea is commonly found in only a minority of patients, be they men or women; most authors quote an incidence of about 30%. In women breast atrophy is not a feature despite the occurrence of estrogen deficiency in some patients. In men the breast often appears normal and gynecomastia is minimal, if present at all. Often there is fat accumulation in the breast. The classic menstrual disorder is amenorrhea and this is more likely to occur when a pituitary tumor is clearly demonstrable and particularly when there is an abnormality of the pituitary fossa on the plain skull film. However, even when pituitary tumors can clearly be demonstrated, oligomenorrhea is often seen and occasionally regular menstruation with infertility due to anovulation or a deficient luteal phase. Men frequently have no features of hypogonadism on examination but simply complain of relative or absolute impotence, with lowering of libido.

Among the common causes of hyperprolactinemia, drugs which interfere with the delivery or efficacy of dopamine, the normal hypothalamic prolactin inhibiting factor, are most frequently found. Dopamine receptor blocking agents such as the major antipsychotic agents and anti-emetics (e.g. metoclopramide) and those drugs which deplete the CNS of dopamine (e.g. reserpine and methyldopa), act to disinhibit prolactin secretion by the normal mammotroph, whereas estrogens increase the number of prolactin secreting cells as well as their secretory activity. Other conditions which have to be excluded are hypothyroidism and chronic renal failure, although the precise mechanisms through which these conditions raise prolactin levels are not clear. It is usually stated that in hypothyroidism the hyperprolactinemia which may be seen must be due to excessive TRH secretion. However, if this were the case hyperprolactinemia would be more or less the rule in primary hypothyroidism whereas in fact it only occurs in about 30% of patients. Also prolactin levels would fall in parallel with TSH on thyroxine replacement therapy and this does not occur since it takes up to 2 or 3 months longer to normalize prolactin than for TSH levels to reach the normal range. Clearly other factors must be present for hyperprolactinemia to occur in hypothyroidism. In chronic renal failure it is known that circulating opiates are elevated, both beta-endorphin and metenkephalin. Since both of these agents will raise prolactin it has sometimes been suggested that this is the cause of the hyperprolactinemia. However, our own experiments have shown that administration of the opiate receptor blocking drug naloxone does not lead to a fall of prolactin in chronic renal failure, so it would appear that it is unlikely that the hyperprolactinemia is opiate-dependent. Successful renal transplantation results in normalization of prolactin levels. In a proportion of patients, lowering of prolactin with dopamine agonist therapy will lead to resolution of the associated hypogonadism, although this will not occur if there is also primary gonadal failure (1).

Once these conditions are excluded the majority of patients appear to have either pituitary tumors or hypothalamic and pituitary stalk lesions. Hypothalamic lesions are dealt with in detail elsewhere, but it must be stated here that small tumors of the hypothalamus such as gliomas and craniopharyngiomas may be clinically and radiologically indistinguishable from pituitary tumors and if the hyperprolactinemia is treated with bromocriptine amenorrhea and other features of hypogonadism as well as galactorrhea may disappear and normal gonadal function ensue just as if there were a primary pituitary tumor secreting prolactin. Care must be taken to avoid diagnosing such patients as having pituitary tumors since such masses do not shrink under dopamine agonist therapy (Fig 1). Final proof of the diagnosis can only be obtained at surgical biopsy. Such cases are examples of "pseudoprolactinoma".

Prolactinomas - pituitary tumors secreting prolactin - are the most common type of pituitary adenoma; they probably constitute at least 40% of tumors previously described as "functionless". High resolution CT scanning, using iv contrast, and reformation in two planes, is usually able to identify accurately and clearly a pituitary tumor. Small pituitary prolactin secreting tumors are characteristically radiolucent under such conditions, although small pituitary cysts and functionless pituitary tumors and areas of necrosis or hemorrhage may be indistinguishable. However, this technique has largely replaced routine pituitary tomography with or without metrizamide or pneumoencephalography. Some patients with hyperprolactinemia still have to be classified as "idiopathic" since there is no associated cause for the hyperprolactinemia and a

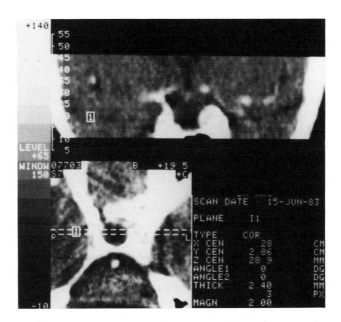

Figure 1. "Pseudoprolactinoma". High resolution GE8800 CT scan, using sagittal reformation and iv contrast, of the hypothalamic and pituitary regions in a patient with secondary amenorrhea and serum prolactin of 1745 mU/l (normal up to 360 mU/l). She had regular menstruation and fully suppressed prolactin levels on bromocriptine 7.5mg /day. Surgical exploration showed the lesion to be craniopharyngioma.

pituitary tumor cannot be distinguished. It may be that some or all of these patients have lesions of the pituitary which are too small to be visualised by current radiological techniques but which would represent small prolactinomas. Patients with small prolactinomas are more often women than men and the most frequent presentation is with symptoms attributable to the high circulating prolactin level. Although prolactinomas are less common in men than women a higher proportion of males present with mass effects of the lesion rather than the consequences of the endocrine disturbance. Mass effects usually present as headache, visual field impairment or oculomotor nerve palsies.

It may not be possible to clearly distinguish those patients who have true prolactin secreting tumors of the pituitary gland from those in whom there is a small functionless pituitary tumor which does not secrete prolactin itself, but which interferes with the vascular supply by which dopamine, the prolactin inhibiting hormone from the hypothalamus, should normally be delivered to the normal pituitary mammotroph. Such small or large non-prolactin secreting masses constitute another cause of "pseudoprolactinoma". Although it is generally true that patients with true prolactinomas have higher prolactin levels than those with pseudoprolactinomas, this is not always the case. Pituitary tumors which do not immunostain for prolactin have occurred in patients with considerable hyperprolactinemia. In a group of 34 patients who had surgery for pituitary macroadenomas, and in whom the tumor did not immunostain for prolactin, mean preoperative serum prolactin levels range from 150 - 5600 mU/l with a median level of 700 mU/l. Our normal range is up to 360mU/1. In 20 other patients similarly operated on but whose tumor did show positive immunostaining, preoperative prolactin levels ranged up to 759,000 mU/l with a median value of 4000 mU/l. One of these patients whose tumor showed positive prolactin immunostaining in a few cells had persistently normal circulating prolactin levels preoperatively. It is unusual for tumors to fail to show significant immunostaining if the preoperative levels are above 2500 mU/l.

CLINICAL MANAGEMENT OF PROLACTINOMAS
AND IDIOPATHIC HYPERPROLACTINEMIA

For the purpose of this discussion it is assumed that appropriate measures have been taken to exclude other causes of hyperprolactinemia. While medical treatment clearly is the treatment of choice for patients in whom no pituitary lesion can be demonstrated, the so-called "idiopathic" cases, the optimal definitive treatment of demonstrable prolactinomas remains controversial. While medical treatment is highly effective, transsphenoidal or transethmoidal hypophysectomy has in the past been the preferred primary treatment in some centres, but even in highly skilled hands surgical cure of the hyperprolactinemia is reported in only 40 - 80% of cases and recurrence of hyperprolactinemia is said to occur in half of these (2,3). Although not a frequent occurrence, there must be a risk of hypopituitarism during this procedure (4,5), particularly of gonadotrophin deficiency and since patients are often young and present with disorders of menstruation or fertility, such an outcome would be particularly discouraging and should be avoided if possible at least during the child-bearing period of life.

MEDICAL MANAGEMENT OF SMALL PROLACTINOMAS

Dopamine agonist therapy in patients with microadenomas (tumors smaller than 1 cm in maximum diameter), small macroadenomas (lesions larger than 1 cm but not producing any mass effects), and idiopathic cases, is highly successful in lowering the elevated prolactin levels and restoring gonadal function to normal both in men and in women. Most experience in the use of dopamine agonist ergot related drugs has been with bromocriptine. Return of circulating prolactin levels to the normal range occurs in over 90% of patients irrespective of the degree of elevation of prolactin before treatment. Occasional patients are encountered in whom there is complete resistance to lowering of prolactin and presumably such tumors lack dopamine receptors. In some patients prolactin levels can be partially lowered but not into the normal range. In about half of these there is partial or complete return of gonadal function despite the persistence of elevated levels on treatment, although such levels are not as high as they were before treatment was started. It seems possible that there has been a change in the form of circulating prolactin to a less biologically active form on bromocriptine as has clearly been shown to occur with growth hormone in the management of acromegaly with this drug (6). Usually within 2 months of the return of regular menstruation, ovulation and adequacy of the luteal phase is encountered and galactorrhea disappears. In men, potency returns to normal and if reduced, the seminal volume also is normalised. Sperm concentrations do not usually change unless there has been associated true gonadotrophin deficiency which resolves as the tumor shrinks under dopamine agonist therapy with the restoration of function of the normal gland within the fossa. The dose of bromocriptine which is usually required lies between 5 and 10 mg per day although occasionally maximum suppression of prolactin can only be achieved with doses of 30 mg, 40 mg or even occasionally more per day. This drug has been shown to directly inhibit secretion by the pituitary lactotrophs through activation of dopamine receptors on the tumor and its action is blocked by dopamine antagonists. High circulating levels of bromocriptine are attained by oral medication and the drug is for the most part metabolized rather than excreted intact.

Bromocriptine may cause nausea and postural hypotension when treatment is started, principally through activation of central receptors. Such side-effects are not encountered when women who are newly delivered are given bromocriptine for puerperal lactation, provided this is started within 48 hours of delivery. In non-puerperal patients the side-effects can always be minimized and usually totally eliminated by starting with low doses of drug, increasing slowly and insisting that the drug is taken during the main part of a meal rather than after food. Once the full therapeutic dose has been achieved, taking the compound in the middle of the meal is less important since tachyphyllaxis is encountered. The first dose of bromocriptine should be 1.25 mg (half a tablet) and should be given at night in the middle of a small snack such as a sandwich and glass of milk as the patient goes to bed. After 3-4 days this dose is increased to 1 tablet (2.5 mg) on retiring and a few days later this dose is moved forward to the middle of the evening meal. The medication is increased at approximately 3 day intervals to 2.5 mg, 2 or 3 times daily during food. If side-effects are still experienced the patient is advised to reduce the dose to that previously found acceptable and then more cautiously increased at less frequent intervals. True intolerance to the drug is rare if this regimen is followed. Other side-effects are extremely unusual on the normal doses used for hyperprolactinemia, although on doses between 30 - 60mg per day as used for Parkinsonism or acromegaly, side-effects such as constipation, erythromelalgia and Raynaud's phenomenon may be encountered. Neuropsychiatric symptoms such as persistent dizziness, insomnia or even precipitation of frank psychosis have been reported. A recent review of 600 patients treated by us for acromegaly or hyperprolactinemia has shown 6 patients who developed dopamine agonist related psychoses, of whom half had predisposition to psychotic disease (7).

MEDICAL MANAGEMENT OF PATIENTS WITH LARGE PROLACTINOMAS

Recently it has become clear that not only are elevated circulating prolactin levels returned to normal by dopamine agonist therapy but in at least two thirds of patients with large tumors there is clear evidence that the tumor mass shrinks concomitantly (8). There is no consistent evidence that functionless pituitary tumors shrink under this treatment, whether they are associated with hyperprolactinemia (pseudoprolactinomas) or not. Conventional doses of bromocriptine, sufficient to lower prolactin levels to nor-

838

mal, or equivalent doses of other dopamine agonists are all that is required. Visual acuity, visual field defects, headache, neighbourhood cranial nerve palsies all resolve if the tumor shrinks. Headache and acuity seem to improve remarkably quickly and often patients report symptomatic change within 48 - 72 hours (Figs. 2 and 3). Frank objective evidence of tumor shrinkage such as obtained from CT scanning may be seen within 10 -14 days although improvement may not be seen for 3 or 4 weeks. In patients with visual field defects, it is our policy to begin treatment under close supervision, with daily monitoring of visual acuity and twice weekly monitoring of visual fields using the Goldman apparatus. The dose of bromocriptine or other dopamine agonist is built up according to the normal regimen but the increments are built up as fast as possible, depending on any side-effects the patient may encounter. If there is no clinical or radiological evidence of tumor shrinkage by 3 months we then refer the patient for hypophysectomy.

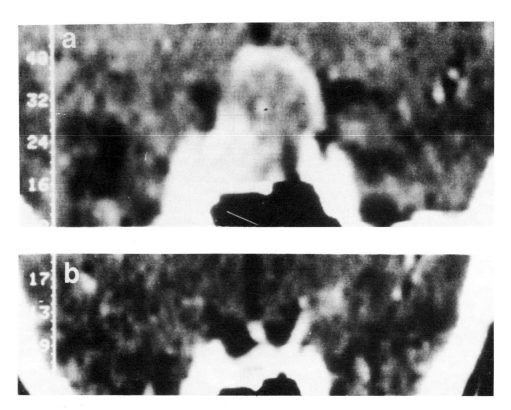

Figure 2. High resolution GE8800 CT scans, using coronal reformation and iv contrast, of hypothalamic and pituitary regions in 16 year old girl with primary amenorrhea, galactorrhea, a 5 year history of severe headaches and bilateral visual defects. Mean serum prolactin before treatment was 50,000 mU/l. (a) Scan before treatment and (b) after 4 months on bromocriptine - the suprasellar extension to the prolactinoma has gone. On treatment headaches disappeared within 24 hrs, vision began to improve after 72 hrs. Visual field changes are shown in Fig. 3. Menarche occurred after 9 months, menses were then regular and ovulatory.

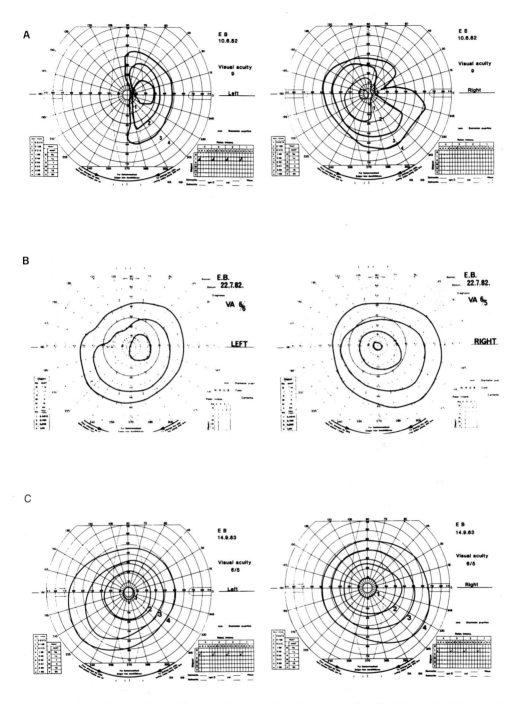

Figure 3. Visual fields by Goldman perimeter of patient referred to in Fig. 2: (a) before and after (b) 5 weeks and (c) 15 months of bromocriptine therapy.

Overall in our experience two thirds of patients with prolactin levels in excess of 1000 mU/l who have macroadenomas with extrasellar extension producing neighborhood compressive symptoms respond by shrinkage of the tumor back into the fossa, thereby avoiding the necessity for surgery. Often this occurs in patients in whom hypophysectomy would clearly fail to cure the patient (Figs. 2 and 3). Once the tumor has shrunk back into the fossa, definitive ablative therapy can be pursued.

In addition to resolution of the neighborhood compressive effects of the tumor mass, in about half of the patients the accompanying hypopituitarism resolves (8). Patients with large pituitary tumors are not hypopituitary because of destruction of the normal pituitary tissue. Most often the normal pituitary is present within the fossa but is functionally disconnected from the hypothalamus by the tumor. The latter impinges on the capillaries of the pituitary stalk or tuber cinereum, preventing delivery of the hypothalamic, hypophysiotropic hormones. When the mass lesion shrinks the hypothalamus can regain functional contact with the normal pituitary and if anterior pituitary function was deficient before treatment, this may then return to normal. We find that pituitary function in terms of vasopressin, ACTH, TSH and gonadotrophin reserve improves in 50% of our macroadenoma patients in whom it was deficient before, as the prolactinoma shrinks (8).

Whether surgery or medical treatment should be used as primary treatment for such massive pituitary lesions is a justifiable source of debate. With microadenomas, clearly transsphenoidal adenomectomy provides the greatest success although recurrence occurs in at least 50% of patients (2,3). With macroadenomas surgery is much less frequently successful in lowering prolactin to normal even transiently and in the majority of patients recurrence occurs (2,3,4). Clearly therefore there is a powerful argument for treating patients with large prolactinomas with medical treatment using ergot-related dopamine agonists such as bromocriptine as first-line treatment. In two thirds of the patients tumor shrinkage will occur (8). In the one third in whom this fails, surgery should be used to at least debulk the tumor. The residual hyperprolactinemia and residual tumor should then be treated with radiotherapy and dopamine agonist therapy (9).

RADIOTHERAPY IN CONJUNCTION WITH DOPAMINE AGONISTS

The use of bromocriptine alone only rarely results in permanent lowering of prolactin levels once treatment is stopped. Clearly there is a case for some additional treatment given in conjunction with dopamine agonist therapy to provide longterm control. Although originally introduced by us to prevent prolactinoma enlargement during pregnancy (10), we have now shown that modern megavoltage radiotherapy is highly effective both in preventing tumor growth and in producing a gradual reduction of circulating prolactin levels to normal. We have recently reviewed 36 women with prolactinomas who have been followed for up to 11 years after radiotherapy (9). Radiotherapy was given using the same technique in all cases. A 4 or 15 MeV linear accelerator delivered a lesion dose of 4,500 cGY (rads) in 25 fractions over 35 days. Individual dose fractions never exceeded 180 cGY. Treatment was planned individually using the smallest target volume compatible with uniform irradiation of the lesion as detected radiologically. With immobilisation in a plastic shell encompassing the whole head and the shoulders,

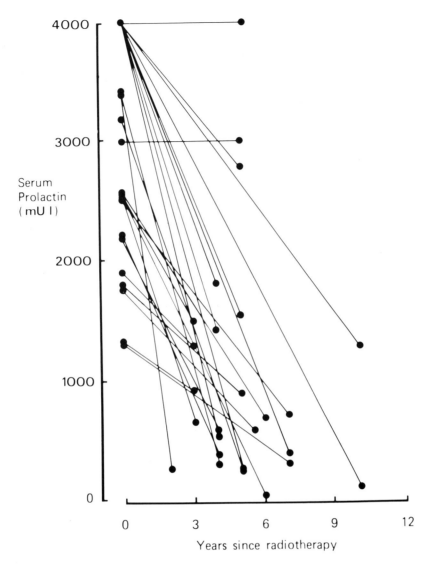

Figure 4. Serial serum prolactin concentrations, after at least 2 months without dopamine agonist treatment, in patients presenting with prolactinomas treated with megavoltage radiotherapy. The open symbols show prolactin values reported as ''greater than'' the value shown. From ref.9.

x-ray simulation and full isodosimetry, a 3-field technique was employed to localize irradiation to the pituitary and minimize the dose to the optic pathways, brain stem, and temporal lobes. Interim dopamine agonist therapy was used in the patients until prolactin levels returned to the normal range. Medical therapy was withdrawn at intervals to determine whether medical treatment was still required when patients had completed their families. Of the 36 women, 16 showed radiological evidence of a macroadenoma before treatment. Of the 36 women, 29 wished to conceive. In them the ovulation rate, as indicated by circulating progesterone concentrations, was 97% and the successful conception rate 86% using this combination of radiotherapy and interim dopamine therapy. No patient had enlargement of their tumor during pregnancy and there were no complications of radiotherapy. No further tumor enlargement was detected in serial skull radiographs and an improvement in the size of the fossa was noted in 45%. When medical treatment was withdrawn (at a mean of 4.2 years, range 1 - 11 years, after radiotherapy) in the 27 patients who had completed their families, the serum prolactin concentration had fallen appreciably in 26, becoming normal later in 8 (Fig. 4).

Only one patient required thyroxine and one needed gonadotrophin replacement. No patient became deficient in ACTH. The incidence of growth hormone deficiency, however, rose from 24% of the whole group before radiotherapy (as assessed by insulin-induced hypoglycemia) to 79% afterwards and this deficiency occurred by 2 years in the majority of the patients. Clearly such growth hormone therapy is of no consequence in this adult group. However, further studies have shown that it is due to failure of secretion or delivery of hypothalamic growth hormone releasing factor to the pituitary cells since the majority of the GH deficient patients still respond to exogenous GHRF after radiotherapy (11). Three patients developed menstrual irregularities more than 5 years after radiotherapy and the pattern suggests a defect of hypothalamic gonadotrophin releasing hormone synthesis or release (9). It is clear the hypopituitarism due to hypothalamic hormone deficiency may occur after a long interval following radiotherapy. However, it seems from our study that the regimen of megavoltage radiotherapy and interim dopamine agonist therapy as outlined, allows women with prolactinomas safely to undergo pregnancy and results in the longterm prospect of tumor shrinkage and control of hyperprolactinemia. If hypopituitarism does develop with longer follow-up, it only appears to occur after passage of sufficient time to allow successful and safe completion of planned families towards the end of the period of normal fertility. Our data agree with the findings of others in suggesting that definitive radiotherapy of prolactinomas, given with a careful technique, obviates the risk of field defects and headache arising during pregnancy. Radiotherapy in patients who do not require fertility in the immediate future should be delayed until plans for conception are definite. An exception to this rule may be made in younger patients who have massive pituitary tumors which shrink back into the fossa on dopamine agonist therapy, and in whom sudden cessation of medical treatment would result in rapid enlargement of macroadenomas. In such patients where successful shrinkage of the tumor into the fossa has been achieved, it is our policy to give radiotherapy at an early stage.

MANAGEMENT OF PATIENTS WITH PROLACTINOMAS DURING PREGNANCY

The normal pituitary gland enlarges significantly during pregnancy. Pituitary tumors also appear to enlarge and there has been controversy as to the precise incidence of this complication. The general consensus is that the risk of tumor enlargement in patients with microadenoma is small, probably of the order of 1%. The reported incidence of tumor enlargement during pregnancy in patients with macroprolactinomas is considerably higher however. The reported incidence varies between 10 - 25% (3); an example is shown in Figure 5. Such a complication may lead to severe headache, visual field or oculomotor nerve palsies. We have even seen this in patients who have had successful clearing of the pituitary fossa after transsphenoidal hypophysectomy, since the original macroadenoma extended into the cavernous sinus and residual tumor was left there. Enlargement of the tumor within the cavernous sinus resulted in nerve pressure affecting the sympathetic nerves around the carotid artery; alternatively the oculomotor or trigeminal nerves might be affected. As discussed above, careful radiotherapy prevents tumor enlargement without adversely affecting fertility. Since prolactin levels fall only slowly after such therapy, despite its protective effect on tumor growth during pregnancy, interim dopamine agonist therapy is used following the radiotherapy; and on this regimen successful conception is achieved (9). Our patients are advised to take mechanical contraceptive precautions following the radiotherapy until 3 regular menstrual cycles have passed and then conception is attempted. Under these circumstances, 50% of the pregnancies are achieved within 2 months. Fertility is clearly not a problem in patients treated with this radiotherapy and dopamine agonist combination; on the contrary, contraception is the problem in this group who are highly fertile on treatment. Our advised method of contraception is an IUCD with spermicidal jelly or use of the low estrogen dose oral contraceptive providing the patient is clearly warned that they must continue bromocriptine whilst taking the oral contraceptive. We have shown that this combination does not result in escape of prolactin levels or evidence of growth of the tumor (12).

Should the patient present with evidence of tumor growth in pregnancy, such as in the patient given bromocriptine without radiotherapy, the clear treatment of choice is to start dopamine agonist therapy forthwith. Estrogen-induced tumor growth is particularly susceptible to shrinkage on bromocriptine at conventional dosage (Fig. 5). Bromocriptine is then continued throughout the pregnancy and radiotherapy is given in the puerperium. Although there is no evidence that bromocriptine is teratogenic, it is not our normal policy to continue bromocriptine throughout the pregnancy unless there is clear evidence of tumor enlargement. Under these circumstances, however, restitution of dopamine agonist therapy is considered mandatory.

DOPAMINE AGONISTS OTHER THAN BROMOCRIPTINE

While use of bromocriptine has the longest and widest experience, newer agents are being introduced. Those under current investigation include lisuride, pergolide and mesulergin (CU32-085). These agents lack the tripeptide component present in bromocriptine and are known as ergolines. Lisuride combines dopamine agonist activity with serotonin antagonist function. Its action lasts as long as that of bromocriptine and the incidence of side-effects appears to be about the same as those of bromocriptine. Pergolide and mesulergin are, however, much longer acting than either of these agents. Both in normal subjects and in patients with hyperprolactinemia our recent studies have suggested that a 2.5 mg dose of bromocriptine is equivalent to 0.5 mg of mesulergin and 50 ug of pergolide. However, at these doses bromocriptine appears to

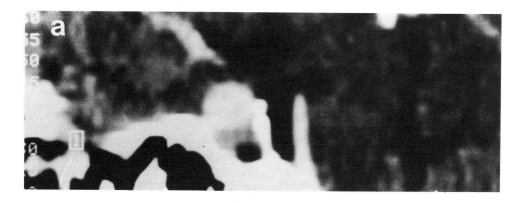

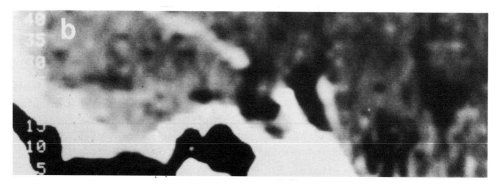

Figure 5. GE9800 CT scans with sagittal reformation after iv contrast (a) at 32 weeks of pregnancy with an expanded radiolucent prolactinoma pushing the pituitary upwards to extend into the suprasellar cistern and (b) at term with shrinkage of the prolactinoma on bromocriptine, and loss of the suprasellar extenstion; CSF extends now into the fossa. The patient's severe frontal and right sided infraorbital headaches were relieved within 12 hours of initiation of bromocriptine therapy.

lower prolactin levels in most subjects for 6 - 8 hours , whereas mesulergin works for a little over 12 hours and pergolide is sometimes still effective 24 hours after administration. Control of hyperprolactinemia in the patients, however, is often possible using mesulergin only once rather than twice a day, but was usual with pergolide. Side-effects with either of the newer agents were much the same as were seen with bromocriptine, however, the tolerance of one of the newer agents in patients intolerant of bromocriptine only rarely occurred.

MECHANISM OF HYPOGONADISM IN HYPERPROLACTINEMIA

The hypogonadism in patients with pituitary causes of hyperprolactinemia is not usually due to gonadotrophin deficiency per se. When tested with gonadotrophin releasing hormone the great majority of patients with hyperprolactinemia showed normal or indeed excessive gonadotrophin responses. Disturbances of pituitary-gonadal function appear to be associated with an alteration of the normal pattern of pulsatility of LH and FSH secretion, abnormality of feedback control and a peripheral gonadal resistance to gonadotrophins. While in amenorrheic patients absence of the normal pulses of gonadotrophins is characteristic, this is by no means always the case (13). In amenorrheic or oligomenorrheic patients before treatment, mean gonadotrophin levels are usually similar to those found in the normal follicular phase. Gonadotrophin pulsatility may be absent or infrequent but of large amplitude (13). The normal surge of LH and FSH seen after a large dose of exogenous estrogen is frequently absent in such patients; there appears to be a defect therefore in positive feedback control of gonadotrophin. Furthermore, high prolactin concentrations have an inhibitory effect on follicular growth and steroidogenesis, suggesting a peripheral resistence to gonadotrophin and this is further supported by absence of an estradiol response in those patients with hyperprolactinemia who do have the infrequent but large surges of gonadotrophins. Reduction of circulating prolactin using dopamine agonists is associated with a rise in estradiol but no change in mean gonadotrophin level. However, the LH positive feedback response rapidly returns and there is restoration of LH pulsatility. In some patients this occurs within a few days of starting bromocriptine, but in others there is a prolonged period of increase in the frequency of the LH pulses and mean LH levels with little initial rise

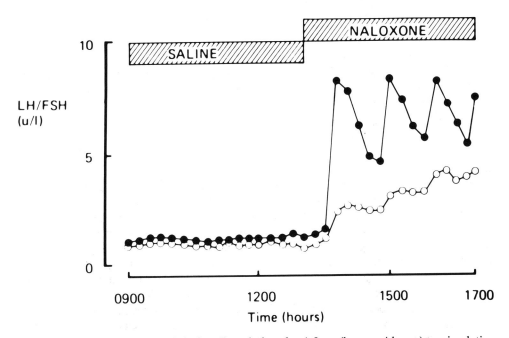

Figure 6. Effects of naloxone infusion (4 mg bolus plus 1.8 mg/hr over 4 hours) on circulating LH and FSH levels in a patient with hyperprolactinemic amenorrhea (from ref. 16).

in estradiol (13). Thus, the defect in ovarian response to endogenous gonadotrophin stimulation may persist for a few weeks after the return of prolactin levels to normal. The restoration of a normal rate of LH pulsatility with bromocriptine therapy can clearly occur without any change in serum estradiol concentration.

The cause of the impaired gonadotrophin pulsatility has not been clear. However, recent evidence suggests that there is an excessive opiate tone in the hypothalamus in hyperprolactinemic patients and that this contributes to the truncation of the LH pulses. Activation of opiate receptors in the median eminence is associated with suppression of the pulsatile release of gonadotrophin releasing hormone and therefore impairment of gonadotrophin secretion. This effect is seen with exogenous opiate alkaloids or peptides and can be blocked with the opiate receptor blocking drug naloxone (14,15). In hyperprolactinemic patients lacking gonadotrophin pulses, administration of naloxone results in the immediate return of gonadotrophin secretion, apparently due to restoration of pulsatile secretion of the gonadotrophin releasing hormone (16) (Fig. 6); this restoration is not seen in patients with anorexia nervosa who also lack pulsatile LH/FSH secretion. The evidence therefore suggests that in hyperprolactinemia there is an excessive opiate tone inhibiting pulsatile release of the gonadotrophin releasing hormone by an action at the median eminence and this must contribute, at least in part, to the disturbance of pulsatile gonadotrophin secretion therefore of the hypogonadism. Restoration of normal prolactin levels results in restoration of normal gonadotrophin secretion and normalisation of gonadal function.

CONCLUSIONS

In the majority of patients who have hypoprolactinemia due to a pituitary cause, the mammotroph cells of evident tumors or in the apparently simply hyperplastic gland, retain dopamine receptors, activation of which lowers prolactin levels to normal. Bromocriptine and similar ergot related dopamine agonist drugs therefore restore prolactin levels to normal; in association with this, gonadal function returns rapidly to normal both in males and females. If bromocriptine is stopped, however, prolactin levels usually rise once more to the pretreatment levels. On dopamine agonist therapy the mass of the pituitary tumor shrinks in at least two thirds of patients, even if these tumors are massive and extend into the neighboring structures outside the pituitary fossa. With the shrinkage of the tumor, resolution of the neighborhood compressive syndromes is seen and in many patients the hypopituitarism resolves. The combination of modern megavoltage radiotherapy with interim dopamine agonist therapy is a highly effective way of providing immediate control of the clinical hyperprolactinemic syndrome. The radiotherapy provides a gradual reduction in prolactin levels so that dopamine agonist therapy may eventually be stopped. Hypopituitarism is a rare association of the radiotherapy; if it does occur, except for growth hormone deficiency which is seen early but is unimportant, it is not seen until many years after the treatment and after the passage of sufficient time to allow successful completion of planned families and towards the end of the period of normal fertility. In patients without evidence of pituitary tumors or who have microadenomas, dopamine agonist therapy alone appears to be the treatment of choice. In patients with macroadenomas associated with prolactin levels above 1000 mU/1 (50 ng/ml) whether there are extrasellar complications or not, an initial trial of dopamine agonist therapy should be given since this will control the prolactin level in over 90% of patients and shrink the tumor back into the fossa in two thirds. Follow-up megavoltage radiotherapy can be safely given then to provide longer term control. In patients with large tumors and a serum prolactin level below 1000 mU/1, bromocriptine is unlikely to produce significant tumor shrinkage. Only in these patients or when dopamine agonist therapy cannot be tolerated or is unavailable, should surgery be performed, but this may be incompletely effective and associated with recurrence. Dopamine agonist therapy can then be used postoperatively with or without radiotherapy as conditions indicate.

In our group of patients with prolactinomas treated with megavoltage radiotherapy, there was no incidence of early or late complications affecting the optic pathways or brain; nor has there been in our total series of 332 patients with pituitary tumors irradiated by us since 1961 using these methods. A lesion dose of 4,500 cGY (rads) given in 25 fractions over 35 days by an isodose planned 3-field technique, using full immobilization of the head, ensures that the dose to vulnerable neural tissue does not exceed 180 cGY (rads) daily; we agree with Sheline (17) that this is an important factor in avoiding such potentially serious complications.

REFERENCES

1. Muir JW, Besser GM, Edwards CRW, Rees LH, Cattell WR, Ackrill P, Baker LRI. (1983): Clin Nephrol 20:308
2. Randall RV, Laws ER, Abboud CF, Ebersold MJ, Kao PC, Scheithauer BW. (1983): Mayo Clin Proc 58:108
3. Serri O, Rasio E, Beauregard H, Hardy J, Somma M. (1983): N Engl J Med 309:280
4. Nabbaro JDN. (1982): Clin Endocrinol 17:129
5. Pelkonen R, Grahne B, Hirvonen E. et al (1981): Clin Endocrinol 14:335
6. Wass JAH, Clemmons DR, Underwood LE, Barrow I, Besser GM, Van Wyke JJ. (1982): Clin Endocrinol 17:369
7. Turner TH, Cookson JC, Wass JAH, Drury PL, Besser GM. (1984): Submitted to Brit Med J
8. Wass JAH, Williams J, Charlesworth M, Kingsley DPE, Halliday AM, Doniach I, Rees LH, McDonald WI, Besser GM. (1982): Brit Med J 284:1908
9. Grossman A, Cohen BL, Charlesworth M, Plowman PN, Rees LH, Wass JAH, Jones AE, Besser GM. (1984): Brit Med J 288:1105
10. Thorner MO, Besser GM, Jones A, Dacie J, Jones AE. (1975): Brit Med J 4:694
11. Grossman A, Lytras N, Savage MO, Wass JAH, Coy DH, Rees LH, Jones AE, Besser GM. (1984): Brit Med J 288:1785
12. Moult PA, Dacie JE, Rees LH, Besser GM. (1982): Brit Med J 284:868
13. Moult PJA, Rees LH, Besser GM. (1982): Clin Endocrinol 17:423
14. Grossman A, Moult P, Gaillard RC, Delitala G, Toff WD, Besser GM. (1981): Clin Endocrinol 14:41
15. Moult PJA, Grossman A, Evans J, Rees LH, Besser GM. (1981): Clin Endocrinol 14:321
16. Grossman A, Moult PJA, McIntyre H, Evans J, Silverstone T, Rees LH, Besser GM. (1982): Clin Endocrinol 17:379
17. Sheline GE. 1982 In: Givens JR (ed) Hormone Secreting Pituitary Tumours. Year Book Medical Publishers Inc. Chicago, p 121

Prolactin. Basic and clinical correlates
R.M. MacLeod, M.O. Thorner and U. Scapagnini (eds.),
Fidia Research Series, vol. I,
Liviana Press, Padova © 1985

Section XI
Clinical and therapeutic
aspects of hyperprolactinemia

THE ROLE OF SURGERY IN THE MANAGEMENT OF PROLACTINOMA

Edward R. Laws, Jr., Michael J. Ebersold, David G. Piepgras, Charles F. Abboud, Raymond V. Randall, and Bernd W. Scheithauer.

Departments of Neurologic Surgery, Endocrinology, and Pathology Mayo Medical School, Mayo Clinic, Rochester MN 55905

Prolactin secreting pituitary adenomas are the most frequently diagnosed and treated pituitary tumors. Currently, they account for 40% of such tumors managed by transsphenoidal selective microsurgery at the Mayo Clinic (1,2). They are more frequently encountered in women than in men, and in our series 83% are in women. The clinical presentation of these tumors reflects endocrine hyperfunction in the majority, producing the Forbes-Albright syndrome (amenorrhea-galactorrhea) with infertility in women, and hypopituitarism and impotence with infertility and, rarely (2%), galactorrhea in men. A smaller percentage present with mass effect producing headache and visual loss (usually bitemporal hemianopsia) in both sexes, but more frequently in men.

The majority (62%) of prolactinomas in our series are microadenomas, defined as tumors 10 mm or less in diameter (65% in women and 2% in men). A small proportion of microadenomas and a large proportion (25%) of macroadenomas are found to be invasive of dura and bone at surgical exploration.

Indications for surgical management continue to be controversial, especially because of the results of medical management with bromocriptine. Because our clinic is a referral center, its criteria for surgical management may differ from those of other centers in the United States and elsewhere. The goals of surgical therapy are several. They include elimination of mass effect, normalization of hyperprolactinemia, preservation of normal pituitary function, and prevention of tumor persistence and recurrence. They also include pathologic confirmation of the presence of a pituitary adenoma, and immunocytological classification.

The preoperative diagnosis of prolactinoma must be made judiciously, as other lesions in and about the sella turcica may produce hyperprolactinemia by interference with the normal physiology of hypothalamic prolactin inhibiting factor (PIF) which exerts a dopaminergic inhibitory control of pituitary prolactin secretion. These lesions have been termed "pseudoprolactinomas" (3) and must be considered in the differential diagnosis of prolactinomas.

Table I. *Surgical Management of Prolactinoma - 100 Women*

Mean Follow-up 5 1/2 Years

Normal Postoperative PRL
microadenoma - 50%
macroadenoma - 25%
overall - 42%

Recurrence
macroadenoma - 27%
microadenoma - 24%
overall - 25%

The ultimate proof of diagnosis of prolactinoma depends upon immunocytochemical analysis of the tumor itself. In our series of 100 presumed prolactinomas (1) 5% proved to be pseudoprolactinomas when subjected to such critical analysis.

This review will focus on the results of surgical management of prolactinoma in women, hoping to provide a firm basis for the role of surgery, its advantages, disadvantages and risks. Criteria for inclusion in this review were: clear evidence from clinical presentation, blood prolactin levels and pathological findings of a prolactinoma (not all patients had immunocytochemical confirmation), and adequate follow-up with serial blood prolactin determinations. This is a consecutive series in that no patient meeting these criteria was excluded, and 100 patients were evaluated, with surgery performed between 1972 and 1980. Excluded from the analysis are those patients without pathologic confirmation of a pituitary adenoma, and a number of patients with proven tumor but inadequate follow-up data.

The ages of our patients ranged from 15-60 years with a mean age of 26.5. The 100 women included 5 with primary amenorrhea, 2 with oligomenorrhea and the remainder with secondary amenorrhea. Galactorrhea was present in 87%. Microadenomas were found and removed in 68, and the remainder had macroadenomas. Visual loss and visual field defects were present in 12 of the women, all with macroadenomas, and one patient with a macroadenoma presented with pituitary apoplexy. Two patients were known to have the Multiple Endocrine Neoplasia Type I syndrome. Prior therapy had been given to a number of these women. One patient had had 2 prior craniotomies, one had craniotomy and radiation, 2 had prior transsphenoidal surgery, and 2 others had radiation therapy. Approximately 20% of the women had been given a trial of bromocriptine therapy.

Surgery was performed using a standard trans-septal transsphenoidal microsurgical technique (4). At surgery 10% of the microadenomas and 25% of the macroadenomas were found to be invasive tumors, involving dura, bone or both. One of these tumors proved to be malignant with metastases and is the subject of a separate report (5).

The results of surgery and subsequent follow-up evaluation are given in Tables I-III. Success for these purposes is defined as prolactin levels below 23 ng/ml at most recent follow-up. Other measures of success include resolution of visual field defects which occurred in all of the 12 women with this problem. Pregnancy was achieved in 44 previously infertile women, representing success in 84% of women for whom fertility was a goal of surgery. As implied by this ability to achieve pregnancy, preservation of normal pituitary function was the rule, and systematic analysis revealed no iatrogenic damage of ACTH or TSH axes and only 2 patients with postoperative impairment of the GH axis. Improvement in preoperative pituitary function other than prolactin occurred in 30% of those with preoperative impairment. Diabetes insipidus lasting more than 72 hours occurred in 2 patients and eventually resolved in both.

Table II. *Macroadenoma - 32 Patients*

	No. of Patients	Mean Preop PRL (ng/ml)
Postop Normal PRL	8	127
Persistent PRL Elevation	21	1787
Recurrences	3	187

COMPLICATIONS

There was no operative mortality in this series. Two patients developed postoperative cerebrospinal rhinorrhea repaired by subsequent transsphenoidal surgery. One woman had a postoperative psychosis which resolved. One developed late visual loss related to prolapse of the optic chiasm into an empty sella; this was surgically corrected. Three patients developed nasal septal complications related to the surgical approach, and one patient had an intraoperative carotid artery injury which was successfully repaired during the operation.

SUBSEQUENT MANAGEMENT

Postoperative radiation therapy was given to 20 patients with large or invasive tumors and persistent hyperprolactinemia. Subsequent surgical approaches for removal

Table III. *Microadenomas - 68 Patients*

	No. of Patients	Mean Preop PRL (ng/ml)
Postop Normal PRL	34	92
Persistent PRL Elevation	23	358
Recurrences	11	211

of persistent or recurrent tumor were undertaken in 2 patients with successful palliation in both. Postoperative bromocriptine therapy has been given to 23 patients.

RECURRENT TUMORS

In this analysis, tumors were considered to be recurrent if the initial postoperative prolactin level was clearly normal and subsequently rose to clearly abnormal levels in women who were neither pregnant nor nursing. The time lapse to detection of recurrence can be distressingly long, ranging from 3 to 59 months in this series, with a mean time to recurrence of 36 months. It is not possible to predict how many more recurrences will develop as the follow-up period is extended. It appears that those patients with preoperative prolactin values greater than 150 are at risk for recurrence, even if initial results suggest cure.

DISCUSSION

This analysis allows for confirmation of prior studies of surgical management of prolactinomas, and also corrects some overly optimistic prior assessments of results based on short follow-up and less than rigorous pathologic criteria. It also permits comparison of this series to others with regard to recurrence (6).

Current methods allow pituitary surgery to be accomplished quite safely with low morbidity and little risk of damage to normal pituitary function. Curative surgical management may be accomplished in many patients with small non-invasive tumors, but this is rarely the case in large or invasive tumors or in those patients with high initial prolactin levels.

Surgical management can play an important role in the restoration of fertility and in ensuring a successful pregnancy. Surgery is effective and prompt in the alleviation of mass effect produced by large prolactinomas.

The results of this study temper somewhat the initial glowing reports of surgery for prolactinomas. The results of long term dopamine agonist therapy are also under continuing review and similar problems may be forthcoming with the critical analysis of medical therapy. There is no substitute for careful review of the results of our practice, and the wisdom that such endeavors can provide.

ACKNOWLEDGMENTS

The authors are grateful to Mrs. Constance B. Hoeft and Mrs. Sandra B. Carpenter for their assistance in the maintenance and review of data and the preparation of the manuscript.

REFERENCES

1. Randall RV, Laws ER Jr, Abboud CF, Ebersold MJ, Kao PC, Scheithauer BW. (1983): Mayo Clinic Proc 58:108
2. Laws ER Jr, Randall RV, Kern EB, Abboud CF (eds). Management of Pituitary Adenomas and Related Lesions with Emphasis on Transsphenoidal Microsurgery. Appleton-Century-Crofts, New York, (1982)
3. Randall RV, Scheithauer BW, Laws ER Jr, Abboud CF. (1982): Trans Am Clin Climatol Assn 94:114
4. Laws ER Jr. (1982): In: Schmidek HH and Sweet WH (eds) Operative Neurosurgical Techniques - Indications, Methods and Results. Grune & Stratton, New York, p 327
5. Scheithauer BW, Randall RV, Laws ER Jr, Kovacs K, Horvath E. Cancer, in press
6. Serri O, Rasio E, Beauregard H, Hardy J, Somma M. (1983): New Eng J Med 309:280

SUBJECT INDEX

Printed in Italy by Biessezeta - Passirana di Rho - Milano
Photosetting by CFP - Padova